Review of Ophthalmology

SECOND EDITION

Commissioning Editor: Russell Gabbedy
Development Editor: Nani Clansey
Editorial Assistant: Emma Cole
Project Manager: Beula Christopher
Design: Charles Gray, Alan Studholme, Miles Hitchen
Illustration Manager: Bruce Hogarth
Illustrator: Merlyn Harvey
Marketing Manager(s) (UK/USA): Gaynor Jones/Helena Mutak

Review of Ophthalmology

SECOND EDITION

William B. Trattler MD
Director of Cornea, Center For Excellence In Eye Care
Department of Ophthalmology
Florida International University Wertheim College of Medicine
Miami, FL, USA

Peter K. Kaiser MD
Chaney Family Endowed Chair for Ophthalmology Research
Professor of Ophthalmology, Cleveland Clinic Lerner College of Medicine
Cole Eye Institute, Cleveland Clinic
Cleveland, OH, USA

Neil J. Friedman MD
Adjunct Clinical Associate Professor,
Department of Ophthalmology, Stanford University School of Medicine
Partner, Mid-Peninsula Ophthalmology Medical Group
Palo Alto, CA, USA
Director, Cataract and Lens Implant Surgery
Pacific Vision Institute
San Francisco, CA, USA

For additional online content visit
www.expertconsult.com

Expert CONSULT

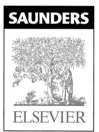

SAUNDERS

ELSEVIER

Edinburgh, London, New York, Oxford, Philadelphia, St Louis, Sydney, Toronto

ELSEVIER
SAUNDERS

First edition 2004

Notices

Knowledge and best practice in this field are constantly changing. As new research and experience broaden our understanding, changes in research methods, professional practices, or medical treatment may become necessary.

Practitioners and researchers must always rely on their own experience and knowledge in evaluating and using any information, methods, compounds, or experiments described herein. In using such information or methods they should be mindful of their own safety and the safety of others, including parties for whom they have a professional responsibility.

With respect to any drug or pharmaceutical products identified, readers are advised to check the most current information provided (i) on procedures featured or (ii) by the manufacturer of each product to be administered, to verify the recommended dose or formula, the method and duration of administration, and contraindications. It is the responsibility of practitioners, relying on their own experience and knowledge of their patients, to make diagnoses, to determine dosages and the best treatment for each individual patient, and to take all appropriate safety precautions.

To the fullest extent of the law, neither the Publisher nor the authors, contributors, or editors, assume any liability for any injury and/or damage to persons or property as a matter of products liability, negligence or otherwise, or from any use or operation of any methods, products, instructions, or ideas contained in the material herein.

British Library Cataloguing in Publication Data
Trattler, Bill.
    Review of ophthalmology. -- 2nd ed.
    1. Ophthalmology.
    I. Title II. Kaiser, Peter K. III. Friedman, Neil J.
    617.7-dc23

ISBN-13: 978-1-4377-2703-6

Working together to grow
libraries in developing countries

www.elsevier.com | www.bookaid.org | www.sabre.org

ELSEVIER   BOOK AID
            International   Sabre Foundation

Printed in China
Last digit is the print number: 9 8 7 6 5 4 3 2

Contents

Preface

Developing an effective textbook that can be used in preparation for written examinations has been a labor of love. We have enjoyed building and designing this book in a way that provides the maximum amount of information in a concise and clear manner. Based on your feedback and reviews, we know we are delivering a text book that can provide the essential information for a comprehensive understanding of each topic, as well as covers the esoteric topics that often appear on tests. We have also updated the material in each chapter to stay current with new information.

The overall goal and layout of Review of Ophthalmology has remained the same. The book is organized into 11 clearly divided chapters which cover the essential topics that ophthalmologists are required to master. We have also included sidebars that focus on the core knowledge base, as well as the results from important clinical trials. New medical and surgical treatments have also been included in the new edition. At the end of each chapter, we have developed additional multiple choice questions that are designed to test your knowledge and to help you prepare for future examinations.

We hope that the improvements and new material contained in this edition will strengthen your review experience, and we wish you success in your future careers.

William B. Trattler, MD
Peter K. Kaiser, MD
Neil J. Friedman, MD

Acknowledgements

Like the first edition, the second edition of Review of Ophthalmology was made possible by the assistance and support of colleagues, family and friends. We owe our thanks to Drs. Dilsher Dhoot, Sumit Sharma, Brian Armstrong, Carlos Buznego, W. Lloyd Clark, and Nicholas Volpe who reviewed the chapters and offered invaluable suggestions.

For their expertise and technical aid, we are also indebted to our editorial and publishing staff led by Russell Gabbedy, Nani Clansey, and Beula Christopher.

Finally, we could not have accomplished this task without the support and love of our families: Jill, Ali, Jeremy, Josh, Henry, Marcia, Peter, Anafu, Christine, Peter Jr, Stephanie, Mae, Jake, Alan, and Diane.

William B. Trattler, MD
Peter K. Kaiser, MD
Neil J. Friedman, MD

1

Optics

PROPERTIES OF LIGHT

Light behaves both as waves and as particles (photons)

Its **speed** (velocity) (v) is directly proportional to wavelength (λ) and frequency (v): $v = \lambda v$

In any given medium, speed of light is constant ($v_{vacuum} = c = 3.0 \times 10^{10}$ cm/s); therefore, wavelength and frequency are inversely proportional

Light slows down in any substance other than air or vacuum, amount of slowing depends on medium; frequency of light remains unchanged, but wavelength changes (becomes shorter) (Figure 1-1)

Its **energy** is directly proportional to frequency and inversely proportional to wavelength: $E = hv = h(c/\lambda)$

Index of refraction (n): ratio of speed of light in a vacuum to speed of light in specific material ($n = c/v$)

Air = 1.00, water = 1.33, aqueous and vitreous = 1.34, cornea = 1.37, crystalline lens = 1.42, intraocular lens (IOL) (silicone = 1.41; polymethyl methacrylate (PMMA) = 1.49; acrylic = 1.55), glass = 1.52, high index lenses = 1.6-1.8

Interference: overlapping of light waves; may be constructive or destructive

Constructive: peaks of 2 waves overlap, resulting in maximum intensity at that wavelength

Destructive: peak of 1 wave overlaps with trough of another, obliterating both waves

Example: antireflective coatings (destructive interference, ¼ wavelength apart); interference filters (allow only green light out of the eye during fluorescein angiography); laser interferometry (retinal function test; optical coherence tomography [OCT])

Coherence: ability of 2 light beams to cause interference (large white source has a coherence close to zero)

Example: OCT

Polarization: each light wave has an electrical field with a particular orientation

Nonpolarized light: electrical field of each wave has a random orientation

Polarized light: all electrical fields have same orientation

Example: Haidinger's brushes (polarizing filter rotated in front of blue background produces rotating image like a double-ended brush or propeller; type of entopic phenomenon; test of macular function), Titmus stereo testing, polarized microscopy, polarizing sunglasses

Diffraction: bending of light waves around edges; change in direction of light wave is related to wavelength (the shorter the wavelength, the less the change in direction); amount of diffraction is related to size of aperture (the smaller the aperture, the greater the diffraction); interference of new waves with original rays forms a diffraction pattern

Example: Airy disc (diffraction pattern produced by a small, circular aperture; occurs when pupil size is <2.5 mm; diameter of central disc increases as pupil size decreases); pinhole (reduces refractive error and improves vision by increasing depth of focus, but limited by diffraction; optimal size is 1.2 mm; may correct for up to 3 D; smaller aperture limits visual acuity; squinting is method of creating a natural pinhole to improve vision; pinhole can also improve vision in eyes with corneal or lenticular irregularities; pinhole can reduce vision in eyes with retinal disorders)

Scattering: disruption of light by irregularities in light path; shorter wavelengths scatter to a greater extent

Example: Opacity (corneal scar or cataract) scatters light, causing glare and image degradation; in atmosphere, scattering involves particles (Rayleigh scattering) and blue light (scattered to the greatest extent; therefore, sky appears blue)

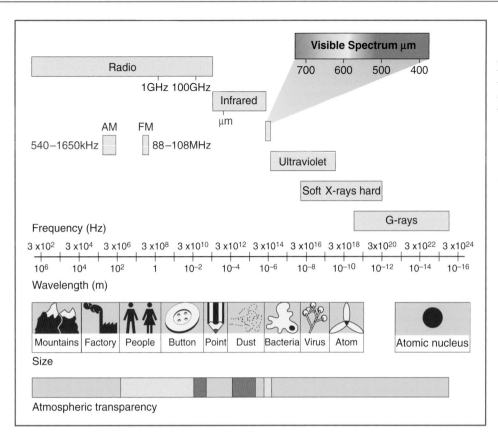

Figure 1-1. The electromagnetic spectrum. The pictures of mountains, people, buttons, viruses, and so forth, are used to produce a real (i.e. visceral) feeling of the size of some of the wavelengths. (From Miller D, Burns SK: Visible light. In: Yanoff M, Duker JS (eds) Ophthalmology, 2nd edn. St Louis, Mosby, 2004.)

Reflection: bouncing of light off optical interfaces; the greater the refractive index difference between the 2 media, the greater is the reflection; also varies with angle of incidence

> **Example:** Asteroid hyalosis (asteroids reflect light back into examiner's eye, creating glare; patient is asymptomatic)

Transmission: percentage of light penetrating a substance (%T); can vary with wavelength

Absorption: expressed as optical density (OD)=log $1/T$

Illumination: measure of incident light

Luminance: measure of reflected or emitted light (lumen/m^2); apostilb=diffusing surface with luminance of 1 lumen/m^2 (used in Humphrey and Goldmann visual field testing)

> **Example:** contrast sensitivity is ability to detect small changes in luminance

Laser: light amplification by stimulated emission of radiation; excited material releases photons of same wavelength and frequency; process is amplified so that released photons are in phase (constructive interference); produces monochromatic, coherent, high-intensity polarized light; power can be increased by increasing energy or decreasing time ($P=E/t$); Q switching and mode locking (types of shutters that synchronize light phase) are methods of increasing laser power by compressing output in time

REFRACTION

Light changes direction when it travels from one material to another of different refractive index (e.g. across an optical interface); direction of refraction is toward the normal when light passes from a medium with a lower index of refraction to a medium with a higher one, and away from the normal when light passes from a more dense to a less dense medium (higher refractive index materials are more difficult for light to travel through, so light takes a shorter path [closer to the normal]); light does not deviate if it is perpendicular to interface (parallel to the normal)

Snell's law: $n \sin (i)=n' \sin (r)$; n=refractive index of material; i=angle of incidence (measured from the normal); r=angle of refraction (measured from the normal) (Figure 1-2)

Critical angle: angle at which incident light is bent exactly 90° away from the normal (when going from medium of higher to lower n) and after which all light is reflected

> **Example:** Glass/air interface has a critical angle of 41°; critical angle of cornea=46.5°

Total internal reflection: angle of incidence exceeds critical angle, so light is reflected back into material with

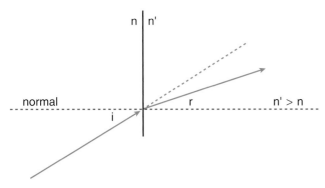

Figure 1-2. Refraction of light ray.

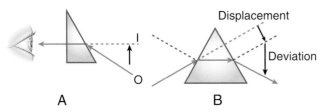

Figure 1-3. **A,** Displacement of image toward apex. **B,** Displacement and deviation of light by prism.

higher index of refraction; $n \sin (i_c) = n' \sin (90°)$; $\sin (i_c) = (n'/n) \times 1$

> **Example:** Gonioscopy lens is necessary to view angle structures owing to total internal reflection of the cornea

PRISMS

Prisms displace and deviate light (because their surfaces are nonparallel); light rays are deviated toward the base; image is displaced toward the apex (Figure 1-3)

Prism diopter (PD, Δ): displacement (in cm) of light ray passing through a prism, measured 100 cm (1 m) from prism

> **Example:** 15 Δ = ray displaced 15 cm at a distance of 1 m
> (1 Δ = 1 cm displacement/1 m); 1° ≈ 2 Δ (this approximation is useful for angles smaller than 45°)

Angle of minimum deviation: total angle of deviation is least when there is equal bending at both surfaces of prism

Plastic prisms are calibrated by angle of minimum deviation: back surface parallel to frontal plane

Glass prisms are calibrated in **Prentice position**: back surface perpendicular to visual axis

Prism placed in front of the eye creates a phoria in the direction of the base

> **Example:** Base-out (BO) prism induces exophoria; to correct, use prism with apex in the opposite direction

Apex is always pointed in direction of deviation: base-out for esotropia, base-in for exotropia, base-down (BD) for hypertropia

Stacking prisms is not additive; 1 prism in front of each eye is additive

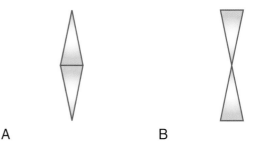

Figure 1-4. **A,** Plus lenses act like 2 prisms base to base. **B,** Minus lenses act like 2 prisms apex to apex.

Risley prism: 2 right-angle prisms positioned back to back, which can be rotated to yield variable prism diopters from 0 to 30 Δ; used to measure prismatic correction for tropias

Fresnel prisms: composed of side-by-side strips of small prisms; prism power is related to apex angle, not the size of the prism; available as lightweight, thin press-on prism to reduce base thickness of the spectacle prism; disadvantage is reflection and scatter at prism interface, causing decreased visual acuity

Prismatic effect of lenses (Figure 1-4): spectacles induce prism; all off-axis rays are bent toward or away from axis, depending on lens vergence

Perceived movement of fixation target when lens moves in front of the eye:

> *Plus lenses:* produce **'against'** motion (target moves in opposite direction from lens)
> *Minus lenses:* produce **'with'** motion (target moves in same direction as lens)

Amount of motion is proportional to the power of the lens

Prismatic effect of glasses on strabismic deviations: $2.5 \times D = \%$ difference; minus lenses make deviation appear larger ('minus measures more'); plus lenses decrease measured deviation

Prentice's rule: prismatic power of lens = $\Delta = hD$ (h = distance from optical axis of lens [cm], D = power of lens [D])

Prismatic power of a lens increases as one moves farther away from optical center (vs power of prism, which is constant)

> **Example:** Reading 1 cm below optical center: OD – 3.00; OS + 1.00 + 3.00 × 90
> OD (*Oculus Dexter* – right eye): prism power = 1 cm × 3 D = 3 Δ BD
> OS (*Oculus Sinister* – left eye): prism power vertical meridian: 1 cm + 1 D = 1 Δ BU (base-up) (Note: power of cylinder in 90° meridian is zero)
> Net prismatic effect = 4 Δ (either BD over OD, or BU over OS)

Treatment of vertical prismatic effect of anisometropia:
1. Contact lenses (optical center moves with eyes)
2. Lower optical centers of lenses (reduce amount of induced prism)
3. Prescribe slab-off prism (technique of grinding lens [done to the more minus of the 2 lenses] to

remove BD prism [to reduce amount of induced prism])
4. Single vision reading glasses

Prismatic effect of bifocal glasses:

Image jump: produced by sudden prismatic power at top of bifocal segment; not influenced by type of underlying lens; as line of sight crosses from optical center of lens to bifocal segment, image position suddenly shifts up owing to base-down prismatic effect of bifocal segment (more bothersome than image displacement; therefore, choose segment type to minimize image jump)

Image displacement: displacement of image by total prismatic effect of lens and bifocal segment; minimized when prismatic effect of bifocal segment and distance lens are in opposite directions

Prismatic effect of underlying lens:
Hyperopic lenses induce BU prism, causing image to move progressively downward in downgaze
Myopic lenses induce BD prism, causing image to move progressively upward in downgaze

Prismatic effect of bifocal segment:
Round top (acts like BD prism): maximum image jump; image displacement less for hyperope than for myope
Flat top (acts like BU prism): minimum image jump; image displacement more for hyperope than for myope
Executive type or progressive lenses: no image jump (optical centers at top of segment)

Plus lens: choose round top

Minus lens: choose flat top or executive type (for myopes, image jump is very difficult to ignore because it is in same direction as image displacement, so avoid round tops in myopes)

Chromatic effects: prismatic effect varies with wavelength

Shorter wavelengths are bent farther, causing chromatic aberration
White light shines through prism: blue rays closer to base (bend farthest), red rays closer to apex
In the eye, blue rays come to focus closer to lens than do red rays; difference between blue and red is 1.5–3 D

Duochrome test: red and green filters create 0.5 D difference; use to check accuracy of refraction

If letters on red side are clearer, focal point is in front of retina (eye is 'fogged' or myopic)
If letters on green side are clearer, focal point is behind retina (eye is overminused or hyperopic)
Technique: start with red side clearer and add minus sphere in 0.25 D steps until red and green sides are equal (focal point on retina); works in colorblind patients because it is based on chromatic aberration rather than color discrimination

Vector addition of prisms: prismatic deviations in different directions are additive, based on pythagorean theorem ($a^2 + b^2 = c^2$) (Figure 1-5)

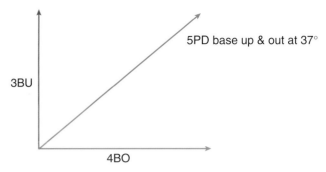

Figure 1-5. Addition of BU and BO prisms.

VERGENCE

The amount of spreading of a bundle of light rays (wavefront) emerging from a point source

Direction of light travel must be specified (by convention, left to right)

Convergence (converging rays): plus vergence; rare in nature; must be produced by an optical system

Divergence (diverging rays): minus vergence

Parallel rays: zero vergence

Diopter: unit of vergence; reciprocal of distance (in meters) to point at which rays intersect; reciprocal of focal length of lens

Lens: adds vergence to light (amount of vergence = power of lens [in diopters])
Plus (convex) lens adds vergence; minus (concave) lens subtracts vergence

Basic lens formula: $U + D = V$ (U = vergence of light entering lens; D = power of lens; V = vergence of light leaving lens)
Power of a spherical surface in a fluid: $D_s = (n' - n)/r$ ($n' - n$ = difference in refractive indices; r = radius of curvature of surface [in meters])
Example: Power of corneal surface: back = −5.7 D; front = +52.9 D (front: n' = 1.37, n = 1.00; back: n' = 1.33, n = 1.37; r = 0.007)
Power of a thin lens immersed in fluid: $D_{air}/D_{fluid} = (n_{lens} - n_{air})/(n_{lens} - n_{fluid})$
Refracting power of a thin lens is proportional to difference in refractive indices between lens and medium

Objects and images:

Object rays: rays that define the object; always on incoming (left) side of lens
Image rays: rays that define the image; always on outgoing (right) side of lens
Objects and images can be on either side of lens: real if on same side as respective rays; virtual if on opposite side from rays (locate by imaginary extension of rays through lens)

If object is moved, image moves in same direction relative to light

Adding power to system also moves image: plus power pulls image against light; minus power pushes image with light

Lenses:

Real (thick) lenses (Figure 1-6):

6 CARDINAL POINTS: 2 principal planes (H and H'); 2 nodal points (N and N'); 2 focal points (F and F')

Refraction occurs at principal planes (U is measured from H; V is measured from H')

Focal lengths are also measured from principal planes

Nodal points coincide with principal planes (exception: if different refractive media are on opposite sides of the lens, then nodal points are both displaced toward the medium with the higher refractive index)

Central ray: passes through both nodal points (tip of object to N, across to N'; then, emerges parallel to original direction)

MENISCUS LENSES: difference between anterior and posterior curvature determines power

Steeper anterior curvature = convergent lens (+power); principal planes displaced anteriorly

Steeper posterior curvature = divergent lens (−power); principal planes displaced posteriorly

Power of lens is measured at posterior surface (posterior vertex power)

Conjugate points: each pair of object-image points in an optical system is conjugate; if direction of light is reversed, position of object and image is exactly reversed

Conjugate planes:

Example: Viewing a slide presentation (image of slide is formed on retina of each person in audience, and very faint image of each person's retina is projected on the screen), direct ophthalmoscope (patient's retina and examiner's retina are conjugate), indirect ophthalmoscope (3 conjugate planes [patient's retina, aerial image plane, examiner's retina]; any object placed at far point [aerial image] will be imaged sharply in focus on patient's retina)

Ideal (thin) lenses: special case of thick lens; as lens gets thinner, principal planes move closer together; in an ideal lens, principal planes overlap at optical center

2 FOCAL POINTS:

PRIMARY (f): object point for image at infinity (point on optical axis at which object is placed so parallel rays emerge from lens)

SECONDARY (f'): image point for object at infinity (point on optical axis at which incident parallel rays are focused)

FOCAL LENGTH: distance between lens and focal points; reciprocal of lens power ($f = 1/D$)

Example: Focal length of +20 D lens is 1/20 = 0.05 m

NODAL POINT (N): point through which light ray passes undeviated; located at center of thin lens (optical center)

RAY TRACING: use to determine image size, orientation, and position

3 PRINCIPAL RAYS:

1. Central ray: undeviated ray passing from tip of object through nodal point of lens (or center of curvature of mirror) to tip of image; gives size and orientation of image (form similar triangles; thus, sizes of object and image are in same ratio as their distances from the lens)

2. Ray from tip of object through F emerges from lens parallel to optical axis

3. Ray from tip of object parallel to optical axis emerges from lens and passes through F' (Figure 1-7)

Lens effectivity: function of lens power and distance from desired point of focus; depends on vertex distance and refractive index of media in which lens is placed ($D_{air} = [n_{IOL} - n_{air}] / [n_{IOL} - n_{aqueous}] \times D_{aqueous}$); moving a lens forward away from eye increases effective plus power, so plus lens becomes stronger and minus lens becomes weaker; when vertex distance decreases, a more plus lens is required to maintain the same distance correction (i.e. as desired point of focus is approached, more plus power is needed); the more powerful the lens, the more significant is the change in position

Vertex distance conversion:

1. Focal point of original lens = far point
2. Distance of new lens from far point = required focal length of new lens
3. Power of new lens = reciprocal of new focal length

Example: +12.50 D spectacle lens at vertex distance of 13 mm; calculate contact lens (CL) power:

1. +12.50 D lens has focal point of 0.08 m = 8 cm = far point
2. Distance of new lens (CL) from far point is 8 cm − 13 mm = 67 mm = required focal length of CL
3. Power of CL = 1/0.067 m = +15 D

Approximation: $D_2 = D_1 + S(D_1)^2$ (S = vertex distance in meters)

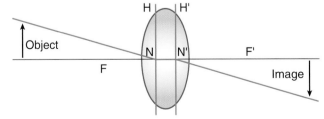

Figure 1-6. Conjugate points of real lens: each pair of object–image points in an optical system is conjugate; if direction of light is reversed, positions of object and image are exactly reversed.

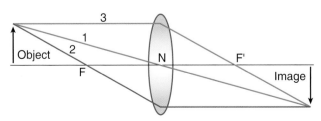

Figure 1-7. Three principal rays of ideal lens.

Pure cylindrical lens: power only in 1 meridian (perpendicular to axis of lens); produces focal line parallel to axis

Spherocylindrical lens: power in 1 meridian greater than other

Spherical equivalent: average spherical power of a spherocylindrical lens; equal to sphere plus ½ the cylinder; places circle of least confusion on retina

Conoid of Sturm: 3-dimensional envelope of light rays refracted by a circular spherocylindrical lens; consists of: vertical line → vertical ellipse → circle (of least confusion) → horizontal ellipse → horizontal line (Figure 1-8)

Circle of least confusion: circular cross section of conoid of Sturm, which lies halfway (dioptrically) between the 2 focal lines at which image is least blurred; dioptrically calculated by spherical equivalent

Interval of Sturm: distance between anterior and posterior focal lines

Cylinder transposition: converting cylinder notation (plus → minus; minus → plus)

New sphere=old sphere+old cylinder

New cylinder=magnitude of old cylinder but with opposite power

New axis=change old axis by 90°

Example: +3.00 +1.50×45 → +4.50 −1.50×135

Power cross diagram: depicts 2 principal meridians of lens with the power acting in each meridian (90° from axis), rather than according to axis (Figure 1-9)

Combining cylinders at oblique axis: complex calculation; therefore, measure with lensometer

Power of cylinder at oblique axis: power of the cylinder +1.00×180° is +1.00 @ 90°; +0.75 @ 60°; +0.50 @ 45°; +0.25 @ 30°; 0 @ 0°

Example:

JACKSON CROSS CYLINDER: special lens used for refraction to determine cylinder power and orientation; combination of plus cylinder in 1 axis and minus cylinder of equal magnitude in axis 90° away; spherical equivalent is zero (e.g.: −1.00 + 2.00×180)

Therefore, does not change the position of the circle of least confusion with respect to the retina; normally, have 0.25 D cross cylinder in phoropter; if patient's acuity is 20/40 or worse, must use larger power cross cylinder so patient can discriminate difference

TIGHT SUTURE AFTER CATARACT OR CORNEAL SURGERY: steepens cornea in meridian of suture, inducing astigmatism

Aberrations

Lenses behave ideally only near optical axis; peripheral to this paraxial region, aberrations occur

Spherical: shape-dependent aberration; periphery of lens has increasing prismatic effect; thus, peripheral rays refracted farther than paraxial ones, producing a blur interval along the optical axis (Figure 1-10)

Produces bull's-eye retinoscopic reflex

Reduce by avoiding biconvex lens shape; use plano-convex, meniscus, or aspheric lens surface

Eye has 3 mechanisms for reducing spherical aberration of lens:

1. Smaller pupil size eliminates a greater number of peripheral rays
2. Cornea progressively flattens in periphery
3. Nucleus of crystalline lens has higher index of refraction

Coma: comet-shaped image deformity from off-axis peripheral rays

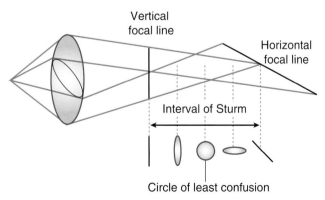

Vertical focal line

Horizontal focal line

Interval of Sturm

Circle of least confusion

Figure 1-8. Conoid of Sturm.

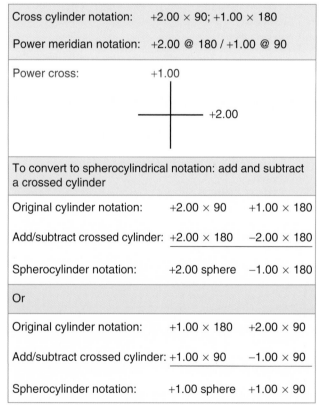

Cross cylinder notation:	+2.00 × 90; +1.00 × 180	
Power meridian notation:	+2.00 @ 180 / +1.00 @ 90	
Power cross:	+1.00 ─┼─ +2.00	
To convert to spherocylindrical notation: add and subtract a crossed cylinder		
Original cylinder notation:	+2.00 × 90	+1.00 × 180
Add/subtract crossed cylinder:	+2.00 × 180	−2.00 × 180
Spherocylinder notation:	+2.00 sphere	−1.00 × 180
Or		
Original cylinder notation:	+1.00 × 180	+2.00 × 90
Add/subtract crossed cylinder:	+1.00 × 90	−1.00 × 90
Spherocylinder notation:	+1.00 sphere	+1.00 × 90

Figure 1-9. Various lens notations.

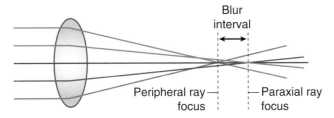

Figure 1-10. Spherical aberration.

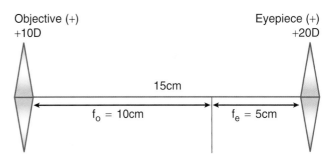

Figure 1-11. Astronomical telescope.

Curvature of field: spherical lens produces curved image of flat object

Astigmatism of oblique incidence: tilting spherical lens induces astigmatism (oblique rays encounter different curvatures at front and back lens surfaces)
> **Example:** pantoscopic tilt (amount of induced sphere and cylinder depends on power of lens and amount of tilt)

Distortion: differential magnification from optical axis to lens periphery alters straight edges of square objects; shape of distortion is opposite of shape of lens (plus lens produces **pincushion** distortion; minus lens produces **barrel** distortion); effect increases with power of lens

Chromatic: light of different wavelengths is refracted by different amounts (shorter wavelengths are bent farther; chromatic interval between blue and red is 1.5-3.0 D)
> **Example:** at night with Purkinje shift, chromatic aberration moves focal point of eye anteriorly, producing myopia

MAGNIFICATION

Transverse (linear or lateral): magnification of image size (away from optical axis); must be able to measure object and image size; ratio of image height to object height (or image distance to object distance); if image is inverted, magnification is negative $M_L = I/O$

Axial: magnification of depth; magnification along optical axis; equal to square of transverse magnification $M_{Ax} = M_L^2$

Angular: magnification of angle subtended by an image with respect to an object; useful when object or image size cannot be measured
> **Example:** moon gazing with telescope
> $M_A = xD = D/4$ (standardized to 25 cm [¼ m], the near point of the average eye)
> **Example:** with direct ophthalmoscope, eye acts as simple magnifier of retina: $M_A = 60/4 = 15\times$ magnification

Size of image seen through glasses:
Shape factors: for any corrective lens, an increase in either front surface curvature or lens thickness will increase the image size (therefore, equalize the front surface curvatures and lens thickness for the 2 lenses)
> **FRONT SURFACE CURVATURE:** every D of change will change image size by ½% (magnification decreases as plus power decreases)

CENTER THICKNESS: every mm of change in thickness will change image size by ½% (magnification decreases as lens thickness decreases)
Power factors:
VERTEX POWER (REFRACTIVE POWER): minus power lenses produce smaller images than do plus lenses
VERTEX DISTANCE: an increase in vertex distance will increase the magnification of plus lenses and decrease the magnification (increase the minification) of minus lenses
> PLUS LENS: every millimeter increase in vertex distance will increase magnification by 0.1% per diopter of lens power
> MINUS LENS: every millimeter increase in vertex distance will decrease magnification by 0.1% per diopter of lens power

Spectacle lens changes retinal image size by 2% per diopter of power at 12 mm vertex distance

Anisometropia: difference in power between the 2 eyes; every 1 D produces approximately 2% of aniseikonia

Aniseikonia: difference in image size between eyes from unequal magnification of correcting lenses
Up to 6–7% is usually well tolerated; corresponds to approximately 3 D of spectacle anisometropia; children can adjust to much larger degrees
> **Example:** unilateral aphakia: 25% enlargement with spectacle lens; 7% with contact lens; 2.5% with IOL

Knapp's rule: when proper corrective lens is positioned at anterior focal point of eye, retinal image size will be equal in both eyes, no matter what the degree of anisometropia (applies only to axial ametropia)

Telescopes: magnify objects by increasing angle that object subtends on retina
Astronomical telescope (Keplerian): combination of 2 plus lenses; focal points coincide in intermediate image plane; distance between lenses is sum of focal lengths; use higher power as eyepiece; inverted image (Figure 1-11)
Galilean telescope: combination of a weak plus lens (objective) and a strong minus lens (eyepiece); distance between lenses is difference of focal lengths; erect image (e.g. surgical loupe) (Figure 1-12)

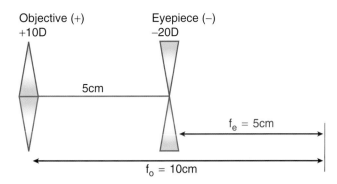

Figure 1-12. Galilean telescope.

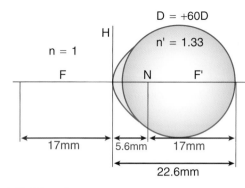

Figure 1-13. Schematic eye.

Angular magnification is the same for both telescopes (power of eyepiece/power of objective): $M_A = -D_e/D_o$

Accommodation through telescope: $A_T = A_N(M_A^2)$
(A_N = normal accommodation)

> **Example:** for monocular aphakia, overcorrect aphakic CL by +3.00 D; then, correct induced myopic error with spectacle of –3.00 D. This produces an inverse Galilean telescope system that results in significantly smaller magnification difference between the 2 eyes than occurs with a CL alone

MIRRORS

Law of reflection: angle of incidence = angle of reflection (measured from the normal)

Objects and images: real if located on left side of mirror, virtual if on right side (inside) of mirror

Focal length: ½ the radius of curvature ($f = r/2$)

Reflecting power: reciprocal of focal length ($D_r = -1/f = -2/r$)

Convex: positive radius of curvature (R); adds minus vergence; produces virtual, erect, minified image ('VErMin')

> **Example:** rear view mirror; cornea (reflecting power of cornea = $-1/f = -2/r = -2/0.0077 = -260$ D [much stronger than refracting power])

Concave: negative r; adds plus vergence; image can be virtual or real, erect or inverted, magnified or minified, depending on object location with respect to center of curvature of mirror:

> At twice focal length (center of curvature): real, inverted, same size
> Between center and focal length: real, inverted, magnified
> At focal length: at infinity
> Inside focal length: virtual, erect, magnified

Plano: no change in vergence; image is virtual, erect, same size; field of view is double the size of the mirror

> **Example:** dressing mirror needs to be only half of body length to provide view of entire self

Central ray: passes through center of curvature of mirror, not center of mirror

Primary and secondary focal points coincide

> *Purkinje-Sanson images*: 4 images from reflecting surfaces of eye

1. Front surface of cornea (image of object at infinity is located at focal point of mirror = $1/-260 = -3.85$ mm; thus, this is a virtual, erect, minified image 3.85 mm posterior to front surface of cornea)

> **Example:** keratometry (see Figure 1-24)

2. Back surface of cornea (virtual, erect, minified image)
3. Front surface of lens (virtual, erect, minified image)
4. Back surface of lens (real, inverted, minified image)

(If patient has intraocular lens [IOL], Purkinje-Sanson images 3 and 4 are taken from front and back surfaces of the IOL, respectively; these are useful in assessment of mild degrees of pseudophacodonesis)

EYE AS OPTICAL SYSTEM

Model Eye

Gullstrand studied the eye's optical system and, based on average measurements (power = +58.64 D; F = 17.05 mm), he created a simplified model: the 'reduced' or 'schematic' eye (Figure 1-13): power = +60 D; F = 17 mm; F' = 22.6 mm

> **Example:** calculate the diameter of the blind spot projected 2 meters in front of the eye (ON = 1.7 mm tall, thus by similar triangles: $1.7/17 = x/2000$; $x = 2000(1.7/17) = 200$ mm)

Vision Measurements

Minimum visible: presence or absence of stimulus; depends on amount of light striking photoreceptors

Minimum discriminable: resolving power of eye; depends on ability to detect differences in light intensity

Minimum separable: smallest angle at which 2 separate objects can be discriminated; detection of a break in a line

Vernier acuity: spatial discrimination; ability to detect misalignment of 2 lines (8 seconds of arc; smaller than diameter of photoreceptor)

Snellen acuity: based on angle that smallest letter subtends on retina; each letter subtends 5 minutes of arc at a specific distance (represented by the denominator [i.e. 20/40 letter subtends 5 minutes at 40 feet, 20/20 letter subtends 5 minutes at 20 feet]; the numerator is the testing distance); each stroke width and space subtends 1 minute (Figure 1-14)

> **Example:** calculate the size of a 20/20 letter at 20 ft (6 m): tan=opposite/adjacent; tan 1'=0.0003 therefore, tan 5'=0.0015=x/6000; x=8.7 mm

ETDRS Chart: 5 letters per line; space between letters is equal to size of letter on that line; geometric proportion of optotype height (changes in 0.1 log unit increments)

Near acuity: must record testing distance

Acuity testing in children: optokinetic nystagmus (OKN), CSM (central, steady, maintain), preferential looking, Allen pictures, HOTV (letter symbols used in pediatric visual acuity testing), visual evoked potential (VEP)

Factors other than disease that reduce measured visual acuity: uncorrected refractive error, eccentric viewing, decreased contrast, smaller pupil size, older age

Legal blindness (in US): visual acuity (VA)=20/200 or worse or visual field (VF) < 20° in better-seeing eye

Visual acuity is influenced by pupil size: larger pupil limits vision owing to spherical and chromatic aberrations; smaller pupil limits vision owing to diffraction; optimal pupil size is 3 mm

Laser inferometer: helium neon laser beam is split and projected onto retina, producing interference fringes; spacing of fringes can be varied; retinal function is estimated by narrowest fringes discernible

Contrast sensitivity: ability to detect changes in luminance

Refractive Error

Secondary focal point (F') of eye is not located on retina (accommodation must be completely relaxed) (Figure 1-15):

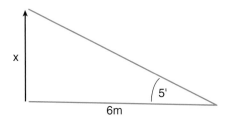

Figure 1-14. Calculation of Snellen letter size.

Emmetropia: focal point on retina
Myopia: focal point in front of retina
Hyperopia: focal point behind retina

total hyperopia =

    manifest hyperopia (absolute and facultative)+

    latent hyperopia (exposed with cycloplegia)

Axial vs refractive:
Axial myopia: length of eye too long (refractive power normal)
Refractive myopia: refractive power too strong (length normal)
Axial hyperopia: length too short (refractive power normal)
Refractive hyperopia: refractive power too weak (length normal)

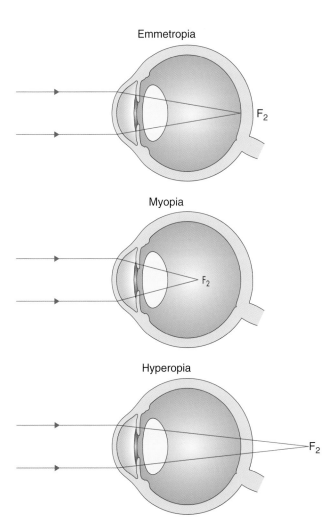

Figure 1-15. Emmetropia, myopia, and hyperopia. In emmetropia, the far point is at infinity and the secondary focal point (F_2) is at the retina. In myopia, the far point is the front of the eye, and the secondary focal point (F_2) is in the vitreous. In hyperopia, the secondary focal point (F_2) is located behind the eye. (Modified with permission from Azar DT, Strauss L: Principles of applied clinical optics. In: Albert DM, Jakobiec FA (eds) Principles and Practice of Ophthalmology, vol 6, 2nd edn. Philadelphia, WB Saunders, 2000.)

Far point: farthest-away eye can see clearly with accommodation completely relaxed (turn light around, start at retina, and trace rays backward through optics of eye; point at which rays intersect is far point)

Myopia: far point is centimeters to infinity in front of eye

Hyperopia: far point is behind eye (virtual far point)

Astigmatism: produces 2 focal lines rather than a single focal point (Table 1-1)

Classification: corneal or lenticular; regular (symmetric [mirror image axis between eyes] or asymmetric) or irregular

'With-the-rule': cornea is steepest in vertical meridian; axis of plus cylinder is 90° (±20°); usually young patients (elastic lids press on top and bottom of cornea)

'Against-the-rule': cornea is steepest in horizontal meridian; axis of plus cylinder is 180° ±20°; older patients

Correction of ametropia: choose lens with focal point that coincides with far point of patient's eye

Acquired hyperopia:

Decreased effective axial length: retrobulbar tumor, choroidal tumor, central serous chorioretinopathy

Decreased refractive power: lens change (posterior lens dislocation, aphakia, diabetes), drugs (chloroquine, phenothiazines, antihistamines, benzodiazepines), poor accommodation (tonic pupil, drugs, trauma), flattening of cornea (contact lens), intraocular silicone oil

Acquired myopia:

Increased lens power: osmotic effect (diabetes, galactosemia, uremia, sulfonamides), nuclear sclerotic cataracts, anterior lenticonus, change in lens position or shape (medication [miotics]), anterior lens dislocation, excessive accommodation)

Increased corneal power: keratoconus, congenital glaucoma, CL-induced corneal warpage

Increased axial length: congenital glaucoma, posterior staphyloma, after scleral buckle, retinopathy of prematurity (ROP)

Night myopia: increased myopia in dark

Pupil dilation: spherical aberration, irregular astigmatism uncovered

Purkinje shift: spectral sensitivity shifts toward shorter wavelengths at lower light levels, and chromatic aberration moves the focal point anteriorly

Dark focus: no accommodative target in dark; therefore, tend to overaccommodate for distance and underaccommodate for near

Length of refraction lane: shorter than 20 feet produces 1/6 D undercorrection (add minus 0.25 D to final refraction)

Acquired astigmatism: lid lesion (tumor, chalazion, ptosis), pterygium, limbal dermoid, corneal degenerations and ectasias, surgery (corneal, cataract), lenticular, ciliary body (CB) tumor

Accommodation

Eye gains plus power when crystalline lens becomes more convex

Accommodation response can be described as:

Amplitude of accommodation: total dioptric amount eye can accommodate

Near point: only for emmetropes

Prince rule: combines reading card with a ruler calibrated in centimeters and diopters to measure amplitude of accommodation

Technique: place +3.00 D lens in front of distance correction to bring far point to $\frac{1}{3}$ mm (33 cm); then, measure how near patient can read and convert into diopters; subtract far point from near point to determine amplitude

Method of spheres: fixate on reading target (e.g. 40 cm), successively increase minus sphere until print blurs, then increase plus sphere until blurring occurs again; absolute difference between the spheres is the amplitude of accommodation

Example: range of –4.00 D to +2.00 D=amplitude of 6 D

Range of accommodation: distance between far point and near point; measured with tape measure or accommodative rule

Far point: point on visual axis conjugate to retina when accommodation is completely relaxed

Near point: point on visual axis conjugate to retina when accommodation is fully active

FOR MYOPIA: near point=amount of myopia+amplitude of accommodation

FOR HYPEROPIA: near point=difference between amplitude of accommodation and amount of hyperopia

Presbyopia: loss of accommodation with age; becomes symptomatic in early 40s with asthenopic symptoms and need for reading glasses

Type	Location of focal lines	Corrective lens	
Compound myopic	Both in front of retina	–sph –cyl; –sph +cyl	(–sphere regardless of notation)
Simple myopic	1 in front, 1 on retina	–sph +cyl; plano –cyl	(–sphere or plano)
Mixed	1 in front, 1 behind	–sph +cyl; +sph –cyl	(–sphere or +sphere depending on notation)
Simple hyperopic	1 on retina, 1 behind	+sph –cyl; plano +cyl	(+sphere or plano)
Compound hyperopic	Both behind retina	+sph +cyl; +sph –cyl	(+sphere regardless of notation)

Table 1-1. Classification of astigmatism

Table 1-2. Donder's table

Age (years):	8	12	16	20	24	28	32	36	40	44	48	52	56	60	64	68
Accommodation (D):	14	13	12	11	10	9	8	7	6	4.5	3	2.5	2	1.5	1	0.5

Theories of accommodation:

Helmholtz: zonular tension decreases, lens becomes more spherical, focusing power increases; presbyopia is due to loss of lens elasticity

Tscherning-Schachar: equatorial zonular tension increases, lens diameter increases, central lens steepens, focusing power increases; lens grows throughout life, decreasing the working distance between lens and ciliary body; presbyopia is due to decreased ciliary muscle effectivity

Donder's table: average accommodative amplitudes for different ages (Table 1-2)

Up to age 40, accommodation decreases by 1 D every 4 years (starting at 14 D at age 8)

At age 40, accommodation is 6.0 D (±2 D)

Between ages 40 and 48, accommodation decreases by 1.5 D every 4 years

Above age 48, accommodation decreases by 0.5 D every 4 years

Conditions that cause asthenopia (eye fatigue with sustained near effort): hypothyroidism, anemia, pregnancy, nutritional deficiencies, chronic illness

Premature presbyopia (subnormal accommodation): debilitating illness, diphtheria, botulism, mercury toxicity, head injury, cranial nerve 3 (CN 3) palsy, Adie's tonic pupil, tranquilizers; treat with reading add, base-in prism (helps convergence)

Color Vision

3 components of color: hue, saturation, brightness

Hue: main component of color perception; depends on which wavelength is perceived as dominant

Saturation: richness of color; vivid colors are saturated; adding white desaturates color (paler) but does not change hue

Brightness: sensation produced by retinal illumination; filters decrease brightness

Example: yellow light; correct mixture of green and red also results in yellow; mixing 2 complements produces white; add white light to yellow, still yellow

Bezold-Brucke phenomenon: as brightness increases, most hues appear to change

At low intensities, blue-green, green, and yellow-green appear greener; at high intensities, they appear bluer

At low intensities, reds and oranges appear redder; at high intensities, they appear yellower

Exception: blue of 478 nm, green of 503 nm, and yellow of 578 nm do not change with changes in intensity

Abney effect: as white is added to any hue, desaturating it, the hue appears to change slightly in color; all colors (except yellow) appear yellower

Luminosity curve: illustrates sensitivity to different wavelengths

Constructed by asking observer to increase luminance of lights of various wavelengths until they appear equal in brightness to a yellow light of fixed luminance

Light-adapted eye: yellow, yellow-green, and orange appear brighter than blues, greens, and reds; peak sensitivity = 555 nm

Dark-adapted: peak sensitivity = 505 nm (blue)

Afterimages: after a color is stared at for 20 seconds, it begins to fade (desaturate)

Then, with gazing at white background, the complement of the color appears (afterimage)

Example: red is perceived when a greater number of red cones are stimulated than green or blue cones; after 20 seconds, red cones fatigue (cannot regenerate pigment fast enough), so color fades; when white background is looked at, there is a relatively greater response by green and blue cones; therefore, a blue-green afterimage is seen (complement of red)

Color perception: white wall appears white because white paint reflects all photons equally well

Charcoal appears black because it absorbs most of the light that strikes it

Blue flower appears blue because it best absorbs red, yellow, and green; blue is absorbed least, so a greater number of blue photons are reflected

Green leaf appears green because chlorophyll absorbs blue and red and reflects green

Incandescent/tungsten light emits a relatively greater number of photons of longer (red) wavelength than shorter (blue) wavelength; conversely, fluorescent light emits a relatively greater number of blue and green wavelengths; therefore, a purple dress may appear redder under incandescent light and bluer under fluorescent light

PRESCRIBING GLASSES

Use cycloplegia in children and hyperopes to uncover full refractive error

Infants average 2 D of hyperopia; myopic shift between ages 8 and 13; most adults are emmetropic

Children (Table 1-3): give full cycloplegic refraction

Table 1-3. Guidelines for prescribing glasses for children

Hyperopia:	≥+5 D
Anisometropia	≥1.5 D
Myopia:	
Up to age 1	≥−5 D
Ages 1–6	≥−3 D
Age >6	≥−1 D
Anisometropia	≥3 D
Astigmatism:	
Up to age 1	≥3 D
Ages 1–6	≥2 D
Age >6	≥1 D
Anisometropia	≥1.5 D

Adults: give manifest refraction; may not accept full astigmatic component, so if cylinder is decreased, adjust sphere to keep spherical equivalent constant; be careful about changing axis

Minus cylinder grinding: placing astigmatic correction on rear surface (closer to eye) is optically preferable
  Astigmatic dial: 12 spokes corresponding to clock hours are projected on screen; spokes parallel to principal meridians of eye's astigmatism are sharp (corresponding with focal lines of conoid of Sturm); the others are blurred

Match base curves: when prescribing new glasses, keep base curve same as that of old lenses
  Geneva lens clock: measures base curve of lens; direct dioptric power of convex, concave, or aspheric lens surface is read on the dial of the clock; calibration is based on the refractive index of crown glass (1.52)

Binocular balance: equally controls accommodation in both eyes (visual acuity must be equal)
  Methods:
  1. *Prism dissociation:* 3 Δ BU over one eye and 3 Δ BD over the other (use Risley prism in phoropter)
  2. *Balanced fogging:* fog both eyes and alternate cover until equally fogged
  3. *Duochrome test:* red–green balance both eyes (vision must be 20/30 or better)

Bifocal add: place segments as high as practical in relation to optical centers of the distance lenses
  Measure accommodation: perform monocularly, then binocularly
  Near point of accommodation (use refractive correction)
  Accommodative amplitude (use Prince rule)
  Determine accommodative requirement for near vision task
  Example: reading at 40 cm=2.5 D
  Hold ½ of measured accommodative amplitude in reserve to prevent asthenopic symptoms
  Example: Prince rule measures 2.0 D of amplitude; thus 1.0 D is available to patient
  Power of add is difference between accommodation (1.0 D) and total amount of accommodation required (2.5 D)

With calculated add in front of distance correction, measure accommodative range (near point to far point of accommodation); if range is too close, reduce add in steps of 0.25 D until correct range found

Kestenbaum's rule: used to estimate strength of plus lens required to read newspaper print without accommodation
  Add power=reciprocal of best distance acuity
  Reciprocal of add power=working distance (in meters)
  Example: 20/80 vision; add=80/20=+4.00 D; working distance=1/4 (0.25 m)

Aphakic spectacles: disadvantages include magnification of 25%, altered depth perception, pincushion distortion, ring scotoma (prismatic effect at edge of lens causes visual field loss of 20%), 'jack-in-the-box' phenomenon (peripherally invisible objects suddenly appear when gaze is shifted)

CONTACT LENSES (CL)

Toric lens: lenses with different radii of curvature in each meridian
  Front toric: anterior surface with 2 different radii of curvature, posterior surface spherical; corrects lenticular astigmatism
  Back toric: cylinder on back surface only; corrects corneal astigmatism
  Bitoric: minus cylinder on posterior surface, plus cylinder on anterior surface; corrects corneal and lenticular astigmatism

Ballasted lens: heavier base to orient lens by gravity; 2 types:
  Prism: 1.5-2 Δ BD prism added
  Truncated: flat along inferior edge

Sagittal depth/apical height: distance between back surface of lens center and a flat surface

Radius of curvature (base curve): curvature of posterior lens surface for a given diameter; the shorter the radius of curvature, the greater is the sagittal depth (the steeper the lens)

Overall diameter: for a given base curve, increasing diameter increases the apical vault
  Example: to tighten a lens, reduce radius of curvature or increase diameter

Oxygen transmission: DK (relative gas permeability) value; D=diffusion coefficient; K=solubility of oxygen in material; oxygen transmissibility=DK/L (L=lens thickness)

Accommodative demand: depends on magnification, which varies with different lens powers and vertex distances
  Hyperopes: decreased accommodative demand when CL are worn compared with spectacles (presbyopic symptoms appear earlier with spectacles)

Myopes: increased accommodative demand when CL are used (presbyopic symptoms appear earlier with CL). In high myopia, spectacles induce base-in prism with near convergence, lessening requirement for convergence

Fitting rigid CL: SAM-FAP rule ('steeper add minus, flatter add plus')

Fit steeper than corneal surface (forms a plus tear meniscus between cornea and CL, which alters required power of CL). Therefore, need to subtract power (add minus) at end of calculation; for each diopter, the base curve is made 'steeper than *K*'; subtract 1 D from the final CL power; if lens is fit flatter than *K*, a minus tear meniscus is formed, so must add plus power

Remember, a rigid lens with base curve of 44 D does not have a power of 44 D; rather, the radius of the CL's central posterior curve is equal to the radius of curvature of a cornea with a calculated power of 44 D

Power calculation: if trial lens not available for overrefraction

1. Measure refraction and keratometry
2. Choose base curve steeper than low *K* (usually +0.50 D steeper to form a tear lens; tear lens prevents apical touch)
3. Convert refraction to minus cylinder form and zero vertex distance; disregard the cylinder (minus cylinder is formed by the tears)
4. Power of CL is sphere from refraction adjusted for tear lens (subtract +0.50); 'SAM-FAP'

Evaluating fit:

Soft lens: evaluate movement (poor movement=too tight [too steep], excessive movement=too flat); choose power based on spherical equivalent

Rigid lens: assess fluorescein pattern (Figures 1-16–1-18)

LOW-VISION AIDS

Kestenbaum's rule: estimates strength of plus lens required to read newspaper print without accommodation

Near devices:

High bifocal add or single vision reading glasses (up to+20 D): large field of view but short reading distance

Magnifiers: handheld (up to +20 D; small field of view) or stand (up to +50 D; bulky)

Loupes: long working distance but small field of view

Electronic displays: high magnification but expensive

Distance devices:

Telescopes: restricted field of view

INTRAOCULAR LENSES (IOL)

Formulas for IOL calculation (see Ch. 10)

Empiric: derived from clinical studies by regression analysis

1ST GENERATION: SRK, Gills-Lloyd

2ND GENERATION: SRK II, Thompson-M, Donzis

Theoretical: derived from optics by vergence formulas

1ST GENERATION: Binkhorst I, Fyodorov, Colenbrander

2ND GENERATION: Binkhorst II, Shamas

3RD GENERATION: Hoffer Q, Holladay 1, SRK/T

4TH GENERATION: Holladay 2, Haigis, Olsen

Newer-generation theoretical formulas are the most accurate

A rough estimation of lens power can be quickly obtained with the *SRK* formula:

IOL power for emmetropia $= P = A - 2.5\,L - 0.9K$

$A = A$ constant (related to lens type)

$L =$ axial length in mm; 1 mm error $= 2.5$ D error in IOL power

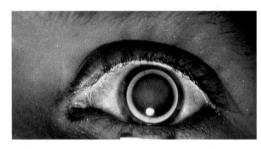

Figure 1-17. Fluorescein pattern of corneal contact lens fitted 'on *K*.' Note the central alignment. (From White P, Scott C: Contact lenses. In: Yanoff M, Duker JS (eds) Ophthalmology. London, Mosby, 1999.)

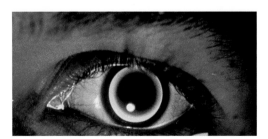

Figure 1-18. Fluorescein pattern of corneal contact lens fitted 1 D flatter than 'flat *K*.' Note the central touch. (From White P, Scott C: Contact lenses. In: Yanoff M, Duker JS (eds) Ophthalmology. London, Mosby, 1999.)

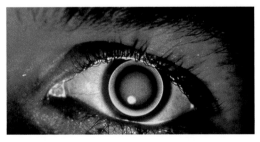

Figure 1-16. Fluorescein pattern of corneal contact lens fitted 1 D steeper than 'flat *K*.' Note the central clearance. (From White P, Scott C: Contact lenses. In: Yanoff M, Duker JS (eds) Ophthalmology. London, Mosby, 1999.)

K = average keratometry value in D; 1.0 D error ≈ 1.25 D error in IOL power

Lens position is important: 1 mm error = 1.0 D change in power

Calculate IOL power for refractive target other than emmetropia: $D_{IOL} = P - (R/1.5)$ (R = desired refractive error)

IOL power for a different lens = original IOL power ± difference in A constants

> **Example:** if instead of +20.0 D IOL with *A* constant of 118, you want to use a different style IOL with *A* constant of 118.5, equivalent power of the new IOL is +20.5 D

OPHTHALMIC INSTRUMENTS

Direct ophthalmoscope (Figure 1-19): coaxial light and lenses to neutralize patient and examiner refractive errors, so retinas become conjugate; examiner uses optics of patient's eye as simple magnifier ($M_A = 60/4 = 15\times$); field of view ~7°

Indirect ophthalmoscope (Figure 1-20): enlarged field of view (25°) with stereopsis by adding condensing lens

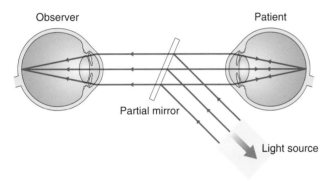

Figure 1-19. Optics of the direct ophthalmoscope. By using a mirror (either half-silvered or with a central aperture), the directions of the light of observation and the light incident to the patient are made concentric (coaxial). (From Miller D, Thall EH, Atebara NH: Ophthalmic instrumentation. In: Yanoff M, Duker JS (eds) Ophthalmology, 2nd edn. St Louis, Mosby, 2004.)

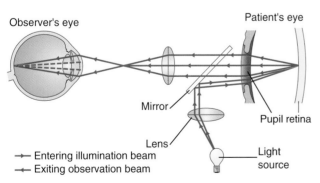

Figure 1-20. Theoretical optics of the indirect ophthalmoscope. The illumination beam enters a small part of the pupil and does not overlap with the observation beam; this minimizes bothersome reflection and backscatter. (From Miller D, Thall EH, Atebara NH: Ophthalmic instrumentation. In: Yanoff M, Duker JS (eds) Ophthalmology, 2nd edn. St Louis, Mosby, 2004.)

between patient and examiner; binocular eyepiece reduces interpupillary distance to 15 mm (~4×); $M_A = D_{eye}/D_{lens} = 60/20 = 3\times$; $M_{Ax} = 3^2 = 9$, but eyepiece reduces depth 4×; therefore $M_{Ax} = 9/4 = 2.25\times$

Retinoscope: instrument to objectively measure refractive state of eye

The blurred image of the filament on the patient's retina is considered a new light source returning to examiner's eye; by observing the characteristics of the reflex, examiner can determine patient's refractive error

If examiner is at far point of patient's eye, all light rays emanating from patient's pupil pass through retinoscope and examiner's pupil, and patient's pupil will appear uniformly illuminated (neutralization)

If far point is between examiner and patient (myopic), reflex moves in direction opposite to retinoscope sweep ('against' motion)

If far point is behind examiner (hyperopia), reflex has 'with' motion

Use correcting lens to determine point of neutralization

Correct for working distance to obtain patient's final refraction (add reciprocal of working distance to final finding)

If poor, irregular retinoscopic reflex, try contact lens overrefraction or stenopeic slit refraction

Slit-lamp biomicroscope (Figure 1-21): illumination and magnification allow stereo viewing of ocular structures; illumination and viewing arms have common pivot point

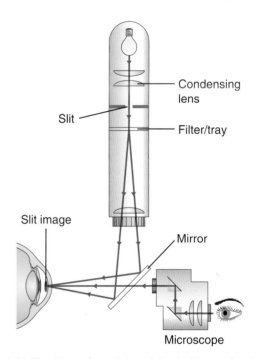

Figure 1-21. The slit lamp. Some slit lamps bring the light to a sharp focus within the slit aperture, and the light within the slit is focused by the condensing lens onto the patient's eyes. The observation system of a modern slit lamp has many potential reflecting surfaces – antireflection coatings on these surfaces help loss of light. (Modified from Spalton DJ, Hitchings RA, Hunter PA: Atlas of Clinical Ophthalmology. New York, Grower Medical, 1985.)

Lensometer: measures power of spectacle or CL using telescope to detect neutralization point; distance measurement is determined from back vertex power; add measurement is taken from front vertex power; prism measurement is derived from displacement of target pattern (Figures 1-22 and 1-23)

Keratometer: measures curvature of anterior corneal surface based on power of reflecting surface; measures only 2 paracentral points 3 mm apart; doubling of image prevents interference from eye movements (Figure 1-24)

Applanation tonometry: direct measure of IOP as force/area with split-field prism; at applanated diameter of 3.06 mm, corneal resistance to deformation and attractive force of tear surface tension cancel each other

A- and B-scan ultrasonography: measure acoustic reflectivity of interfaces to provide 2-dimensional picture of ocular structures

Ocular coherence tomography (OCT): measures optical reflectivity to provide cross-sectional image of ocular structures

EQUATIONS

Vergence formula:

$$U + D = V$$

U=object vergence, D=lens power, V=image vergence

Lens power (diopters):

$$D = 1/f$$

f=focal length (meters)

Snell's law:

$$n\sin(i) = n'\sin(r)$$

n=refractive index, i=angle of incidence, r=angle of refraction

Prismatic power:

$$\Delta = \frac{\text{image deflection (cm)}}{\text{meters}} = 100\tan(\beta)$$

β=angle of deviation

Prentice's rule:

$$\Delta = hD$$
h=distance from optical axis (cm), D=lens power

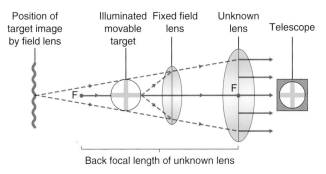

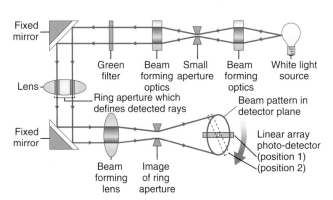

Position of target image by field lens — Illuminated movable target — Fixed field lens — Unknown lens — Telescope

Back focal length of unknown lens

Figure 1-22. The lensometer resembles an optical bench. The movable illuminated target sends light to the field lens, with the target in the end-point position. Because the focal point of the field coincides with the position of the unknown lens, all final images are of the same size. (From Miller D, Thall EH, Atebara NH: Ophthalmic instrumentation. In: Yanoff M, Duker JS (eds) Ophthalmology, 2nd edn. St Louis, Mosby, 2004.)

Figure 1-23. Optics of a typical automated lensometer. Parallel light strikes unknown lens. The refracted light rays (which are confined to a pencil beam within an annulus) ultimately strike an array of electronic photoreceptors. (From Miller D, Thall EH, Atebara NH: Ophthalmic instrumentation. In: Yanoff M, Duker JS (eds) Ophthalmology, 2nd edn. St Louis, Mosby, 2004.)

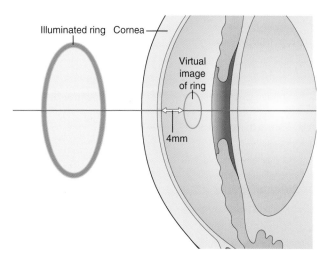

Figure 1-24. Keratometer principle. An illuminated ring is placed in front of the cornea, which acts as a convex mirror and produces a virtual image of the ring approximately 4 mm behind the cornea. (From Miller D, Thall EH, Atebara NH: Ophthalmic instrumentation. In: Yanoff M, Duker JS (eds) Ophthalmology, 2nd edn. St Louis, Mosby, 2004.)

Reduced schematic eye (calculations of retinal image size):

$$\frac{I}{17\ \text{mm}} = \frac{O}{X}$$

I=retinal image size, O=object size, X=distance to object

Spherical equivalent:

spherical equivalent = sphere + (cylinder / 2)

Refracting power of a spherical surface:

$$Ds = \frac{n'-n}{r}$$

n'=refractive index to right, n=refractive index to left, r=radius of curvature of surface (m), (+=convex; −=concave)

Reflecting power of a spherical mirror:

$$Dr = \frac{-1}{f} = \frac{-2}{r}$$

f=focal length of mirror, r=radius of curvature of mirror, (−=convex; +=concave)

Power of a thin lens immersed in fluid:

$$\frac{D_{\text{air}}}{D_{\text{aqueous}}} = \frac{n_{\text{IOL}} - n_{\text{air}}}{n_{\text{IOL}} - n_{\text{aqueous}}}$$

Power of lens at new vertex distance:

$$D_2 = D_1 = S(D_1)^2$$

D_1=original dioptric power of lens, D_2=new dioptric power, S=difference in location (m)

Linear magnification:

$$M_L = I/O$$

I=image distance or height, O=object distance or height

Axial magnification:

$$M_{\text{ax}} = (M_L)^2$$

Angular magnification:

$$M_A = xD$$

x=distance, D=dioptric power of lens

Simple magnifier:

$$M_A = D/4$$

(divide by 4 because distance set as reading distance of 0.25 m)
Example: 1× magnifier=+4 lens; 2× magnifier=+8 lens

Telescope (Galilean and astronomical):

$$M_A = -D_e / D_o$$

D_e=power of eyepiece, D_o=power of objective

Total accommodation through telescope:

$$A_T = A_N(M_A)^2$$

A_N=normal accommodation required, M_A=telescope magnification

IOL power (SRK):

$$P = A - 2.5L - 0.9K$$

A=A constant for type of IOL, L=axial length, K=average keratometry value

AC/A ratio (accommodative converge/accommodation): (see Ch. 5, Strabismus)

normal = 3 : 1 to 5 : 1 (expressed as PD of deviation per D of accommodation)

Calculations:
HETEROPHORIA METHOD: measure deviation with fixation target at 6 m and at ⅓ m

$$AC/A = \frac{\text{deviation at near} - \text{deviation at distance}}{\text{accommodative demand}} + PD$$

PD=interpupillary distance (cm)

LENS GRADIENT METHOD: stimulate accommodation by measuring deviation with target at 6 m, then remeasuring with −1 D sphere in front of both eyes; or, relax accommodation by measuring deviation with target at ⅓ m, then remeasuring with +3 D sphere in front of both eyes

$$AC/A = \frac{\text{deviation with lens} - \text{deviation without lens}}{\text{lens power}}$$

REVIEW QUESTIONS (Answers start on page 355)

1. Prince's rule is helpful in determining all of the following except
   a. amplitude of accommodation
   b. near point of accommodation
   c. far point of accommodation
   d. accommodative convergence
2. A myope who pushes his spectacles closer to his face and tilts them is
   a. decreasing effectivity, increasing cylinder
   b. decreasing effectivity, decreasing cylinder
   c. increasing effectivity, decreasing cylinder
   d. increasing effectivity, increasing cylinder

3. The Prentice position refers to
   a. glass prism perpendicular to visual axis
   b. glass prism in frontal plane
   c. plastic prism perpendicular to visual axis
   d. plastic prism in frontal plane
4. The purpose of Q-switching a laser is to
   a. increase energy, increase power
   b. decrease energy, increase power
   c. decrease energy, decrease power
   d. increase energy, decrease power
5. A 50-year-old woman with aphakic glasses wants a new pair of spectacles to use when applying make-up. How much power should be added to her distance correction so that she can focus while sitting 50 cm in front of her mirror?
   a. −2.00 D
   b. −1.00 D
   c. +1.00 D
   d. +2.00 D
6. How far from a plano mirror must a 6-ft-tall man stand to see his whole body?
   a. 2 feet
   b. 3 feet
   c. 6 feet
   d. 12 feet
7. A 33-year-old woman with a refraction of −9.00 +3.00×90 OD at vertex distance 10 mm and keratometry readings of 46.00@90/43.00@180 is fit for a rigid gas-permeable (RGP) contact lens 1 D steeper than flattest K. What power lens is required?
   a. −5.00 D
   b. −6.00 D
   c. −7.00 D
   d. −8.00 D
8. What is the size of a 20/60 letter on a standard 20-ft Snellen chart (tangent of 1 minute of arc=0.0003)?
   a. 9 mm
   b. 15 mm
   c. 18 mm
   d. 27 mm
9. A Galilean telescope with a +5 D objective and a −20 D eyepiece produces an image with what magnification and direction?
   a. 4×, erect
   b. 4×, inverted
   c. 100×, erect
   d. 100×, inverted
10. An object is placed 33 cm in front of an eye. The image formed by reflection from the front surface of the cornea (radius of curvature equals 8 mm) is located
    a. 4 mm in front of cornea
    b. 4 mm behind cornea
    c. 8 mm in front of cornea
    d. 8 mm behind cornea
11. A convex mirror produces what type of image?
    a. virtual, inverted, magnified
    b. real, inverted, minified
    c. real, erect, magnified
    d. virtual, erect, minified
12. In general, the most bothersome problem associated with bifocals is

a. image jump
b. image displacement
c. induced prism
d. anisophoria

13. A refraction with a stenopeic slit gives the following measurements: +1.00 at 90° and −2.00 at 180°. The corresponding spectacle prescription is
    a. −2.00+1.00×90
    b. −2.00+1.00×180
    c. −2.00+3.00×180
    d. +1.00+3.00×90
14. A point source of light is placed ⅓ of a meter to the left of a +7 D lens. Where will its image come to focus?
    a. 25 cm to the right of the lens
    b. 25 cm to the left of the lens
    c. 10 cm to the right of the lens
    d. 10 cm to the left of the lens
15. What is the equivalent sphere of the following cross cylinder: −3.00×180 combined with +0.50×90?
    a. −1.00
    b. −1.25
    c. −1.50
    d. −1.75
16. What is the size of a letter on a standard 20-ft Snellen chart if it forms an image of ½ mm on a patient's retina?
    a. 59 cm
    b. 30 cm
    c. 25 cm
    d. 18 cm
17. The image of a distant object is largest in which patient?
    a. aphake with contact lens
    b. hyperope with spectacles
    c. emmetrope
    d. myope with spectacles
18. What type of image is produced if an object is placed in front of a convex lens within its focal length?
    a. erect and real
    b. erect and virtual
    c. inverted and real
    d. inverted and virtual
19. What is the correct glasses prescription if retinoscopy performed at 50 cm shows neutralization with a plano lens?
    a. −2.00
    b. −1.50
    c. plano
    d. +2.00
20. An anisometropic patient experiences difficulty while reading with bifocals. Which of the following is not helpful for reducing the induced phoria?
    a. dissimilar segments
    b. slab-off lens
    c. progressive lenses
    d. fresnel 'press-on' prisms
21. A Geneva lens clock is used to measure what?
    a. thickness
    b. power
    c. index of refraction
    d. base curve

22. What is the induced prism when a 67-year-old woman reads 10 mm below the upper segment optical center of her bifocals, which measure +2.50+1.00×90 OD and −1.50+1.50×180 OS add +2.50 OU
    a. 4.0 Δ
    b. 3.5 Δ
    c. 2.5 Δ
    d. 2.0 Δ

23. The optimal size of a pinhole for measuring pinhole visual acuity is approximately
    a. 2.50 mm
    b. 2.00 mm
    c. 1.25 mm
    d. 0.75 mm

24. A person looking at an object 5 m away through a 10 Δ prism placed base-in over the right eye would see the image displaced
    a. 20 cm to the right
    b. 50 cm to the right
    c. 20 cm to the left
    d. 50 cm to the left

25. Calculate the soft contact lens power for a 40-year-old hyperope who wears +14.00 D glasses at a vertex distance of 11 mm.
    a. +15.00 D
    b. +16.00 D
    c. +17.00 D
    d. +18.00 D

26. After cataract surgery, a patient's refraction is −0.75+1.75×10, in what meridian should a suture be cut to reduce the astigmatism?
    a. 180°
    b. 100°
    c. 90°
    d. 10°

27. What is the appropriate correction in the IOL power if the A constant for the lens to be implanted is changed from 117 to 118?
    a. decrease IOL power by 1.0 D
    b. increase IOL power by 1.0 D
    c. decrease IOL power by 0.5 D
    d. increase IOL power by 0.5 D

28. An IOL labeled with a power of +20 D has a refractive index of 1.5. If this lens were removed from the package and measured with a lensometer, what power would be found?
    a. +10 D
    b. +13 D
    c. +30 D
    d. +59 D

29. The total cylindrical power of a 0.50 D cross cylinder is
    a. plano
    b. 0.25 D
    c. 0.50 D
    d. 1.00 D

30. To minimize image displacement in a hyperope, the best type of bifocal segment style is
    a. flat top
    b. progressive
    c. round top
    d. executive

31. The logMAR equivalent to 20/40 Snellen acuity is
    a. 0.4
    b. 0.3
    c. 0.2
    d. 0.1

32. A patient who is pseudophakic in one eye and phakic in the other eye will have what amount of aniseikonia
    a. 1%
    b. 2.5%
    c. 5%
    d. 7%

33. A patient with 20/80 vision is seen for a low-vision evaluation. What add power should be prescribed so the patient does not have to use accommodation to read the newspaper
    a. +3
    b. +4
    c. +8
    d. +16

34. The spherical equivalent of a −2.00+1.50×90 lens is
    a. +0.50
    b. −0.50
    c. −1.25
    d. −3.50

35. After extracapsular cataract extraction a patient is found to have 2 D of with-the-rule astigmatism and a tight suture across the wound at 12 o'clock. Corneal topography is obtained and the placido disc image shows an oval pattern with the mires closest together at
    a. 12 o'clock with the short axis at 90°
    b. 12 o'clock with the short axis at 180°
    c. 6 o'clock with the short axis at 90°
    d. 6 o'clock with the short axis at 180°

36. A 57-year-old woman has a 0.25 mm macular hole in her left eye. The size of the corresponding scotoma on a tangent screen at 1 m is approximately
    a. 1.0 cm
    b. 1.5 cm
    c. 2.5 cm
    d. 3.0 cm

37. During retinoscopy, when neutralization is reached, the light reflex is
    a. narrowest and slowest
    b. narrowest and brightest
    c. widest and slowest
    d. widest and fastest

38. A patient undergoing fogged refraction with an astigmatic dial sees the 9 to 3 o'clock line clearer than all the others. At what axis should this patient's minus cylinder correcting lens be placed?
    a. 30°
    b. 45°
    c. 90°
    d. 180°

39. Myopia is associated with all of the following conditions except
    a. nanophthalmos
    b. pigment dispersion syndrome
    c. spherophakia
    d. nuclear sclerotic cataract

40. What is the ratio of the magnification from a direct ophthalmoscope to the magnification from an indirect ophthalmoscope with a 20 D lens at a distance of 25 cm if the patient and examiner are both emmetropic?
    a. 15:2
    b. 10:3
    c. 5:1
    d. 4:1

41. A patient with anisometropia wears glasses with a prescription of +5.00 OD and +1.25 OS. Which of the following actions will not reduce the amount of aniseikonia?
    a. decrease base curve of right lens
    b. decrease center thickness of left lens
    c. decrease vertex distance of the glasses
    d. fit the patient with contact lenses

42. The principal measurement determined by a Prince's rule and +3 D lens in front of the patient's eye is the
    a. range of accommodation
    b. amplitude of accommodation
    c. near point of accommodation
    d. accommodative convergence

43. The 10× eyepiece of the slit-lamp biomicroscope is essentially a simple magnifier. Using the standard reference distance of 25 cm, what is the dioptric power of the 10× eyepiece?
    a. +2.5 D
    b. +10 D
    c. +25 D
    d. +40 D

44. When refracting an astigmatic patient with a Lancaster dial, the examiner should place the
    a. circle of least confusion on the retina
    b. posterior focal line on the retina
    c. anterior focal line behind the retina
    d. entire conoid of Sturm in front of the retina

45. To increase the magnification of the image during indirect ophthalmoscopy, the examiner should:
    a. move closer to the condensing lens
    b. move the eyepiece prisms farther apart
    c. use a higher dioptric power condensing lens
    d. remove the plus lens in the eyepiece

SUGGESTED READINGS

American Academy of Ophthalmology: Optics, Refraction, and Contact Lenses, vol 3. San Francisco, AAO, 2012.

Benjamin WJ: Borish's Clinical Refraction, 2nd edn. Philadelphia, Elsevier, 2006.

MacInnes BJ: Ophthalmology Board Review: Optics and Refraction. St Louis, Mosby, 1994.

Milder B, Rubin ML, Weinstein GW: The Fine Art of Prescribing Glasses Without Making a Spectacle of Yourself. Gainesville, Triad Scientific Publications, 1991.

Rubin ML: Optics for Clinicians. Gainesville, Triad Scientific Publications, 1993.

2

Pharmacology

OCULAR PHARMACOLOGY

Pharmacodynamics: the study of the biochemical and physiologic effects of drugs and their mechanisms of action.

Pharmacokinetics: the study of the factors that determine the relationship between drug dosage and the change in concentration over time in a biological system.

Bioavailability: amount of drug absorbed (penetration into ocular tissues)
Depends on concentration, rate of absorption, tissue binding, transport, metabolism, and excretion
Methods of improving bioavailability:
INCREASE CONCENTRATION: limited by solubility and tonicity (hypertonicity causes reflex tearing, which dilutes and washes drug from the eye)
SURFACTANTS: surface-active agents alter cell membranes, increasing permeability of the corneal epithelium
OSMOTICS: alter tonicity
INCREASE PH: increases nonionized (lipid-soluble) form of drug, increasing corneal penetration (pH of tears = 7.4)
INCREASE VISCOSITY: viscous additives (methylcellulose, polyvinyl alcohol) increase contact time and therefore penetration
INCREASE CONTACT TIME: gels and oil-based ointment formulations (mineral oil, petrolatum), polymer matrix (DuraSite); must be able to release drug

Therapeutic index: method of comparing potency of different antibiotics. A measure of relative effective (therapeutic) concentration of antibiotic at target site against a target organism.

Inhibitory quotient (IQ):
The most potent antibiotic has the lowest minimum inhibitory concentration (MIC) (or highest IQ).

ROUTES OF ADMINISTRATION

Topical: absorption related to corneal penetration
1 drop = 50 μL (20–40 drops in most bottles)
Conjunctival cul-de-sac holds only 10 μL (20% of drop)
Drop diluted by reflex tearing and normal tear turnover:
only ~50% of drug that reaches the cul-de-sac is present 4 minutes later (10% of drop)
Corneal barriers to penetration:
TIGHT JUNCTIONS (epithelium and endothelium): limit passage of hydrophilic drugs
STROMA (water rich): limits passage of lipophilic drugs
Methods of increasing absorption:
1. Add surfactants (disrupts epithelial integrity; e.g. benzalkonium chloride, topical anesthetic).
2. Promote punctal occlusion (decreases drainage).
3. Close eyelid after drops are placed.
4. Increase lipid solubility of drug (increases pH); more important than water solubility.
5. Increase frequency of drops.
Topical medications have systemic adverse effects because the drugs bypass hepatic 'first-pass' metabolism (cul-de-sac → nasolacrimal duct → mucosa → bloodstream)

Examples of other delivery systems:

PRODRUG: dipivalyl epinephrine (Propine; prodrug of epinephrine, less toxicity), nepafenac (Nevanac; prodrug of amfenac)

OINTMENT: drugs that have better uptake in ointment form, including tetracycline, chloramphenicol, and fluorometholone

SUSTAINED RELEASE GEL: pilocarpine (Pilopine HS; decreased dosing)

INSERT: pilocarpine (Ocusert; membrane-controlled system; slow release over 1 week); hydroxypropyl cellulose (Lacrisert; artificial tear slow-release pellet); collagen shield (bandage contact lens presoaked in antibiotic)

Subconjunctival/sub-Tenon's: increases duration and concentration, bypasses conjunctival and corneal barriers, avoids systemic toxicity; useful if poor compliance

Retrobulbar/peribulbar: used for anesthesia; alcohol or chlorpromazine (to kill pain fibers and optic nerve [ON] in blind, painful eye)

Intraocular: direct ocular effects; beware toxicity (particularly from preservatives), retinal tear, retinal detachment (RD), endophthalmitis; used intraoperatively (intracameral, intravitreal) and in retinal diseases (intravitreal) including macular edema, choroidal neovascularization (CNV), endophthalmitis, cytomegalovirus (CMV) retinitis

Systemic: must cross blood–ocular barrier (blood–aqueous for anterior segment, blood–retinal for posterior segment); penetrance is improved with decreased molecular size, decreased protein binding, and increased lipid solubility

Concentration

1% solution = 1 g/100 mL = 10 mg/mL

Example: How much atropine is contained in 5 mL of a 2% solution?

2% = 2 g/100 mL = 20 mg/mL = 100 mg in 5 mL

ANESTHETICS

Mechanism: reversible blockade of nerve fiber conduction (block sodium channels); pH dependent (less effective at low pH [inflamed tissue])

Structure: 2 classes; do not necessarily have allergic cross-reactivity

Ester: hydrolyzed by plasma cholinesterase and metabolized in liver; cocaine, tetracaine (amethocaine), proparacaine, procaine, benoxinate

Amide: longer duration and less systemic toxicity; metabolized in liver; lidocaine, mepivacaine, bupivacaine

Topical: disturb intercellular junction of corneal epithelium (increase permeability)

Proparacaine (Ophthaine): 10- to 30-minute duration, corneal toxicity; may cause allergic dermatitis (also common with atropine and neomycin); does not necessarily have allergic cross-reactivity with tetracaine

Tetracaine (Pontocaine): similar to proparacaine but longer duration and more toxic to corneal epithelium

Benoxinate: similar to proparacaine; combined with fluorescein (Fluress) for tonometry

Cocaine: greatest epithelial toxicity; excellent anesthesia, sympathomimetic effect (test for Horner's syndrome)

Parenteral: may be used with epinephrine (1 : 100,000) to increase duration by preventing systemic absorption; also decreases bleeding; hyaluronidase (Wydase) 150 IU increases tissue penetration, but decreases duration. Side effect of retrobulbar anesthesia = respiratory depression, bradycardia

Toxicity: hypotension, convulsions, nausea, vomiting

Lidocaine (Xylocaine): 1-hour duration (2 hours with epinephrine); used for local anesthesia : akinesia

Procaine (Novocain): 30- to 45-minute duration

Mepivacaine (Carbocaine): 2-hour duration

Bupivacaine (Marcaine): 6-hour duration

General: all agents decrease IOP except ketamine, chloral hydrate, N_2O, and ether

Malignant hyperthermia: rare, autosomal dominant condition that occurs after exposure to inhalation agents (most commonly halothane, also succinylcholine, haloperidol); more common in children and males; thought to be due to calcium-binding disorder in sarcoplasmic reticulum that causes increased intracellular calcium, which stimulates muscle contraction

Interference with oxidative phosphorylation causes hypermetabolic crisis

FINDINGS: tachycardia (1st sign), elevated CO_2 levels, tachypnea, unstable BP, arrhythmias, cyanosis, sweating, increased temperature (later sign), muscle contractions; later, heart failure and disseminated intravascular coagulation (DIC) develop; laboratory tests show respiratory and metabolic acidosis and increased K, Mg, myoglobin, creatine phosphokinase (CPK), hypoxemia, hypercarbia, myoglobinuria

SCREENING: elevated CPK, muscle biopsy/contracture test, platelet bioassay (decreased adenosine triphosphate [ATP] in platelet exposed to halothane)

TREATMENT: stop anesthesia, hyperventilate with 100% oxygen, give sodium bicarbonate, cool patient (iced saline IV and lavage; surface cooling), mannitol and furosemide (Lasix), IV dantrolene (prevents release of calcium from sarcoplasmic reticulum), procainamide, insulin (do not use lactated Ringer's solution, which increases potassium)

PROGNOSIS: 50-60% mortality

AUTONOMIC SYSTEM

Sympathetic

Extensive system for mass response ('fight or flight') (Table 2-1)
Synapses near cord (superior cervical ganglion)
Long postganglionic nerves

Adrenergic receptors:

α_1: smooth muscle contraction (arteries [decrease aqueous production by reducing ciliary body blood flow], iris dilator, Müller's muscle)

α_2: feedback inhibition, ciliary body (decreases production and/or increases outflow)

β_1: cardiac stimulation

β_2: pulmonary and GI smooth muscle relaxation, ciliary body/trabecular meshwork (increase aqueous production, increase outflow facility)

Neurotransmitter: acetylcholine (ACh) at preganglionic terminal, epinephrine and norepinephrine (NE) at postganglionic terminal

Monoamine oxidase (MAO) breaks down NE in nerve terminal; blocked by MAO inhibitors (avoid with phenylephrine, epinephrine, and pseudoephedrine-based cold remedies)

Catechol-O-methyltransferase (COMT) breaks down NE in effector cell

Reserpine prevents storage of NE in nerve terminal

Cocaine, tricyclics block reuptake of NE by nerve terminal (thus potentiate its action)

Hydroxyamphetamine increases release of NE from nerve terminal

Parasympathetic

More limited system for discrete response (homeostatic)
Synapses near end organ (ciliary ganglion)
Short postganglionic nerves

Cholinergic receptors:

Nicotinic: somatic motor and preganglionic autonomic nerves (extraocular muscles, levator, orbicularis [outside eye])

Muscarinic: postganglionic parasympathetic nerves (iris sphincter, ciliary muscle [inside eye])

Neurotransmitter: ACh
Acetylcholinesterase (AChE) breaks down ACh

Cholinergic Drugs

Direct-acting agonists: act on end organ; therefore, do not need intact innervation; cause shallowing of anterior chamber (AC); disruption of blood–aqueous barrier, miosis, brow ache, and decrease in IOP

Acetylcholine (miochol: very short-acting, unstable, used intracamerally), methacholine, carbacholine (carbamylcholine, carbachol; direct and indirect acting), pilocarpine (less potent than ACh, but resistant to AChE; no miosis if IOP >40 mmHg)

Indirect-acting agonists: anticholinesterases (AChE inhibitor); strongest agents; cause miosis and decrease in IOP (contract longitudinal fibers of ciliary muscle=increased outflow of trabecular meshwork [TM]).

Reversible: carbacholine, physostigmine (eserine; treat lid lice), edrophonium (Tensilon; for diagnosis of myasthenia gravis): can cause bradycardia, treat with atropine

Irreversible: echothiophate (Phospholine Iodide; treat glaucoma and accommodative esotropia [ET]; may cause iris cysts and subcapsular cataracts), isofluorophate (very long-acting, not used clinically), demecarium

Adverse effects: cataract, RD, pupillary block, blocks metabolism of succinylcholine (prolonged respiratory paralysis) and ester anesthetics, can mimic acute abdomen (GI effects); antidote is pralidoxime (PAM) or atropine

Muscarinic antagonists: anticholinergics; cause deepening of AC, stabilization of blood–aqueous barrier, mydriasis, and cycloplegia

Atropine (1- to 2-week duration; most allergenic, supersensitivity seen in Down syndrome), scopolamine (hyoscine; 1-week duration; greater CNS toxicity than atropine), homatropine (1- to 3-day duration), cyclopentolate (Cyclogyl; 24-hour duration; beware CNS side effects with 2% solution, especially in children), tropicamide (Mydriacyl; 4- to 6-hour duration)

Toxicity: mental status changes, hallucinations, tachycardia, urinary retention, dry mouth/skin, fever

Antidote: physostigmine (1-4 mg IV)

Nicotinic antagonists:

Nondepolarizing agents: gallamine, pancuronium; do not cause muscle contraction

Depolarizing agents: succinylcholine, decamethonium; cause muscle contraction and elevated IOP; contraindicated for ruptured globe (extraocular muscle [EOM] contraction can cause extrusion of intraocular contents)

Organ/Function	Sympathetic (fight/flight)	Parasympathetic (homeostasis)
HR	Increase	Decrease
BP	Increase	Decrease
GI motility	Decrease	Increase
Bronchioles	Dilate	Constrict
Bladder	Constrict	Dilate
Vessels	Constrict	Dilate
Sweat	Decrease	Increase
Pupils	Dilate	Constrict
Eyelids	Elevate	Normal

Table 2-1. Autonomic system responses

Adrenergic Drugs

Sympathomimetics: may cause mydriasis, vasoconstriction, decreased IOP

Direct-acting α-agonists: epinephrine, phenylephrine, dipivefrin, clonidine, apraclonidine (iopidine), brimonidine, methyldopa, naphazoline (Naphcon), oxymetazoline (Afrin), tetrahydrozoline (Visine)

Direct-acting β-agonists: epinephrine, isoproterenol, terbutaline, dopamine, albuterol (salbutamol)

Indirect-acting agonists: cocaine, hydroxyamphetamine (Paredrine), ephedrine

Sympatholytics: may cause decreased IOP

General blockers: guanethidine, bethanidine, protriptyline, 6-hydroxydopamine

α-blockers: thymoxamine, dibenamine, phentolamine, prazosin, labetalol, dapiprazole (Rev-Eyes; miosis)

β-blockers: timolol, levobunolol, betaxolol, metipranolol, carteolol, propranolol, metoprolol, atenolol, nadolol, pindolol

OCULAR HYPOTENSIVE (GLAUCOMA) MEDICATIONS

β-Blockers

Mechanism: reduce aqueous production (inhibit Na^+/K^+ pump) by decreasing cyclic adenosine monophosphate (cAMP) production in ciliary epithelium; around 20% IOP reduction

Loss of effectiveness over time due to downregulation of β-receptors (long-term drift)

Adverse effects: dry eye syndrome (decreased corneal sensitivity), bradycardia, heart block, bronchospasm, impotence, lethargy, depression, headache, rarely diarrhea and hallucinations, alopecia, dermatitis; may mask hypoglycemia

Nonselective ($β_1$ and $β_2$): timolol (Timoptic), levobunolol (Betagan), metipranolol (Optipranolol), carteolol (Ocupress)

10% do not show a therapeutic effect; inhibit lipoprotein lipase (break down chylomicrons and VLDL) and cholesterol acyltransferase (incorporate cholesterol into HDL); may cause decreased HDL levels

Carteolol has intrinsic sympathomimetic activity

Cardioselective ($β_1 \gg β_2$): betaxolol (Betoptic)

Fewer pulmonary adverse effects

Indications: patients with pulmonary problems who cannot tolerate nonselective β-blockers; often used for normal tension glaucoma; may not cause as much vasoconstriction of vessels supplying ON

α₂-Agonists

Apraclonidine (Iopidine), brimonidine (Alphagan P)

Mechanism: reduce aqueous production by decreasing episcleral venous pressure

Adverse effects: allergy, superior lid retraction, dry mouth, blanching of conjunctival vessels, miosis, lethargy, headache, stomach cramps; avoid in children especially <3 years of age: increased risk of somnolence, seizures, apnea due to CNS penetration

Dipivefrin (Propine): prodrug of epinephrine (converted into epinephrine in cornea by esterases), lower concentration and increased solubility vs epinephrine (penetrates cornea 17× better); thus less toxicity and fewer adverse effects

Mechanism: improves aqueous outflow, slightly reduces aqueous production

Adverse effects: allergy, cystoid macular edema (CME) in aphakia, hypertension, tachycardia (fewer systemic adverse effects than epinephrine)

Epinephrine: 1–2% is equivalent to Propine 0.1%; 3 salt forms: hydrochloride, borate, bitartrate (1st two are equivalent, 2% bitartrate is equivalent to 1% hydrochloride or borate)

Mechanism: improves aqueous outflow, slightly reduces aqueous production

Adverse effects: allergy, CME in aphakia (reversible), hypertension, tachycardia, arrhythmias, adrenochrome (black) deposits in conjunctiva

Miotics

Mechanism: increase aqueous outflow (contraction of ciliary muscle opens trabecular meshwork), decrease uveoscleral outflow

Pilocarpine: only direct cholinergic agonist; peak action at 2 hours, 8-hour duration

Beware for treatment of angle closure: causes shallowing of AC and narrowing of angle, but miosis pulls peripheral iris away from angle, balancing out the other effects

Adverse effects: headache, brow ache, accommodative spasm, increased range of accommodation, miosis (dimming, reduction of vision), induced myopia (forward shift of lens–iris diaphragm), pupillary block, follicular conjunctivitis, dermatitis, nyctalopia, rarely retinal tear or even RD

Other effects: breakdown of blood–aqueous barrier, reduction of uveoscleral outflow

Carbachol: direct and indirect cholinergic agonist; stronger effect and longer duration of action; poor corneal penetration; needs corneal surface disrupter (benzalkonium chloride); intraocular formulation (Miostat) used during surgery for pupillary miosis

Echothiophate (phospholine iodide): indirect cholinergic agonist (cholinesterase inhibitor); 3-week duration; also used in accommodative esotropia

Adverse effects: greater orbicularis, ciliary, and iris muscle spasm; cataracts in adults (therefore, use only in aphakic or pseudophakic patients); iris cysts in children (proliferation of iris pigment epithelium;

phenylephrine prevents cyst formation); decreased serum pseudocholinesterase activity (can accentuate succinylcholine effects during general anesthesia)

Carbonic Anhydrase Inhibitors (CAIs)

Mechanism: decrease bicarbonate formation in ciliary body epithelium; bicarbonate formation is linked to Na+ and fluid transport, so CAIs reduce aqueous production

Carbonic anhydrase catalyzes the reaction: $CO_2 + H_2O \leftrightarrow H_2CO_3$
Amount of carbonic anhydrase is 100× that needed for aqueous production; so, >99% must be inhibited to achieve IOP decrease
Sulfonamide derivative (do not administer to patients with sulfa allergy)

Oral: acetazolamide (Diamox; PO/IV), methazolamide (Neptazane, PO; more lipid soluble, less toxicity)
   Adverse effects: dry eye syndrome (decreased tear production), metabolic acidosis (IV administration causes greater metabolic acidosis), kidney stones (reduced excretion of urinary citrate or magnesium), hypokalemia (especially when used with other diuretics; very dangerous with digoxin), paresthesias (hands/feet/lips), GI upset, diarrhea, lethargy, loss of libido, weight loss, metallic taste, aplastic anemia, Stevens-Johnson syndrome; transient myopia

Topical: dorzolamide (Trusopt), brinzolamide (Azopt)
   Adverse effects: metallic taste, paresthesias, malaise, weight loss, depression, skin rash, corneal endothelial decompensation/toxicity (consider stopping prior to cataract surgery)

Prostaglandin Analogues/Prostanoids

Mechanism: increase uveoscleral outflow, around 30% IOP reduction

Latanoprost (Xalatan), **bimatoprost** (Lumigan), **travoprost** (Travatan), **unoprostone** isopropyl (Rescula): prostaglandin $F_{2\alpha}$ analogues
   Adverse effects: flu-like symptoms, hyperemia, eyelash growth, periocular skin and iris pigmentation (increases number of melanosomes, but not melanocytes), CME, reactivation of herpes simplex virus (HSV) keratitis

Hyperosmotic Agents

Mechanism: low-molecular-weight substances that increase serum osmolality to draw fluid out of eye (reduces vitreous volume)
   Adverse effects: headache, thirst, nausea, vomiting, diarrhea, diuresis, dizziness, and rebound IOP elevation; IV agents can cause subarachnoid hemorrhage

Urea (IV; 30% solution): not commonly used; extravasation causes tissue necrosis

Mannitol (Osmitrol; IV; 20% solution): most potent; may exacerbate congestive heart failure

Glycerin (Osmoglyn; PO; 50% solution): may cause hyperglycemia in diabetics (metabolized by liver into glucose)

Isosorbide (Ismotic; PO): not metabolized (can be used in diabetics); secreted 95% unchanged in urine

Other hyperosmotic agents: used topically for corneal edema
   Glycerin (Ophthalgan; topical; 100% solution): used to clear corneal edema for examination or laser procedure
   Muro 128 (hypertonic saline; topical; drops or ointment; 2.5% or 5% strength): used to reduce epithelial edema of cornea, especially in treatment of recurrent erosions

Order of Allergy

Greatest to least: iopidine > epinephrine > Propine > brimonidine > β-blocker > pilocarpine

ANTI-INFLAMMATORY DRUGS

The Inflammatory Pathway (Figure 2-1)

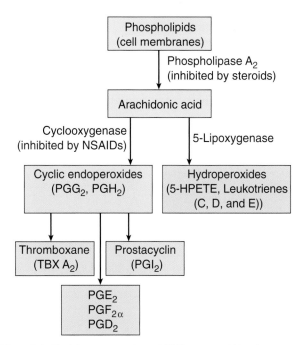

Figure 2-1. The inflammatory pathway. NSAIDs, nonsteroidal anti-inflammatory drugs; PG, prostaglandin; 5-HPETE, 5-hydroperoxyeicosatetraenoic acid.

Nonsteroidal Anti-inflammatory Drugs (NSAIDs)

Mechanism: inhibit cyclooxygenase pathway

Classes:

Salicylates: acetylsalicylic acid (ASA), diflunisal, salicylamide

Acetic acids: indomethacin (indometacin), diclofenac (Voltaren), sulindac, etodolac, ketorolac (Acular, Toradol), nepafenac (Nevanac), bromfenac (Xibrom, Bromday)

Phenylalkanoic acids: ibuprofen, suprofen (Profenal), flurbiprofen (Ocufen), naproxen, fenoprofen, ketoprofen

Cyclooxygenase-2 inhibitors: celecoxib (Celebrex)

Indications:

Prevent miosis during intraocular surgery: Profenal, Ocufen

Allergic conjunctivitis, corneal pain, postsurgical inflammation, CME: Voltaren, Acular, Nevanac, Xibrom, Bromday

Scleritis, uveitis: oral agents

Steroids

Mechanism: anti-inflammatory and immunosuppressive by inhibiting release of arachidonic acid, inhibiting release of lysosomal enzymes, preventing macrophage migration, interfering with lymphocyte function, decreasing fibroblast activity, inhibiting neovascularization, and reducing capillary permeability

Classes:

Ester: loteprednol

Ketone: all others

Preparations (ketones):

Phosphate: hydrophilic; poor penetration of intact corneal epithelium (improved penetration with epithelial defect)

Alcohol: biphasic; penetrate intact cornea

Acetate: more biphasic; best corneal penetration

Potency: increased by 1–2 double bond(s), 9 fluorination, 6 methylation, O at C11; IOP elevation from deoxygenation at C21 (Table 2-2)

Derivatives of progesterone (weaker): FML, medrysone

Subconjunctival/sub-Tenon's injection (Table 2-3): produces higher ocular concentration and longer duration; beware in IOP responder

Other routes of administration: oral, IV, intraocular

Oral dose of 7.5 mg dexamethasone results in intravitreal concentration of therapeutic levels

Indications: conjunctivitis, keratitis, scleritis, uveitis, hyphema, CME, macular edema, CNV, endophthalmitis

Adverse effects:

Systemic: adrenal insufficiency, hyperglycemia, hypertension, hypokalemia, peptic ulcers, delayed wound healing, superinfection, emotional lability, psychosis, growth retardation, muscle atrophy, osteoporosis, aseptic necrosis of the hip, hirsutism, weight gain, cushingoid appearance, pseudotumor cerebri

Ocular: posterior subcapsular cataract (PSC), elevated IOP, delayed wound healing/corneal re-epithelialization, secondary infections (e.g. HSV, fungal)

IOP-elevating potential: dexamethasone > prednisolone > fluorometholone > hydrocortisone > tetrahydrotriamcinolone > medrysone (after 6 weeks of dexamethasone therapy, 42% have IOP >20 mmHg; 6% have IOP >31)

Steroids with less IOP-elevating potential: rimexolone (Vexol), loteprednol (Lotemax, Alrex)

Table 2-2. Relative potencies of steroids

Steroid	Relative potency
Hydrocortisone	1 (the standard)
Cortisone	0.8
Triamcinolone	4
Prednisone	4
Prednisolone	5
Dexamethasone	25–30
Betamethasone	25–30
Fluorometholone	40–50
Fluocinolone	240

Table 2-3. Common ophthalmic steroids

Generic name	Trade name
Topical	
Prednisolone acetate 1%	Pred Forte, Omni Pred
Fluorometholone acetate 0.1%	Flarex
Dexamethasone alcohol 0.1%	Maxidex
Fluorometholone alcohol 0.1%	FML
Prednisolone phosphate 1%	Inflamase
Dexamethasone phosphate 1%	Decadron
Difluprednate 0.05%	Durezol
Loteprednol etabonate 0.5%	Lotemax
Loteprednol etabonate 0.2%	Alrex
Subconjunctival	
Dexamethasone phosphate	Decadron
Methylprednisolone acetate	Solumedrol, Depomedrol
Prednisolone acetate	Durapred
Triamcinolone acetonide	Kenalog
Betamethasone	Celestone
Intravitreal	
Triamcinolone acetonide	Kenalog, Triesence

ANTIALLERGY MEDICATIONS

Antihistamines/Vasoconstrictors (over-the-counter)

Naphazoline hydrochloride/pheniramine maleate: (OcuHist, Opcon-A, Naphcon-A), **naphazoline hydrochloride/antazoline phosphate** (Vasocon-A): vasoconstrictor naphazoline temporarily removes redness, but can cause rebound redness with chronic use

Mast Cell Stabilizer

Cromolyn (cromoglicate; Crolom; Opticrom): reduces permeability of mast cell plasma membrane, preventing release of histamine; reduces phosphodiesterase activity (facilitator of mast cell degranulation); inhibits activation of neutrophils, monocytes, and eosinophils; does not interfere with binding of antigen to previously sensitized cells; no antihistamine activity therefore useful for chronic allergies, not for acute symptomatic relief

Mast Cell Stabilizer + Eosinophil Suppressor

Lodoxamide (Alomide): 2500 times more potent than cromolyn; also inhibits eosinophil activation

H₁-Blockers (Antihistamines)

Levocabastine (Livostin), **emedastine** (Emadine): pure H₁-specific receptor antagonists; bind to histamine receptors (inhibit itching and hyperemia)

H₁-Blockers + Mast Cell Stabilizers

Nedocromil (Alocril), **pemirolast** (Alamast), **ketotifen** (Zaditor, Alaway), **olopatadine** (Patanol, Pataday), **azelastine** (Optivar), **epinastine** (Elestat), **bepotastine** (Bepreve), alcaftadine (Lastacaft): stabilize mast cells and binds to H₁ receptors (inhibits itching); binds to H₂ receptors at low level (inhibits hyperemia)

IMMUNOSUPPRESSIVE AGENTS

Cytotoxic Antimetabolites

Inhibit purine ring biosynthesis

Methotrexate: folate analogue; inhibits folate metabolism; inhibits synthesis of deoxythymidine monophosphate nucleotide; inhibits enzyme dehydrofolate reductase; inhibits T-cell function
> *Adverse effects:* leukopenia, thrombocytopenia, hepatotoxicity, lung or renal toxicity; teratogenic; periorbital edema, hyperemia

Azathioprine (Imuran): purine analogue that inhibits purine synthesis

Cytotoxic Alkylating Agents

Create cross linkage between DNA strands, resulting in inhibition of transcription of mRNA and prevention of DNA synthesis

Chlorambucil (Leukeran): interacts with 7-guanine of DNA, resulting in strand breakage or cross linkage
> *Adverse effects:* sterility, bone marrow suppression

Cyclophosphamide (Cytoxan):
> *Adverse effects:* hemorrhagic cystitis (oral > IV), renal transitional cell cancer, sterility, bone marrow suppression
> Prevent hemorrhagic cystitis with high water intake (IV or oral)

Cytostatic Anti-Inflammatories

Steroids
(see earlier)

Immunomodulator

Cyclosporine: blocks production of interleukin-2 (IL-2) and IL-2 receptors, inhibits proliferation of lymphocytes, inhibits T-cell activation and recruitment, interferes with production of IL-2 by T cells, prevents formation of IL-2 receptors by T cells; natural product of fungi
> *Indications:*
> **TOPICAL:** necrotizing scleritis, Sjögren's syndrome/dry eye syndrome, ligneous conjunctivitis, atopic keratoconjunctivitis
> **SYSTEMIC:** Mooren's ulcer, uveitis in Behçet's or sympathetic ophthalmia, prevention of corneal transplant rejection; also used in ocular cicatricial pemphigoid (OCP) and thyroid-related ophthalmopathy
> *Adverse effects* (systemic administration only): renal toxicity (renal tubular atrophy, interstitial fibrosis), hypertension, paresthesia, peripheral neuropathy, elevated erythrocyte sedimentation rate (ESR), hypertrichosis, hepatotoxicity, hyperuricemia

Others

Colchicine: inhibits leukocyte migration; prevents recurrence of Behçet's

Oncolytic agents:
> *Antineoplastics:* bleomycin, dactinomycin, mitomycin (topically in glaucoma, corneal and pterygium surgery), daunorubicin (daunomycin), doxorubicin (hydroxydaunorubicin, Adriamycin)
> **ADVERSE EFFECTS:** anemia, Stevens-Johnson syndrome (SJS), decreased vision, conjunctivitis, tearing
> *Alkylating agents:* busulfan, carmustine, chlorambucil, cyclophosphamide
> **ADVERSE EFFECTS:** rare
> *Vinca alkaloids:* vincristine, vinblastine
> **ADVERSE EFFECTS:** diplopia, nystagmus, ptosis, CN palsies

Antiestrogen: tamoxifen
   ADVERSE EFFECTS: corneal opacities, retinopathy
Heavy metals: cisplatin
   ADVERSE EFFECTS: papilledema, optic neuritis
Antimetabolites: methotrexate, 5-fluorouracil (5-FU; topically in glaucoma surgery)
   ADVERSE EFFECTS: periorbital edema, conjunctival hyperemia, photophobia, tearing; corneal epithelial erosions

ANTI-INFECTIVE DRUGS

Antibiotics

Inhibitors of Intermediary Metabolism

Sulfonamides: static; sulfacetamide, sulfadiazine, sulfisoxizole, sulfamethoxazole; resistance is problem
   Mechanism: inhibit folic acid synthesis
   Spectrum: Gram-positives and Gram-negatives; also, toxoplasmosis, *Chlamydia, Actinomyces, Pneumocystis*
   Indications: blepharitis, conjunctivitis, toxoplasmosis
   Adverse effects: allergy (SJS syndrome), transient myopia
   Pyrimethamine (Daraprim):
      ADVERSE EFFECTS: bone marrow depression (anemia, thrombocytopenia; prevent with use of folinic acid [Leucovorin])
   Dapsone:
      INDICATIONS: OCP, leprosy
      CONTRAINDICATIONS: patients allergic to sulfa or with G6PD deficiency

Trimethoprim: blocks next step in folate metabolism; often combined with sulfamethoxazole (Bactrim)
   Spectrum: Gram-positives and Gram-negatives (*Staphylococcus, Streptococcus, Serratia, Proteus, Haemophilus, Enterobacter, Escherichia coli, Klebsiella*)
   Indications: conjunctivitis

Inhibitors of Cell Wall Synthesis

β-Lactams (cidal)

Penicillins (PCN): least toxic; variable protein binding
   Adverse effects: allergy, diarrhea
   Penicillin G:
      SPECTRUM: *Streptococcus* and non–penicillinase-producing *Staphylococcus, Neisseria, Treponema pallidum*
      INDICATIONS: syphilis
   Isoxazolyl PCNs: penicillinase-resistant; methicillin, nafcillin, oxacillin, cloxacillin, dicloxacillin
      SPECTRUM: extended to *Staphylococcus aureus*
   Amino PCNs: broader spectrum; ampicillin, amoxicillin
      SPECTRUM: Gram-positives (except staph), *Neisseria, Haemophilus, Proteus, Shigella, Salmonella, Listeria, E. coli*
      INDICATIONS: preseptal cellulitis
   Carboxy PCNs: antipseudomonal; carbenicillin, ticarcillin
      SPECTRUM: extended to Gram-negatives (*Pseudomonas* and Enterobacteriaceae) and anaerobes (*Bacteroides*)

Ureido PCNs: antipseudomonal; piperacillin, mezlocillin, azlocillin
   SPECTRUM: extended to Gram-negatives (*Pseudomonas* and Enterobacteriaceae) and anaerobes (*Bacteroides*)
β-Lactamase Inhibitors: combined with PCNs to increase spectrum of activity; clavulanate (amox/clavulanate=Augmentin), sulbactam (amp/sulbactam = Unasyn)

Cephalosporins: more resistant to β-lactamases; 20% cross react with PCN-allergic patients
   1st generation: cefazolin (Ancef, Kefzol), cefalexin (cephalexin, Keflex), cephalothin (Keflin), cefaclor (Ceclor)
      SPECTRUM: Gram-positives (staph, strep) and some Gram-negatives
      INDICATIONS: cefazolin for keratitis, endophthalmitis
   2nd generation: cefamandole (cephamandole, Mandol), cefonicid (Monocid), cefotetan (Cefotan), cefoxitin (Mefoxin), cefuroxime (Zinacef)
      SPECTRUM: better Gram-negative but less Gram-positive, anaerobic (cefoxitin, cefotetan), *Haemophilus influenzae* and *Neisseria* (cefuroxime)
   3rd generation: cefoperazone (Cefobid), cefotaxime (Claforan), ceftazidime (Tazidime), ceftizoxime (Cefizox), ceftriaxone (Rocephin), moxalactam (Moxam)
      SPECTRUM: even better Gram-negative, *Pseudomonas* (ceftazidime)

Monobactams (aztreonam): aerobic Gram-negatives

Carbapenems (imipenem): β-lactamase resistant; very broad activity (almost all Gram-positives, Gram-negatives, and anaerobes); does not cover methicillin-resistant *S. aureus* (MRSA)

Non β-Lactams (cidal)

Polymyxin B: basic peptides; act as detergents and disrupt cell membrane
   Spectrum: Gram-negatives (*Haemophilus, Enterobacter, E. coli, Klebsiella, Pseudomonas*)
   Indications: conjunctivitis (combined with trimethoprim [Polytrim])

Bacitracin: polypeptides; often used in combination with neomycin or polymyxin to broaden activity
   Spectrum: Gram-positives, *Neisseria, Haemophilus, Actinomyces*
   Indications: blepharitis, conjunctivitis

Vancomycin: glycopeptide
   Spectrum: very good for Gram-positives; staph (including MRSA), strep (including PCN- resistant strains), *Bacillus, Propionibacterium acnes, Clostridium difficile*
   Indications: keratitis, endophthalmitis
   Adverse effects: systemic administration is associated with ototoxicity and nephrotoxicity

Inhibitors of Protein Synthesis

Aminoglycosides: cidal; inhibit 30S ribosome; poor GI absorption

Gentamycin (gentamicin [better for *Serratia*]), tobramycin (Tobrax [better for *Pseudomonas*]), amikacin (best for *Pseudomonas* and *Mycobacterium*; less nephrotoxic than gent), streptomycin (TB, *Streptococcus viridans*), neomycin (*Acanthamoeba*; allergy common), paromomycin (*Acanthamoeba*), kanamycin

Spectrum: Gram-negative bacilli and some staph (gent and tobra are active against *S aureus* and *Staphylococcus epidermidis*)

Indications: conjunctivitis, keratitis, endophthalmitis

Adverse effects: systemic administration is associated with ototoxicity and nephrotoxicity, allergy

Spectinomycin: cidal; inhibits 30S ribosome; not an aminoglycoside; used for *Neisseria*

Tetracyclines: static; inhibit 30S ribosome; take on empty stomach (chelates calcium, antacids; iron, causing decreased absorption); use with caution in woman of childbearing age; also decreases efficacy of oral contraceptive medications

Tetracycline, doxycycline, minocycline, meclocycline

Spectrum: Gram-positive and Gram-negative, *Chlamydia*, *Rickettsia*, *Mycoplasma*

Indications: prophylaxis and treatment of ophthalmia neonatorum, *Chlamydia*; also rosacea, meibomianitis, scleral melting (due to anti-inflammatory and anticollagenolytic properties)

Adverse effects: GI upset, phototoxic dermatitis, tooth discoloration in children <8 years of age, teratogenic, nephrotoxicity and hepatotoxicity, decreased prothrombin activity (potentiates warfarin sodium [Coumadin])

Macrolides: static; inhibit 50S ribosome

Erythromycin, azithromycin (Zithromax), clarithromycin (Crixan, Biaxin)

Spectrum: Gram-positives and a few Gram-negatives, *Chlamydia*, *Mycoplasma*, *Legionella*

Indications: blepharitis, conjunctivitis, *Chlamydia*

Adverse effects: GI upset

Chloramphenicol: static; inhibits 50S ribosome

Spectrum: Gram-positives and Gram-negatives, anaerobes, *Chlamydia*, *Rickettsia*, *Mycoplasma*, spirochetes

Adverse effects: aplastic anemia and reversible bone marrow suppression

Clindamycin: static; inhibits 50S ribosome

Spectrum: Gram-positives and anaerobes, toxoplasmosis

Indications: toxoplasmosis

Adverse effects: may cause pseudomembranous colitis (due to overgrowth of *C difficile*; treat with oral vancomycin or metronidazole [Flagyl])

Others

Fluoroquinolones: cidal; analogues of nalidixic acid; inhibitors of genetic replication; inhibit DNA gyrase (topoisomerase II) and topoisomerase IV

2nd generation: ciprofloxacin (Ciloxan), ofloxacin (Ocuflox), norfloxacin (Chibroxin)

3rd generation: levofloxacin (Quixin, Iquix)

4th generation: gatifloxacin (Zymar, Zymaxid), moxifloxacin (Vigamox, Moxeza), besifloxacin (Besivance)

Spectrum: aerobic Gram-negatives and some Gram-positives (*H. influenzae*, *Pseudomonas*, Enterobacteriaceae, *S aureus*); also, *Chlamydia*, *Rickettsia*, *Mycoplasma*, and *Mycobacterium*. 4th generation agents have extended spectrum with enhanced activity against Gram-positives, fluoroquinolone-resistant organisms, and atypical mycobacteria

Indications: conjunctivitis, keratitis, surgical prophylaxis; prophylaxis in penetrating trauma (oral cipro achieves high levels in vitreous)

Adverse effects: GI upset; cartilage damage in children

Anti-TB Agents

Isoniazid: cidal; inhibits cell wall synthesis of mycobacteria

Adverse effects: hepatotoxicity, vitamin B_6 deficiency

Rifampin: inhibits RNA polymerase of mycobacteria

Adverse effects: hepatotoxicity, turns body fluids orange-red

Pyrazinamide: unknown mechanism; analogue of nicotinamide

Adverse effects: hepatotoxicity, gout

Ethambutol: chelates metals

Adverse effects: optic neuropathy

Fumagillin: treatment of microsporidia keratoconjunctivitis

Antivirals

Mechanism: static; inhibit genetic replication; most are nucleotide analogues

Topical: treatment of HSV keratitis

Idoxuridine (IDU, Stoxil): can cause follicular conjunctivitis, corneal epitheliopathy, punctal stenosis

Vidarabine (Vira-A): adverse effects less severe than IDU

Trifluorothymidine (Viroptic): inhibits thymidylate synthetase (virus-specific enzyme)

Ganciclovir (Zirgan): guanosine analogue; activated only by thymidine kinase (virus-specific enzyme) and selectively interferes with viral DNA replication. Similar efficacy as topical acyclovir (not available in US); more effective than Viroptic, and less toxic to cornea; best tolerated

Systemic:

Acyclovir (acycloguanosine, Zovirax; guanosine analogue; activated only by thymidine kinase (virus-specific enzyme)), **valacyclovir** (Valtrex; prodrug of acyclovir), **penciclovir**, **famciclovir** (Famvir; prodrug of penciclovir)

INDICATIONS: treatment of HSV and varicella zoster virus (VZV)
    ADVERSE EFFECTS: may cause GI upset; high doses can cause nephrotoxicity and neurotoxicity
Ganciclovir (Cytovene): treatment of CMV
    ADVERSE EFFECTS: bone marrow suppression (cannot use with azidothymidine [AZT])
Foscarnet (Foscavir): treatment of CMV
    ADVERSE EFFECTS: nephrotoxicitiy, less myelosuppression, electrolyte abnormalities

Antifungals

Mechanism: disrupt cell membranes

Classification:
Yeasts: form pseudohyphae; *Candida, Cryptococcus*
Molds: filamentous; form hyphae
    SEPTATE: *Fusarium, Aspergillus, Penicillium, Curvularia, Paecilomyces, Phialophora*
    NONSEPTATE: *Phycomycetes, Rhizopus, Mucor*
Dimorphic fungi: grow as yeast or mold; *Histoplasma, Blastomyces, Coccidioides*

Polyenes: bind to ergosterol; damages fungal membranes
Amphotericin B: systemic
    SPECTRUM: broad (especially *Candida*; also, *Cryptococcus, Blastomyces, Histoplasma, Coccidioides,* mucormycosis; not as good for *Aspergillus, Fusarium*)
    INDICATIONS: keratitis, endopthalmitis (intravenous drug abuse [IVDA], immunosuppression, hyperalimentation)
    ADVERSE EFFECTS: fever, hypotension, headache, phlebitis, GI upset, nephrotoxicity, anemia
Natamycin (pimaricin): topical only; too toxic for IV use, toxic to retina intravitreally
    SPECTRUM: filamentous fungi (especially *Aspergillus, Fusarium*), not as good for *Candida*; not effective against *Mucor* (nonseptate, branching hyphae)
    INDICATIONS: keratitis (removal of epithelium improves penetration)

Azoles: inhibit ergosterol synthesis; second-line agents to amphotericin; also used for *Acanthamoeba*
Adverse effects: GI upset, headache, rash
Imidazoles:
    MICONAZOLE (topical, IV, intravitreal): broad spectrum (filamentous fungi and yeast)
        ADVERSE EFFECTS: may cause corneal erosions, anemia
    KETOCONAZOLE (topical, oral): broad spectrum
        ADVERSE EFFECTS: reversible hepatotoxicity
    CLOTRIMAZOLE (oral): good for *Aspergillus*
        ADVERSE EFFECTS: hepatotoxicity
Triazoles: safer
    ITRACONAZOLE (oral): broad spectrum
    FLUCONAZOLE (oral): broad spectrum

Antimetabolites: most fungi are resistant, except *Cryptococcus* and some *Candida*

Flucytosine: converted to 5-FU, disrupts DNA synthesis
    ADVERSE EFFECTS: myelosuppression, nausea, vomiting, diarrhea

Antiamoebics

Mechanism: cidal (amoebae and cysts); cationic surface-active properties; interfere with cell membranes and inhibit enzymes

Indications: topical for *Acanthamoeba* keratitis

Biguanides: polyhexamethylene biguanide (PHMB), chlorhexidine; first-line agents, less corneal toxicity

Diamidines: propamidine (Brolene), hexamidine; synergistic effect with biguanides, corneal toxicity

Antihelmintics

Mebendazole, thiabendazole, albendazole: inhibit glucose uptake and microtubule synthesis
Adverse effects: GI upset

Pyrantel pamoate: neuromuscular junction blocker
Adverse effects: nausea, vomiting, headache, rash

Diethylcarbamazine: enables phagocytosis of microfilaria

Ivermectin: increases gamma-aminobutyric acid (GABA) release paralyzing microfilaria
Adverse effects: fever, headache, rash

Praziquantel: causes calcium loss, paralyzing worm
Adverse effects: GI upset, fever

MISCELLANEOUS

Aminocaproic acid (Amicar): synthetic amino acid similar to lysine
Mechanism: antifibrinolytic; stabilizes blood clot, delays lysis, decreases secondary hemorrhages
Indications: hyphema
Contraindications: hypercoagulable states, pregnancy, renal disease, liver disease, patients at risk for myocardial infarction (MI), pulmonary embolism, cerebrovascular accident (CVA)
Adverse effects: nausea, vomiting, diarrhea, hypotension, rash

Botulinum toxin (Botox): neurotoxin that blocks release of acetylcholine from nerve terminal; paralyzes muscle (1–3 months)
Indications: blepharospasm, hemifacial spasm, strabismus
Adverse effects: ptosis, diplopia, exposure keratopathy

Fluorescein dye: IV for fluorescein angiography
Adverse effects: nausea, vomiting, dizziness, headache, dyspnea, hypotension, skin necrosis, phototoxic reactions, anaphylaxis

Indocyanine green (ICG) dye: IV for ICG angiography; contraindicated in patients allergic to iodine
 Adverse effects: GI upset, hypotension, urticaria, anaphylaxis

OCULAR TOXICOLOGY (TABLE 2-4)

Anticholinergics (atropine, scopolamine, Donnatal): toxicity causes flushing, agitation, tachycardia, somnolence, dry mouth, dry eye, mydriasis, cycloplegia, blurry vision, angle closure; increased sensitivity in albinism, Down syndrome, and neonates

Antihistamines: dry eye, mydriasis, cycloplegia, blurry vision, angle closure

Antibiotics:
 Aminoglycosides: intraocular administration may cause macular infarction (intravenous fluorescein angiography [IVFA]: pruned tree appearance of retinal vasculature)
 Chloramphenicol: optic neuropathy; peripheral neuritis can precede visual complaints by 1–2 weeks
 Penicillin and tetracycline: pseudotumor
 Sulfonamides: conjunctivitis, transient myopia, angle closure, optic neuropathy
 Isoniazid, rifampin, ethambutol: optic neuropathy

Antimalarials (chloroquine/hydroxychloroquine): cornea verticillata, fine pigmentary macular changes (bull's-eye maculopathy); patients may complain of halos around lights; visual acuity usually unchanged; dose related

Quinine: overdose can result in acute visual loss (to no light perception [NLP]), tinnitus, weakness, confusion

Barbiturates (phenobarbital): nystagmus, diplopia, ptosis, conjunctivitis

Phenothiazines (chlorpromazine, thioridazine): pigmentary retinopathy, corneal deposits, cataracts, angle closure

Tricyclic antidepressants: mydriasis, cycloplegia, dry eye, angle closure

Dilantin: diplopia, nystagmus, papilledema

Gold: deposits in inferior corneal stroma and anterior lens capsule (chrysiasis)

Talc: multiple tiny yellow-white glistening particles scattered through posterior pole with macular edema, venous engorgement, hemorrhages, arterial occlusion, retinal nonperfusion, and peripheral neovascularization (NV)

Amiodarone (Cordarone): cornea verticillata, occasionally anterior subcapsular opacities

Digoxin: changes in color vision (xanthopsia [yellow vision]), optic neuropathy

Diuretics (hydrochlorothiazide): xanthopsia, transient myopia, angle closure

Table 2-4. Ocular toxicology

Ocular structure	Effect	Drug
Extraocular muscles	Nystagmus, diplopia	Anesthetics, sedatives, anticonvulsants, propranolol, antibiotics, phenothiazines, pentobarbital, carbamazepine, MAO inhibitors
Lid	Edema	Chloral hydrate
	Discoloration	Phenothiazines
	Ptosis	Guanethidine, propranolol, barbiturates
Conjunctiva	Hyperemia	Reserpine, methyldopa
	Allergy	Antibiotics, sulfonamides, atropine, antivirals, glaucoma medications
	Discoloration	Phenothiazines, chlorambucil, phenylbutazone
Cornea	Keratitis	Antibiotics, phenylbutazone, barbiturates, chlorambucil, steroids
	Deposits	Chloroquine, amiodarone, tamoxifen, indomethacin, gold
	Pigmentation	Vitamin D
Increased IOP	Open angle	Anticholinergics, caffeine, steroids
	Narrow angle	Anticholinergics, antihistamines, phenothiazines, tricyclic antidepressants, haloperidol, sulfonamides (Topamax)
Lens	Opacities/cataract	Steroids, phenothiazines, ibuprofen, allopurinol, long-acting miotics
	Myopia	Sulfonamides, tetracycline, prochlorperazine, autonomic antagonists, duloxetine (Cymbalta)
Retina	Edema	Chloramphenicol, indomethacin, tamoxifen, carmustine
	Hemorrhage	Anticoagulants, ethambutol
	Vascular damage	Oral contraceptives, oxygen, aminoglycosides, talc, carmustine, interferon
	Pigmentary degeneration	Phenothiazines, indomethacin, nalidixic acid, ethambutol, isotretinoin, chloroquine, hydroxychloroquine
Optic nerve	Neuropathy	Ethambutol, isoniazid, sulfonamides, digitalis, imipramine, streptomycin, busulfan, cisplatin, vincristine, chloramphenicol, disulfiram
	Papilledema	Steroids, vitamin A, tetracycline, phenylbutazone, amiodarone, nalidixic acid, isotretinoin

Phosphodiesterase 5 inhibitors (Viagra, Cialis, Levitra): decreased retinal blood flow by up to −30%; altered color and light perception; possibly ischemic optic neuropathy

Carmustine: retinal infarction, RPE changes, arterial occlusions, hemorrhages, macular edema, glaucoma, optic neuritis, INO

Narcotics (opiates): miosis

NSAIDs (indomethacin): corneal deposits, diplopia, optic neuritis, pigmentary macular changes; may have changes in vision, dark adaptation, and visual fields

Corticosteroids: posterior subcapsular cataracts, increased IOP, delayed wound healing, secondary infections, pseudotumor cerebri

Oral contraceptives: dry eye, vascular occlusions, perivasculitis, optic neuritis, pseudotumor cerebri

Tamoxifen: deposits in cornea and macula, may have macular edema

Isotretinoin: impairment of dark adaptation

Interferon: reversible vaso-occlusive disease

REVIEW QUESTIONS (Answers start on page 357)

1. Which antibiotic results in the highest intravitreal concentration when administered orally?
   a. ciprofloxacin
   b. penicillin
   c. bactrim
   d. clindamycin
2. Which anesthetic agent would most interfere with an intraocular gas bubble?
   a. isoflurane
   b. propofol
   c. sodium thiopental
   d. nitrous oxide
3. Which of the following is not an adverse effect of CAIs?
   a. death
   b. paresthesias
   c. iris cysts
   d. Stevens-Johnson syndrome
4. Which β-blocker has the least effect on β_2 receptors?
   a. levobunolol
   b. betaxolol
   c. carteolol
   d. timolol
5. Which drug has the least effect on uveoscleral outflow?
   a. atropine
   b. latanoprost
   c. pilocarpine
   d. dorzolamide

6. Which enzyme is inhibited by steroids?
   a. cyclooxygenase
   b. phospholipase A_2
   c. lipoxygenase
   d. endoperoxidase
7. Which of the following steroid formulations has the best corneal penetrability?
   a. prednisolone acetate
   b. dexamethasone phosphate
   c. prednisolone phosphate
   d. dexamethasone alcohol
8. Adverse effects of foscarnet include all of the following except
   a. seizures
   b. infertility
   c. electrolyte abnormalities
   d. myelosuppression
9. Which glaucoma medication is not effective when IOP is >60 mmHg?
   a. acetazolamide
   b. timolol
   c. pilocarpine
   d. apraclonidine
10. Which medicine is not associated with OCP-like conjunctival shrinkage?
   a. phospholine iodide
   b. pilocarpine
   c. epinephrine
   d. timolol
11. Which β-blocker is β_1-selective?
   a. carteolol
   b. timolol
   c. betaxolol
   d. levobunolol
12. The most appropriate treatment for neurosyphilis is
   a. penicillin G
   b. erythromycin
   c. penicillin VK
   d. tetracycline
13. The correct mechanism of action of botulinum toxin is
   a. it prevents release of acetylcholine
   b. it blocks acetylcholine receptors
   c. it inhibits reuptake of acetylcholine
   d. it is an acetylcholinesterase inhibitor
14. Fluoroquinolones are least effective against
   a. *Klebsiella*
   b. *H. influenzae*
   c. anaerobic cocci
   d. *Serratia*
15. Hydroxychloroquine toxicity depends most on
   a. patient age
   b. cumulative dose
   c. patient race
   d. daily dose
16. Calculate the amount of cocaine in 2 mL of a 4% solution
   a. 2 mg
   b. 8 mg
   c. 20 mg
   d. 80 mg

17. NSAIDs block the formation of all of the following substances except
    a. thromboxane
    b. leukotrienes
    c. prostaglandins
    d. prostacyclin
18. Systemic effects of steroids may include all of the following except
    a. papilledema
    b. hirsutism
    c. potassium depletion
    d. renal tubular acidosis
19. Which drug does not produce decreased tear production?
    a. pilocarpine
    b. diphenhydramine (Benadryl)
    c. timolol
    d. atropine
20. Natamycin is a
    a. diamine
    b. imidazole
    c. polyene
    d. aminoglycoside
21. Which glaucoma medicine does not decrease aqueous production?
    a. aproclonidine
    b. pilocarpine
    c. acetazolamide
    d. timolol
22. β-blockers may cause all of the following except
    a. constipation
    b. impotence
    c. alopecia
    d. depression
23. Idoxuridine may cause all of the following except
    a. filamentary keratitis
    b. punctal stenosis
    c. corneal hypesthesia
    d. nonhealing epithelial erosion
24. Which of the following antifungal agents has the broadest spectrum against yeast-like fungi?
    a. miconazole
    b. natamycin
    c. ketoconazole
    d. amphotericin
25. All of the following medications are combination antihistamine and mast cell stabilizers except
    a. Alomide
    b. Zaditor
    c. Optivar
    d. Patanol
26. The antidote for atropine toxicity is
    a. endrophonium
    b. physostigmine
    c. carbacholine
    d. pilocarpine
27. Which of the following agents is contraindicated for ruptured globe repair?
    a. gallamine
    b. halothane
    c. pancuronium
    d. succinylcholine
28. The duration of action of 1 drop of proparacaine is
    a. 5 minutes
    b. 20 minutes
    c. 45 minutes
    d. 1 hour
29. Which of the following medications is not commercially available as a topical formulation?
    a. ganciclovir
    b. azithromycin
    c. cyclosporine
    d. vancomycin
30. All of the following are complications of carbonic anhydrase inhibitors except
    a. hypokalemia
    b. aplastic anemia
    c. metabolic alkalosis
    d. kidney stones
31. Topiramate is associated with
    a. open-angle glaucoma
    b. normal tension glaucoma
    c. angle-closure glaucoma with pupillary block
    d. angle-closure glaucoma without pupillary block
32. A patient with ocular hypertension and an allergy to sulfonamides should not be treated with
    a. bimatoprost
    b. dorzolamide
    c. timolol
    d. brimonidine
33. Infectious keratitis due to *Candida albicans* is best treated with topical
    a. amphotericin B
    b. natamycin
    c. fluconazole
    d. clotrimazole
34. Which of the following oral agents should be used to treat a patient with ocular cicatricial pemphigoid?
    a. pyrazinamide
    b. 5-fluorouracil
    c. cyclophosphamide
    d. flucytosine
35. The glaucoma medication contraindicated in infants is
    a. timolol
    b. brimonidine
    c. latanoprost
    d. dorzolamide
36. Which systemic antibiotic is used to treat *Chlamydia* during pregnancy?
    a. doxycycline
    b. ceftriaxone
    c. penicillin
    d. erythromycin
37. The local anesthetic with the longest duration of action is
    a. mepivacaine
    b. procaine
    c. bupivacaine
    d. lidocaine
38. A 33-year-old man has had follicular conjunctivitis with a watery discharge for 5 weeks. Elementary bodies are

present on a conjunctival smear, therefore, the most appropriate treatment is
a. oral azithromycin
b. oral acyclovir
c. topical cromolyn
d. topical prednisolone

39. The most appropriate treatment for *Fusarium* keratitis is topical
a. tobramycin
b. pimaricin
c. chloramphenicol
d. ciprofloxacin

40. All of the following are associated with vitamin A toxicity except
a. CN 6 palsy
b. retinal hemorrhages
c. papilledema
d. band keratopathy

SUGGESTED READINGS

Doughty M: Ocular Pharmacology and Therapeutics: A Primary Care Guide. Philadelphia, Butterworth-Heinemann, 2001.

Fraunfelder FT, Fraunfelder FW, Randall JA: Drug-Induced Ocular Side Effects, 5th edn. Philadelphia, Butterworth-Heinemann, 2001.

Fraunfelder FT, Roy FH: Current Ocular Therapy, 5th edn. Philadelphia, WB Saunders, 2000.

Grant WM, Schuman JS: Toxicology of the Eye, 4th edn. Springfield, IL, Charles C. Thomas, 1993.

Greenbaum S: Ocular Anesthesia. Philadelphia, WB Saunders, 1997.

Physicians' Desk Reference for Ophthalmic Medicines. Montvale, NJ, Medical Economics, 2012.

Zimmerman TJ: Textbook of Ocular Pharmacology. Philadelphia, Lippincott-Raven, 1997.

3

Embryology / Pathology

Embryology

Formation of eye: embryonic plate → neural plate → optic pits → optic vesicles → optic cups

Embryonic plate (Figure 3.1):
1. Ectoderm (forms eye and brain): neural ectoderm, surface ectoderm, and neural crest
2. Mesoderm
3. Endoderm

Optic pit: forms at day 23 of gestation

Optic vesicle: anterolateral outpouching of primitive brain stem; evaginates on day 25 and becomes the globe

Optic vesicle induces the lens placode at day 27

Abnormalities of evagination: may result in anophthalmia, cyclopia (synophthalmia), congenital cystic eye, congenital nonattachment of the retina. Apical forebrain lesions such as synophthalmia are associated with arrhinencephaly, proboscis, ethmocephaly, trisomy 13

Optic cup (Figure 3.2): develops embryologically as an anterolateral evagination of the forebrain

Inner layer becomes the retina

Outer layer becomes the retinal pigment epithelium

Potential space between the two becomes the subretinal space (which was the cavity of the neural tube and optic vesicle)

Cells at anterior margin of optic cup form the posterior pigment epithelium of the iris

Cells between the future iris and the future retina form the ciliary body

Embryonic fissure: on undersurface of optic cups; closes on day 33 allowing pressurization of globe

Closure occurs first in midzone/equator, then extends posteriorly and anteriorly

Serves as portal for mesoderm to enter eye (i.e. hyaloid artery)

Coloboma: failure of closure of embryonic fissure; sporadic or autosomal dominant (AD); typical (located in inferonasal quadrant) or atypical (located elsewhere)

May involve retina and choroid (associated with basal encephalocele, cleft palate, and CHARGE syndrome), iris, and/or optic nerve

An eyelid coloboma is not related to closure of embryonic fissure

Microphthalmos with cyst: small, abnormal eye with cystic expansion extending posteriorly into orbit

Arises in area of and external to a choroidal coloboma; cyst usually contains dysplastic neuroectodermal tissue and may not directly connect with the eye

Optic pit: considered an atypical coloboma; associated with basal encephalocele

Hyaloid artery (Figure 3-3): enters through embryonic fissure and forms vasa hyaloidea propria (blood supply to primary vitreous)

Intravitreal portion regresses by $8\frac{1}{2}$ months; intraneural portion becomes central retinal artery

Posterior tunica vasculosa lentis supplies the posterior lens

Retinal vascular development begins during 16th week: mesenchymal cells next to hyaloid artery form capillary network, then form arteries and veins;

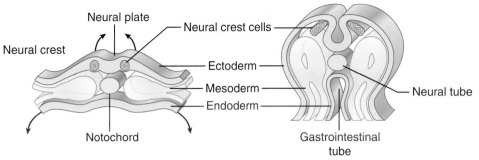

Figure 3-1. Neural tube formation.

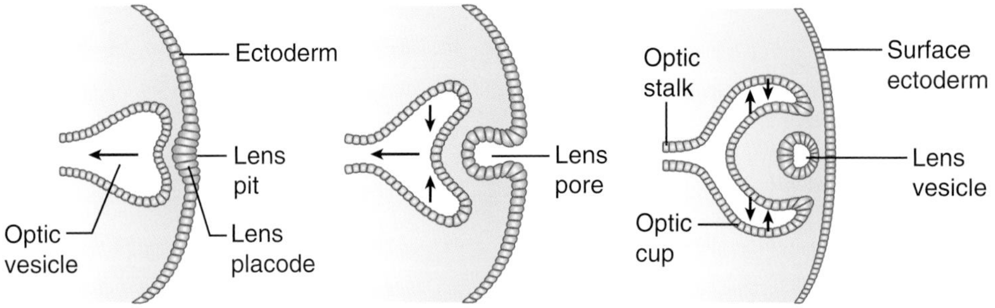

Figure 3-2. Optic cup formation.

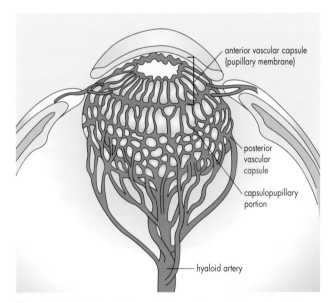

Figure 3-3. Hyaloid vasculature and primary vitreous during embryologic ocular development. (From Dass AB, Trese MT: Persistent hyperplastic primary vitreous. In: Yanoff M, Duker JS (eds): Ophthalmology. London, Mosby, 1999.)

vessels grow centrifugally from optic disc, reach nasal ora serrata during 8th month and temporal ora 1–2 months later

3% of normal neonates have a patent hyaloid artery

Remnants of hyaloid vasculature system:

    BERGMEISTER'S PAPILLAE: at optic nerve head; glial sheath of Bergmeister envelops posterior third of hyaloid artery and begins to atrophy during 7th month; epipapillary veil results if it does not fully regress

    PERIPAPILLARY LOOP: vascular loop extending from optic nerve head; risk of artery obstruction or vitreous hemorrhage

    MITTENDORF'S DOT: small opacity on posterior lens capsule at which hyaloid artery is attached to posterior tunica vasculosa lentis

    PERSISTENT PUPILLARY MEMBRANE: thin iris strands bridging pupil; may attach to anterior lens capsule; remnants of anterior tunica vasculosa lentis

Primitive epithelial papillae: cells from inner layer of optic cup at superior end of embryonic fissure, which becomes the optic disc

    Ganglion cell axons grow through

    Myelination starts centrally, reaching the chiasm at $7\frac{1}{2}$ months and lamina cribrosa at birth; complete approximately 1 month after birth

    Inner limiting membrane of Elschnig: covers ON, contiguous with ILM

    ON may show deceptively exaggerated cupping because nerve fibers posterior to lamina cribrosa are incompletely myelinated at birth

    ON hypoplasia is associated with DeMorsier's syndrome; 13% have pituitary abnormalities

Vitreous: produced by lens, retina, and walls of hyaloid artery; contains mesenchymal cells

    Primary vitreous: formed by hyaloid vascular system (vasa hyaloidea propria, which includes hyaloid canal, hyaloid vessels, and posterior portions of tunica vasculosa lentis); eventually replaced by secondary vitreous; failure to regress causes persistent hyperplastic primary vitreous (PHPV) (Figure 3-4)

    Secondary vitreous: formed by retina

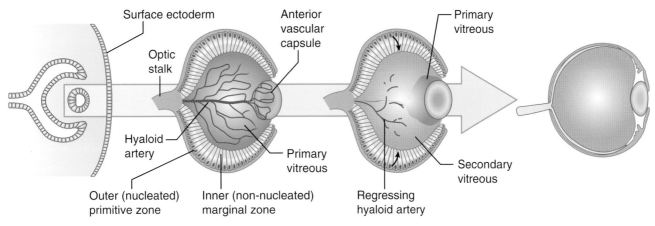

Figure 3-4. Posterior segment development.

Area of Martegiani: extends from disc into vitreous to become Cloquet's canal

Cloquet's canal: junction of primary and secondary vitreous

Tertiary vitreous: zonule fibers formed from ciliary processes and lens capsule

Berger's space: retrolental space

Retina: neuroectoderm; vascularization begins at 4 months; temporal periphery is last portion to become vascularized

Development of fovea is not complete until 4 or more weeks after birth

Retinal dysplasia: abnormal proliferation of developing retina produces tubular structures with a rosette-like appearance; represents nonspecific response to disorganizing influence during development; associated with maternal LSD ingestion, Patau's syndrome (trisomy 13), microphthalmos, congenital glaucoma, Peter's anomaly, uveal and optic nerve colobomas, cyclopia, and synophthalmia

Choroid: requires RPE for development

Stroma is from neural crest cells

Vascular endothelium is from mesoderm

Vessel walls are from neural crest cells

Sclera: neural crest cells and mesoderm (temporal aspect)

Blue hue at birth due to thinness (see underlying uveal pigment)

Cornea: neural crest cells (2 waves)

1st wave grows between epithelium and lens, forming double layer of corneal endothelium

2nd wave grows between epithelium and endothelium; this zone is rich in hyaluronic acid and collagen fibrils

At 4 months, Descemet's membrane develops

At 5 months, Bowman's membrane develops

Angle: neural crest cells from peripheral cornea differentiate into chamber angle during 7th week

In 4th month, Schlemm's canal forms

In 7th month, angle moves posteriorly

In 8th month, formation is complete; trabecular meshwork appears just before birth

Lens: at 27 days, surface ectoderm adjacent to optic vesicle enlarges to form lens placode (lens plate)

Circular indentation then occurs on lens plate, forming lens pit, which invaginates the wall of the optic vesicle until it closes to form a sphere

Basement membrane of the surface ectoderm forms the surface of the sphere (the lens vesicle) and subsequently becomes the lens capsule

Lens epithelial cells on posterior aspect of this sphere elongate and migrate first (primary lens fibers); these cells fill the core of the lens vesicle at approximately 40 days (embryonal nucleus)

At 7 weeks, anterior cells migrate toward equator and proliferate to form secondary lens fibers that encase the embryonal nucleus and form the Y sutures; Y sutures represent the meeting of embryonal and fetal nuclei (upright anteriorly, inverted posteriorly)

After 3 months, zonules of Zinn (zonular fibers) develop (Figure 3-5)

Summary

3 weeks	lens placode from surface ectoderm
6 weeks	lens vesicle; further development requires normal neuroretina
12 weeks	tunica vasculosa lentis
28–38 weeks	degeneration of tunica vasculosa lentis

Lens of a newborn is more spherical than that of an adult; therefore, anterior chamber appears shallow

Iris: rim of optic cup grows around lens and forms iris

Epithelial layers (iris pigment epithelium [IPE]; anterior pigmented and posterior nonpigmented) are from inner and outer layers of the optic cup (neuroectoderm); forms part of the blood–aqueous barrier

In 7th week, stroma forms from neural crest cells, and tunica vasculosa lentis forms

In 6th month, sphincter and dilator muscles form from neuroectoderm

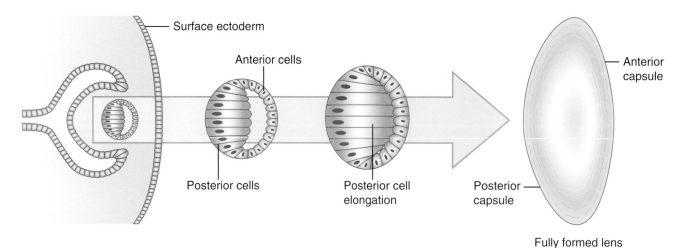

Figure 3-5. Lens development.

In 7th month, blood vessels enter iris

In 9th month, tunica vasculosa lentis disappears

Newborn iris is usually gray-blue; development of iris color takes weeks to months, as stromal chromatophores (dendritic melanocytes from neural crest) complete their migration into uvea shortly after birth

Iris dilator muscle is immature, causing relative miosis in infancy

Retinal pigment epithelium (RPE) and posterior pigment epithelium of the iris form from the outer layer of the optic cup (have mature coloration because pigment granules develop very early in gestation)

Ciliary body (CB): formation begins in 3rd month; fold in optic cup becomes epithelial layers of ciliary processes

In 4th month, filaments from surface cells form zonules; the major arterial circle of the iris (located in CB), the longitudinal ciliary muscle, and the ciliary processes develop

In 5th month, pars plana develops, and ciliary body stroma and ciliary muscle develop from neural crest cells adjacent to cornea

In 7th month, circular fibers of ciliary muscle differentiate

Patient's age can be determined by analysis of CB cellularity

Nasolacrimal system: at 6 weeks, surface ectoderm is buried in mesoderm, between maxillary and lateral nasal processes

During 3rd month, the cord canalizes

Defects: may result in imperforate valve of Hasner; rarely, absent puncta or canaliculi

Eyelids: at 8 weeks, upper lids form by fusion of medial and lateral frontonasal processes; lower lids by fusion of maxillary processes and medial nasal processes

At 12 weeks, lid folds fuse

At 24 weeks, separation begins from nasal side

Embryologic tissues and their components:

Neural ectoderm: sensory retina, RPE, nonpigmented ciliary body epithelium, pigmented CB epithelium (extension of RPE), IPE, iris sphincter and dilator muscle, optic nerve (neural and glial elements), sympathetic ganglion, lateral geniculate body, ocular pigment granules (RPE, CB, IPE), peripheral nerves related to eye function, erector pili muscle associated with hair follicles of the skin

Surface ectoderm: crystalline lens, corneal and conjunctival epithelium, lid epithelium, lacrimal gland, nasolacrimal system

Surface and neural ectoderm: vitreous, zonules

Neural crest cells: corneal stroma and endothelium, iris stroma, TM, chamber angle, Schlemm's canal, sclera (except temporal portion), sheaths and tendons of extraocular muscles, ciliary muscle (nonpigmented layer of ciliary body), choroidal stroma, melanocytes, meningeal sheaths, orbital bones, connective tissue of orbit, muscular and connective tissue layers of blood vessels

S-100 STAIN: specific for neural crest–derived structures

3 WAVES OF NEURAL CREST CELL MIGRATION (during 7th week): corneal and TM endothelium, keratocytes (corneal stroma), iris stroma

ANTERIOR SEGMENT DISORDERS DUE TO NEURAL CREST ABNORMALITIES:

ABNORMAL MIGRATION: congenital glaucoma, posterior embryotoxin, Axenfeld-Rieger syndrome, Peter's anomaly, sclerocornea

ABNORMAL PROLIFERATION: iridocorneal endothelial (ICE) syndromes

ABNORMAL TERMINAL INDUCTION: corneal endothelial dystrophies

Mesoderm: blood vessel endothelium, anterior chamber angle outflow apparatus, sclera (small area temporally), EOM, Schlemm's canal, portion of vitreous

Mesenchyme: primitive connective tissue; originates from neural crest cells and mesoderm (Figure 3-6)

Period after conception	Event	Period after conception	Event
22nd day	Optic groove appears	3rd month	Differentiation of precursors of rods and cones
25th day	Optic vesicle forms from optic pit		Ciliary body develops
26th day	Primordia of superior rectus, inferior rectus, medial rectus, and inferior oblique appear		Appearance of limbus
			Anterior chamber appears as a potential space
27th day	Formation of lens plate from surface ectoderm		Sclera condenses
	Primordium of lateral rectus appears		Eyelid folds lengthen and fuse
28th day	Embryonic fissure forms	4th month	Formation of retinal vasculature begins
	Cells destined to become retinal pigment epithelium acquire pigmentation		Beginning of regression of hyaloid vessels
			Formation of physiologic cup of optic disc
29th day	Primordium of superior oblique appears		Formation of lamina cribrosa
5th week	Lens pit forms and deepens into lens vesicle		Major arterial circle of iris forms
	Hyaloid vessels develop		Development of iris sphincter muscle
	Primary vitreous develops		Development of longitudinal ciliary muscle and processes of ciliary body
	Osseous structures of the orbit begin to develop		
6th week	Closure of embryonic fissure		Formation of tertiary vitreous
	Corneal epithelial cells develop interconnections		Bowman's membrane forms
	Differentiation of retinal pigment epithelium		Canal of Schlemm appears
	Proliferation of neural retinal cells		Eyelid glands and cilia form
	Formation of secondary vitreous	5th month	Photoreceptors differentiate
	Formation of primary lens fibers		Eyelid separation begins
	Development of periocular vasculature	6th month	Cones differentiate
	Appearance of eyelid folds and nasolacrimal duct		Ganglion cells thicken in macula
	Ciliary ganglion appears		Differentiation of dilator pupillae muscle
7th week	Migration of ganglion cells toward optic disc		Nasolacrimal system becomes patent
	Formation of embryonic lens nucleus	7th month	Rods differentiate
	Development of choroidal vessels from periocular mesenchyme		Ora serrata forms
			Migration of ganglion cells to form nerve fiber layer of Henle
	Three waves of neural crest migration: first wave: formation of corneal and trabecular endothelium second wave: formation of corneal stroma third wave: formation of iris stroma		Choroid becomes pigmented
			Circular ciliary muscle fibers develop
			Myelination of optic nerve
			Posterior movement of anterior chamber angle
	Formation of tunica vasculosa lentis		Orbicularis muscle differentiation
	Sclera begins to form	8th month	Completion of anterior chamber angle formation
			Hyaloid vessels disappear
		9th month	Retinal vessels reach the temporal periphery
			Pupillary membrane disappears
		After birth	Development of macula

Figure 3-6. Time line of ocular embryogenesis. (From Azar NJ, Davis EA: Embryology in the eye. In: Yanoff M, Duker JS (eds): Ophthalmology, 2nd edn. St. Louis, Mosby, 2004.)

Pathology

MICROBIAL STUDIES

Stains

Gram: bacteria, fungi

Giemsa: *Acanthamoeba*, fungi, and cytology; best for intranuclear inclusion bodies

Acid fast (Ziehl-Neelsen): *Mycobacterium, Nocardia*

Periodic acid-Schiff (PAS): fungi

Gomori's methenamine silver: fungi

Calcofluor white: fungi and *Acanthamoeba* (binds to cell wall, visible with fluorescent microscopy)

KOH: fungi

Culture Media

Blood agar: most bacteria; very good for atypical *Mycobacterium*

Blood agar in 5–10% carbon dioxide: *Moraxella*

Chocolate (contains hemin and nicotinamide adenine dinucleotide [NAD]): *Haemophilus, Neisseria*

Thioglycolate: anaerobes

Sabouraud's: fungi

Löwenstein-Jensen: *Mycobacterium tuberculosis, Nocardia*

Loeffler's: *Corynebacteria*

Non-nutrient agar with *E. coli* overgrowth: *Acanthamoeba*

Cytology

Intracytoplasmic basophilic inclusions (Giemsa stain): *Chlamydia*

Intranuclear eosinophilic inclusions (Papanicolaou stain): herpes (Tzanck smear)

TISSUE STAINS

Hematoxylin and eosin (H&E): hematoxylin is specific for nucleic acids within nuclei and stains blue (basophilic); eosin is specific for most cytoplasmic organelles (such as mitochondria) and stains pink (eosinophilic)

Periodic acid-Schiff (PAS): stains basement membrane material magenta (Descemet's, lens capsule, Bruch's membrane, ILM [internal limiting membrane], gutattae, drusen); also stains glycogen, fungi, conjunctival goblet cells (useful for differentiation of corneal from conjunctival epithelium)

Masson trichrome: stains collagen blue and hyaline red; used for granular dystrophy

Congo red: stains amyloid orange; used for lattice dystrophy

Crystal violet: stains amyloid red-purple; used for lattice dystrophy

Alcian blue: stains acid mucopolysaccharide blue; used for macular dystrophy

Colloidal iron: stains acid mucopolysaccharide blue; used for macular dystrophy

Oil red O: stains neutral lipids red-orange in frozen section; must be used on fresh tissue because formalin leaches out lipid

Sudan black: stains phospholipids; myelin in ON

Luxol fast blue: stains myelin blue; demyelinated plaques lose affinity for stain

Bodian: stains nerve fibers black

Mucicarmine: stains mucus pink/red; mucus-secreting adenocarcinomas (i.e. GI, breast)

Verhoeff Van Gieson: stains elastic tissue black; used for elastotic degeneration

Movat's pentachrome: stains elastic tissue black

Wilder: stains reticulin fibers black

Alizarin red: stains calcium red-orange

von Kossa: stains calcium black; used for band keratopathy

Prussian blue: stains iron (hemosiderin, ferric ions) blue

Fontana-Masson: stains melanin black; used for amelanotic melanoma

S-100 protein: stains nevi, melanomas, schwannomas, neurofibromas, and other heterologous cell lines

Polarizing filters: for evaluating structures or deposits that have a regular molecular structure (amyloid, calcium oxalate crystals), as well as suture granulomas and vegetable foreign bodies

TISSUE FIXATION

Orientation of globe: identify superior oblique (SO) (tendinous insertion) and inferior oblique (IO) (muscular insertion) muscles

Paraffin: embedding process for histologic examination: water is removed, organic solvents leach out lipids; PMMA is dissolved completely; to preserve lipids, fresh or frozen tissue specimens are used; paraffin must be removed before different stains are applied

Glutaraldehyde: for electron microscopy

Formalin and Bouin's fixative: for light microscopy; 10% buffered formalin (formalin = 40% solution of formaldehyde in water); formalin stabilizes protein, lipid, and carbohydrates, and prevents postmortem enzymatic destruction of tissue

Ethyl alcohol: cytology

Fixation artifacts:

Lange's fold: fold at ora serrata in newborn eyes probably caused by unequal shrinkage of retinociliary tissues during fixation

Artifactual RD: common histologic finding, differentiated from true retinal detachment by lack of subretinal fluid, preservation of photoreceptors, and pigment attached to outer surface of rods and cones (Figure 3-7)

Clefts in corneal stroma: clear spaces within stroma; obliterated in corneal edema

HYPERSENSITIVITY REACTIONS (COOMBS AND GELL CLASSIFICATION)

Type I: anaphylactic/immediate hypersensitivity (IgE)
Example: hay fever, vernal, atopic, giant papillary conjunctivitis (GPC)

Type II: cytotoxic hypersensitivity (complement mediated)
Example: OCP, Mooren's ulcer

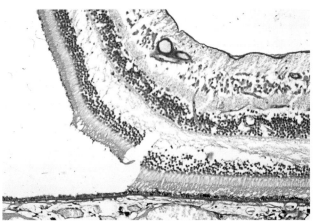

A

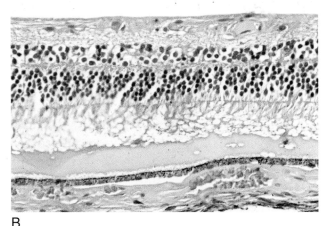

B

Figure 3-7. A, Artifact RD with no fluid, pigment adherent to photoreceptors, and normal retinal architecture. B, True RD with material in subretinal space and degeneration of outer retinal layers. (From Yanoff M, Fine BS: Ocular pathology, 5th edn. St Louis, Mosby, 2002.)

Type III: immune complex deposition (Ag–Ab complex)
Example: Stevens-Johnson, marginal infiltrates, disciform keratitis, subepithelial infiltrates, Wessely ring, scleritis, retinal vasculitis, phacoanyphlaxis

Type IV: cell-mediated, delayed hypersensitivity (CD4 lymphocytes)
Example: phlyctenule, graft reaction, contact dermatitis, interstitial keratitis, granulomatous disease (TB, syphilis, leprosy), sympathetic ophthalmia, Vogt-Koyanagi-Harada (VKH) syndrome

Type V: stimulating antibody
Example: Graves' disease, myasthenia gravis

IMMUNOGLOBULINS

IgG: most abundant; crosses the placenta; binds complement

IgA: second most abundant; monomeric or joined by J chain; important against viral infection; found in secretions

IgM: largest; binds complement; important in primary immune response

IgD: present in newborns; not in tear film

IgE: sensitizes mast cells and tissue leukocytes; role in atopy

Table 3-1. HLA associations

Uveitis	
A29	Birdshot retinochoroidopathy (90%)
B7, DR2	Presumed ocular histoplasmosis syndrome (80%)
B8, B13	Sarcoidosis
B8, B51, DR2, DR15	Intermediate uveitis
B27 (1-5% of population)	Adult iridocyclitis (usually unilateral): Reiter's syndrome (75%), ankylosing spondylitis (90%), inflammatory bowel disease (90%), psoriatic arthritis, juvenile rheumatoid arthritis (JRA) (subtype V)
B51	Behçet's disease (70%)
DR4	Sympathetic ophthalmia, Vogt-Koyanagi-Harada syndrome
DR15	Pars planitis
DQ7	Acute retinal necrosis (50%)
External disease	
B5, DR3, DR4	HSV keratitis
B8, DR3	Sjögren's syndrome
B12	Ocular cicatricial pemphigoid
B15	Scleritis
DR3	Thygeson's superficial punctate keratitis (SPK)
Neuro-ophthalmology	
A1, B8, DR3	Myasthenia gravis (MG)
B7, DR2	Multiple sclerosis (MS)
DR3	Graves' disease

HLA (HUMAN LEUKOCYTE ANTIGEN) SYSTEM

Major histocompatibility complex (MHC) proteins found on surfaces of all nucleated cells

In humans, MHC proteins are the HLA molecules

Gene loci are located on chromosome 6
    Class I: antigen presentation to cytotoxic T cells (CD8 positive); loci A, B, C
    Class II: antigen presentation to helper T cells (CD4 positive); loci DR, DP, DQ

INFLAMMATION

Tissue infiltration by inflammatory cells

Types of Inflammatory Cells

Neutrophils: polymorphonuclear leukocytes (PMNs)
    Primary cell in acute inflammation; phagocytosis
    Multilobed nucleus
    Abscess: focal collection of PMNs
    Pus: PMNs and tissue necrosis

Eosinophils:
    Allergic and parasite-related reactions ('worms, wheezes, weird diseases'); modulation of mast cell reactions, phagocytosis of Ag–Ab complexes
    Bilobed nucleus, granular cytoplasm

Mast cells: tissue basophils
    IgE bound to surface; Ag causes degranulation with release of histamine and heparin
    Example: anaphylaxis, allergic conjunctivitis
    Looks like plasma cell

Lymphocytes:
    Main cell in humoral and cell-mediated immune reactions

Types: B cells, T cells (helper, suppressor, cytotoxic, killer, null cells)
Scanty cytoplasm

Plasma cells: activated B cells
    Synthesis and secretion of antibodies
    Eccentric 'cartwheel' nucleus, basophilic cytoplasm
    Plasmacytoid cell: granular eosinophilic cytoplasm
    Russell body: immunoglobulin crystals

Macrophages: histiocytes, monocytes (Figure 3-8)
    Primary phagocytic cell; second line of cellular defense; regulation of lymphocytes via Ag presentation and monokine production
    Transformation into epithelioid and giant cells
    Kidney-shaped nucleus

Epithelioid histiocyte: activated macrophage with vesicular nucleus and eosinophilic cytoplasm; cells resemble epithelium; hallmark of granulomatous inflammation; fuse to form giant cells

Giant cells: 3 types
    Langhans': nuclei arranged around periphery in ring/horseshoe pattern
    Example: TB, sarcoidosis
    Touton: midperipheral ring of nuclei; central eosinophilic cytoplasm; nuclei are surrounded by clear zone of foamy lipid
    Example: juvenile xanthogranuloma (JXG)
    Foreign body: nuclei randomly distributed; surrounds or contains foreign body

Types of Inflammation

Acute:
Suppurative: neutrophils
Nonsuppurative: lymphocytes

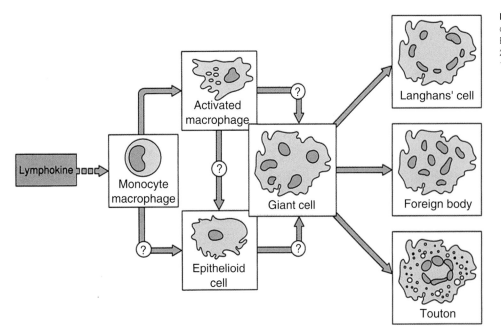

Figure 3-8. Macrophage differentiation. (Modified from Roitt IM, Brostoff J, Male DK: Immunology, 2nd edn. London, Gower Medical, 1989.)

Chronic:

Nongranulomatous: lymphocytes and plasma cells
Granulation tissue in reparative phase; exuberant response causes pyogenic granuloma
Granulomatous: epithelioid histiocytes; 3 patterns
    DIFFUSE: epithelioid cells distributed randomly against background of lymphocytes and plasma cells
        Example: sympathetic ophthalmia, fungal infection, JXG, lepromatous leprosy
    DISCRETE: epithelioid cells form nodules with giant cells, surrounded by rim of lymphocytes and plasma cells
        Example: sarcoidosis, miliary TB, tuberculoid leprosy
    ZONAL: palisaded giant cells surround central nidus
        Example: phacoantigenic endophthalmitis (phacotoxic uveitis is nongranulomatous); rheumatoid scleritis (nidus = scleral collagen); chalazion
Endophthalmitis: inflammation involving at least one ocular coat and adjacent cavity, sclera is not involved
Panophthalmitis: suppurative endophthalmitis also involving sclera and orbit

Sequelae of Inflammation

Cornea: scarring
Calcific band keratopathy: basophilic granules in Bowman's membrane
Inflammatory pannus: subepithelial fibrovascular and inflammatory ingrowth with destruction of Bowman's membrane
    Example: trachoma
Degenerative pannus: fibrous tissue between epithelium and intact Bowman's membrane
    Example: chronic corneal edema

Anterior chamber: organization of hypopyon; retrocorneal fibrous membranes
Peripheral anterior synechiae (PAS): seclusio pupillae (if 360°)
Pupillary membrane: occlusio pupillae

Lens:
Anterior subcapsular cataract: fibrous plaque beneath folded anterior capsule, secreted by irritated metaplastic anterior epithelial cells
Posterior subcapsular cataract: bladder cells adjacent to capsule

Ciliary body:
Cyclitic membrane: retrolental collagenous membrane attached to CB; contraction leads to detachment of pars plana, ciliary muscle remains adherent to scleral spur attachment; due to organization and scarring of vitreous, metaplastic ciliary epithelium, organized inflammatory residua

Retina:
CME: retinal vascular leakage or Müller cell edema
RPE changes: hypertrophy, hyperplasia, and migration (pseudoretinitis pigmentosa); fibrous metaplasia (collagen and basement membrane material deposited on Bruch's membrane, contain lacunae of RPE cells [pseudoadenomatous proliferation]); intraocular bone from osseous metaplasia
Reactive gliosis

Phthisis: rectus muscle traction on hypotonous globe causes squared-off appearance; thickened sclera, high incidence of retinal detachment and disorganization, calcareous degeneration of lens

EYELID EPITHELIAL CHANGES

Hyperkeratosis: thickening of the keratin layer; clinically appears as white, flaky lesion (leukoplakia)

Parakeratosis: thickening of the keratin layer with retention of nuclei; indicates shortened epidermal regeneration time; granular layer is thin or absent

Dyskeratosis: keratin formation within the basal cell layer or deeper

Acanthosis: thickening of the squamous cell layer due to proliferation of prickle cells

Acantholysis: loss of cohesion between epidermal cells with breakdown of intercellular junctions, creating spaces within the epidermis; occurs in pemphigus and produces intraepithelial bullae

Dysplasia: disorderly maturation of epithelium with loss of polarity, cytologic atypia, and mitotic figures found above the basilar layer
    Mild: <50% epidermal thickness involved
    Severe: >50% involved

Carcinoma in situ (CIN): full-thickness replacement of epithelium by malignant cells without invasion through the basement membrane

Squamous cell carcinoma: malignant epithelial cells invade below basement membrane

Anaplasia: cytologic malignancy with pleomorphism, anisocytosis, abnormal nuclei, and mitotic figures

Papillomatosis: proliferation of dermal papillae, causing surface undulation

Pseudoepitheliomatous hyperplasia: inflammatory response with hyperplasia of epithelium, which mimics carcinoma; acanthosis with protrusion of broad tongues of benign epidermis into the dermis

Elastosis: actinic damage; seen as blue staining (normally pink) of superficial dermal collagen with H&E stain; damaged collagen stains with elastic tissue stains but is not susceptible to digestion with elastase (Figure 3-9)

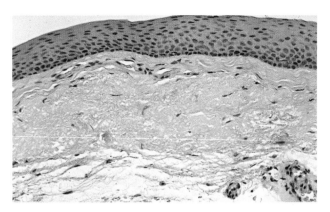

Figure 3-9. Elastosis demonstrating basophilic degeneration of conjunctival substantia propria in a pinguecula. (From Yanoff M, Fine BS: Ocular pathology, 5th edn. St Louis, Mosby, 2002.)

AGING CHANGES

Cornea: Hassal-Henle warts (excrescences and thickenings of Descemet's membrane in corneal periphery)

Ciliary epithelium: hyperplasia and proliferation

Pars plana and pars plicata: clear (teardrop) cysts

Retina: loss of retinal cells and replacement with glial tissue; chorioretinal adhesions and pigmentary lesions in periphery; peripheral microcystoid degeneration (Blessig-Iwanoff cysts): located in outer plexiform layer; bubbly appearance just behind ora serrata; lined by Müller cells; contain mucopolysacharides

WOUNDS

Wound Healing

Cornea: stromal healing is avascular; fibrosis; neutrophils arrive via tears in 2–6 hours; wound edges swell and glycosaminoglycans (keratan sulfate, chondroitin sulfate) disintegrate at edge of wound; activated fibroblasts migrate across wound and produce; takes 4–6 weeks to return to full corneal thickness collagen and fibronectin; anterior surface re-epithelializes; endothelium migrates and regenerates Descemet's membrane

Sclera: does not heal itself; it is avascular and acellular; ingrowth of granulation tissue from episclera and choroid

Iris: no healing

Retina: scars are produced by glial cells rather than fibroblasts

Wound Complications

Epithelial ingrowth: sheet of multilayered nonkeratinized squamous epithelium over any intraocular surface; may form cyst (free-floating or attached to iris); implanted cells tend to be 2–4 cell layers thick and have conjunctival characteristics (more than corneal)

Fibrous downgrowth: proliferating fibroblasts originate from episcleral or corneal stroma; contraction can occur; can occur with a puncture wound if there is a break in Descemet's membrane

Hemorrhage:

Corneal blood staining: hemoglobin (Hgb) breakdown products are forced through endothelial cells by increased intraocular pressure (IOP); Hgb molecules are removed by phagocytic and biochemical processes

Hemosiderosis bulbi: hemosiderin contains iron; can damage essential intracellular enzyme systems

Ochre membrane: hemorrhage that accumulates on posterior surface of detached vitreous

Synchysis scintillans: accumulation of cholesterol within vitreous following breakdown of red blood cell (RBC) membranes; angular, birefringent, flat crystalline particles with golden hue located in dependent portions of globe; cholesterol dissolves during preparation of tissues in paraffin; cholesterol clefts are negative image of cholesterol crystals, surrounded by serous fluid

---

Box 3-1. Differential diagnostics of intraocular calcification

Retinoblastoma

Choroidal osteoma

Choroidal hemangioma

Phthisis

Osseous choristoma

Box 3-2. Differential diagnostics of intraocular cartilage

PHPV (retrolental plaque)

Medulloepithelioma

Teratoma

Trisomy 13 (Figure 3-10)

Complex choristoma of conjunctiva

Box 3-3. Collagen

Type 1: normal corneal stroma; Bowman's membrane (highly disorganized type 1, basal lamina has type 4)

Type 2: vitreous

Type 3: stromal wound healing

Type 4: basement membranes

OCULAR INJURIES

Blunt Trauma

Scleral rupture (weak spots):
1. Limbus (on opposite side from trauma)
2. Posterior to rectus muscle insertions

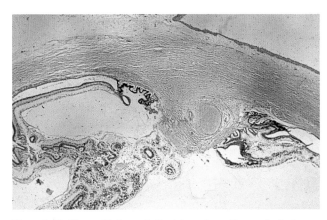

Figure 3-10. Trisomy 13 demonstrating intraocular cartilage and retinal dysplasia. (Reported in Hoepner J, Yanoff M: Ocular anomalies in Trisomy 13–15: an analysis of 13 eyes with two new findings. Am J Ophthalmol 74:729-37, 1972.)

3. Equator
4. Lamina cribrosa (ON)

Uveal tract is connected to sclera in 3 places:
1. Scleral spur
2. Internal ostia of vortex veins
3. Peripapillary tissue

Cyclodialysis: disinsertion of longitudinal fibers of ciliary muscle from scleral spur

Angle recession: rupture of face of ciliary body; plane of relative weakness at ciliary body face extending posteriorly between longitudinal fibers and more central oblique and circular fibers; oblique and circular muscles atrophy, changing cross-sectional shape of ciliary body from triangular to fusiform

Iridodialysis: disinsertion of iris root from ciliary body

Vossius ring: compression and rupture of IPE cells against anterior surface of lens deposit ring of melanin concentric to pupil

Lens capsule rupture: capsule is thinnest at posterior pole; cataract can form immediately; epithelium may be stimulated by trauma to form anterior lenticular fibrous plaque

Descemet's rupture: causes acute edema (hydrops); due to minor trauma (keratoconus) or major trauma (forceps injury)

Choroidal rupture: often concentric to optic disc; risk of CNV

Sclopoteria: choroidal rupture with overlying necrosis of retina

Retinal dialysis: retina anchored anteriorly to nonpigmented epithelium of pars plana and reinforced by vitreous base, which straddles the ora serrata;

circumferential tear of retina at point of attachment of ora or immediately posterior to vitreous base attachment

Commotio retinae: temporary loss of retinal transparency; due to disruption of photoreceptor elements, not true retinal edema

Penetrating Trauma

Penetration: partial-thickness wound (into)

Perforation: full-thickness wound (through) (globe penetration is due to perforation of the cornea or sclera; globe perforation is a double penetrating injury)

Sequelae of Trauma

Phthisis bulbi:
Atrophia bulbi without shrinkage: initially, size and shape of eye are maintained; with loss of nutrition: cataract develops, retina atrophies and separates from RPE by serous fluid accumulation, synechiae cause increased IOP
Atrophia bulbi with shrinkage: eye becomes soft owing to ciliary body dysfunction; internal structures are atrophic but histologically recognizable; globe becomes smaller with squared-off shape (because of tension of rectus muscles); anterior chamber (AC) collapses; corneal endothelial cell damage leads to corneal edema and opacification
Atrophia bulbi with disorganization (phthisis bulbi): globe shrinks to average diameter of 16–19 mm; most ocular contents are disorganized; calcification of Bowman's layer, lens, retina, and drusen; bone formation in uveal tract

Intraocular Foreign Body

Copper:
≥85%: noninfectious suppurative endophthalmitis
<85% (chalcosis): copper deposits in basement membranes (Kayser-Fleisher ring, sunflower cataract, retinal degeneration)

Steel (contains iron): siderosis bulbi; follow with electroretinogram (ERG) (early increased a wave, normal b wave; later decreased b wave leading to extinguished)

Organic (vegetable matter): severe granulomatous foreign body response

Chemical Injury

Acid: precipitates proteins; zone of coagulative necrosis acts as barrier to deeper penetration

Alkali: denatures proteins and lyses cell membranes; no effective barrier is created – therefore deeper penetration; vascular occlusion, ischemia, corneal damage during healing phase owing to collagenase released by regenerating tissue; limbal bleaching in severe cases (if limbal stem cells are depleted the corneal surface is repopulated with conjunctival cells)

Radiation

Nonionizing: depends on wavelength

Microwave: cataract

Infrared: true exfoliation of lens capsule (glassblower's cataract)

Ultraviolet: keratitis (welder's flash)

Ionizing: tissue damage is direct (actively reproducing cells) or indirect (blood vessels); epithelial atrophy and ulceration, dermatitis of eyelids, dysfunction of adnexa, destructive ocular surface disease with keratinization, cataract; retinal necrosis, ischemia, neovascularization, optic atrophy (retina is relatively radioresistant, but retinal blood vessels are vulnerable)

Infection (Table 3-2)

Table 3-2. Most common cause of infections

Endophthalmitis:	
Acute postoperative (<6 weeks)	Coagulase-negative *Staphylococcus*, *Staphylococcus aureus*
Delayed postoperative	*Propionibacterium acnes*, coagulase-negative *Staphylococcus*
From filtering bleb	*Streptococcus pneumoniae, Staphylococcus, Haemophilus influenzae*
Post-traumatic	*Staphylococcus* species, *Bacillus cereus*, Gram-negative organisms
Endogenous (IVDA)	*Candida*
Dacryocystitis	*S. pneumoniae, Staphylococcus*
Dacryadenitis	*Staphylococcus*
Canaliculitis	*Actinomyces*
Orbital cellulitis (children)	*S. aureus*
Preseptal cellulites	*S. aureus*
Angular blepharitis	*Staphylococcus, Moraxella*

Tumors (Box 3-4)

Box 3-4. Tumors

Congenital:

Hamartoma: composed of tissues normally found in that area

Example: hemangioma

Choristoma: composed of tissues not normally found in that area

Example: choroidal osteoma

Most common primary malignant intraocular tumor in adults: uveal melanoma

Second most common primary malignant intraocular tumor in adults: lymphoma

Most common primary malignant intraocular tumor in children: retinoblastoma

Second most common primary malignant intraocular tumor in children: medulloepithelioma

Most common malignant lacrimal gland tumor: adenocystic carcinoma

Most common benign orbital tumor in adults: cavernous hemangioma

Most common benign orbital tumor in children: capillary hemangioma

Most common primary malignant orbital tumor in children: rhabdomyosarcoma

Most common metastasis to orbit in children: neuroblastoma

REVIEW QUESTIONS (Answers start on page 358)

1. Which stain is the most helpful in the diagnosis of sebaceous cell carcinoma?
   a. Giemsa
   b. hematoxylin and eosin
   c. oil-red-O
   d. methenamine silver

2. Pagetoid spread is most commonly associated with
   a. malignant melanoma
   b. squamous cell carcinoma
   c. sebaceous cell carcinoma
   d. Merkel cell tumor

3. A melanoma occurring in which of the following locations has the best prognosis?
   a. iris
   b. ciliary body
   c. choroid, anteriorly
   d. choroid, posterior pole

4. Calcification in retinoblastoma is due to
   a. RPE metaplasia
   b. necrosis
   c. hemorrhage
   d. metastasis

5. The type of organism that causes Lyme disease is a
   a. bacillus
   b. spirochete
   c. protozoan
   d. tick

6. Characteristics of ghost cells include all of the following except
   a. khaki colored
   b. rigid
   c. Heinz bodies
   d. biconcave

7. A moll gland is best categorized as
   a. mucin
   b. apocrine
   c. sebaceous
   d. holocrine

8. Which of the following is not a Gram-positive rod?
   a. *Corynebacterium*
   b. Bacillus
   c. Serratia
   d. Listeria

9. Trantas' dots are composed of what cell type?
   a. macrophage
   b. neutrophil
   c. eosinophil
   d. mast cell

10. Types of collagen that can be found in the cornea include all of the following except
    a. I
    b. II
    c. III
    d. IV

11. Lens nuclei are retained in all of the following conditions except
    a. Leigh's syndrome
    b. Lowe's syndrome
    c. rubella
    d. Alport's syndrome

12. Vogt-Koyanagi-Harada syndrome is best described by which type of hypersensitivity reaction?
    a. I
    b. II
    c. III
    d. IV

13. Lacy vacuolization of the iris occurs in which disease?
    a. central retinal vein occlusion
    b. diabetes
    c. central retinal artery occlusion
    d. hypercholesterolemia

14. Antoni A and B cells occur in which tumor?
    a. neurilemmoma
    b. meningioma
    c. glioma
    d. neurofibroma

15. Which tumor is classically described as having a 'Swiss cheese' appearance?
    a. rhabdomyosarcoma
    b. adenoid cystic carcinoma
    c. benign mixed tumor
    d. meningioma

16. Which iris nodule is correctly paired with its histopathology
    a. JXG, inflammatory cells
    b. Lisch nodule, neural crest hamartoma
    c. Koeppe nodule, stromal hyperplasia
    d. Brushfield spot, histiocytes and Touton giant cells

17. Which of the following statements is true concerning immunoglobulin
    a. IgG crosses the placenta
    b. IgA binds complement
    c. IgM is present in newborns
    d. IgD is the second most abundant

18. A retinal detachment caused by fixation artifact can be differentiated from a true RD by all of the following except
    a. a fold at the ora serrata
    b. no subretinal fluid
    c. normal retinal architecture
    d. pigment adherent to photoreceptors

19. Which of the following epithelial changes in the eyelid refers to thickening of the squamous cell layer
    a. parakeratosis
    b. acanthosis
    c. dysplasia
    d. papillomatosis

20. Intraocular hemorrhage may cause all of the following sequelae except
    a. synchysis scintillans
    b. ochre membrane
    c. asteroid hyalosis
    d. hemosiderosis bulbi

21. Intraocular calcification may occur in all of the following except
    a. retinoblastoma
    b. medulloepithelioma
    c. choroidal hemangioma
    d. phthisis

22. The histopathology of which tumor is classically described as a storiform pattern of tumor cells
    a. rhabdomyosarcoma
    b. plasmacytoma
    c. neurilemoma
    d. fibrous histiocytoma

23. Which of the following findings is a histologic fixation artifact
    a. Lange's fold
    b. Mittendorf's dot
    c. Berger's space
    d. Cloquet's canal

24. The corneal stroma is composed of
    a. surface ectoderm
    b. neural crest cells
    c. mesoderm
    d. neural ectoderm

25. *Neisseria* is best cultured with which media
    a. Loeffler's
    b. Sabaroud's
    c. thioglycolate
    d. chocolate agar

26. Which of the following stains is used to detect amyloid
    a. colloidal iron
    b. Alcian blue
    c. crystal violet
    d. Masson trichrome

27. HLA-B7 is associated with
    a. Behçet's disease
    b. presumed ocular histoplasmosis syndrome
    c. iridocyclitis
    d. sympathetic ophthalmia

28. Which of the following conjunctival lesions should be sent to the pathology lab as a fresh unfixed tissue specimen?
    a. lymphoma
    b. squamous cell carcinoma
    c. Kaposi's sarcoma
    d. melanoma

29. Subepithelial infiltrates in the cornea from epidemic keratoconjunctivitis are thought to be
    a. lymphocytes and dead adenovirus
    b. polymorphonuclear leukocytes surrounding live adenovirus
    c. macrophages containing adenoviral particles
    d. lymphocytes and polymorphonuclear leukocytes

30. Which is the correct order of solutions for performing a Gram stain?
    a. iodine solution, crystal violet stain, ethanol, safranin
    b. crystal violet stain, safranin, ethanol, iodine solution
    c. iodine solution, safranin, ethanol, crystal violet stain
    d. crystal violet stain, iodine solution, ethanol, safranin

SUGGESTED READINGS

Embryology

Mann I: The Development of the Human Eye. New York, Grune & Stratton, 1964.

Pathology

Apple DJ: Ocular Pathology: Clinical Applications and Self-Assessment, 5th edn. St Louis, Mosby, 1998.

Char PH: Tumors of the Eye and Ocular Adnexa. Hamilton, Ontario, Canada, BC Decker, 2001.

Eagle RC: Eye Pathology: An Atlas and Basic Text, 2nd edn. Philadelphia, Lippincott Williams & Wilkins, 2011.

Spencer WH: Ophthalmic Pathology: An Atlas and Textbook, 4th edn. Philadelphia, WB Saunders, 1996.

Yanoff M, Sassani JW: Ocular Pathology, 6th edn. Philadelphia, Mosby, 2008.

4

Neuro-ophthalmology

ANATOMY OF THE VISUAL PATHWAY

Optic nerve → chiasm → optic tract → lateral geniculate body → optic radiation → occipital lobe (Figure 4-1)

Optic nerve: composed of 1.2 million nerve fibers; approximately 1.5 mm in diameter, enlarges to 3.5 mm posterior to lamina cribrosa due to myelin sheath; located 3–4 mm from fovea; causes absolute scotoma (blind spot) 15° temporal to fixation and slightly below horizontal meridian; approximately 45-50 mm in length (1 mm intraocular, 25 mm intraorbital, 9 mm intracanalicular, 10–15 mm intracranial) (Figure 4-2); acquires myelin posterior to lamina cribrosa

Surrounded by 3 layers of meninges: dura mater (outer layer; merges with sclera), arachnoid layer, pia mater (inner layer, fused to surface of nerve); space between arachnoid and pia contains cerebrospinal fluid (CSF)

ON runs through annulus of Zinn (ring of tendinous origins of the rectus muscles) and enters the optic canal

Optic canal: 9 mm long and 5–7 mm wide; thinnest medially, adjacent to ethmoid and sphenoid sinuses; dura of ON fuses with periosteum of canal

Intracranial ON: above are found the frontal lobe, olfactory tract, and anterior cerebral and anterior communicating arteries; laterally, the internal carotid artery emerges from the cavernous sinus

Blood supply (Figure 4-3)

ORBITAL PORTION: ophthalmic artery with meningeal anastomoses

INTRACANALICULAR PORTION: pial branches from ophthalmic artery; possibly internal carotid artery (ICA)

INTRACRANIAL PORTION: small vessels from ICA, anterior cerebral and anterior communicating arteries

Chiasm: 10 mm above pituitary gland

55% of ON fibers cross in chiasm: nasal retinal fibers cross in chiasm to contralateral optic tract (decussating nasal fibers); temporal fibers remain uncrossed; macular fibers run posteriorly (posterior compression leads to bitemporal defect)

'Knee of von Willebrand': inferonasal retinal fibers cross in chiasm and course anteriorly approximately 4 mm into contralateral ON before running posteriorly; produces junctional scotoma

Carotid arteries course on either side of chiasm (Figure 4-4)

Blood supply: ICA; occasionally by anterior cerebral and anterior communicating arteries

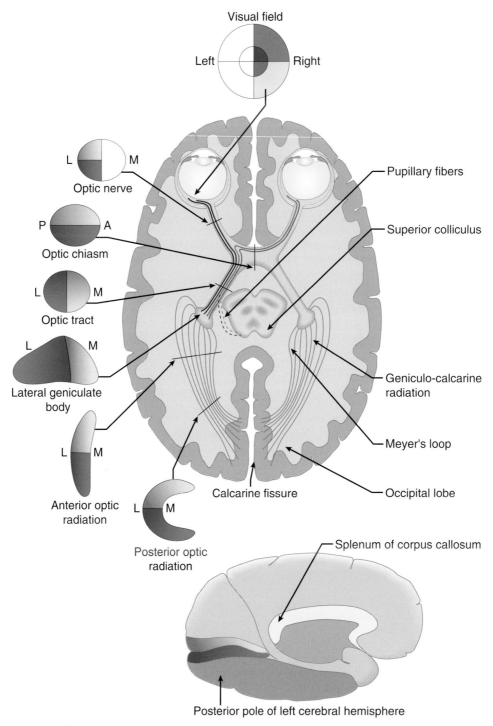

Figure 4-1. Visual pathway.

Optic tract: lower fibers lie laterally (90° rotation of fibers); tract courses laterally around cerebral peduncle

Damage to optic tract results in contralateral relative afferent pupillary defect (RAPD) because 55% of fibers cross (greater quantity of nasal fibers [nasal to foveal]), including the large monocular crescent (which corresponds with the extreme nasal retina)

Special fibers run to the hypothalamus, contributing to neuroendocrine systems that control diurnal rhythms

A major projection leaves the optic tract just before the lateral geniculate body (LGB) to form the brachium of the superior colliculus (also called *optic tectum*)

Superior colliculus: involved in foveation reflexes (receives input from pupillary fibers); injury disrupts eye movements but does not cause visual field (VF) defect

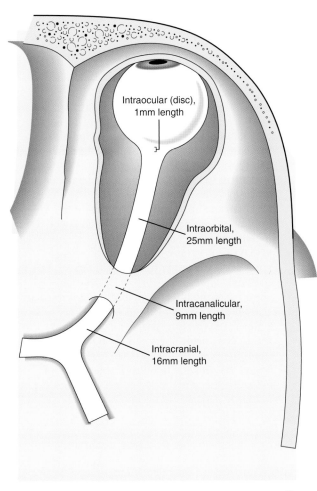

Figure 4-2. The 4 portions of the optic nerve. The lengths are given. (From Sadun AA: Anatomy and physiology. In: Yanoff M, Duker JS (eds) Ophthalmology, 2nd edn. St Louis, Mosby, 2004.)

Pupillary fibers pass through brachium of superior colliculus to pretectal area, which innervates both Edinger-Westphal subnuclei of CN 3

Optic tract provides retinal input to visual nucleus (pulvinar) in the thalamus

Blood supply: anterior choroidal artery; branches from posterior communicating artery

Lateral geniculate body: part of the thalamus (Figure 4-5)

Lower fibers lie laterally in optic tract and LGB (90° rotation of fibers)

Crossed fibers (contralateral eye): project to layers 1, 4, and 6

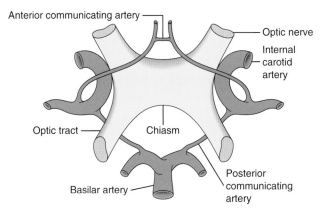

Figure 4-4. Relationship of the optic chiasm, optic nerves, and optic tracts to the arterial circle of Willis. The chiasm passes through the circle of Willis and receives its arterial supply from the anterior cerebral and communicating arteries from above, and the posterior communicating, posterior cerebral, and basilar arteries from below. (Adapted from Reed H, Drance SM: The Essentials of Perimetry: Static and Kinetic, 2nd edn. London, Oxford University Press, 1972.)

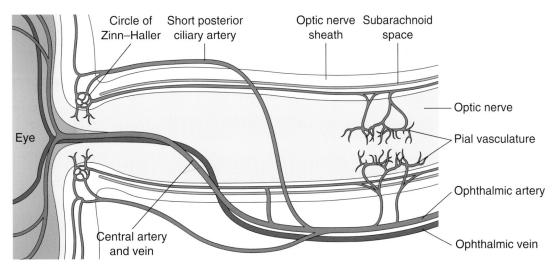

Figure 4-3. Anterior optic nerve. The sheath and the vascular supply to the intraocular and intraorbital portions are shown. (From Sadun AA: Anatomy and physiology. In: Yanoff M, Duker JS (eds) Ophthalmology, 2nd edn. St Louis, Mosby, 2004.)

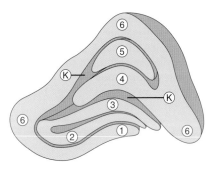

Figure 4-5. Lateral geniculate body section. The layers are numbered from ventral to dorsal in this posterior view. K fibers travel between the lamellae. (From Lawton AW: Retrochiasmal pathways, higher cortical function, and nonorganic visual loss. In: Yanoff M, Duker JS (eds) Ophthalmology, 2nd edn. St Louis, Mosby, 2004.)

Uncrossed fibers (ipsilateral eye): project to layers 2, 3, and 5
Layers of LGB can also be categorized by neuronal size:
   MAGNOCELLULAR NEURONS (M cells): layers 1 and 2; subserve motion detection, stereoacuity, and contrast sensitivity; project to layer 4C alpha of visual cortex
   PARVOCELLULAR NEURONS (P cells): layers 3 to 6; subserve fine spatial resolution and color vision; project to layer 4C beta of visual cortex
   KONIOCELLULAR NEURONS (K cells): sit in interlaminar zones and superficial layers; receive input from both retinas and the superior colliculus; may modulate information among other pathways
   BLOOD SUPPLY: anterior communicating artery and choroidal arteries

Optic radiation: myelinated nerve fibers; connect LGB to occipital cortex
   Superior retinal fibers (inferior VF): travel in white matter underneath parietal cortex to occipital lobe
   Inferior retinal fibers (superior VF): travel around ventricular system into temporal lobe (Meyer's loop); Meyer's loop is about 5 cm from tip of temporal lobe; temporal lobe injury causes incongruous homonymous superior quadrantanopia, or a 'pie-in-the-sky' VF defect
   Macular fibers: travel more centrally than do inferior retinal fibers
   Blood supply: middle cerebral arteries

Primary visual cortex (striate cortex, V1, Brodmann's area 17): medial face of occipital lobe, divided horizontally by calcarine fissure
   Visual cortex contains a topographic map of the contralateral hemifield; central portion of VF is highly magnified
   Macular region is posterior, extending slightly onto lateral aspect of occipital lobe
   Peripheral VF is located anteriorly along calcarine fissure
   Temporal crescent in each VF (from 55° to 100°) is seen only by nasal retina of ipsilateral eye; located most anteriorly; only site posterior to chiasm that if injured would cause a monocular VF defect; temporal crescent

may also be the only portion of VF spared after occipital lobe damage
   Blood supply: middle and posterior cerebral arteries

Visual association areas: areas 18 and 19

Other areas:
   Ganglia:
   1. **CILIOSPINAL CENTER OF BUDGE:** sympathetic fibers from hypothalamus synapse; located at level C8–T2
   2. **SUPERIOR CERVICAL:** 2nd-order sympathetic fibers synapse
   3. **CILIARY:** small parasympathetic ganglion; 1 cm from optic foramen between ON and lateral rectus muscle
      RECEIVES 3 ROOTS:
      Long sensory: sensory from cornea, iris, and ciliary body
      Short parasympathetic (synapse): motor to ciliary body and iris sphincter
      Sympathetic (do not synapse): conjunctival vasoconstrictor fibers and iris dilator
   4. **GENICULATE:** traversed by CN 7; contains cell bodies that provide taste from anterior ⅔ of tongue
   5. **SPHENOPALATINE:** parasympathetic fibers to lacrimal gland
   Horizontal gaze center: controls gaze to ipsilateral side; located in paramedian pontine reticular formation (PPRF) at level of CN 6 nucleus; projects to ipsilateral CN 6 nucleus and (via medial longitudinal fasciculus [MLF]) to contralateral CN 3 nucleus (Figure 4-6)
   Medial longitudinal fasciculus: extends from anterior horn cells of the spinal cord to the thalamus; connects CN 3 nuclei and gaze centers (ipsilateral CN 3 and contralateral CN 6)
   Vertical gaze center: originates in frontal eye fields or in superior colliculus; requires bilateral cortical input; projections travel to rostral interstitial nucleus of the MLF (riMLF) located behind red nucleus in midbrain; fibers travel to nuclei of CN 3 and 4 (Figure 4-7)
      UPGAZE (lateral portion of riMLF): stimulates CN 3 nucleus (superior rectus (SR) and inferior oblique (IO))
      DOWNGAZE (medial portion of riMLF): stimulates CN 3 nucleus (inferior rectus (IR)) and CN 4 nucleus
      TORSIONAL MOVEMENTS: via interstitial nucleus of Cajal
   Glial cells:
      OLIGODENDROCYTES: myelination (begins at LGB and reaches lamina cribrosa after birth)
      ASTROCYTES: support and nutrition
      MICROGLIAL CELLS: phagocytosis

PHYSIOLOGY

Testing

Color vision tests: Ishihara pseudoisochromatic or Hardy-Rand-Ritter plates; Farnsworth tests

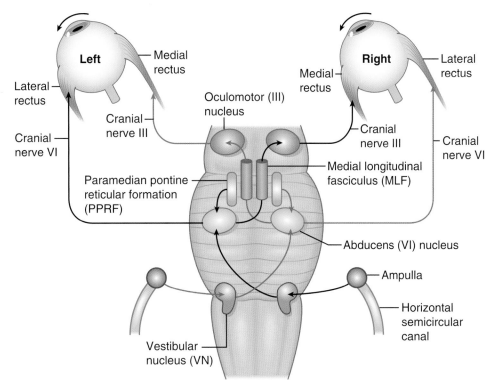

Figure 4-6. Horizontal eye movement pathways. (From Bajandas FJ, Kline LB: Neuro-Ophthalmology Review Manual. Thorofare, NJ, Slack, 1988.)

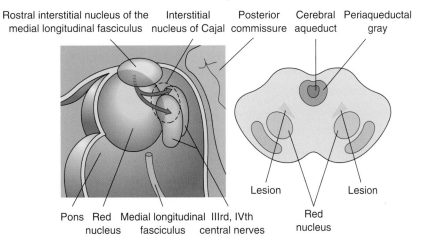

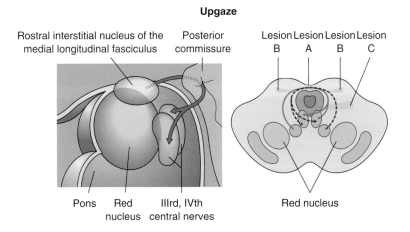

Figure 4-7. Pathways for vertical gaze. Upgaze pathways originate in the rostral interstitial nucleus of the medial longitudinal fasciculus and project dorsally to innervate the oculomotor and trochlear nerves, traveling through the posterior commissure. Lesions to both axon bundles are necessary to produce upgaze paralysis (lesions B or C). Upgaze paralysis is a feature of the dorsal midbrain syndrome as a result of the lesion's effect on the posterior commissure (lesion A). Downgaze pathways also originate in the rostral interstitial nucleus of the medial longitudinal fasciculus but probably travel more ventrally. Bilateral lesions also are needed to affect downgaze and usually are located dorsomedial to the red nucleus. (From Donahue SP, Lavin PJM: Disorders of supranuclear control of ocular motility. In: Yanoff M, Duker JS (eds) Ophthalmology. London, Mosby, 1999.)

Congenital defects: usually red/green

Acquired macular disease: may diminish blue/yellow in early stages (blue cones concentrated in perifoveal ring)

Fovea has mostly red/green cones, so red/green defects are detected in optic nerve diseases. Perception of red object indicates gross macular function

Photostress recovery test: determine best-corrected vision, shine bright light into eye for 10 seconds, record time for vision to recover within 1 line of best-corrected vision; test each eye separately; invalid for eyes with vision worse than 20/80

Optic nerve disease: normal recovery time (<60 seconds)

Macular disease: prolonged time (>90 seconds)

Contrast sensitivity: Pelli-Robson chart; Regan contrast sensitivity chart; VectorVision chart

Visually evoked cortical potentials/responses

(VEP, VER): measure macular visual function, integrity of primary and secondary visual cortex, and continuity of optic nerve and tract radiations; fovea has large area in occipital cortex, close to recording electrodes; smaller area representing more peripheral retina lies deep within calcarine fissure (Figure 4-8)

Can measure vision in preverbal infants

Flash VER: strobe light

Pattern VER: checkerboard pattern or bar grating (amacrine and ganglion cell layer of retina)

P100 wave: positive deflection at 100 ms; amplitude is height from peak to trough, latency is time from onset of flash to peak of wave

Toxic or compressive optic neuropathies: reduction of amplitude more pronounced than prolongation of latency

Demyelination: latency is prolonged; amplitude may be only mildly reduced

Amsler grid: tests central 10° of the visual field (held at 35 cm); 10 cm × 10 cm grid composed of 5-mm squares; primarily used to evaluate foveal pathology

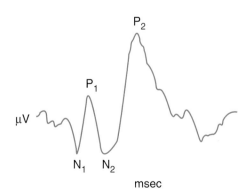

Figure 4-8. Normal visual evoked cortical response. (Reprinted with permission from Slamovits TL: Basic and clinical science course. Section 12: Retina and Vitreous. San Francisco, American Academy of Ophthalmology, 1993.)

Optokinetic nystagmus (OKN): presence suggests visual input is present; slow phase is noted in direction of moving stimulus

Parieto-occipital area controls slow pursuit, frontal lobe controls saccades

Pathway in visual association area terminates in ipsilateral pontine gaze center, resulting in pursuit movements to the same side (i.e. right visual association area controls pursuit to the right)

Can use to diagnose functional visual loss

Normal (symmetric) OKN response: occipital lobe, temporal lobe, LGB, or optic tract lesions do not interfere with pursuit

Deficient pursuit movements to side of lesion (asymmetric OKN): parietal lobe lesion

Cogan's dictum (for homonomous hemianopia): asymmetric OKN indicates parietal lobe lesion; symmetric OKN indicates occipital lobe lesion

Reversal of OKN response: 60% of patients with congenital motor nystagmus

Dorsal midbrain syndrome: downward moving OKN drum causes convergence–retraction nystagmus

Congenital ocular motor apraxia: loss of voluntary horizontal gaze (vertical gaze intact); abnormal OKN (fast phase absent); maintained tonic deviation; requires neuroimaging

Red glass test: evaluation of diplopia

Potential acuity meter (PAM): projects image of letter chart onto retina to test macular potential in patients with media opacities

Purkinje vascular phenomena and blue field entopic test: visualization of retinal vasculature; indicates gross retinal function

Visual Field (VF) Defects (Figure 4-9)

Types:

Blind spot: physiologic due to ON; 15° temporal to fixation and slightly below horizontal midline

Baring of blind spot: glaucoma, normal patients

Cecocentral scotoma: involves blind spot and macula (within 25° of fixation); can occur in any condition that produces a central scotoma, dominant optic atrophy, Leber's optic atrophy, toxic/nutritional optic neuropathy, optic pit with serous retinal detachment, optic neuritis

Central scotoma: unilateral (optic neuritis, compressive lesion of ON, retinal lesion [macular edema, disciform scar]); bilateral (toxic optic neuropathy, nutritional deficiency, macular lesions)

Arcuate scotoma: glaucoma, optic neuritis, anterior ischemic optic neuropathy (AION), branch retinal artery occlusion (BRAO), branch vein occlusion (BVO), ON drusen

Altitudinal defect: damage to upper or lower pole of optic disc; optic neuritis, AION, hemiretinal artery or vein occlusion

Spiraling of VF: suggests malingering/functional visual loss

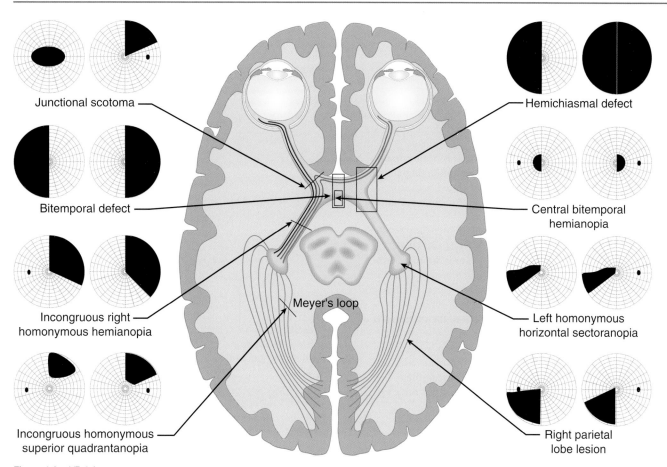

Figure 4-9. VF defects.

Pseudobitemporal hemianopia (slope and cross-vertical meridian): uncorrected refractive error, tilted optic disc, enlarged blind spot (papilledema), large central or cecocentral scotoma, sector retinitis pigmentosa (nasal quadrant), overhanging lid, coloboma

Binasal defect: most nasal defects due to arcuate scotomas (glaucoma); also, pressure on temporal aspect of ON and anterior angle of chiasm, aneurysm, pituitary adenoma, infarct

Constricted field (ring scotoma): retinitis pigmentosa, advanced glaucoma, thyroid-related ophthalmopathy, ON drusen, vitamin A deficiency, occipital stroke, panretinal photocoagulation, functional visual loss

Neurologic defect: bilateral and respects vertical midline

Localizing VF defects:
Nerve fiber layer: arcuate, papillomacular, temporal wedge
Chiasm: bitemporal hemianopia (junctional scotoma if involving Willebrand's knee)
Optic tract: incongruous homonymous hemianopia
Temporal lobe (Meyer's loop): 'pie-in-the-sky' (denser superiorly, spares central)
Parietal lobe: denser inferiorly
Occipital lobe: congruous; ±macular sparing

Neurologic VF defects:
Congruity of VF defect (retrochiasmal lesions): the more congruous the defect, the more posterior is the lesion
Superior field: anterior retinal ganglion cells → lateral portion of optic tract → temporal lobe (Meyer's loop) → inferior bank of calcarine fissure
Vision not reduced by unilateral lesion posterior to the chiasm (20/20 acuity with macula-splitting hemianopia)
Chiasm: pituitary tumor, pituitary apoplexy, craniopharyngioma, meningioma, ON glioma, aneurysm, trauma, infection, metastatic tumor, MS, sarcoid
ANTERIOR CHIASMAL SYNDROME: lesion at junction of ON and chiasm; involves fibers in Willebrand's knee (contralateral nasal retinal loop); causes **junctional scotoma** (central scotoma in 1 eye and superotemporal defect in the other)
BODY OF CHIASM: bitemporal hemianopia; vision may be preserved
POSTERIOR CHIASM: bitemporal hemianopia; primarily involves crossing macular fibers
LATERAL COMPRESSION (very rare): binasal hemianopia (more commonly caused by bilateral ON or retinal lesions)
Optic tract: posterior sellar or suprasellar lesions; homonymous hemianopia, contralateral RAPD

Retro-LGB lesions: 90% of isolated homonymous hemianopias due to stroke

Optic radiations:

TEMPORAL LOBE (Meyer's loop): 'pie-in-the-sky' (superior homonymous hemianopia), formed visual hallucinations, seizures

PARIETAL LOBE: inferior homonymous hemianopia, hemiparesis, visual perception difficulty, agnosia, apraxia, OKN asymmetry

GERSTMANN'S SYNDROME: lesion of dominant parietal lobe; acalculia, agraphia, finger agnosia, left–right confusion, associated with inferior homonymous hemianopia if optic radiation involved

Occipital lobe:

HOMONYMOUS HEMIANOPIA WITH MACULAR SPARING: suggests infarct in area supplied by posterior cerebral artery; macular region receives dual supply from both middle cerebral artery and posterior cerebral artery

BILATERAL CONGRUOUS CENTRAL ISLANDS WITH VERTICAL STEP: equivalent to homonymous hemianopia with macular sparing; vertical step does not occur in retinal or optic nerve lesions

CHECKERBOARD FIELD: bilateral incomplete homonymous hemianopias, superior on 1 side and inferior on opposite side (left upper and right lower homonymous quadrant defects)

BILATERAL HOMONYMOUS ALTITUDINAL DEFECTS: infarction or trauma to both occipital lobes, above or below calcarine fissure

MONOCULAR TEMPORAL CRESCENT DEFECT: anterior occipital infarct; far temporal field is seen by only 1 eye

Cortical blindness: bilateral occipital lobe destruction; pupillary response intact, blindsight (rudimentary visual capacity), unformed visual hallucinations, **Riddoch phenomenon** (perceive moving targets but not stationary ones); may deny blindness (**Anton's syndrome**)

Eye Movements under Supranuclear Control

Horizontal gaze center (Figures 4-10, 4-11):

Saccades: contralateral frontal eye fields (frontal lobe) → superior colliculus → pontine paramedian reticular formation (PPRF) → horizontal gaze center (CN 6 nucleus) → ipsilateral lateral rectus l (LR) and contralateral medial rectus (MR) (via MLF)

Smooth pursuit: ipsilateral parieto-occipital lobe → superior colliculus (SC) → PPRF → horizontal gaze center → ipsilateral LR and contralateral MR (via MLF)

Saccadic system: generates fast eye movements (FEM) (refixation); 300-700°/s

Tests: refixation, rotation, calorics, and optokinetic nystagmus (fast saccadic return phase)

Abnormalities: progressive external ophthalmoplegia, myasthenia gravis, Wilson's disease, Huntington's

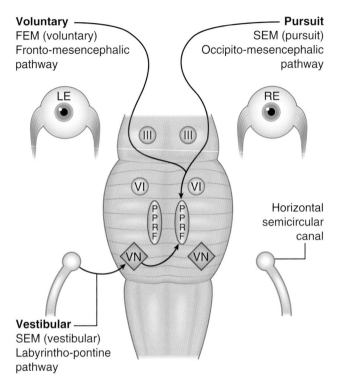

Voluntary — FEM (voluntary) Fronto-mesencephalic pathway

Pursuit SEM (pursuit) Occipito-mesencephalic pathway

Horizontal semicircular canal

Vestibular — SEM (vestibular) Labyrintho-pontine pathway

Figure 4-10. FEM (voluntary), SEM (pursuit), and SEM (vestibular). Pathways all converge on PPRF for horizontal eye movements. VN, vestibular nuclei. (From Bajandas FJ, Kline LB: Neuro-Ophthalmology Review Manual. Thorofare, NJ, Slack, 1988.)

disease, ataxia-telangiectasia, spinocerebellar degeneration, progressive supranuclear palsy, olivopontocerebellar atrophy, Whipple's disease, Gaucher's disease, MS, Pelizaeus-Merzbacher disease

Ocular motor apraxia: failure to initiate a saccade

Smooth pursuit system: slow eye movements (SEM); following movements; ipsilateral parieto-occipital junction (horizontal); interstitial nucleus of Cajal (vertical)

Tests: Doll's head, rotation, OKN (pursuit movement)

Abnormalities: demyelination (young patients), microvascular disease (older patients)

Vergence system: maintains foveal fixation on approaching object; controlled by frontal and occipital lobes, and possibly midbrain

Types: voluntary, accommodative, fusional

Test: look from distance to near

Position maintenance system (vestibulo-ocular reflex [VOR]): maintains specific gaze position during head movements

Teleologically oldest eye movement system; also fastest (shortest latency)

Semicircular canals → CN 8 → vestibular nucleus → contralateral horizontal gaze center → EOMs

Test: calorics; rotation

Abnormalities cause oscillopsia

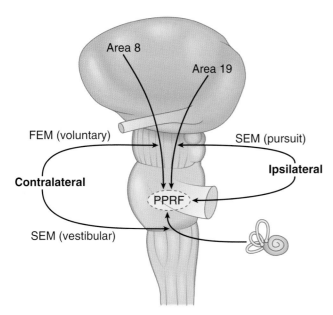

Figure 4-11. Composite reminder of the course and lateralization of the 3 conjugate horizontal eye movement pathways. (From Bajandas FJ, Kline LB: Neuro-ophthalmology Review Manual. Thorofare, NJ, Slack, 1988, p 55.)

Nonoptic reflex systems: integrate eye movements with body movements

Normal caloric and Doll's head responses when nuclear and internuclear connections are intact

Calorics: irrigate water into ears and observe induced eye movements; mnemonic COWS (cold opposite, warm same) refers to direction of fast phase of nystagmus in awake patient (jerk nystagmus); in comatose patient, get tonic deviation in opposite direction of mnemonic (sustained slow phase movement only (Figure 4-12))

Bilateral cold water irrigation produces nystagmus with fast phase upward in awake patient and downward tonic deviation in comatose patient; opposite effects with warm water

PATHWAY: vestibular nuclei → contralateral CN 6 nuclei → ipsilateral LR and contralateral MR (via MLF); no connection to the PPRF

Doll's head (oculocephalic reflex): turn head and observe direction of eye movements; vestibular system moves eyes; use when patient cannot voluntarily move eyes

Eyes should have tonic movement in direction opposite head rotation

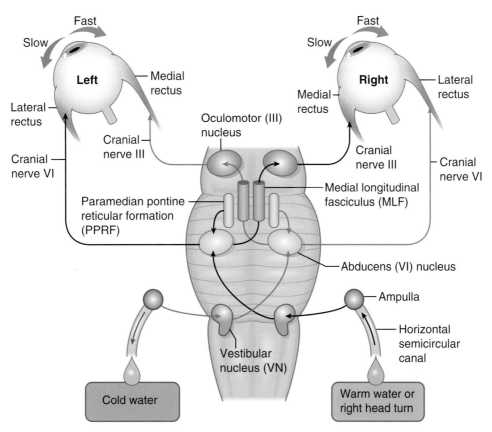

Figure 4-12. Vestibulo-ocular reflex demonstrating right beating nystagmus. Right COWS = cold opposite, warm same. (Calorics should be performed with head back 60°.) (From Bajandas FJ, Kline LB: Neuro-Ophthalmology Review Manual. Thorofare, NJ, Slack, 1988.)

INTACT DOLL'S HEAD: supranuclear lesion (cranial nerve pathways to muscles are intact) (i.e. progressive supranuclear palsy)

ABNORMAL DOLL'S HEAD: lesion is infranuclear paresis or restrictive disease (perform forced ductions)

Bell's phenomenon: upward turning of eyes with forced closure of eyelids

INTACT BELL'S PHENOMENON: supranuclear lesion

DIPLOPIA

Types:

Comitant: amount of deviation same in all fields of gaze

Incomitant: amount of deviation varies in different fields of gaze

Etiology:

Monocular: high astigmatism, chalazion or lid mass, corneal abnormality, iris atrophy, polycoria, cataract, subluxed crystalline lens, decentered IOL, posterior capsular opacity, retinal pathology, functional

Binocular: neuropathic (cranial nerve palsies, MS), myopathic (thyroid-related ophthalmopathy, orbital pseudotumor), neuromuscular junction (MG)

Differential diagnosis (DDx):

Supranuclear (due to inadequate convergence): skew deviation, progressive supranuclear palsy, Parkinson's disease, Huntington's disease, dorsal midbrain syndrome

Intermittent: MG, MS, migraine, thyroid-related ophthalmopathy, convergence spasm, decompensated phoria, convergence-retraction nystagmus, ocular myotonia

Vertical: MG, MS, thyroid-related, orbital disease (tumor, trauma, inflammation), CN 3 or CN 4 palsy, Brown's syndrome, skew deviation

Aberrant regeneration: Duane's syndrome, Marcus Gunn jaw-winking syndrome

Restrictive syndromes: IOP elevation >4 mmHg when eyes directed into restricted field (thyroid, trauma, inflammatory orbital disease, neoplastic process)

EYE MOVEMENT DISORDERS

Central Disorders (Supranuclear)

(Figure 4-13)

Often no symptoms or complaints

Horizontal Gaze Palsies

Congenital

Must distinguish between supranuclear and infranuclear causes; often abnormality of CN 6 or interneurons; vertical movements usually unaffected

Möbius' Syndrome

Horizontal gaze palsy with CN 6, 7, 8, and 9 palsies (facial diplegia, deafness, abnormal digits)

Ocular Motor Apraxia

Saccadic palsy; impairment of voluntary horizontal eye movements with preservation of reflex movements; male > female; congenital or acquired (**Balint's syndrome**); extensive bilateral cerebral disease involving supranuclear pathways (usually bilateral frontoparietal); usually benign and resolves in congenital disease

Associations: Gaucher's disease, spinocerebellar degeneration, MR, ataxia-telangiectasia, Wilson's disease, hypoplasia of corpus callosum, hydrocephalus; rarely cerebellar mass lesion (perform magnetic resonance imaging [MRI])

Findings:

Head thrusting: patient must move head to look at objects; head thrust toward desired direction of gaze results in contralateral slow eye movement so patient

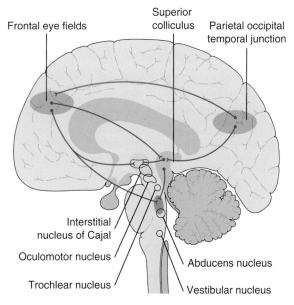

Rostral interstitial nucleus of the medial longitudinal fasciculus
Paramedian pontine reticular formation

Figure 4-13. Supranuclear control of eye movements. The pontine horizontal gaze center (blue) and the vertical gaze center in the midbrain (yellow) receive input from the frontal eye fields to initiate saccades, and from the parietal occipital temporal junction to control pursuit. These gaze centers control ocular motility by synapsing upon the ocular motor nerve nuclei (III, IV, and VI). (From Lavin PJM, Donahue SP: Disorders of supranuclear control of ocular motility. In: Yanoff M, Duker JS (eds) Ophthalmology, 2nd edn. St Louis, Mosby, 2004.)

must overshoot target; lessens with age; may resolve by age 20; patient may also blink to break fixation
Abnormal OKN: fast phase absent
Abnormal vestibular nystagmus: fast phase absent
Normal pursuits
Normal vertical saccades

Acquired

Frontoparietal lesion (stroke, trauma, or infection): tonic deviation of eyes to side of lesion (contralateral area 8 unopposed); seizure will move eyes *away* from lesion

Doll's head testing and calorics: can turn eyes contralateral to lesion (intact vestibular pathway)

Parieto-occipital lesion: ipsilateral pursuit palsy (cogwheel pursuit)

Tegmental lesion: ipsilateral pursuit and saccadic palsy

Pontine lesion (PPRF): ipsilateral horizontal gaze palsy

Parkinson's disease: reduced blinking, reduced saccades, reduced glabellar reflex suppression, blepharospasm, oculogyric crisis

Huntington's chorea
  Metabolic disorders: hyperglycemia, Wernicke's encephalopathy, Wilson's disease

Drug-induced: tricyclic antidepressants, phenytoin, phenothiazines

Pseudogaze palsies: myasthenia gravis, chronic progressive external ophthalmoplegia (CPEO), Duane's syndrome

Internuclear ophthalmoplegia (INO) (Figure 4-14): lesion of MLF; inability to adduct ipsilateral eye with nystagmus of fellow eye; may have skew deviation, vertical diplopia, and gaze-evoked, upbeat nystagmus; rule out myasthenia gravis
  Unilateral: ischemia (young), demyelination (older patients), tumor, infection (meningitis, encephalitis), trauma, compression
  Bilateral (involves both MLF near junction with the 3rd nerve nucleus in midbrain): demyelination/MS (most common), trauma, ischemia, infection, Chiari malformation, toxicity (amitriptyline, ethanol, benzodiazepine)
  Types:
    ANTERIOR (midbrain): preserved convergence
    POSTERIOR (pons): impaired convergence (WEBINO = wall-eyed bilateral INO)

One-and-a-half syndrome (Fisher syndrome) (Figure 4-15): lesion of CN 6 nucleus and ipsilateral MLF; causes ipsilateral gaze palsy and INO; only movement is abduction of contralateral eye (with nystagmus); supranuclear lesion therefore convergence intact; called paralytic pontine exotropia when patient appears exotropic;

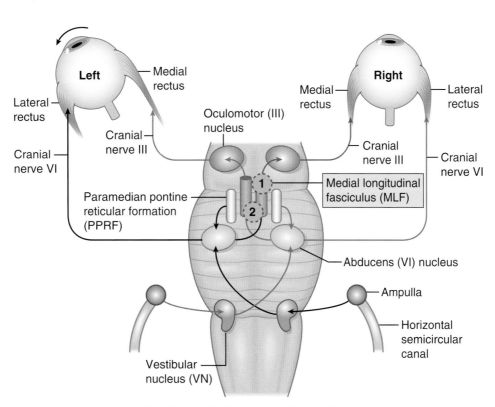

Figure 4-14. 1. Right internuclear ophthalmoplegia (INO) 2. Bilateral INO. (From Bajandas FJ, Kline LB: Neuro-Ophthalmology Review Manual. Thorofare, NJ, Slack, 1988.)

59

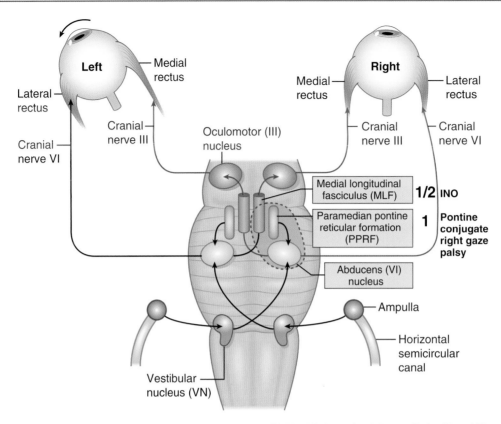

Figure 4-15. Right acute 1½ syndrome (paralytic pontine exotropia). (From Bajandas FJ, Kline LB: Neuro-Ophthalmology Review Manual. Thorofare, NJ, Slack, 1988.)

patients with recovery from 1½ syndrome may develop oculopalatal myoclonus

> *Etiology:* stroke (most common), MS, basilar artery occlusion, pontine metastases

Vertical Gaze Abnormalities

Parinaud's Syndrome (Dorsal Midbrain Syndrome)

Supranuclear gaze palsy with nuclear CN 3 palsy

Etiology: 90% due to pineal tumor; also, demyelination, infarction, trauma

Findings: supranuclear paresis of upgaze (Doll's head intact), bilateral mid-dilated pupils, convergence-retraction nystagmus on attempted upgaze (synchronous backward jerking movements of both eyes due to cocontraction of horizontal recti), light-near dissociation, vertical OKN, skew deviation, lid retraction (Collier's sign)

Diagnosis: MRI; human chorionic gonadotropin (Hcg) level

Treatment: radiation therapy (XRT)

Progressive Supranuclear Palsy (Steele-Richardson-Olszewski Syndrome)

Progressive vertical (early) and horizontal (late) gaze palsy (downward gaze usually affected first); no Bell's phenomenon; doll's head maneuver gives full range of movement (ROM), indicating supranuclear nature of disorder; eventually frozen globe to all stimuli, spasm of fixation, decreased blink rate, blepharitis, blepharospasm; occasionally, apraxia of eye opening; also, axial rigidity, dysarthria, and dementia

Skew Deviation

Vertical misalignment of visual axes due to imbalance of prenuclear inputs; comitant or incomitant

Vertical tropia, hyperdeviation usually increases on ipsilateral downgaze, no cyclodeviation; hypodeviated eye usually ipsilateral to lesion, except when associated with INO in which hyperdeviated eye is ipsilateral; may occur with other brain stem symptoms or cerebellar disease; MRI of posterior fossa recommended

Etiology: brain stem infarct, MS, increased intracranial pressure (ICP), pseudotumor cerebri, vestibulo-ocular imbalance, cerebellar disease; vertebral–basilar insufficiency may cause transient skew deviation

Treatment: often transient and requires observation only; chronic deviations may be treated with prism spectacles or surgery

Whipple's Disease

Oculomasticatory myorhythmia (vertical eye movements and facial activity similar to myoclonus)

Olivopontocerebellar Atrophy

Hereditary or sporadic; onset early adulthood; unsteady gait, slurred speech, dementia, optic atrophy, retinal degeneration

Eye movements progressively slow in all directions, finally complete external ophthalmoplegia

Pathology: cerebellar and pontine atrophy

Kernicterus

Progressive loss of eye movements
Also, metabolic diseases (maple syrup disease, Wernicke's encephalopathy), drug-induced

NYSTAGMUS

Rhythmic involuntary oscillations of the eyes due to disorder of SEM system. Direction named after fast phase (brain's attempt to correct problem), even though abnormality is noted with slow phase

Etiology: abnormal slow eye movement, high gain instability (SEM is working at high gain), vestibular tone imbalance, integrator leak (gaze-evoked nystagmus), OKN abnormality

Characteristics: may be fast or slow, pendular or jerk (designated by direction of rapid phase), unidirectional or multidirectional, symmetric or asymmetric, congenital or acquired

    Gain: eye moves 15° (output) in response to a retinal image position error of 15° (gain = 1)
    Foveation: bring an image onto, or maintain an image on, the fovea
    Frequency: oscillations per second (Hz)
    Amplitude: excursion of oscillation
    Intensity: product of amplitude and frequency
    Null point: position in which intensity of nystagmus is least
    Neutral point: position in which a reversal of the direction of jerk nystagmus occurs

Childhood Nystagmus

Most commonly, congenital, latent, sensory, and spasmus nutans (see Ch. 5, Pediatrics/Strabismus)

Physiologic Nystagmus

Several forms of nystagmus, including end-gaze, optokinetic, caloric, and rotational

Acquired Nystagmus

Pattern helps localize pathology, may have oscillopsia

Bruns'

Combination of gaze-paretic nystagmus when looking toward lesion (fast phase toward the lesion), and vestibular imbalance nystagmus when looking away from lesion (fast phase away from lesion) (i.e., with right-sided lesion: high-amplitude, low-frequency, right-beating nystagmus on right gaze; low-amplitude, high-frequency, left-beating nystagmus on left gaze)

Gaze-paretic component is of high amplitude and low frequency (because of impairment of horizontal gaze mechanism on side of lesion)

Vestibular component is of low amplitude and high frequency, with fast phase away from damaged vestibular nuclei on side of lesion

Due to cerebellopontine angle mass (usually acoustic neuroma or meningioma)

Convergence-Retraction

Cocontraction of lateral recti produces convergence movement (abnormal saccades) on attempted upgaze

Due to periaqueductal gray matter or dorsal midbrain lesion (Parinaud's syndrome, pinealoma, trauma, brain stem arteriovenous malformation [AVM], MS)

Dissociated

Asymmetric between the 2 eyes (different direction, amplitude, frequency, etc); always pathologic
Due to posterior fossa disease, MS

Downbeat

Eyes drift upward with corrective saccade downward; worsens in downgaze, improves in upgaze; oscillopsia

Due to lesion that affects pathways responsible for downgaze; cervicomedullary junction lesion (Arnold-Chiari malformation, tumor, syrinx: 33%), spinocerebellar degeneration, intoxication, lithium, paraneoplastic cerebellar degeneration, 50% with no identifiable cause

Treatment: clonazepam

Gaze-Evoked

Nystagmus in direction of gaze, absent in primary position, fast phase toward lesion (cerebellar)

Due to extra-axial mass compressing brain stem (acoustic neuroma, cerebellar hemisphere tumor), intoxication (alcohol or anticonvulsant medications)

If asymmetric, must obtain neuroimaging

Waveform: exponentially decreasing

Periodic Alternating Nystagmus (PAN)

Changes horizontal direction; jerks right 90 seconds, 5- to 10-second pause, jerks left 90 seconds, repeats; remains horizontal in vertical gaze; usually acquired

Due to disease of vestibulocerebellar system (albinism, cranio-cervico junction lesion [Arnold-Chiari malformation], MS, syphilis, tumor, vascular, dilantin, spinocerebellar degeneration)

Treatment: baclofen; surgery (large recession of all 4 recti muscles)

Seesaw

Vertical and torsional nystagmus with 1 eye rising and intorting while fellow eye falls and excyclotorts, then reverses

Due to suprasellar lesions, CVA, or trauma, or is congenital (craniopharyngioma)

MRI: rule out large parasellar tumors expanding into third ventricle

Treatment: baclofen

Upbeat

Eyes drift downward with corrective saccade upward

Due to medullary lesions, midline cerebellar (vermis) lesions, medulloblastoma, cerebellar degeneration, MS

Vestibular

Horizontal, rotary, jerk nystagmus in primary gaze; same in all fields of gaze; slow component is linear; remains horizontal in vertical gaze

Due to vestibular disease, infection (labrynthitis), Ménière's disease, vascular, trauma, toxicity

Peripheral vestibular disease: fast phase toward good side; slow phase toward lesion; associated with tinnitus, vertigo, deafness; fixation inhibits vertigo and nystagmus; direction of Romberg fall changes with head turning

Central vestibular disease: nonlocalizing; no tinnitus or deafness

Voluntary

Unsustainable for longer than 30 seconds; associated with hysteria and malingering

Other Eye Movement Disorders

Ocular Bobbing

Intermittent conjugate rapid downward eye movements followed by slow return to primary position

Often secondary to hemorrhage; patient usually comatose

Ocular Dipping

Opposite of ocular bobbing; intermittent rapid upward eye movements followed by slow return to primary position

Ocular Myoclonus

Vertical pendular nystagmus associated with synchronous palatal (uvula) beating

Due to bilateral pseudohypertrophy of inferior olives in medulla, lesion in myoclonic triangle (red nucleus, ipsilateral inferior olive, contralateral dentate nucleus)

Opsoclonus (Saccadomania)

Rapid, chaotic eye movements in all directions; persists in sleep

Associated with dancing hands and feet
Abnormality of pause cells (normally suppress burst cells of PPRF)

Due to remote, paraneoplastic effect on cerebellum from metastatic neuroblastoma (check urine vanillylmandelic acid [VMA]), occasionally with encephalitis

Waveform: no slow phase; repetitive, random; no intersaccadic interval

Oscillopsia

Illusion of movement in the seen world

Usually occurs in SO myokymia and acquired nystagmus; rarely in congenital nystagmus

Due to vestibulo-ocular reflex abnormality

CRANIAL NERVE PALSIES (FIGURE 4-16)

Oculomotor Nerve (CN 3) Palsy

Anatomy: nucleus in rostral midbrain; fascicle travels ventrally through midbrain, traversing red nucleus and corticospinal tract in cerebral peduncle; nerve enters subarachnoid space, passes between posterior cerebral and superior cerebellar arteries, then courses lateral to posterior communicating artery and enters lateral wall of cavernous sinus; receives sympathetics from internal carotid plexus; passes through superior orbital fissure and divides into superior (supplies SR and levator) and inferior (supplies IR, MR, IO, iris sphincter, and ciliary muscle) divisions.

Only 1 subnucleus (midline location) supplies both levator palpebrae superioris; fibers from superior rectus (SR) subnucleus supply contralateral SR; Edinger-Westphal nucleus supplies both pupils (Figure 4-18)

Types: complete, partial, pupil sparing

Findings: ptosis, hypotropia, exotropia; may involve pupil (fixed and dilated); may cause pain

7 syndromes (Figure 4-17):
Nuclear CN 3 palsy (Figure 4-17, ①): extremely rare; contralateral SR paresis and bilateral ptosis; pupil involvement is both or neither

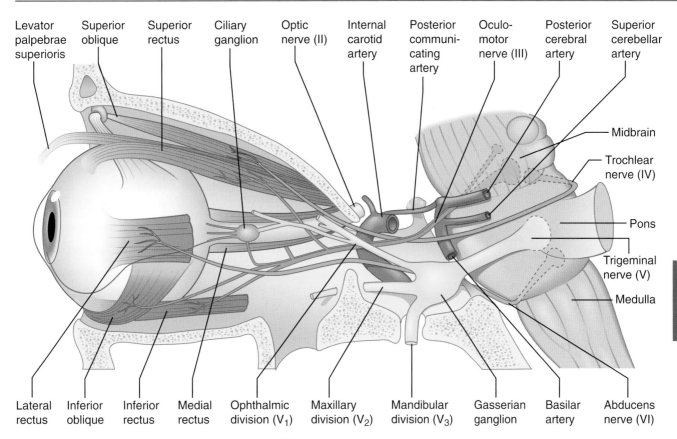

Figure 4-16. Cranial nerve pathways. (Copyright Peter K. Kaiser, MD.)

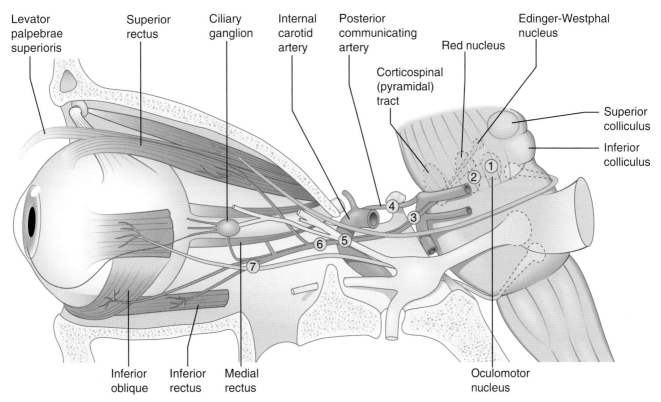

Figure 4-17. Seven syndromes of CN 3 palsy. (Copyright Peter K. Kaiser, MD.)

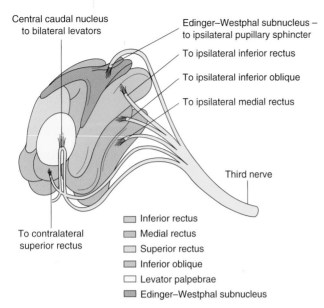

Central caudal nucleus to bilateral levators

Edinger–Westphal subnucleus – to ipsilateral pupillary sphincter

To ipsilateral inferior rectus

To ipsilateral inferior oblique

To ipsilateral medial rectus

Third nerve

To contralateral superior rectus

☐ Inferior rectus
☐ Medial rectus
☐ Superior rectus
☐ Inferior oblique
☐ Levator palpebrae
☐ Edinger–Westphal subnucleus

Figure 4-18. Anatomy of the 3rd nerve nucleus. The 3rd nerve nucleus consists of a single, central, caudally located nucleus for the levator palpebrae, paired bilateral subnuclei with crossed projections that innervate the superior recti, and paired bilateral subnuclei with uncrossed projections that innervate the medial recti, inferior recti, and inferior oblique muscles. Parasympathetic input to the ciliary body and iris sphincter arises from the Edinger-Westphal nucleus. (Redrawn from Warwick R: Representation of the extraocular muscles in the oculomotor nuclei of the monkey. J Comp Neurol 98:449--503,1953.)

Fascicle syndromes (see Figure 4-17, ②): ischemic, infiltrative (tumor), or inflammatory (rare)

NOTHNAGEL'S SYNDROME: lesion of fascicle and superior cerebellar peduncle that causes ipsilateral CN 3 paresis and cerebellar ataxia

BENEDIKT'S SYNDROME: lesion of fascicle and red nucleus that causes ipsilateral CN 3 paresis, contralateral hemitremor (resting and intentional), and contralateral decreased sensation

WEBER'S SYNDROME: lesion of fascicle and pyramidal tract that causes ipsilateral CN 3 paresis and contralateral hemiparesis

CLAUDE'S SYNDROME: combination of Nothnagel's and Benedikt's syndromes

Uncal herniation (see Figure 4-17, ③): supratentorial mass may cause uncal herniation compressing CN 3

Posterior communicating artery (PCom or PCA) aneurysm (see Figure 4-17, ④): most common nontraumatic, isolated, pupil involving CN 3 palsy; aneurysm at junction of PCom and carotid artery compresses nerve, particularly external parasympathetic pupillomotor fibers; usually painful

Cavernous sinus syndrome (see Figure 4-17, ⑤): associated with multiple CN palsies (3, 4, V$_1$, 6) and Horner's; CN 3 palsy often partial and pupil sparing; may lead to aberrant regeneration

Orbital syndrome (see Figure 4-17, ⑥): tumor, trauma, pseudotumor, or cellulitis; associated with multiple CN palsies (3, 4, V$_1$, 6), proptosis, chemosis, injection; ON can appear normal, swollen, or atrophic

After passing through the superior orbital fissure, CN 3 splits into superior and inferior divisions; therefore, CN 3 palsies distal to this point may be complete or partial

Pupil-sparing isolated CN 3 palsy (see Figure 4-17, ⑦): small-caliber parasympathetic pupillomotor fibers travel in outer layers of nerve closer to blood supply (but more susceptible to damage by compression); fibers at core of nerve are compromised by ischemia; may explain pupil sparing in 80% of ischemic CN 3 palsies and pupil involved in 95% of compressive CN 3 palsies (trauma, tumor, aneurysm)

ETIOLOGY:

ADULTS: vasculopathic/ischemic (diabetes mellitus [DM], hypertension [HTN]), trauma, giant cell arteritis (CGA), occasionally tumor, aneurysm (very rare)

CHILDREN: congenital, trauma, tumor, aneurysm, migraine

14% of PCom aneurysms initially spare pupil

20% of diabetic CN 3 palsies involve pupil

Microvascular CN 3 palsies usually resolve in 3 to 4 months

Myasthenia gravis may mimic CN 3 palsy

Aberrant regeneration: IR and/or MR fibers may innervate levator and/or iris sphincter; sign of previous CN 3 palsy caused by aneurysm or tumor (occasionally trauma); never occurs after vasculopathic injury

Findings:

LID-GAZE DYSKINESIS: lid retracts on downgaze (pseudo–von Graefe's sign) and/or adduction

PUPIL-GAZE DYSKINESIS: more pupillary constriction with convergence than to light (pseudo-Argyll-Robertson pupil) and/or pupillary constriction on downgaze

2 forms:

PRIMARY: no preceding acute CN 3 palsy; insidious development of CN 3 palsy with accompanying signs of misdirection; due to intracavernous lesion (meningioma, aneurysm, neuroma)

SECONDARY: occurs months after CN 3 palsy from trauma, aneurysm (carotid-cavernous [C-C]), or tumor compression, but never after vasculopathic/ischemic lesion

Other causes of CN 3 palsy:

Congenital: variable degrees of aberrant regeneration; 75% have smaller pupil on involved side (due to aberrant regeneration); ptosis and anisocoria

TREATMENT: muscle surgery to straighten eye in primary gaze

Ophthalmoplegic migraine: onset in childhood; positive family history of migraine; paresis of CN 3 occurs as headache abates; usually resolves in 1 month (can be permanent)

Cyclic oculomotor palsy: usually at birth or early childhood; very rare; occurs after complete CN 3 palsy, can be due to diabetic ischemia

FINDINGS: spastic movements of muscles innervated by CN 3 occur at regular intervals for 10–30

seconds (spasms of lid elevation, adduction, miosis)

MRI: rule out aneurysm

Workup:

If < age 11: MRI/MRA

If aged 11–50: MRI/MRA and medical workup

If > age 50:

    WITH PUPIL INVOLVEMENT: MRI/MRA; if normal, cerebral angiography (catheter)

    WITH PUPIL SPARING: usually microvascular; no invasive investigation needed initially; check BP (HTN), blood glucose (DM), ESR, C-reactive protein (giant cell arteritis), complete blood count (CBC), antinuclear antibody (ANA), Venereal Disease Research Laboratory (VDRL), fluorescent treponemal antibody absorption (FTA-ABS); if it persists >3 months, MRI/MRA (magnetic resonance angiography) with cerebral angiography (aneurysm) if negative

Trochlear Nerve (CN 4) Palsy

Anatomy: nucleus in caudal mesencephalon at level of inferior colliculus; decussates in anterior medullary velum next to aqueduct of Sylvius; fascicle passes between posterior cerebral artery and superior cerebellar artery; nerve travels in lateral wall of cavernous sinus, enters orbit via superior orbital fissure outside annulus of Zinn; innervates superior oblique muscle

Longest intracranial course (75 mm); only CN that exits dorsally from brain stem; only CN that decussates (except for CN 3 subnucleus that innervates SR); most commonly injured CN following closed head injury (owing to long course)

Etiology: congenital (most common in kids); in adults: 40% trauma, 30% ischemia, 20% miscellaneous or undetermined, 10% aneurysm

Findings: ipsilateral hypertropia (due to superior rectus overaction)

5 syndromes (Figure 4-19):

Nuclear/fascicular syndrome (see Figure 4-19, ①): hemorrhage, infarction, demyelination, trauma; may have contralateral Horner's or INO

Subarachnoid space syndrome (see Figure 4-19, ②): injury as nerve emerges from dorsal surface of brain stem; trauma (contracoup forces transmitted to brain stem by free tentorial edge), tumor (pinealoma, tentorial meningioma), meningitis, neurosurgical trauma

Cavernous sinus syndrome (see Figure 4-19, ③): multiple CN palsies (3, 4, V$_1$, 6) and Horner's

Orbital syndrome (see Figure 4-19, ④): multiple CN palsies (3, 4, V$_1$, 6) and Horner's; proptosis, chemosis, injection

Isolated CN 4 palsy (see Figure 4-19, ⑤):

    CONGENITAL: most common; may occur in elderly due to decompensation; large, vertical fusion amplitudes (10–15 Δ); check old photos for head tilt

    ACQUIRED: acute onset of vertical diplopia; head position (chin down, face turn to opposite side, head tilt to opposite shoulder)

DDx of vertical diplopia: myasthenia gravis, thyroid-related ophthalmopathy, orbital disease (tumor, trauma, inflammation), CN 3 palsy, CN 4 palsy, Brown's syndrome, skew deviation, MS

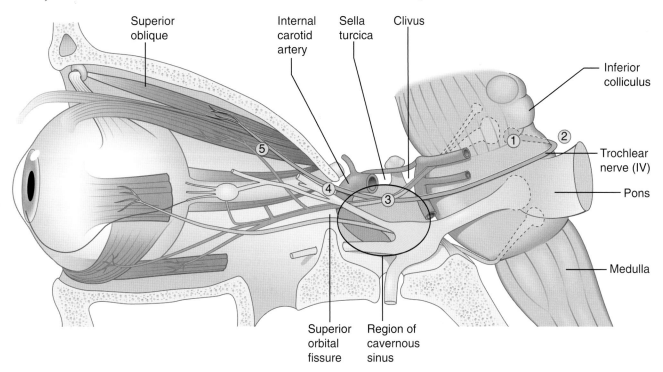

Figure 4-19. 5 syndromes of CN 4 palsy. (Copyright Peter K. Kaiser, MD.)

Diagnosis: Parks-Bielschowsky 3-step test (used for hypertropia due to weakness of a single muscle)

Step 1: Which eye is hypertopic?

LEFT HYPER: paresis of OD elevators (RSR or RIO) or OS (*oculus sinister*, left eye) depressors (LIR or LSO)

Step 2: Worse on right or left gaze?

If hyper, is worse in left gaze:

Problem with OS muscles that have greatest vertical action during abduction (SR and IR)

Problem with OD muscles that have greatest vertical action during adduction (SO and IO)

SR and IR work best when eye is ABducted

So if left hyper is worse on gaze left: LIR

SO and IO work best when eye is ADducted

So if left hyper is worse on gaze left: RIO

If L hyper is worse on gaze right: RSR or LSO

Step 3: Worse on right or left head tilt?

With head tilt, eyes undergo corrective torsion (with right head tilt, OD intorts and OS extorts)

If 1 of the intorters is the cause of the hyper, then tilting head will worsen hyper on side of head tilt

If worse hyper on left head tilt, problem with left intorters (LSR, LSO) or right extorters (RIR, RIO)

Bilateral CN 4 palsies: usually due to severe head trauma (contusion of anterior medullary velum)

Vertical deviation in primary gaze may or may not be present

RHT in left gaze; LHT in right gaze

Either eye can be hyper on step 3 of 3-step test

V-pattern esotropia (ET >25 Δ)

>10° of torsion with double Maddox rod test

Workup: check BP, blood glucose, CBC, ESR, VDRL, FTA-ABS, ANA; neuroimaging if history of head trauma or cancer, signs of meningitis, young age, other neurologic findings, or isolated palsy that does not improve after 3–4 months

Treatment:

Glasses: occlude lens or prisms for diplopia

Muscle surgery:

KNAPP'S PRINCIPLES FOR CN 4 PALSY: strengthen (tuck) the palsied SO, weaken the antagonist (ipsilateral IO), or weaken the yoke (contralateral IR) to correct hyperdeviation

HARADA-ITO PROCEDURE: anterior and lateral displacement of palsied muscle to correct excyclotorsion

Abducens Nerve (CN 6) Palsy

Anatomy: nucleus in dorsal pons medial to CN 7; travels anterior and lateral to PPRF, then through pyramidal tract, and exits lower pons in pontomedullary groove in subarachnoid space; climbs over clivus (vulnerable to elevated ICP) over petrous ridge, along base of skull, through Dorello's canal, under Gruber's ligament; enters cavernous sinus and then orbit through superior orbital fissure; passes laterally to supply lateral rectus

Second most common CN to be injured following closed head injury

CN 6 lesions occur in conditions that cause increased ICP

6 syndromes (Figure 4-20):

Brain stem syndromes (see Figure 4-20, ①):

MILLARD-GUBLER SYNDROME: lesion of CN 6 and 7 fascicles and pyramidal tract causing CN 6 and 7 palsies with contralateral hemiparesis

RAYMOND'S SYNDROME: lesion of CN 6 and pyramidal tract causing CN 6 palsy and contralateral hemiparesis

FOVILLE'S SYNDROME: lesion of CN 6 nucleus, CN 5 and 7 fascicles, and sympathetics causing ipsilateral 5, 6, and 7 palsies, horizontal conjugate gaze palsy, and ipsilateral Horner's

MÖBIUS' SYNDROME: associated with CN 7 lesion, supernumerary digits, skeletal abnormalities, mental retardation

Subarachnoid space syndrome (see Figure 4-20, ②): increased ICP can cause downward displacement of brain stem with stretching of CN 6 (tethered at exit from pons and Dorello's canal); occurs in 30% of patients with pseudotumor cerebri; also hemorrhage, meningitis, inflammation (sarcoidosis), infiltration (lymphoma, leukemia, carcinoma)

Petrous apex syndrome (see Figure 4-20, ③): portion of CN 6 within Dorello's canal is in contact with tip of petrous pyramid and is susceptible to processes affecting the petrous bone

GRADENIGO'S SYNDROME: localized inflammation or extradural abscess of petrous apex (mastoiditis) following otitis media; CN 6 palsy with ipsilateral decreased hearing, facial pain, and facial paralysis

PSEUDO-GRADENIGO'S SYNDROME: various etiologies:

NASOPHARYNGEAL CA: obstruction of Eustachian tube can cause serous otitis media, can invade cavernous sinus causing CN 6 palsy

CEREBELLOPONTINE ANGLE TUMOR: CN 5, 6, and 7 palsies; decreased hearing, papilledema

PETROUS BONE FRACTURE: may have CN 5, 6, 7, or 8 lesions, hemotympanum, Battle's sign (bruising over mastoid bone), CSF otorrhea

BASILAR ANEURYSM

CLIVUS CHORDOMA

Cavernous sinus syndrome (see Figure 4-20, ④):

ETIOLOGY: trauma, vascular (diabetes, migraine, aneurysms, arteriovenous [AV] fistula), tumor, inflammation, granuloma

FINDINGS: CN 3, 4, V₁, Horner's, ON, chiasm, and pituitary involvement

Orbital syndrome (see Figure 4-20, ⑤):

ETIOLOGY: trauma, tumor, orbital pseudotumor, cellulitis

FINDINGS: proptosis, chemosis, conjunctival injection; may have ON edema or atrophy; CN V₁ may be involved

Isolated CN 6 palsy (see Figure 4-20, ⑥):

CHILDREN: often postviral (resolves over weeks), associated with otitis media; consider tumor (pontine glioma), trauma

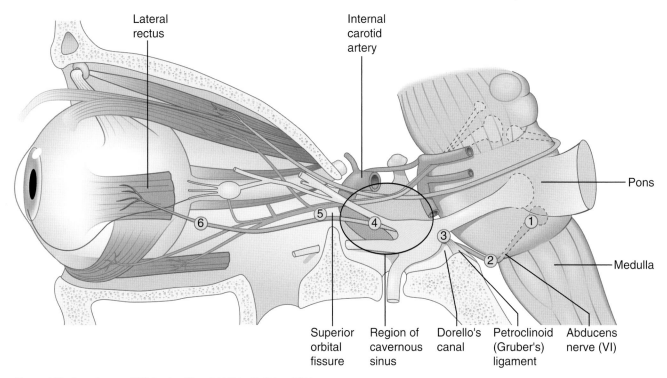

Lateral rectus

Internal carotid artery

Pons

Medulla

5

4

6

3

2

1

Superior orbital fissure

Region of cavernous sinus

Dorello's canal

Petroclinoid (Gruber's) ligament

Abducens nerve (VI)

Figure 4-20. 6 syndromes of CN 6 palsy. (Copyright Peter K. Kaiser, MD.)

ADULTS: vasculopathic, undetermined, MS, tumor (nasopharyngeal CA, cavernous sinus meningioma, chordoma), trauma, temporal arteritis, syphilis

Pseudo–CN 6 palsy: thyroid-related ophthalmopathy, convergence spasm, strabismus, medial wall fracture, myasthenia gravis, orbital myositis, Miller Fisher syndrome

Workup:
Congenital: usually resolves by 6 weeks
Acquired: same as for CN 4 palsy; consider lumbar puncture (LP) and Tensilon test

Trigeminal Nerve (CN 5) Palsy

Anatomy: nerve emerges from ventral pons; passes below tentorium to ganglion; divides into 3 divisions (Figure 4-21)
Ophthalmic (V_1): passes through lateral wall of cavernous sinus; divides into lacrimal, frontal, and nasociliary nerves
Maxillary (V_2): passes through lateral wall of cavernous sinus; exits cranium through foramen rotundum
Mandibular (V_3): exits cranium through foramen ovale
Supplies sensory to face and eye, motor to muscles of mastication (Figure 4-22)

Trigeminal neuralgia (tic douloureux): due to compression of CN 5 at root (superior cerebellar artery aneurysm or tumor); facial pain involves entire CN 5 division; lasts seconds; 95% unilateral; usually involves maxillary or mandibular distribution, ophthalmic distribution alone is rare

Diagnosis: neuroimaging

Treatment: medical (carbamazepine) or surgical (radiofrequency destruction of trigeminal ganglion through foramen ovale)

Facial Nerve (CN 7) Palsy

Anatomy: passes around CN 6 nucleus; exits brain stem ventrally at cerebellopontine angle; enters internal auditory canal (of petrous portion of temporal bone) with nervus intermedius and cochlear and vestibular nerves; enters facial nerve canal; exits temporal bone via stylomastoid foramen; branches in parotid gland.

Supplies facial muscles and lacrimal and salivary glands; posterior ⅔ of tongue; external ear sensation; dampens stapedius
Lacrimal gland innervation (parasympathetic): originates in superior salivatory nucleus, fibers leave brain with nervus intermedius (glossopalatine) and travel with CN 7 through geniculate ganglion, emerges from petrous portion of sphenoid bone as greater superficial petrosal nerve; enters pterygoid canal and enters sphenopalatine ganglion, where primary parasympathetic fibers synapse and second-order fibers join zygomatic nerve, which sends a branch to lacrimal gland.
Frontal lobe (precentral motor cortex) provides input to CN 7 nuclei in pons (control voluntary facial movements); upper face innervation is bilateral (from both supranuclear motor areas), lower face innervation is mainly from contralateral supranuclear motor area (Figure 4-23)

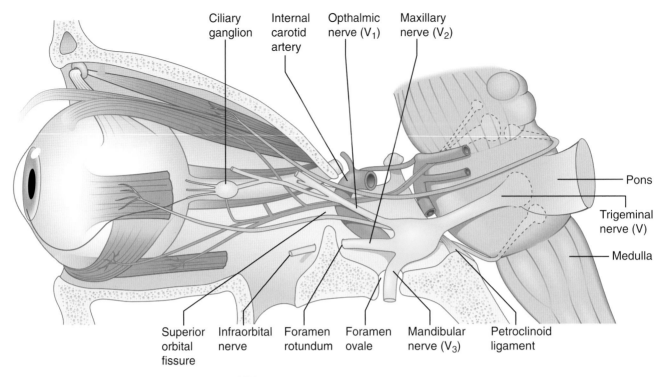

Figure 4-21. CN 5 pathway. (Copyright Peter K. Kaiser, MD.)

Ciliary ganglion

Internal carotid artery

Opthalmic nerve (V₁)

Maxillary nerve (V₂)

Pons

Trigeminal nerve (V)

Medulla

Superior orbital fissure

Infraorbital nerve

Foramen rotundum

Foramen ovale

Mandibular nerve (V₃)

Petroclinoid ligament

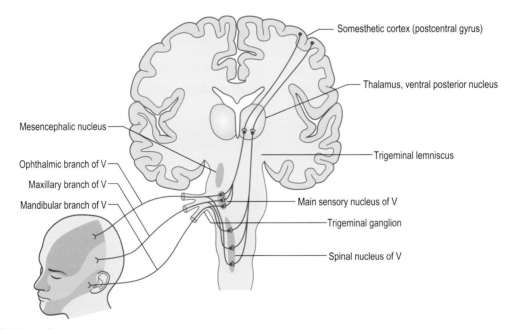

Figure 4-22. CN 5 innervation.

Somesthetic cortex (postcentral gyrus)

Thalamus, ventral posterior nucleus

Mesencephalic nucleus

Trigeminal lemniscus

Ophthalmic branch of V

Maxillary branch of V

Mandibular branch of V

Main sensory nucleus of V

Trigeminal ganglion

Spinal nucleus of V

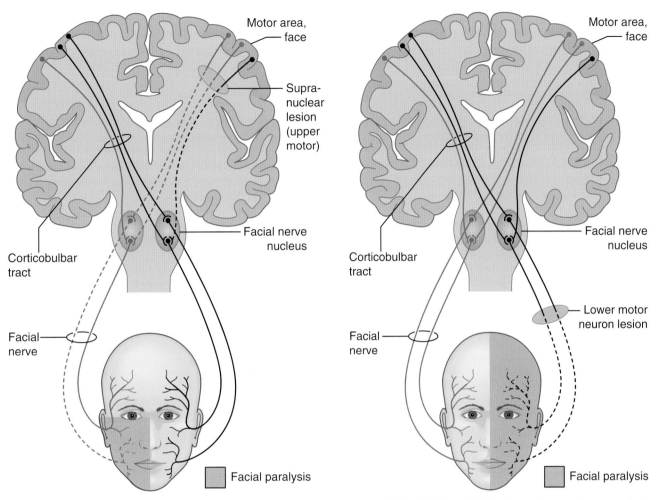

Figure 4-23. Facial weakness due to upper and lower motor neuron lesions. (From Bajandas FJ, Kline LB: Neuro-Ophthalmology Review Manual. Thorofare, NJ, Slack, 1988.)

Supranuclear palsy: lesion in precentral gyrus of cerebral cortex results in contralateral paralysis of volitional facial movement involving lower face more severely than upper

Emotional and reflex movements (smiling, spontaneous blinking) are preserved (extrapyramidal)

Brain stem lesion (pons): ipsilateral facial weakness involving both upper and lower face; due to tumor, vascular causes

Associated with CN 5 and 6 palsies, lateral gaze palsy, cerebellar ataxia, and contralateral hemiparesis

With CN 5 palsy: cerebellopontine angle tumors, infratemporal fossa tumors

With CN 6 palsy: brain stem injury or injury near anteromedial portion of temporal bone (Gradenigo's syndrome)

Peripheral CN 7 lesion: acute unilateral facial nerve palsy is most common cranial neuropathy

Bell's palsy: idiopathic facial nerve palsy; may be preceded by preauricular or mastoid pain

Facial weakness progressing to paralysis over months
Associated with progressive twitching or facial spasm; suggests neoplasm; most common between ages 15 and 45; 10% have positive family history
TREATMENT: consider oral steroids
PROGNOSIS: 70% have complete recovery in 6 weeks; 85% will fully recover; 10% recurrence (ipsilateral or contralateral)
POOR PROGNOSTIC SIGNS: complete facial paralysis at presentation, impairment of lacrimation, advanced age; if incomplete recovery, aberrant regeneration is common
Trauma: fracture of temporal bone
FINDINGS: hearing loss, vertigo, hemotympanum, perforated tympanic membrane, Battle's sign (bruising over mastoid bone)
Delayed onset or incomplete paralysis usually due to nerve contusion or swelling
Complete facial paralysis immediately after head trauma suggests nerve transection
BIRTH TRAUMA WITH FORCEPS: congenital CN 7 lesion; tends to resolve

Infection:

RAMSAY-HUNT SYNDROME: herpes zoster virus (HZV) oticus (infection of outer ear and nerves of inner auditory canal); 20% have sensorineual hearing loss and dizziness

Preauricular or mastoid pain precedes facial paralysis by 1–3 days; associated with a vesicular rash of outer ear or on tympanic membrane

TREATMENT: acyclovir and prednisone

PROGNOSIS: poor; only 10% recovery in patients with complete paralysis; 66% recovery with partial paralysis

May develop postherpetic neuralgia

Also HIV, Lyme disease, otitis media, malignant otitis externa (usually elderly diabetics; can progress to cellulitis of inner ear canal and osteomyelitis of temporal bone; usually caused by *Pseudomonas*)

Sarcoidosis: most frequent cause of bilateral 7th due to infiltration of CN 7, usually at parotid gland

Erosive cholesteatoma: pressure on segment of CN 7 that travels through middle ear

Tumor: most intracranial and bone tumors that cause facial paralysis are benign (including acoustic neuroma, meningioma, glomus tumors [triad of facial paralysis, pulsatile tinnitus, and hearing loss]); tumors of parotid gland are usually malignant (adenoid cystic carcinoma)

Guillain-Barré syndrome (Miller Fisher variant): facial diplegia can occur with ophthalmoplegia and ataxia; absent deep tendon reflexes; CSF protein elevated with normal cell count; often bilateral

Melkersson-Rosenthal syndrome: recurrent facial paralysis with chronic facial swelling and lingua plicata (furrowing of tongue); unilateral or bilateral; occurs in childhood or adolescence

Aberrant facial innervation:

MARCUS-GUNN JAW WINKING: activation of muscles of mastication induces orbicularis oculi contraction

CROCODILE TEARS: lacrimation evoked by chewing

Other findings: lacrimation (damage to greater superficial petrosal nerve), impaired stapedius muscle reflex (damage to stapedial nerve), impaired taste (damage to chorda tympani nerve), swelling of parotid gland or cervical lymphatics (suggests malignant tumor or inflammatory condition of parotid [sarcoidosis, TB])

Disorders of CN 7 overactivity:

Benign essential blepharospasm: frequent bilateral blinking proceeds to involuntary spasms and forceful contractures of orbicularis; may cause functional blindness; unknown etiology; usually affects women over age 50; absent during sleep

TREATMENT: botulinum toxin (Botox) injections, rarely surgery (orbicularis myomectomy)

Hemifacial spasm: unilateral contractions of facial muscles; usually due to vascular compression of CN 7 at brain stem; rarely caused by tumor; present during sleep; obtain MRI

Facial myokymia: fasciculations of facial muscles; if multifocal and progressive, consider MS

Eyelid myokymia: benign fasciculations of eyelid

Multiple CN Palsies

CN 3, 4, and 5: due to lesion of brain stem, cavernous sinus (Figure 4-24), and/or superior orbital fissure

DDx: AV fistula, cavernous sinus thrombosis, metastases to cavernous sinus, skin malignancy with perineural spread to cavernous sinus, meningioma, mucormycosis, HZV, Tolosa-Hunt syndrome, mucocele, nasopharyngeal CA, carcinomatous meningitis, pituitary apoplexy (headache with bilateral signs and decreased vision)

Herpes zoster ophthalmicus: CN 3, 4, and 6 palsies occur in about 15%; pain and skin eruption in trigeminal distribution, decreased corneal sensation, pupil may be involved (tonic pupil)

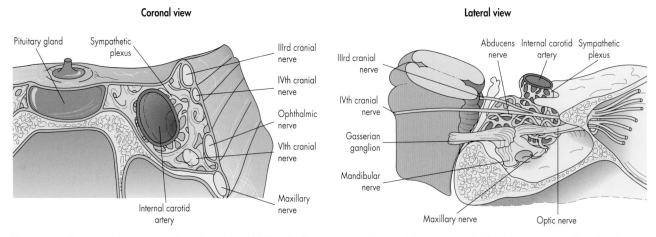

Figure 4-24. Anatomy of the cavernous sinus. (From Moster M: Paresis of isolated and multiple cranial nerves and painful ophthalmoplegia. In: Yanoff M, Duker JS (eds) Ophthalmology. London, Mosby, 1999.)

Hutchinson's rule: if tip of nose involved (nasociliary nerve), eye will probably (but not always) be involved

Mimics of multiple cranial nerve palsies: MG, CPEO, orbital lesions (thyroid, pseudotumor, tumor), progressive supranuclear palsy, Guillain-Barré syndrome

PUPILS

Innervation (Figure 4-25)

Iris Sphincter

Parasympathetic innervation from Edinger-Westphal nucleus

Pathway of pupillary light reflex: optic nerve → chiasm (fibers split) → optic tract → pretectal nucleus (synapse) → cross to both EW nuclei (synapse) → travel via CN 3 though subarachnoid space and cavernous sinus, then travel in inferior division of CN 3 to ciliary ganglion → postganglionic fibers travel via short ciliary nerves to ciliary body and iris sphincter

Iris Dilator

Sympathetic innervation

Pathway: posterior hypothalamus → down spinal cord → synapse in ciliospinal center of Budge (C8–T2 level) → second-order neuron ascends sympathetic chain → over apex of lung → synapse at superior cervical ganglion → third-order neuron ascends with ICA and joins CN 6 in cavernous sinus → enters orbit via long ciliary nerve (through superior orbital fissure next to CN V_1) to iris dilator and Müller's muscle

Disorders

Relative Afferent Pupillary Defect (RAPD; Marcus-Gunn Pupil)

Large retinal lesion, asymmetric optic nerve disease, chiasm lesion, optic tract lesion (contralateral RAPD)

No RAPD: cataract, acute papilledema, amblyopia, refractive error, functional visual loss, lesions posterior to lateral geniculate body

Light-Near Dissociation

Pupil does not react to light but near response intact

Etiology: syphilis (Argyll-Robertson), Adie's pupil, familial dysautonomia (Riley-Day syndrome), Parinaud's

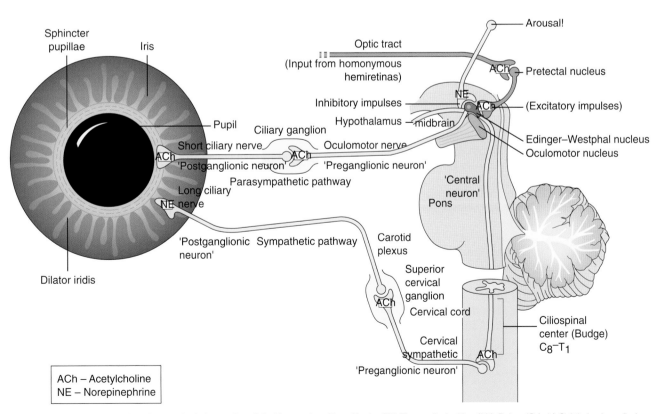

Figure 4-25. Parasympathetic and sympathetic innervation of the iris muscles. (From Kardon RH: The pupils. In: Yanoff M, Duker JS (eds) Ophthalmology, 2nd edn. St Louis, Mosby, 2004.)

syndrome, RAPD, physiologic, severe retinal disease, aberrant regeneration of CN 3, diabetes, myotonic dystrophy, encephalitis, alcoholism, herpes zoster ophthalmicus (HZO)

Abnormal Light and Near Response

Pharmacologic, trauma, CN 3 palsy

Anisocoria

Pupils of unequal size

Miosis: small pupil
  DDx: Horner's syndrome, pharmacologic (pilocarpine, brimonidine, narcotics, insecticides), Argyll-Robertson pupil, iritis, diabetes, spasm of near reflex, senescence

Mydriasis: large pupil
  DDx: CN 3 palsy, Adie's tonic pupil, pharmacologic (mydriatics, cycloplegics, cocaine), iris damage (trauma, ischemia, surgery (Urrets-Zavalia syndrome)), Hutchinson's pupil
  Both Horner's and Adie's are examples of denervation hypersensitivity (sympathetic tone loss in Horner's, parasympathetic tone loss in Adie's)

Horner's Syndrome

Sympathetic lesion causing ptosis, miosis, and anhidrosis; anhidrosis often present in both first- and second-order lesions; may also have facial numbness, diplopia, and vertigo; may have mild inverse ptosis of lower lid, dilation lag; anisocoria most pronounced in dim light; congenital (forceps injury, shoulder dystocia); can cause iris heterochromia (ipsilateral lighter iris)

Preganglionic: from hypothalamus to superior cervical ganglion
  First-order neuron (central Horner's): hypothalamus to spinal cord level C8-T2 (ciliospinal center of Budge)
    ETIOLOGY:
      MIDBRAIN: neuron located near CN 4 nucleus in dorsolateral tegmentum; lesion at this level (usually ischemia) causes Horner's and superior oblique palsy
      PONS: near CN 6 nucleus; ischemia, tumor, demyelination, polio, syringomyelia, and inflammation, Foville's syndrome (lesion of CN 5, 6, and 7 and Horner's)
      MEDULLA: lateral medullary syndrome of Wallenberg (stroke of vertebral artery or PICA causing lateral medullary infarction; ipsilateral lesion of CN 9, 10, and 11; Horner's, vertigo, cerebellar signs, skew deviation, ipsilateral decreased pain/temperature sensation of face, contralateral decreased pain/temperature sensation of trunk and limbs); no extremity weakness
      VERTEBROBASILAR STROKES AND VERTEBRAL ARTERY DISSECTION
      CERVICAL DISC DISEASE: arthritis, demyelination, inflammation, tumors

SYRINGOMYELIA: spinal cord cavities surrounded by gliosis involving spinothalamic tracts; causes ipsilateral loss of pain/temperature sensation but preservation of touch; muscle wasting and weakness (especially small hand muscles); Charcot's arthropathy (35%)
  Second-order neuron: majority of preganglionic Horner's; ciliospinal center of Budge to superior cervical ganglion
    ETIOLOGY: mediastinal or apical tumor (neuroblastoma [most common], Pancoast's), thyroid disease, neurofibroma, pneumothorax, cervical infections, upper respiratory tract tumors, brachial plexus syndromes, carotid artery dissection, aneurysm, trauma

Postganglionic: superior cervical ganglion to iris dilator
  Third order neuron: anhidrosis limited to ipsilateral forehead
    ETIOLOGY:
      INTERNAL CAROTID ARTERY DISSECTION: transient ischemic attack (TIA), stroke, neck pain, amaurosis, dysacusia, bad taste in mouth
      LESIONS INVOLVING MECKEL'S CAVE OR CAVERNOUS SINUS: associated with CN 3, 4, V_1, V_2, and 6 palsies
      TRIGEMINAL HERPES ZOSTER
      HEADACHE SYNDROMES: migraine, cluster headaches, Raeder's syndrome (middle-aged men with Horner's and daily unilateral headaches)
      TUMOR OF PAROTID GLAND, NASOPHARYNX, SINUSES
      TRAUMA

Diagnosis: pharmacologic testing
  Cocaine test: topical cocaine (4%, 10%) blocks reuptake of norepinephrine (NE), causing pupil dilation
    Determines presence of Horner's syndrome
    Functioning neuron will release NE, and pupil will dilate
    ABNORMAL RESULT: no pupil dilation
  Hydroxyamphetamine 1% (Paredrine) test: releases NE from nerve terminal
    Distinguishes between preganglionic and postganglionic lesions
    POSITIVE IN PREGANGLIONIC LESIONS: pupil dilates because postganglionic neuron is intact
    NEGATIVE IN POSTGANGLIONIC LESIONS: pupil does not dilate because neuron does not have NE

Treatment: ptosis surgery to shorten Müller's muscle (Putterman procedure [conjunctival–Müller's muscle resection], Fasanella-Servat procedure [tarsoconjunctival resection])

Adie's Tonic Pupil

Dilated, tonic pupil due to postganglionic parasympathetic pupillomotor damage; 90% women; 20–40 years of age; 80% unilateral

Findings: initially, pupil is dilated and poorly reactive; later becomes miotic; segmental contraction of pupil (vermiform movements); light-near dissociation with slow (tonic) redilation after near stimulus

Adie's syndrome: Adie's pupil and decreased deep tendon reflexes; orthostatic hypotension

Pathology: loss of ganglion cells in ciliary ganglion, degenerated axons in short ciliary nerves

DDx: HZV, giant cell arteritis (GCA), syphilis, orbital trauma, diabetes, alcoholism, and dysautonomia associated with cancer and amyloidosis

Diagnosis: dilute pilocarpine (0.125%) or mecholyl 2.5% will constrict the tonic pupil but not the normal pupil; false-positive test can occur in CN 3 palsy

Argyll-Robertson Pupil

Bilateral small, irregular pupils with light-near dissociation caused by tertiary syphilis

Hutchinson's Pupil

Unilateral dilated, poorly reactive pupil in comatose patient due to ipsilateral supratentorial mass causing displacement of hippocampal gyrus (uncal herniation) entrapping CN 3; pupillomotor fibers travel in peripheral portion of nerve and are susceptible to early damage from compression

Simple Anisocoria

Most common cause of relative difference (<1 mm) between pupils; occurs in up to 20% of general population

OCULAR MUSCLE DISORDERS

Ophthalmoplegia

Static

Agenesis of extraocular muscles, congenital fibrosis syndrome, congenital myopathies

Progressive

Chronic Progressive External Ophthalmoplegia (CPEO)

Mitochondrial disease, several types

Kearns-Sayre syndrome: ophthalmoplegia with ptosis, retinal pigment degeneration, heart block

Oculopharyngeal Dystrophy (AD)

Onset in 5th–6th decade; French-Canadian ancestry; progressive dysphagia followed by ptosis; most develop CPEO

Pathology: vacuolar myopathy

Myotonic Dystrophy (AD)

Mapped to chromosome 19; myotonia of peripheral muscles; worsens with cold, excitement, fatigue

Findings: Christmas tree cataract (presenile cataract with polychromatic subcapsular cortical crystals), mild pigmentary retinopathy, ptosis, lid lag, light-near dissociation, miotic pupils, may develop ocular hypotony

Other findings: myotonia, testicular atrophy, frontal baldness, cardiac abnormalities (myopathy, conduction defects), bilateral facial weakness, insulin resistance, mental retardation

Diagnosis: ERG (low voltage), electromyogram (EMG) (myotonic discharge)

Inflammatory Disorders

Thyroid-related ophthalmopathy, orbital pseudotumor, amyloidosis

Others

Vitamin E deficiency, muscle tumors

Episodic

Familial periodic paralysis, trauma, ischemia, vasculitis, disorders of neuromuscular junction (myasthenia gravis, Eaton-Lambert syndrome, organophosphate poisoning, botulism)

Myasthenia Gravis (MG):

Weakness of voluntary muscles due to autoimmunity to motor end plates (antibodies block ACh receptors), hallmark is fatigability; 90% have eye symptoms, 50% present with eye symptoms; females > males; onset aged 15-50; 80% with ocular presentation will develop generalized disease; 15% spontaneously resolve; does not affect pupillary fibers

Neonatal form: transplacental transfer of ACh receptor antibody

Congenital form: genetic defect in ACh receptor

Types:
   Ocular: consists of ptosis and extraocular weakness only
   Systemic: other skeletal muscles involved; 5% of patients develop Graves' disease

Associations: thymic hyperplasia (70%), thymoma (occurs in 10% of MG patients; 30% of people with thymoma have MG), other autoimmune diseases (rheumatoid arthritis, lupus, thyroid disease)

Drugs that exacerbate MG: steroids, antibiotics (aminoglycosides, clindamycin, erythromycin), β-blockers, D-penicillamine, phenytoin, curare, methoxyflurane, lidocaine

Findings: asymmetric ptosis, seesaw ptosis ('curtaining'; when more ptotic lid is lifted, other lid falls owing to Hering's law), Cogan's lid twitch (when patient looks from downgaze to primary position, lid will overshoot), facial muscle weakness, ophthalmoplegia, pseudo-INO, nystagmus (on extreme gaze)

Other findings: jaw weakness, dysphagia, dysarthria, dyspnea, muscle bulk usually preserved until late

DDx: Myotonic dystrophy, CPEO, involutional ptosis, toxins (snake, arthropod, bacteria [botulism])

> *Eaton-Lambert syndrome*: paraneoplastic syndrome consisting of profound proximal muscle pain and weakness, dysarthria, dysphagia; associated with small cell lung cancer
>> MECHANISM: impaired presynaptic release of ACh; 50% demonstrate specific antibodies against presynaptic voltage-gated calcium channels
>> DIAGNOSIS: muscle strength and reflexes are enhanced with exercise; no improvement with edrophonium
>> EMG: increased muscle action potentials with repeated nerve stimulation

Diagnosis:

> *Tensilon test* (edrophonium [IV]; AChE inhibitor that prolongs action of ACh, resulting in stronger muscle contraction): positive 80–90% of the time, but high false-negative rate; may cause bradycardia – therefore, give test dose of 1–2 mg first; other adverse effects include sweating, nausea, vomiting, salivation, fever, elevated IOP; antidote is atropine sulfate (0.5 mg); alternative test is neostigmine methylsulfate (Prostigmine [IM]: useful in children and adults without ptosis, requires longer observation period [20–45 minutes])
> *ACh receptor antibody*: 3 types (binding Ab, blocking Ab, modulating Ab); 50% sensitive in ocular MG, 80% sensitive in general MG, 90% positive in MG with thymoma, 99% specific; seronegative MG due to antigen excess, ocular-specific Ab; Ab against other components of ACh receptor
> *EMG*: fatigue with repetitive nerve stimulation; single-fiber EMG is best
> *Photos*: check old photos; morning versus evening for variability in lid position
> *Rest test*: rest with eyes closed for 30 minutes; positive if improvement in ptosis occurs
> *Ice test*: neuromuscular transmission improves in cold; therefore, apply ice pack for 2 minutes; positive if improvement occurs
> *Others*: chest CT/MRI, thyroid function and lupus tests

Treatment: pyridostigmine (Mestinon [AChE inhibitor]), steroids, plasmapheresis, IV gamma globulin, cyclosporine (ciclosporin), azothioprine, thymectomy (33% resolve, 33% improve, 33% no benefit); prism spectacles and consider surgery for stable strabismus (>6–12 months)

Primary Overaction Syndromes

Convergence Spasm

Miosis with increasing esodeviation

Superior Oblique Myokymia

Episodic repetitive firing of SO causes intermittent oscillopsia, shimmering vision, and vertical and/or torsional diplopia; chronic; unknown etiology; treat with carbamazepine (Tegretol) or propranolol; consider simultaneous weakening of ipsilateral SO and IO

Ocular Neuromyotonia

Failure of muscle to relax; occurs after radiation therapy to parasellar lesions; may affect CN 3 or 6; diagnose by having patient look in direction of action of muscle (up and in for CN 3, laterally for CN 6); treat with carbamazepine (Tegretol)

Oculogyric Crisis

Bilateral tonic supraduction of eyes and neck hyperextension due to acute effect of phenothiazine overdose; also described with postinfectious Parkinson's disease

EYE MOVEMENTS IN COMA

Normal Eye Movements and Pupils

Bilateral cerebral depression

Limited Eye Movements and Normal Pupils

Metabolic, drugs

Horizontal Limitation

Eyes straight: pontine damage

Eyes deviated to side: cerebral damage

Bilateral horizontal limitations (gaze palsy, INO, CN 6 palsy): pontine damage

Ipsilateral horizontal deviation with contralateral limb weakness: basal ganglia damage

Contralateral horizontal deviation without limb weakness: cerebellar lesions

Vertical Limitation

Eyes straight: midbrain or pretectal damage

Upward deviation: hypoxic encephalopathy (severe cerebellar damage), lithium toxicity, phenothiazine overdose, heatstroke

Downward deviation (more common and more ambiguous than upward deviation): pretectal, metabolic, thalamic hemorrhage; tentorial herniation; pineal tumors; meningitis; hepatic encephalopathy

Vertical-gaze paresis and bilateral CN 3 palsy: midbrain damage

Total Ophthalmoplegia

Midbrain stroke, pituitary apoplexy, meningitis

Skew Deviation

Posterior fossa dysfunction

Bilateral Lid Retraction

Pretectal dysfunction

Nystagmus

Upbeat (structural), downbeat (hypoxic, Arnold-Chiari malformation, toxic [lithium], paraneoplastic), convergence-retraction (dorsal midbrain)

Calorics

Water irrigated into ear produces nystagmus; direction of nystagmus (fast phase) is COWS (cold opposite, warm same); jerk nystagmus in awake patient; tonic deviation in comatose patient in opposite direction of mnemonic; bilateral cold water irrigation produces upbeat nystagmus in awake patient; downward tonic deviation in comatose patient

OPTIC NERVE

Developmental Anomalies

(See Ch. 5, Pediatrics/Strabismus.)

Optic Disc Swelling

Nerve fibers anterior to lamina cribrosa swell due to obstruction of axoplasmic flow at level of lamina choroidalis or lamina scleralis
Orthograde transport (ganglion cells to LGB): slow component = 2 mm/day; fast component = 500 mm/day
Retrograde transport (LGB to ganglion cells)

Mechanism: ischemia, inflammation, increased intracranial pressure, compression

Findings: elevated hyperemic nerve head (3 diopters = 1 mm), blurred disc margins, loss of physiologic cup, peripapillary NFL edema, chorioretinal folds, dilated/tortuous veins, peripapillary flame-shaped hemorrhages, exudates, cotton wool spots (nerve fiber layer [NFL] infarcts)

Chronic swelling may cause Paton's lines (radial or concentric folds of peripapillary retina), gliosis, high water marks, pale disc, disc pseudodrusen, attenuated vessels, vision loss

DDx of optic disc edema/pseudoedema:
papilledema, ischemic optic neuropathy, optic neuritis, central retinal vein occlusion (CRVO), diabetic papillitis, malignant hypertension, neuroretinitis (cat-scratch disease), infiltration of the optic disc (sarcoidosis, tuberculosis, leukemia, metastases), optic disc drusen, optic nerve head tumors (astrocytic hamartoma, gliomas, capillary hemangioma), orbital disease/compressive optic neuropathy (thyroid-related ophthalmopathy, orbital pseudotumor, orbital mass), inflammatory diseases (syphilis, acute posterior multifocal placoid pigment epitheliopathy [APMPPE], Vogt-Koyanagi-Harada [VKH] syndrome), Leber's hereditary optic neuropathy

Papilledema

Disc edema due to increased intracranial pressure

Findings: disc edema (may be asymmetric); loss of spontaneous venous pulsations (absent in 20% of normals); transient visual obscurations (visual blackouts lasting <10 seconds associated with postural changes); diplopia (due to unilateral or bilateral CN 6 palsies); normal color vision, acuity, and pupils; enlarged blind spot on VF; headache, nausea, vomiting
  Chronic cases: pale atrophic nerve, arteriolar attenuation, poor vision, VF loss, refractile small hyaline bodies on the disk

DDx: intracranial tumor (posterior fossa in children), meningitis, carcinomatous meningitis, pseudotumor cerebri (IIH, see below)

Diagnosis: check blood pressure; brain CT/MRI, if no mass, perform lumbar puncture (measure opening pressure)

Idiopathic Intracranial Hypertension (IIH; Pseudotumor Cerebri)

Papilledema with normal neuroimaging and CSF
90% female, mean age = 33 years old; associated with obesity

Findings: headache, nausea, vomiting, optic disc edema (may be asymmetric), transient visual obscurations, photopsias, VF defect (enlarged blind spot, constriction, or arcuate scotoma), retrobulbar pain, pulsatile intracranial noises; may have visual loss, positive RAPD, diplopia (CN 6 palsy)
  In children: irritability; no disc swelling if fontanelles open

Associations: endocrine disorder (Addison's; steroid withdrawal), chronic obstructive lung disease, thrombosis of dural sinus (trauma, childbirth, middle ear infection, hypercoagulable state); use of steroids, birth control pills, vitamin A, tetracycline, nalidixic acid, isotretinoin; may be exacerbated with pregnancy

DDx: (see optic disc swelling above)

Diagnosis: normal brain MRI, elevated CSF pressure with normal composition (diagnosis of exclusion)

Treatment:

No vision loss: headache treatment and weight loss
Mild vision loss: acetazolamide (Diamox), furosemide, weight loss
Advanced VF loss: ON sheath decompression, serial lumbar punctures (temporary relief), lumbar–peritoneal shunt

Optic Neuritis

Inflammation of optic nerve; idiopathic or associated with systemic disease; most common optic neuropathy in people <45 years old; female preponderance

Findings: acute unilateral visual loss (can evolve over 1st week, then spontaneous improvement over weeks [70% regain 20/20]), ocular pain exacerbated by eye movements, decreased color vision and contrast sensitivity, positive RAPD, VF defect (50% diffuse, 20% central scotoma, rarely altitudinal), optic nerve appears normal or swollen (35%), disc pallor late

Other findings:

Pulfrich phenomenon: motion of pendulum appears elliptical owing to altered depth perception from delayed conduction in the demyelinated nerve
Uhthoff's symptom: worsening of symptoms with heat or exercise; present in 50% after recovery
Phosphenes: flashes of light induced by eye movements or sound
Auditory clicks: CN 7 innervates stapedius, and patient hears click with effective transmission

DDx: idiopathic, MS, syphilis, sarcoidosis, Lyme disease, Wegener's granulomatosis, systemic lupus erythematosus (SLE), Devic's syndrome (bilateral optic neuritis and transverse myelitis)

Treatment:

Controlled High-risk Avonex Multiple Sclerosis Prevention Study (CHAMPS): randomized trial of interferon beta-1a (Avonex) for the prevention of MS after acute demyelinating episode and abnormal MRI
3-YEAR RESULTS: risk of MS lower and fewer MRI lesions in treatment group

MAJOR CLINICAL STUDY

Optic Neuritis Treatment Trial (ONTT)

Objective: to evaluate the role of corticosteroids in the treatment of unilateral optic neuritis
Methods: patients with unilateral optic neuritis were randomly assigned into 3 treatment groups:
1. *IV steroids:* 250 mg IV methylprednisolone qid × 3 days, followed by oral prednisone (1 mg/kg/day) × 11 days
2. *Oral steroids:* prednisone (1 mg/kg/day) × 14 days
3. *Oral placebo:* 14 days

Results:

IV steroids: more rapid recovery of visual acuity at 2 weeks; did not reduce risk of subsequent attacks; decreased incidence of MS at 2 years vs placebo, but no difference at 3 years
Oral prednisone: associated with higher rate of new attacks in either eye at 1 year; highest relapse rate of optic neuritis at 5 years (41% vs 25% for IV and placebo groups)
Brain MRI: periventricular white matter lesions were associated with MS
Lesions in 50% of patients with first attack of optic neuritis
5-YEAR RESULTS: 30% risk of developing MS regardless of treatment group
WITH NO LESIONS: 16% developed MS
3 OR MORE LESIONS: 51% developed MS
Increased risk of developing MS if previous neurologic symptoms (regardless of MRI status)
10-YEAR RESULTS:
WITH NO LESIONS: 22% developed MS
WITH ¹1 LESION: 56% developed MS
If normal MRI, no previous neurologic findings or fellow eye involvement: decreased risk of MS if optic neuritis was painless, if disc swelling was present and vision loss was only mild
No patients developed MS who had normal MRI with peripapillary hemorrhage or macular exudates
Abnormal MRI: 43% progress to MS by 3 years; progression to MS at 1 year was 7.5% with IV steroids, 14.7% with oral steroids, and 16.7% with placebo

Conclusions:

In general, about 30% develop MS within 4 years and 38% develop MS by 10 years (risk is higher in women than men)

Consider treating optic neuritis with IV steroids; do not initiate treatment with oral steroids

Regardless of MRI status, there is a higher risk of developing MS if the patient has previous neurologic symptoms or a history of optic neuritis in the fellow eye

Optic Neuropathies

Anterior Ischemic Optic Neuropathy (AION)

Infarction of optic nerve head just posterior to lamina cribrosa due to inadequate perfusion by posterior ciliary arteries; results in acute visual loss

2 forms: arteritic (giant cell arteritis); nonarteritic (ischemic)

Findings: decreased color vision and acuity, positive RAPD, VF loss (altitudinal or arcuate defects most common, central scotomas also occur), unilateral optic disc edema (often involving 1 sector), contralateral disc appears crowded (small C/D ratio)

Arteritic: due to giant cell (temporal) arteritis (inflammatory vasculopathy affecting medium-sized to large vessels) affecting the posterior ciliary arteries; female > male (2 : 1); aged >55 years; may have amaurosis fugax or diplopia

> *Other findings:* scalp tenderness, jaw or tongue claudication, polymyalgia rheumatica (PMR), fever, malaise, anorexia, weight loss, anemia, headache, tender temporal artery, neck pain, brain stem stroke (due to involvement of vertebral artery); cotton wool spots, choroidal ischemia (seen as patchy choroidal filling on fluorescein angiography (FA))

> *Pathology:* granulomatous inflammation with epithelioid cells, lymphocytes, giant cells; disruption of internal elastic lamina and proliferation of intima with aneurysm formation (Figure 4-26)

> *Diagnosis:* elevated ESR (for men > [age/2]; for women > [(age +10)/2]; may be normal in 10%), C-reactive protein (above 2.45 mg/dL), low hematocrit (anemia of chronic illness), FA (patchy choroidal filling, nonperfusion), temporal artery biopsy (inflammation in artery wall with disruption of internal elastica lamina, skip lesions [specimen at least 3 cm], perform within 2 weeks of steroid treatment)

> *Treatment* (emergent): steroids (prednisone 60–120 mg orally; consider IV initially [1 g for 3 days]) to prevent fellow eye involvement (65% risk of involvement of fellow eye without treatment; usually affected within 10 days); some patients lose vision despite treatment

Nonarteritic (NAION) (ischemic): no associated symptoms; usually aged 50–75 years; associated with microvascular disease (diabetes, hypertension) and collagen vascular disorders; recurrence in same eye is rare; 25–40% risk of fellow eye involvement; normal ESR; NAION may be mimicked by amiodarone and phosphodiesterase-5 inhibitors

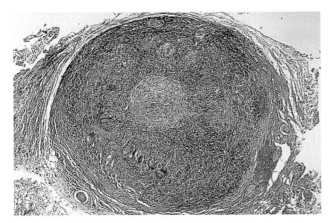

Figure 4-26. Arteric AION demonstrating vasculitis of all coats of temporal artery with giant cells. (Courtesy of MM Rodrigues. From Yanoff M, Fine BS 2002 Ocular Pathology, 5th edn. Mosby, St Louis.)

Treatment: none

> **ISCHEMIC OPTIC NEUROPATHY DECOMPRESSION TRIAL** (IONDT): optic nerve sheath fenestration is not effective

> Smokers had earlier mean onset (age 64) than nonsmokers (age 70)

> 43% of control patients regained 3 or more lines of vision at 6 months (vs 34% of those having surgery)

> Surgery had higher risk of loss of 3 lines of vision (24% vs 12% with observation)

Pseudo Foster-Kennedy syndrome: AION is the most frequent cause of unilateral disc edema and contralateral optic atrophy; disc not hyperemic like true Foster-Kennedy syndrome

Retrobulbar Optic Neuropathy (Posterior Ischemic Optic Neuropathy)

Rare; usually bilateral; occurs with severe anemia and hypotension (i.e. major blood loss from surgery, trauma, GI bleed, dialysis); associated with medications (antibiotics [ethambutol, isoniazid, sulfonamides, chloramphenicol], anticancer drugs [cisplatin, vincristine, busulfan])

Findings: disc swelling may occur if ischemic process extends anteriorly

Treatment: treat acute cause (prompt reversal of hypotension, blood transfusion)

Compressive Optic Neuropathy

Intraorbital, intracanalicular, or intracranial (prechiasmal)

Etiology: ON tumor, pituitary tumor or apoplexy, thyroid-related ophthalmopathy

Findings: slow progressive vision loss, decreased color vision, positive RAPD, VF defect (central scotoma that extends to periphery), proptosis; disc may be normal, pale, or swollen; may have endocrine abnormalities (parachiasmal lesions), chemosis and restricted motility (thyroid)

Diagnosis: orbit CT/MRI

Infiltrative Optic Neuropathy

Etiology: leukemia, lymphoma, multiple myeloma, plasmacytoma, metastatic carcinoma (breast and lung most common), sarcoidosis, TB, cryptococcus, toxoplasmosis, toxocariasis, CMV, coccidiomycosis

Findings: disc may appear grayish-white with associated hemorrhages; mass may be visible

Toxic/Nutritional Optic Neuropathy

Painless symmetric progressive vision loss

Etiology: ethanol, methanol, digoxin, ethambutol, chloramphenicol, isoniazid, rifampin, lead toxicity, tobacco-alcohol amblyopia, thiamine and B_{12} deficiency, cisplatin

Findings: decreased vision (20/200 or worse), VF loss (cecocentral scotomas), disc hyperemia then pallor

Traumatic Optic Neuropathy

ON contusion or compression due to trauma

Findings: decreased vision, VF defects, positive RAPD

CT scan: rule out canal fracture, orbital hematoma, ON hematoma

Treatment: lateral canthotomy for tense orbit, drain subperiosteal hematoma
> *IV steroids* (methylprednisolone): 30 mg/kg loading dose, then 5.4 mg/kg/h × 48 hours
> If vision improves, switch to 80 mg oral, and taper by 20 mg every 2–3 days; if vision worsens on oral steroids, restart high-dose IV and consider surgical decompression of canal
> Consider surgical decompression of optic canal if no response to steroids after 48 hours
> If no improvement in vision after 3 days, stop steroids

Hereditary Optic Neuropathy

(See Ch. 5, Pediatrics/Strabismus.)

Optic Atrophy

Pale white appearance of ON head caused by injury to any part of pathway from retinal ganglion cells to LGB

Etiology: optic neuropathy, optic neuritis, glaucoma, central retinal artery occlusion (CRAO), tumors, aneurysms

Pathology: increased number of astrocytes (gliosis) within nerve; normal parallel architecture of glial columns seen in sagittal sections is lost; widened space between nerve and meninges; loss of myelin; thickened pial septa

ON Tumors

ON Glioma (Figure 4-27)

Low-grade astrocytoma: usually in children aged <10 years

'Benign' but 14% mortality rate (highest with hypothalamus involvement)

10–50% have neurofibromatosis (15% of patients with NF have ON gliomas)

50% intraorbital, 50% intracranial
> *Findings:* vision loss, strabismus, nystagmus, disc edema or atrophy; may have proptosis (intraorbital ON glioma); can spread to chiasm and contralateral ON
> *MRI:* fusiform thickening and kinking of ON

Malignant ON glioma (glioblastoma multiforme): occurs in adults
Painful vision loss; becomes bilateral; death in 3–9 months

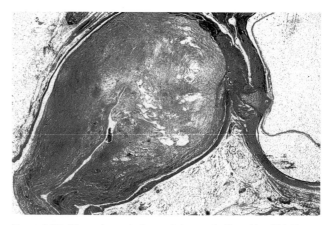

Figure 4-27. Glioma demonstrating central necrosis. (From Yanoff M, Fine BS 2002 Ocular Pathology, 5th edn. Mosby, St Louis.)

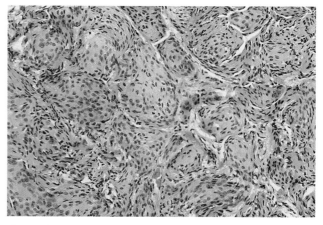

Figure 4-28. Meningioma demonstrating proliferation of meningothelial cells. (From Yanoff M, Fine BS 2002 Ocular Pathology, 5th edn. Mosby, St Louis.)

ON Meningioma

Derived from outer arachnoid; may arise from ectopic nests of meningeal cells; female > male (3:1)

Findings: triad of decreased vision, optic atrophy, optociliary shunt vessels; also proptosis, ON edema, retinal vascular occlusions

Sphenoid wing meningioma: fullness of temporal orbital fossa and orbit

Pathology: psammoma bodies and whorls of concentrically packed spindle cells (Figure 4-28)

CT/MRI: railroad track sign (due to calcification)

CHIASM COMPRESSION

Chiasm anatomy: location with respect to pituitary gland
> *Prefixed:* chiasm is forward; pituitary tumor will compress the optic tracts

Normal: chiasm is aligned with pituitary; pituitary tumor will compress chiasm

Postfixed: chiasm is behind; pituitary tumor will compress optic nerves

Etiology: pituitary tumor (most common), pituitary apoplexy, craniopharyngioma, meningioma, glioma, aneurysm, trauma, infection, metastasis, MS, sarcoidosis

VF defects: central scotoma, bitemporal hemianopia, incongruous homonymous hemianopia, junctional scotoma (ipsilateral central scotoma with contralateral superotemporal defect due to lesion at junction of ON and chiasm)

DDx of bitemporal VF defect: sector retinitis pigmentosa, coloboma, tilted disc

Pituitary Tumor

Most commonly chromophobe (often prolactinoma); can also secrete adrenocorticotropin (ACTH) (Cushing's disease); basophil can secrete ACTH; eosinophil can secrete growth hormone (GH) (acromegaly); secreting tumors usually present with endocrine dysfunction, except prolactin-secreting tumor in males (presents with signs of chiasmal compression); 30% nonsecreting (present with vision loss)

Findings: VF defect (bitemporal hemianopia), hormone imbalance, optic atrophy

Diagnosis: X-ray shows large pituitary fossa, double floor sign, bony erosion

Treatment: dopamine antagonist (bromocriptine) for prolactinoma, hormone replacement, transsphenoidal surgery for nonsecreting tumor, XRT

Meningioma

Derived from meningothelial cells of arachnoid; often at sphenoid ridge; occurs in adults, especially middle-aged women

Tuberculum sellae meningioma: compression of optic nerve just before chiasm, may cause unilateral VF defect
Findings: optic atrophy, hyperostosis

Pathology: whorled cellular pattern; may see psammoma bodies

Pituitary Apoplexy

Acute hemorrhage and expansion of a pituitary tumor, usually secondary to ischemic necrosis

Findings: headache, decreased vision, ocular motility disturbance; progresses to no light perception (NLP) and complete ophthalmoplegia

Sheehan's Syndrome

Panhypopituitarism in pregnancy due to hemorrhage

Craniopharyngioma

Usually causes compression of chiasm from above and behind; occurs in children and young adults

Findings: initial damage to upper nasal fibers (inferior bitemporal field defect); later, upper temporal defect papilledema, optic atrophy

MRI: calcification

DDx of calcification of sella turcica: craniopharyngioma, supraclinoid aneurysm, meningioma, AV malformation, glioma of chiasm (very rare), chordoma (extremely rare)

Glioma

Occurs in children and adults; may extend into both optic nerves causing bilateral vision loss with complicated bilateral VF defects

Aneurysm

ICA and anterior cerebral artery; middle-aged adults; present with vision loss, ophthalmoplegia

Subfrontal Mass Lesion

Slow progressive asymmetric bilateral visual loss, late ON pallor

Other Chiasmal Lesions

MS, trauma, basal meningitis, sphenoid sinus mucocele or carcinoma

RETROCHIASMAL DISORDERS

Cause homonymous VF defects (see Figure 4-9)

Cogan's Dictum: causes homonymous hemianopia
With asymmetric OKN = parietal lobe lesion (usually mass)
With symmetric OKN = occipital lobe lesion (usually infarction)

Optic Tract

Vascular, craniopharyngioma extending posteriorly

Findings: incongruous homonymous hemianopia, bilateral optic atrophy (bow-tie appearance), contralateral RAPD

LGB

Very rare

Findings: incongruous homonymous hemianopia or congruous homonymous sectoranopia (sectoral optic atrophy), normal pupils

Temporal Lobe

Glioma, vascular

Findings: 'Pie-in-the-sky' VF defect (inferior macular fibers do not travel as far anteriorly into Meyer's loop)

Other findings: déjà vu symptoms, foul odors; may have formed visual hallucinations

Parietal Lobe

Gioma, meningioma, metastases, middle cerebral artery thrombosis

Findings: affect fibers from superior retina first (contralateral inferior homonymous quadrantanopia) or contralateral inferior homonymous hemianopia denser inferiorly; spasticity of conjugate gaze (tonic deviation of eyes to opposite side of parietal lesion); OKN asymmetry (nystagmus dampened when stimuli moved in direction of damaged parietal lobe); may have contralateral motor paresis

Gerstmann's syndrome: lesion of dominant parietal lobe (inferior homonymous hemianopia, acalculia, agraphia, finger agnosia, left–right confusion)

Occipital Lobe

Vascular (90%), tumors, trauma

Findings:
Central homonymous hemianopia (periphery spared): fibers from macula terminate at tip of occipital lobes
Macula sparing: fibers from retinal periphery terminate on mesial surface of occipital lobe (supplied by PCA)
Temporal crescent: homonymous hemianopia with sparing of far temporal periphery (supplied by nasal retina and travels to most anterior portion of mesial surface of contralateral occipital lobe)

Other findings: unformed visual hallucinations, paliopia (perseveration in homonymous field), prosopagnosia (inability to recognize faces; bilateral medial occipitotemporal lesion), Riddoch phenomenon (ability to perceive moving objects but not stationary ones)

Disconnection syndrome: dominant occipital lobe and splenium of corpus callosum; usually due to posterior artery stroke (right homonymous hemianopia with alexia [cannot read] but not agraphia [can write])

CORTICAL LESIONS

Cause disorders of visual integration

Visual information from LGB goes to primary visual cortex (V1) of both occipital lobes; further processing occurs in areas V2–V5

To read, information travels from visual cortex to angular gyrus in parietal lobe of dominant hemisphere (usually on left side); visual information from right hemifield is transmitted directly from left occipital lobe to ipsilateral angular gyrus, and information from left hemifield is transmitted through splenium of corpus callosum to contralateral angular gyrus

Disorders

Alexia

Inability to read despite normal vision

Pseudoalexia

Can be caused by inability to read, hemianopias with split fixation, and expressive (Broca's) or conduction aphasias

Alexia with Agraphia (Inability to Write)

Parietal lesions involving angular gyrus

Alexia without Agraphia

Large left occipital lesions that also disrupt fibers crossing in splenium of corpus callosum from right occipital cortex to left angular gyrus; information from left VF cannot travel to left parietal lobe (angular gyrus); patient is blind in right visual field, can see and write but not read, even what they have just written

Dyslexia

Central nervous system problem in which letters appear reversed; male > female (3 : 1).; visual training does not improve academic abilities of dyslexic or learning disabled children

Visual Neglect

Patient ignores 1 side of visual space

Visual Extinction

Patient ignores 1 side of visual space when presented with simultaneous stimuli to both visual fields; occurs more often with right parietal lesions

Visual Agnosia

Bilateral lesions of occipitotemporal area; inability to recognize objects by sight, although can recognize by touch, language, and intellect

Anomia

Inability to name objects

Prosopagnosia

Bilateral infero-occipital lesions; inability to recognize faces

Cerebral Achromatopsia

Unilateral or bilateral lesion in infero-occipital area; loss of color vision in opposite hemifield

DISORDERS DURING PREGNANCY

Occur more commonly with eclampsia and preeclampsia

Conditions: central serous retinopathy (CSR), hypertensive retinopathy, Purtscher's-like retinopathy, RD, cerebral venous thrombosis, CRAO, carotid cavernous fistula, Sheehan's syndrome (postpartum pituitary infarct causing panhypopituitarism; secondary hemorrhage can cause CN 2-6 palsies)

Conditions that worsen during pregnancy: uveal melanoma, pituitary adenoma, meningioma, DM, Graves' disease, orbital and choroidal hemangiomas

Conditions that improve during pregnancy: MS, optic neuritis, sarcoidosis, lupus

Migraines: may improve or worsen

Preeclampsia: transient visual loss in 50%, cerebral blindness in 1–5%; ischemic cerebrovascular complication risk increases 13× during pregnancy and postpartum due to hypercoagulable state
  Arterial abnormalities: occur in 60-90%; most common during 2nd and 3rd trimesters and 1st week postpartum
  Venous abnormalities: during first 6 weeks postpartum (venous sinus thrombosis presents with headache and papilledema).

BRAIN TUMORS

(Table 4-1)

Foster-Kennedy Syndrome

Frontal lobe mass (usually olfactory or sphenoid ridge meningioma) causing anosmia (loss of smell), ipsilateral optic atrophy (tumor compression), and contralateral ON edema (elevated ICP)

Pseudo–Foster-Kennedy syndrome: bilateral AION (pale nerve from old AION and fellow nerve edema from new AION)

Cerebellopontine Angle Tumors

Usually acoustic neuroma; associated with neurofibromatosis; peripheral CN 7 lesion (orbicularis weakness, inability to wrinkle forehead), CN 6 lesion, CN 5 lesion (decreased corneal sensation), nystagmus (vestibular to contralateral side, gaze paretic to ipsilateral side)

Table 4-1. Classification of brain tumors

By origin:	
Glial (gliomas)	Astrocytoma
Neuronal	Neuroblastoma, medulloblastoma
Connective tissue	Sarcoma
Lymphoreticular	Primary (non-Hodgkin's) CNS lymphoma
Blood vessels	Hemangioma, angioma
Bone	Osteoma
Neural crest	Meningioma (arachnoid cells), primary
Congenital rests:	CNS melanoma
Notochord	Chordoma
Adipose cells	Lipoma
Ectodermal derivatives	Craniopharyngioma, teratoma, dermoid
Glands:	Adenoma
Pituitary gland	Pineocytoma, pineoblastoma, germ cell
Pineal gland	tumors
By age:	
<20 years old	CNS tumors are second most common type of malignancy (leukemia is first); approximately 66% located in posterior fossa; gliomas of cerebellum, brain stem, optic nerve; pinealomas; primitive neuroectodermal tumors; craniopharyngiomas
20–60 years old	Meningiomas, gliomas of cerebral hemispheres, pituitary tumors
>60 years old	Malignant gliomas, metastases

Posterior Fossa Tumors

Cause most severe papilledema because encroach on cerebral aqueduct and 4th ventricle with rapid rise in ICP

Metastases

In order of frequency at autopsy: melanoma, lung, breast, renal, colorectal, ovarian

HEADACHES

(Figure 4-29)

Migraines

Etiology: cerebral vasospasm; slow-moving concentric wave of suppressed electrical activity

Types:
  Common (without aura): male=female; any age; little or no prodrome; throbbing headache, photophobia, nausea
  Classic (with aura) (20%): male=female; any age; trigger factors; visual prodrome followed by hemicranial pain, nausea, vomiting, dizziness, photophobia
    Scintillating scotoma (5–30 minutes, half visual field; may have macropsia, micropsia, hallucinations, achromatopsia); may have tingling on 1 side of face and/or ipsilateral hand; rarely, hemiparesis, vertigo, mood changes, distortion of hearing and smell

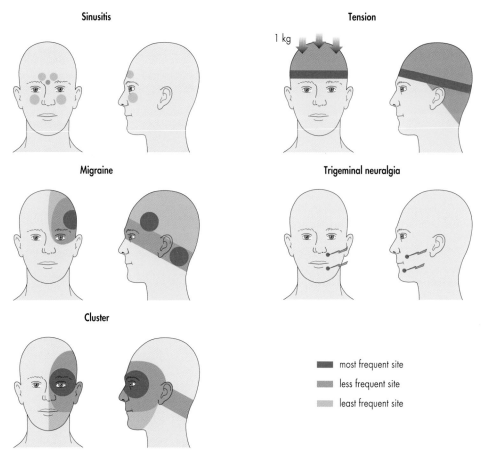

Sinusitis

Tension

1 kg

Migraine

Trigeminal neuralgia

Cluster

■ most frequent site
■ less frequent site
■ least frequent site

Figure 4-29. Location of pain for the common headache syndromes. (From Weinstein JM: Headache and facial pain. In: Yanoff M, Duker JS (eds) Ophthalmology. London, Mosby, 1999.)

Complicated: hemiplegic or hemiparetic; mostly children

OPHTHALMOPLEGIC: headache and recurrent paresis of 1 or more ocular motor nerves (usually CN 3) May last longer than 1 week; rarely, permanent ophthalmoplegia

Childhood: brief attacks of nausea/vomiting; usually no headache

Acephalgic (migraine equivalent): aura without headache Most common after age 40; history of migraines with or without aura; rule out TIA

Retinal: temporary scotoma or monocular blindness; headache may precede or occur within an hour Examination during attack reveals venous constriction

Migraine infarction: focal signs persist for longer than 1 week; corresponding lesion on neuroimaging

Status migrainosus: attack lasting longer than 72 hours (with or without treatment); continuous headache or intermittent with interruptions at less than 4 hours

Precipitating factors:

Diet: tyramine (bananas, avocado, yogurt, aged cheese), phenylethylamine (chocolate, cheese, wine), sodium nitrite (preservatives, food coloring, processed meats and fish), monosodium glutamate (Chinese food, processed meats, frozen dinners, canned soup), caffeine, alcohol, artificial sweeteners

Lifestyle: excessive sleep, fasting or dieting, exertion, fatigue, stressful events, depression

Hormonal: supplemental estrogen, menses, oral contraceptives, ovulation

Environmental: sun exposure, loud noise, bright lights, glare, flickering lights, strong odors

Treatment:

General: alter diet, lifestyle, hormonal and environmental factors

Abortive: ice pack, cold shower, exercise, massage, local scalp pressure; analgesics; oral ergotamine or dihydroergotamine (DHE); antiemetics; sumatriptan ([Imitrex], serotonin agonist; works on peripheral trigeminal nerve terminals that supply pain-sensitive vascular and meningeal structures; also causes constriction of certain intracranial blood vessels; oral and injectable forms; 83% obtain relief within 4 hours, 45% have recurrence 24 hours later; adverse effects include flushing or tingling, chest pain)

Prophylactic: consider if attacks occur once every 2 months or more often, if severity limits normal activity, or if acute therapies have failed or are contraindicated

β-BLOCKERS: reduce frequency of attacks by half (in 70% of patients)

TRICYCLIC ANTIDEPRESSANTS: amitriptyline, nortriptyline, imipramine, and doxepin

SEROTONIN REUPTAKE INHIBITORS: fluoxetine

CALCIUM CHANNEL BLOCKERS: decrease frequency of attacks, do not affect severity

Tension Headaches

Dull, persistent pain like tight band around head

Cluster Headaches

Severe, unilateral, orbital, supraorbital, and/or temporal pain lasting from 15 minutes to 3 hours; may awaken patient from sleep; usually occur in men 30–40 years of age; more common in smokers; attacks occur in groups and last weeks or months

Findings (ipsilateral): conjunctival injection, lacrimation, nasal congestion, rhinorrhea, forehead/facial sweating, miosis, ptosis, and/or eyelid edema; may develop postganglionic Horner's syndrome

Glossopharyngeal Neuralgia

Unilateral pain in region of larynx, tongue, tonsil, and ear; may have hoarseness and coughing; can be stimulated by swallowing or pungent tastes

Treatment: carbamazepine, baclofen, phenytoin

Carotidynia

Pain arising from cervical carotid artery, radiates to ipsilateral face and ear; rule out carotid dissection

Temporomandibular Joint (TMJ) Syndrome

Unilateral ear or preauricular pain, radiates to temple, jaw, or neck; worse with chewing

Findings: limitation of normal jaw movement, audible click on jaw opening

Other Causes of Headache/Facial Pain

Acute: subarachnoid hemorrhage, meningitis, encephalitis, focal scalp inflammation, sinusitis, dental disease, acute uveitis, acute glaucoma, scleritis, HZV, cervical spondylitis, GCA

Recurrent: asthenopia, cerebral aneurysm or angioma, severe hypertension

Chronic: muscle tension, depression, cerebral tumor, pituitary or nasopharyngeal tumor, metastatic carcinoma, Paget's disease, increased intracranial pressure, chronic subdural hemorrhage, postherpetic neuralgia, trigeminal neuralgia (tic douloureux), Costen's syndrome (temporomandibular osteoarthritis)

VISUAL DISTURBANCES

Functional Visual Loss

Diagnosis of exclusion; trick patient with visual tests

Bottom-up acuity: start with 20/20 line and slowly progress up chart

Deception of eye tested: fogging with phoropter; trial frame with 2 high-power cylinders of opposite sign in same axis (so net power is zero), then spin 1 of the cylinders thus fogging good eye; red-green glasses used with duochrome filter of projection chart (red letters are seen with eye behind red lens)

Stereoacuity: minimum amount of acuity is needed to distinguish different stereo images

Binocular integrated multicolored vision assessment test (BIMVAT): red and blue filters placed over near correction in trial frame; blue filter over 'bad' eye, then show letters made up of orange, brown, and blue components (orange components seen through blue filter but not red filter); some letters designed so that they can be read as 2 different letters (e.g. P or R) depending on what components are seen, so any letter with all orange components read correctly was read by the 'bad' eye

Visual field testing: spiral field

With complete blindness: OKN, signature (truly blind patients can do this without difficulty), touch nose or other finger (patient may mistake this for a visual task and be unable to perform), ERG

Transient Visual Loss

Visual Obscurations

Last seconds; occur in papilledema (change in posture or eye movement) or optic disc drusen

Amaurosis Fugax

Monocular loss or dimming of vision lasting from 2 to >30 minutes; commonly due to carotid or cardiac disease, also occurs in temporal arteritis, vertebrobasilar insufficiency (bilateral), hypotension, hyperviscosity (anticardiolipin), migraine, eclampsia; brief episodes may indicate impending CRAO

Uhthoff's Phenomena

Blurring of vision with activity or heat; due to optic neuritis

Scintillating Scotoma

Ocular migraine

Whiteout of Vision or 'Chicken-Wire' Pattern

Occipital ischemia

Gradual Peripheral Constriction of Vision with Visual Phenomena

Cerebrovascular disease or occipital migraine

Other Visual Phenomena

Visual Hallucinations

Release hallucinations (Charles Bonnet syndrome): formed (faces, objects) or unformed (flashes of light); occur in areas of absent vision; usually continuous and variable; common in age-related macular degeneration (AMD) and patients with large VF defects; associated with lesions anywhere in visual pathway; stop with eye movement

Ictal hallucinations: stereotyped, paroxysmal visual hallucinations; unformed (occipital lobe lesion) or formed (associated with strange odor; temporal lobe lesion)

Palinopsia: abnormal perseveration of visual images; occurs with evolving lesions, more commonly in right hemisphere

Phosphenes

Unstructured flashes of light

Photopsias

Structured geometric figures

VASCULAR DISORDERS

Cerebral Aneurysm

Occurs in 5% of population; rarely symptomatic before age 20; associated with hypertension

Risk factors: HTN, AV malformation, coarctation of the aorta, polycystic kidney disease, fibromuscular dysplasia, Marfan's syndrome, Ehlers-Danlos syndrome

Types: fusiform or saccular ('berry'; most common at arterial bifurcations; 90% supratentorial; >10 mm have highest risk of rupture)

Location:
Internal carotid artery (85%): main trunk (PCA, ophthalmic artery, cavernous sinus), anterior communicating artery, middle cerebral artery (MCA) trifurcation, anterior cerebral artery. Most common site is at origin of posterior communicating artery lading to 3rd CN palsy with pupil involvement
Basilar artery (5%)
Vertebral artery (5%)

Findings:
Anterior communicating artery: ON compression, chiasm compression, paraplegia
Origin of PCA: sudden-onset severe headache, complete CN 3 palsy
Bifurcation of MCA: hemiparesis, aphasia
Bifurcation of ICA: ON compression, chiasm compression, hemiparesis
Subarachnoid hemorrhage: neurosurgical emergency; severe headache ('worst headache of life'), nausea, vomiting, stiff neck; **Terson's syndrome** (vitreous and subarachnoid hemorrhages [when ICP in ON sheath exceeds ocular venous pressure])
Sentinal bleed: headache with transient neurologic symptoms before major rupture

Diagnosis:
Cerebral arteriogram: 4-vessel study of both carotid and vertebral arteries
MRI: detects aneurysms >5 mm in size
Magnetic resonance angiography (MRA): can detect 3-mm aneurysm
CT scan: acutely to screen for subarachnoid and intraparenchymal bleed; unacceptable screen for unruptured aneurysms (if negative, perform LP to determine presence of subarachnoid blood)

Treatment:
Medical (symptomatic, unruptured): stabilize, lower ICP with hyperventilation and mannitol; prevent vasospasm with calcium channel blockers and blood volume expansion; control blood pressure
Surgery: clip aneurysm; if unable, may need to ligate feeding artery
Prognosis: risk of bleed is 1%/year
30% mortality at time of rupture; if untreated, 33% mortality at 6 months; survivors have neurologic deficits
Rebleed risk is highest in first 24 hours; untreated patients have 25% risk of rebleed during first 2 weeks
Vasospasm is major cause of morbidity and death; 30% within first 2 weeks, highest risk between days 4 and 10

Arteriovenous Malformation (AVM)

Congenital, may be familial; symptoms usually before age 20; 90% supratentorial, 70% cortical, 20% deep, 10% in posterior fossa or dura mater; 6% have intracranial aneurysm

Findings: intracranial bleed (50%), sometimes with subarachnoid hemorrhage; neurologic symptoms before bleed (50%) (seizures, headaches, other neurologic deficits); may hear bruit
Cortical AVM in occipital lobe: visual symptoms and migraines
Hemispheric AVM: can get homonymous hemianopia
Brain stem AVM: diplopia, nystagmus, gaze palsy, pupil abnormality

Diagnosis:
CT scan: hemorrhage; calcified AVMs visible on plain X-ray
MRI: better for small AVMs
Cerebral angiogram: demonstrate anatomy

Treatment: resection, ligation of feeding vessel, embolization, stereotactic radiosurgery

Prognosis: 20% mortality when bleeding begins; rebleed rate is 2.5%/year

Carotid Artery Dissection

Intracranial or extracranial

Etiology:
Trauma: blunt (head, neck), carotid artery compression, hanging, manipulative neck therapy, surgery, carotid artery cannulation during angiography
Spontaneous: fibromuscular dysplasia, Marfan's syndrome, Ehlers-Danlos, polycystic kidney disease, syphilis, atherosclerosis, moyamoya, idiopathic

Findings:
Traumatic: ipsilateral headache and ophthalmic signs, contralateral neurologic deficits; may hear bruit
Symptoms can be delayed (weeks to months); severe cases can present with cerebral ischemia and coma
Spontaneous: transient or permanent neurologic defects; amaurosis fugax, monocular visual loss, or ipsilateral Horner's syndrome; intracranial extension may cause CN palsies, diplopia, tongue paralysis, facial numbness
Visual loss from embolic occlusion of ophthalmic artery, central retinal artery, or short posterior ciliary arteries
Rarely, ocular ischemia from reduced blood flow

Diagnosis: MRI

Treatment: controversial

Vertebrobasilar Dissection

40% of all dissecting aneurysms; basilar more common than vertebral

General findings: headache, neck pain, signs of brain stem and cerebellar dysfunction
Basilar artery dissection: ocular motor palsies, progresses to coma and death

Vertebral artery dissection (various presentations): fatal brain stem infarction (usually young adults); subarachnoid hemorrhage; aneurysmal dilation with brain stem and lower cranial nerve signs from mass effect; chronic dissection with recurrent TIAs, strokes, and subarachnoid hemorrhages

Vertebrobasilar Insufficiency (VBI)

Posterior circulation ischemia; vertebrobasilar system (vertebral, basilar, posterior cerebral arteries) supplies occipital cortex and areas involved with ocular motility in brain stem and cerebellum

Etiology: thrombus, emboli, hypertension, arrhythmias, arterial dissection, hypercoagulable state, subclavian steal syndrome

Findings: ataxia, vertigo (may also have tinnitus, deafness, or vomiting), dysarthria, dysphagia, hemiparesis, hemiplegia, drop attack (patient suddenly drops to ground without warning, no loss of consciousness), bilateral dimming of vision lasting seconds to minutes, photopsias, homonymous VF loss without other neurologic findings

Cerebral blindness/cortical blindness

Bilateral occipital lobe lesions; pupils react normally; may deny blindness (Anton's syndrome)

Cerebral Venous and Dural Sinus Thrombosis

Occlusion of cortical and subcortical veins produces neurologic symptoms; most commonly, cavernous sinus, lateral sinus, and superior sagittal sinus

Etiology: inflammation (Behçet's, SLE), infection, trauma, invasion of vessel wall by tumor (leukemia, lymphoma, meningioma), altered blood flow (hypoperfusion, hematologic disorders, venous emboli, hypercoagulability, oral contraceptives, pregnancy, sickle cell disease, protein C or S deficiency, antithrombin III deficiency, lupus anticoagulant)

Cavernous sinus thrombosis: aseptic or septic (infection of sinus or face; rarely otitis or orbital cellulitis)
Findings: usually unilateral; orbital congestion, lacrimation, chemosis, eyelid swelling, ptosis, proptosis, ophthalmoplegia (CN 6 most common); may have corneal anesthesia, facial numbness, Horner's syndrome
Other findings: headache, nausea, vomiting, somnolence, fever, chills, evidence of meningitis or sepsis
Treatment: antibiotics, anticoagulants, corticosteroids, surgery

Lateral sinus thrombosis: usually septic from chronic otitis media
Findings: CN 6 palsy most common (severe facial pain [Gradenigo's syndrome] if compressed against petroclinoid ligament), papilledema
Other findings: symptoms of infection, neck pain, tenderness of ipsilateral jugular vein, retroauricular edema; may have facial weakness

Superior sagittal sinus (SSS) thrombosis: usually aseptic
Aseptic: occurs during pregnancy, immediately postpartum, or with oral contraceptives; risk factors include vasculitis and systemic inflammatory disorders

Septic: most commonly from meningitis; also paranasal sinus infection, pulmonary infection, tonsillitis, dental infection, pelvic inflammatory disease, and otitis media

Findings:

THROMBOSIS OF ANTERIOR THIRD OF SINUS: mild symptoms

THROMBOSIS OF POSTERIOR SINUS: may cause pseudotumor cerebri (headaches and papilledema; consider in pseudotumor that occurs in thin patients), seizures, altered mental status, focal neurologic signs; may be fatal from brain hemorrhage and herniation

Treatment: anticoagulation, fibrinolytic agents, ICP-lowering agents

Diagnosis: CT, MRI, MRA (venous phase)

INTRACRANIAL ARACHNOID CYST

Congenital malformation: CSF-filled cyst most commonly in middle cranial fossa (Sylvian fissure)

Findings: seizures, headaches, CN palsy, exophthalmos, hydrocephalus (compression of foramen of Munroe, aqueduct, or 4th ventricle), increased intracranial pressure, papilledema

Cyst rupture may cause subdural hematoma

Treatment: fenestration, shunt

NEURO-OPHTHALMIC MANIFESTATIONS OF AIDS

CNS Lymphoma

High-grade B-cell non-Hodgkin's lymphoma; second most common malignancy in AIDS

Findings: diplopia (from CN 3, 4, 6 involvement; may have disc swelling from infiltration of orbit and optic nerve)

Progressive Multifocal Leukencephalopathy (PML)

Papovavirus destroys oligodendrocytes; gray matter relatively spared; can affect central visual pathway and ocular motor fibers

Findings: ataxia, altered mental status, dementia, hemiparesis, focal neurologic defects

Diagnosis: MRI (demyelination; usually parieto-occipital areas, typically involves subcortical white matter with focal or confluent lesions; may see focal enhancement with contrast)

Treatment: none; death common within 6 months

1. The visual field defect most characteristic of optic neuritis is
   a. altitudinal
   b. central
   c. centrocecal
   d. arcuate

2. Which cranial nerve is most prone to injury in the cavernous sinus?
   a. 3
   b. 4
   c. 5
   d. 6

3. Which of the following agents is least toxic to the optic nerve?
   a. isoniazid
   b. dapsone
   c. methanol
   d. ethambutol

4. Seesaw nystagmus is produced by a lesion located in which area?
   a. chiasm
   b. posterior fossa
   c. suprasellar
   d. cervicomedullary junction

5. What is the location of a lesion that causes an ipsilateral Horner's syndrome and a contralateral CN 4 palsy?
   a. midbrain
   b. pons
   c. cavernous sinus
   d. orbit

6. The least useful test for functional visual loss is
   a. confrontation VF
   b. OKN
   c. HVF
   d. tangent screen at 1 m and 2 m

7. Optociliary shunt vessels may occur in all of the following conditions except
   a. chronic glaucoma
   b. CVO
   c. meningioma
   d. ischemic optic neuropathy

8. Which is not a symptom of pseudotumor cerebri?
   a. diplopia
   b. entoptic phenomena
   c. visual obscurations
   d. headache

9. A 63-year-old woman reports sudden onset of jagged lines in the right peripheral vision. She has experienced 3 episodes in the past month, which lasted approximately 10–20 minutes. She denies headaches and any history or family history of migraines. The most likely diagnosis is
   a. vertebrobasilar insufficiency
   b. occipital AVM
   c. migraine variant
   d. posterior vitreous detachment

10. A 60-year-old man with optic disc swelling in the right eye and left optic atrophy most likely has
    a. ischemic optic neuropathy
    b. left sphenoid ridge meningioma
    c. Leber's hereditary optic neuropathy
    d. left optic nerve glioma
11. Which of the following findings may not be present in a patient with an INO?
    a. dissociated horizontal nystagmus
    b. limitation of adduction
    c. absent convergence
    d. abnormal abduction saccades
12. A paradoxical pupillary reaction is not found in which condition?
    a. achromatopsia
    b. albinism
    c. Leber's congenital amaurosis
    d. optic nerve hypoplasia
13. Inheritance of Leber's optic neuropathy is
    a. sporadic
    b. autosomal dominant
    c. mitochondrial DNA
    d. X-linked recessive
14. An OKN strip moved to the left stimulates what part of the brain?
    a. right frontal, left occipital
    b. right frontal, right occipital
    c. left frontal, left occipital
    d. left frontal, right occipital
15. The smooth pursuit system does not involve the
    a. PPRF
    b. prestriate cortex
    c. occipital motor area
    d. frontal motor area
16. Dorsal midbrain syndrome is not associated with
    a. absent convergence
    b. gaze palsy
    c. light-near dissociation
    d. nystagmus
17. The location of Horner's syndrome is best differentiated by which drug?
    a. cocaine
    b. hydroxyamphetamine (Paredrine)
    c. pilocarpine 0.125%
    d. pilocarpine 1%
18. The blood supply to the prelaminar optic nerve is
    a. meningeal arteries
    b. ophthalmic artery
    c. short posterior ciliary arteries
    d. central retinal artery
19. Optic nerve hypoplasia is associated with all of the following except
    a. paradoxical pupillary response
    b. midline abnormalities
    c. maternal ingestion of LSD
    d. spasmus nutans
20. A lesion in the pons causes
    a. anisocoria
    b. miosis
    c. light-near dissociation
    d. mydriasis
21. Which of the following syndromes is characterized by abduction deficit and contralateral hemiplegia?
    a. Foville's
    b. Gradenigo's
    c. Millard-Gubler
    d. Weber's
22. All of the following are features of progressive supranuclear palsy except
    a. hypometric saccades
    b. loss of oculovestibular reflex
    c. full motility with doll's head maneuver
    d. limitation of downgaze
23. Pituitary apoplexy is characterized by all of the following except
    a. nystagmus
    b. facial numbness
    c. headache
    d. diplopia
24. Which of the following is most likely to produce a junctional scotoma?
    a. craniopharyngioma
    b. multiple sclerosis
    c. pituitary adenoma
    d. meningioma
25. All of the following are characteristics of an optic tract lesion except
    a. relative afferent pupillary defect
    b. decreased vision
    c. homonymous hemianopia
    d. optic nerve pallor
26. The saccade system does not involve the
    a. occipital motor area
    b. premotor cortex
    c. frontal motor area
    d. PPRF
27. A 22-year-old man sustains trauma resulting in a transected left optic nerve. Which of the following is true regarding the right pupil?
    a. it is larger than the left pupil
    b. it is smaller than the left pupil
    c. it is equal in size to the left pupil
    d. it reacts consensually
28. Characteristics of spasmus nutans include all of the following except
    a. spontaneously disappears within 3 years
    b. may mimic chiasmal glioma
    c. begins before 1 year of age
    d. signs present during sleep
29. A congenital CN 4 palsy can be distinguished from an acquired palsy by
    a. vertical fusional amplitude >10 Δ
    b. incyclotropia of 5°
    c. excyclotropia of 5°
    d. spontaneous head tilt to the opposite side
30. Characteristics of a diabetic CN 3 palsy may include all of the following except
    a. pain
    b. spontaneous recovery within 90 days
    c. sluggish pupillary response
    d. aberrant regeneration

31. A CN 3 lesion may cause all of the following except
    a. contralateral ptosis
    b. ipsilateral ptosis
    c. bilateral ptosis
    d. no ptosis
32. Optic nerve drusen is associated with all of the following except
    a. RP
    b. CRAO
    c. CME
    d. CNV
33. A lesion causing limited upgaze with an intact Bell's phenomenon is located where?
    a. supranuclear
    b. nuclear
    c. tract
    d. cavernous sinus
34. An acute subarachnoid hemorrhage due to a ruptured aneurysm may produce all of the following except
    a. ptosis
    b. orbital hemorrhage
    c. vitreous hemorrhage
    d. afferent pupillary defect
35. The length of the canalicular portion of the optic nerve is approximately
    a. 5 mm
    b. 10 mm
    c. 15 mm
    d. 20 mm
36. Findings in ocular motor apraxia include all of the following except
    a. abnormal OKN response
    b. abnormal pursuits
    c. head thrusting
    d. abnormal vestibular nystagmus
37. Which of the following statements is true regarding the optic chiasm?
    a. 55% of temporal retinal fibers remain uncrossed in the ipsilateral optic tract
    b. 45% of temporal retinal fibers cross to the contralateral optic tract
    c. 55% of nasal retinal fibers cross to the contralateral optic tract
    d. 45% of nasal retinal fibers cross to the contralateral optic tract
38. Which of the following statements is false regarding the lateral geniculate body (LGB)?
    a. M cells are important for stereoacuity
    b. LGB is part of the thalamus
    c. There is a 90° rotation of optic nerve fibers in the LGB
    d. P cells are important for motion detection
39. A patient with a homonymous hemianopia is found to have an asymmetric OKN response. The location of the lesion is
    a. parietal lobe
    b. occipital lobe
    c. temporal lobe
    d. lateral geniculate body

40. The only intact eye movement in 1½ syndrome is
    a. abduction of ipsilateral eye
    b. adduction of ipsilateral eye
    c. abduction of contralateral eye
    d. adduction of contralateral eye
41. A pineal tumor is most likely to cause
    a. Ballint's syndrome
    b. Fisher syndrome
    c. Nothnagel's syndrome
    d. Parinaud's syndrome
42. Metastatic neuroblastoma is most likely to be associated with
    a. opsoclonus
    b. ocular bobbing
    c. ocular dipping
    d. ocular myoclonus
43. Which of the following statements regarding pupillary innervation is true?
    a. sympathetic innervation of the iris sphincter involves 3 neurons from the Edinger-Westphal nucleus
    b. parasympathetic innervation of the iris sphincter involves 2 neurons and the ciliospinal center of Budge
    c. parasympathetic innervation of the iris dilator involves 2 neurons from the Edinger-Westphal nucleus
    d. sympathetic innervation of the iris dilator involves 3 neurons and the ciliospinal center of Budge
44. The most important test to order in a patient with chronic progressive external ophthalmoplegia is
    a. ERG
    b. electrocardiogram (EKG/ECG)
    c. EMG
    d. ESR
45. Pseudotumor cerebri is most likely to cause a palsy of which cranial nerve?
    a. 3
    b. 4
    c. 5
    d. 6
46. CT scan of a patient with visual loss shows a railroad-track sign. The most likely diagnosis is
    a. optic nerve glioma
    b. pituitary adenoma
    c. optic nerve meningioma
    d. craniopharyngioma
47. The most likely etiology of homonymous hemianopia with macular sparing is
    a. vascular
    b. infectious
    c. neoplastic
    d. traumatic
48. All of the following findings are associated with optic neuritis except
    a. abnormal color perception
    b. abnormal depth perception
    c. flashes of light with eye movements
    d. metamorphopsia

49. Which of the following findings is not associated with an acoustic neuroma
    a. lagophthalmos
    b. light-near dissociation
    c. decreased corneal sensation
    d. nystagmus
50. A superior oblique muscle palsy is most commonly caused by
    a. tumor
    b. multiple sclerosis
    c. aneurysm
    d. trauma
51. A 29-year-old obese woman with headaches, papilledema, and a normal head CT scan is diagnosed with idiopathic intracranial hypertension. All of the following findings are consistent with her diagnosis except
    a. visual obscurations
    b. homonymous hemianopia
    c. enlarged blind spot
    d. incomitant esotropia
52. Transection of the left optic nerve adjacent to the chiasm results in
    a. visual field defect in the right eye
    b. decreased corneal sensation in the right eye
    c. afferent pupillary defect in the right eye
    d. pseudoproptosis of the right eye
53. The Amsler grid viewed at 30 cm tests how many degrees of central vision?
    a. 5
    b. 10
    c. 15
    d. 30
54. Aberrant regeneration of CN 3 may cause all of the following except

a. lid elevation on abduction
b. pupillary constriction on adduction
c. monocular dampening of the OKN response
d. lid elevation on down gaze

55. A 42-year-old woman admitted to the hospital with severe headache and neck stiffness suddenly becomes disoriented and vomits. On examination her left pupil is dilated and does not react to light. She most likely has
    a. encephalitis
    b. meningitis
    c. brainstem herniation
    d. subarachnoid hemorrhage

SUGGESTED READINGS

American Academy of Ophthalmology: Neuro-ophthalmology, vol 5. San Francisco, AAO, 2012.

Burde RM, Savino PJ, Trobe JD: Clinical Decisions in Neuro-ophthalmology, 3rd edn. Philadelphia, Mosby, 2002.

Kline LB, Bajandas F: Neuro-ophthalmology Review Manual, 6th edn. Thorofare, NJ, Slack, 2007.

Liu GT, Volpe NJ, Galetta S: Neuro-ophthalmology Diagnosis and Management. Philadelphia, WB Saunders, 2001.

Loewenfeld IE, Lowenstein O: The Pupil Anatomy: Physiology and Clinical Applications, 2nd edn. Philadelphia, Butterworth-Heineman, 1999.

Milder B, Rubin ML, Weinstein GW: The Fine Art of Prescribing Glasses Without Making a Spectacle of Yourself. Gainesville, FL, Triad Scientific Publications, 1991.

Miller NR, Newman NJ: Walsh & Hoyt's Clinical Neuro-ophthalmology, 5th edn. Baltimore, MD, Lippincott Williams and Wilkins, 1999.

Walsh TJ: Neuro-ophthalmology: Clinical Signs and Symptoms, 4th edn. Baltimore, MD, Williams and Wilkins, 1997.

5

Pediatrics / Strabismus

Pediatrics

ANATOMY

At birth, diameter of eye is 66% that of adult eye

Eye enlarges until 2 years of age, then further growth in puberty (Table 5-1)

Infants have variable levels of astigmatism

Majority of children are hyperopic; increases up to 7 years of age, then diminishes

Eye color darkens during first few months of life

Dilator pupillae poorly developed at birth

Fovea matures during first few months of life
Myelinization of optic nerve completed shortly after birth

PHYSIOLOGY

Visual acuity levels (see Strabismus section)
  Documented by visual evoked potentials in infancy and preferential looking tests in first months of life

Premature infants reach landmarks later
Decreased vision in infants and children

History: family history, complications in pregnancy, perinatal problems

Examination: visual response (assess each eye independently), pupillary reactions (paradoxical response suggests achromatopsia, congenital stationary night blindness (CSNB), optic nerve hypoplasia), ocular motility (strabismus, nystagmus, torticollis), cycloplegic refraction, fundus examination

Additional tests: optokinetic (OKN) response, forced preferential looking, electroretinogram (ERG), visual evoked response (VEP, VER), ultrasonography, imaging studies

Differential diagnosis of infant with poor vision and normal ocular structures: Leber's congenital amaurosis, achromatopsia, blue cone monochromatism, CSNB, albinism, optic nerve hypoplasia, optic atrophy, congenital infection (TORCH syndrome), cortical visual impairment (due to extensive occipital lobe damage), delay in visual maturation

Table 5-1. Changes in ocular measurements with age		
Ocular dimensions	**Infant (mm)**	**Adult (mm)**
Axial length	17	24
Corneal diameter	9.5–10.5	12
Corneal radius of curvature	6.6–7.4	7.4–8.4
Scleral thickness	Half of adult	

ORBITAL DISORDERS

Congenital Anomalies

Anophthalmos

Bilateral absence of eye due to failure of primary optic vesicle to form; extremely rare

Findings: hypoplastic orbits

Buphthalmos

Large eye due to increased intraocular pressure in congenital glaucoma

Cryptophthalmos

Failure of differentiation of lid and anterior eye structures

Partial or complete absence of the eyebrow, palpebral fissure, eyelashes, and conjunctiva

Attenuation of the levator, orbicularis, tarsus, and conjunctiva

Often associated with severe ocular defects

Microphthalmos

Small, disorganized eye

Disruption of ocular development occurs after budding of optic vesicle

Usually unilateral

Microphthalmos with Cyst

Due to failure of embryonic fissure to close

Usually blue mass of lower lid

Associated with congenital rubella, congenital toxoplasmosis, maternal vitamin A deficiency, maternal thalidomide ingestion, trisomy 13, trisomy 15, and chromosome 18 deletion

Nanophthalmos

Small eye with normal features

Normal-sized lens and thickened sclera

Associated with hyperopia and angle-closure glaucoma

Increased risk of choroidal effusion during intraocular surgery

Infections

Preseptal Cellulitis

Infection anterior to orbital septum; spares globe

Largest risk factor is recent skin trauma

Most common organism: *Staphylococcus aureus*

Findings: lid edema, erythema, and pain; may have fever; may progress to orbital cellulitis

Treatment: systemic antibiotics (IV in severe cases, children <5 years old, and failed oral treatment)

Orbital Cellulitis

Infection posterior to orbital septum; involves globe

Most common cause of proptosis in children

Usually secondary to sinusitis (ethmoid sinus is most common)

Associated with subperiosteal abscesses

Etiology: extension of infection from periorbital structures, sinusitis, dacryocystitis, dacryoadenitis, endophthalmitis, dental infections, intracranial infections, trauma or previous surgery, endogenous (bacteremia with septic embolization)

Organisms: *S. aureus* (most common organism in children), *Streptococcus pneumoniae*, fungi (Phycomycetes, most aggressive)

Findings: fever, decreased vision, positive RAPD, proptosis, restriction of ocular motility, pain on eye movement, periorbital swelling, chemosis, optic disc swelling

CT scan: diagnosis, localization, and involvement of adjacent structures

Treatment: IV antibiotics, surgical drainage

Complications: subperiosteal abscess, cavernous sinus thrombosis, or intracranial extension causing blindness or death

Benign Lesions

Dermoid Cyst (Choristoma)

Arises from dermal elements (neural crest origin)

Lined by keratinizing epithelium with dermal appendages

Most common orbital mass in childhood

Usually located in superotemporal quadrant near brow, often adjacent to bony suture

Often filled with keratin

Generally do not enlarge after 1 year of age

May induce bony erosion

Rupture can cause intense inflammatory reaction

CT scan: well circumscribed with bony molding

Treatment: complete excision, remove en bloc because contents may cause granulomatous inflammation

Epidermoid Cyst (Choristoma)

Arises from epidermal elements

Lined by epidermis only (no dermal appendages)

Usually filled with keratin

Rupture can lead to an acute inflammatory process

Lipodermoid

Solid tumor usually located beneath the conjunctiva over lateral surface of globe

May appear similar to prolapsed orbital fat, prolapsed lacrimal gland, or lymphoma

Usually no treatment is needed

Difficult to excise completely

Teratoma

Rare, cystic tumor arising from 2 or more germinal layers

Usually composed of ectoderm along with either endoderm or mesoderm (or both)

Can cause dramatic proptosis at birth

Rarely malignant

Capillary Hemangioma

Most common benign tumor of the orbit in children

Often manifests in the first few weeks of life and enlarges over the first 6 to 12 months, with complete regression by age 5–8 years in 80% of cases

Spontaneous involution over the next few years

Predilection for the superior nasal quadrant of the orbit and medial upper eyelid

Female > male (3:2)

Diffuse irregular mass of plump endothelial cells and small vascular channels

High-flow lesion

Findings:
Strawberry nevus: skin involvement; appears as red, irregularly dimpled, elevated surface; blanches with direct pressure (port wine stain does not blanch)
Orbital location: can present with proptosis; bluish appearance of eyelids and conjunctiva

Pathology: numerous blood-filled channels lined by endothelium; little contribution from larger vessels or stroma; unencapsulated (Figure 5-1)

CT/MRI scan: well-circumscribed lesion

Treatment: required if tumor causing ptosis or astigmatism with resultant anisometropia, strabismus, or amblyopia. Options include observation, intralesional steroid injection, systemic steroids, interferon, laser, radiation, or excision

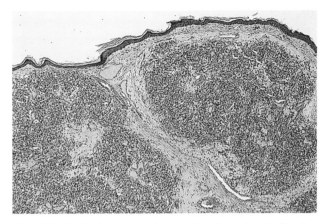

Figure 5-1. Capillary hemangioma demonstrating abnormal proliferation of blood vessels and endothelial cells. (From Yanoff M, Fine BS: Ocular Pathology, 5th edn, St Louis, Mosby, 2002.)

Complications:
Eyelid involvement may cause: ptosis with occlusion amblyopia, astigmatism and anisometropia with refractive amblyopia, strabismus with strabismic amblyopia
Kassabach-Merritt syndrome: consumptive coagulopathy with platelet trapping, resulting in thrombocytopenia and cardiac failure; acute hemorrhage is possible; mortality approximately 30%
High-output congestive heart failure can occur with multiple visceral capillary hemangiomas
Respiratory compromise with subglottic hemangiomas

Lymphangioma

Rare, lymphatic-filled choristoma

Often superonasal

Appears in first decade of life

Involves the eyelids, conjunctiva, and deeper orbital tissues
Lesion waxes and wanes, but does not involute

Findings: acute pain, proptosis (often increasing with upper respiratory infection), bluish hue to overlying lid, may hemorrhage into channels (chocolate cyst)

Pathology: lymph-filled vascular channels lined by endothelium; unencapsulated (Figure 5-2)

CT scan: may show layered blood in a lobular, cystic mass with infiltrative pattern

MRI: infiltrating pattern with indistinct margins

Treatment: observation (spontaneous regression common); rarely surgical evacuation because complete excision difficult and recurrence common

Complications: anisometropia, amblyopia, strabismus

Varix

Most common vascular abnormality

Dilations of preexisting venous channels

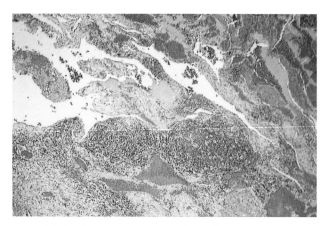

Figure 5-2. Lymphangioma demonstrating lymph-filled spaces, some with blood. (From Yanoff M, Fine BS: Ocular Pathology, 5th edn, St Louis, Mosby, 2002.)

Findings: proptosis (increases with crying or straining; can occur when head is in a dependent position), orbital hemorrhage (especially after trauma), motility disturbance (usually restricted upgaze), disc swelling, optic atrophy

Radiograph: phlebolith present in 30% of cases

Treatment: surgery
  Indications: cosmetic, severe proptosis, optic nerve compression, pain; surgery is often difficult because of intertwining of normal structures and direct communication with cavernous sinus

Fibrous Dysplasia

Tumor of fibrous connective tissue, cartilage, and bone
Progressive disease of childhood and young adulthood
Monostotic (in young adults) or polyostotic

Orbital involvement: usually monostotic; frontal (most common), sphenoid, and ethmoid bones; causes unilateral proptosis during first 2 decades of life

Polyostotic: multiple bones involved; can cause narrowing of optic canal and lacrimal drainage system

Albright's syndrome: polyostotic fibrous dysplasia, short stature, premature closure of epiphysis, precocious puberty, and hyperpigmented macules
  Findings: diplopia, proptosis, headaches, facial asymmetry, decreased visual acuity (compromised optic canal), hearing loss (compromised external ear canal)
  Pathology: normal bone is replaced by immature woven bone and osteoid in a cellular fibrous matrix, stroma of the bone is highly vascularized, no osteoblasts present

Neurofibroma

Hamartoma
18% have neurofibromatosis (NF) type 1
Nearly all adults with NF 1 have neurofibromas

Plexiform neurofibroma: most commonly involves the upper lid; tortuous, fibrous cords infiltrate orbital tissues

Nodular: firm and rubbery consistency

Findings: often involves eyelid or causes proptosis, may cause glaucoma

Pathology: well-circumscribed, nonencapsulated proliferation of Schwann cells, perineural cells, and axons; stains with S-100 (specific for neural crest–derived structures) (Figure 5-3)

Treatment: surgical excision

Optic Nerve Glioma (Grade I Astrocytoma)

Considered pilocytic astrocytoma of the juvenile type
Slow-growing hamartoma derived from interstitial cells, astroglia, and oligodendroglia
Usually does not metastasize
Usually appears during first decade of life
Associated with neurofibromatosis (25–50%)

Findings: unilateral proptosis, loss of vision, strabismus, and papilledema; may develop retinal vascular occlusions, optociliary shunt vessels; orbital tumors may cause chorioretinal folds, optic disc swelling, or atrophy; chiasmal tumors may cause pituitary or hypothalamic dysfunction, and nystagmus and head nodding from compression of 3rd ventricle

Pathology: circumscribed astrocytic tumor from neural crest tissue, glial hypercellularity, Rosenthal fibers, myxomatous, arachnoid hyperplasia; reactive meningothelial hyperplasia may occur, which can lead to a false diagnosis of meningioma

CT scan: fusiform enlargement of ON, enlargement of optic foramen, bony erosion

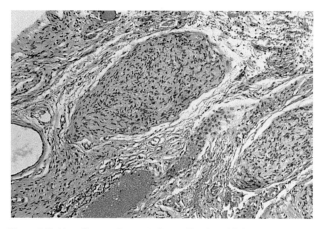

Figure 5-3. Neurofibroma demonstrating proliferation of Schwann cells. (From Yanoff M, Fine BS: Ocular Pathology, 5th edn, St Louis, Mosby, 2002.)

Treatment: observation; consider surgery if tumor spreads posteriorly into the chiasm

Prognosis: in adults, tumor is malignant with death occurring in 6–12 months; better prognosis in children or in adults with neurofibromatosis

Idiopathic Orbital Inflammation (Orbital Pseudotumor [IOI])

Idiopathic inflammatory disorder of orbit

Commonly bilateral with episodic recurrence

Findings: decreased vision, diplopia, red eye, headache; acute, painful presentation in children; resembles orbital cellulitis

Other findings: constitutional symptoms in 50%

Treatment: systemic steroids

Graves' Disease

(Occasionally occurs in adolescents; see Ch. 6, Orbit/Lids/Adnexa.)

Malignant Neoplasms

Rhabdomyosarcoma

Most common primary orbital malignancy of children

Most common soft tissue malignancy of childhood

Most common mesenchymal tumor of orbit

Malignant spindle cell tumor with loose myxomatous matrix

Average age at diagnosis is 8 years old (90% before age 16)

Cell of origin is an undifferentiated, pluripotent cell of the soft tissue; does *not* originate from the extraocular muscles

Unilateral; tends to involve superonasal portion of orbit

More common in males (5:3)

Aggressive local spread through orbital bones; hematogenous spread to lungs and cervical lymph nodes; most common location for metastasis is chest

Findings: rapidly progressive proptosis, reddish discoloration of eyelid; may have ptosis; later develop tortuous retinal veins, choroidal folds, and optic nerve edema

Types:
Embryonal: most common (70%), usually occurs in children; tumor appears circumscribed, but often there is microscopic evidence of invasion of nearby structures
   PATHOLOGY: elongated spindle cell with central hyperchromatic nucleus, eosinophilic granular

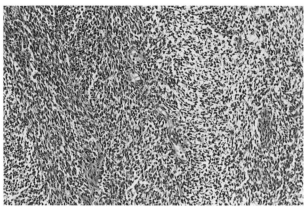

A

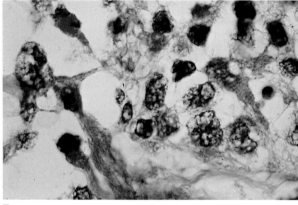

B

Figure 5-4. A, Embryonal type demonstrating primitive rhabdomyoblasts. **B,** Cross-striations in cytoplasm of some cells. (From Yanoff M, Fine BS: Ocular Pathology, 5th edn, St Louis, Mosby, 2002.)

   cytoplasm; cells arranged in parallel palisading bands; obvious cross-striations are rare (Figure 5-4)
Botryoid: subtype of embryonal; can occur in anterior orbit, embryonal rhabomyosarcoma abutting a mucosal surface, multiple polypoid masses protruding from hollow viscera
Pleomorphic: least common, usually occurs in adults, rare involvement of orbit, most differentiated, best prognosis
   PATHOLOGY: dense spindle cell arrangement with enlarged cells containing hyperchromatic nuclei, deeply eosinophilic cytoplasm; may see cross-striations on microscopic examination
Alveolar: poorest prognosis, usually found in inferior orbit, generally arises in extremities (adolescents)
   PATHOLOGY: dense cellular proliferations of loosely cohesive small round cells separated by connective tissue septa; lack of cohesiveness may explain metastatic potential

CT scan: well-circumscribed orbital mass with possible extension into adjacent orbital bones or sinuses, bony destruction

A-scan ultrasound: orbital mass with medium internal reflectivity

Treatment: urgent biopsy, radiation (100% local control with 6000 cGy; 30% mortality due to metastases), chemotherapy for any microscopic metastases, surgical debulking

Prognosis: with chemotherapy and XRT, 3-year survival = 90%; cure rate close to 100% with localized orbital tumor; 60% if invasion of adjacent structures

Tumors arising in the orbit, bladder, and prostate: 77% disease-free survival at 2 years
Intrathoracic tumors: worst prognosis, 24% disease-free survival at 2 years

Neuroblastoma

Most common metastatic orbital tumor of childhood

Usually originates in the adrenal gland or sympathetic ganglion chain, also mediastinum or neck

40% develop orbital metastases

Average age of presentation with metastatic neuroblastoma to orbit is 2 years old
Spontaneous regression is rare

Findings: sudden proptosis and periorbital ecchymosis (raccoon eyes); may have ipsilateral Horner's syndrome and opsoclonus (better prognosis)

Paraneoplastic syndrome associated with metastatic neuroblastoma: opsoclonus (saccadomania; random, rapid eye movements in all directions that disappear during sleep)

Pathology: sheets of indiscrete round cells with scant cytoplasm and high mitotic figures, areas of tumor necrosis; can have bony invasion; usually positive for neuronal markers (synaptophysin and neuron-specific enolase) (Figure 5-5)

CT scan: bony destruction

Treatment: chemotherapy and local XRT

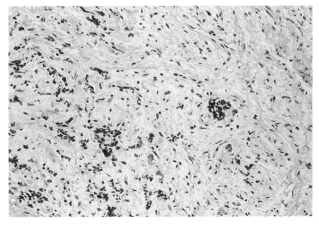

Figure 5-5. Neuroblastoma. (Case presented by Dr E. Torcynski at the meeting of the Eastern Ophthalmic Society, 1994. From Yanoff M, Fine BS: Ocular Pathology, 5th edn, St Louis, Mosby, 2002.)

Prognosis: poor if age of onset is over 1 year with metastases to bone; however, metastases to just liver, bone marrow, or spleen can be associated with a survival rate as high as 84%

Accounts for 15% of all childhood cancer deaths

In adults, neuroblastoma usually metastasizes to the uveal tract

Ewing's Sarcoma

Second most frequent metastatic tumor to the orbit

Primary intermedullary malignancy of bone; originates in long bones of extremities or axial skeleton

Frequently metastasizes to bone and lungs

Occurs in 2nd-3rd decade of life

Findings: acute proptosis, hemorrhage, and inflammation from tumor necrosis

Treatment: chemotherapy

Granulocytic Sarcoma ('Chloroma')

Patients with myelogenous leukemia may present with orbital signs before hematologic evidence of leukemia

Findings: proptosis, may have subcutaneous periocular mass

Pathology: infiltration of involved tissues by leukemic cells

Treatment: radiotherapy, chemotherapy

Histiocytosis X

Group of disorders resulting from abnormal proliferation of histiocytes (Langerhans' cells) that may involve orbit

Spectrum of disease, from isolated bone lesions with excellent prognosis (eosinophilic granuloma) to systemic spread with rapid death (Letterer-Siwe disease)

Children under age 2 with multifocal disease have a poor prognosis (50% survival rate)

Findings: most frequent orbital presentation is lytic defect of orbital roof causing progressive proptosis

Pathology: granulomatous histiocytic infiltrate, Birbeck granules (central, dense core, and thick outer shell), stains positively for S-100 and vimentin

Eosinophilic granuloma: Benign, local, solitary bone lesion
Most likely to involve superior temporal bony orbit in childhood or adolescence
CT SCAN AND X-RAY: sharply demarcated osteolytic lesions
TREATMENT: incision and curettage, intralesional steroids, or radiotherapy

Hand-Schüller-Christian disease:
Triad of proptosis, lytic skull defects, and diabetes insipidus

More aggressive

Multifocal bony lesions; frequently involves orbit, usually superolaterally

TREATMENT: systemic steroids and chemotherapy

PATHOLOGY: good

Letterer-Siwe disease:

Most severe and malignant

Progressive and fatal

Multisystem involvement

Rarely ocular/orbital involvement

PATHOLOGY: systemic steroids and chemotherapy

Burkitt's Lymphoma

Primarily affects the maxilla in black children, with secondary invasion of the orbit

Related to Epstein-Barr virus infection

Findings: proptosis and bony destruction

Pathology: malignant B cells, 'starry sky' appearance due to histiocytes interspersed among uniform background of lymphocytes

CRANIOFACIAL DISORDERS

Structural development of head and face occur during 4th–8th week of gestation

Ocular motility disturbances occur in 75% of patients with craniofacial disorders

Craniofacial cleft syndromes: 1 or more facial fissures fail to close during the 6th–7th week of gestation

Ocular complications: Corneal exposure from proptosis or lid defects

Refractive errors from lid anomalies

Ocular motility disturbances, most commonly exotropia

Papilledema and optic atrophy from increased intracranial pressure (ICP) or fibrous dysplasia involving optic canal

Ocular anomalies from embryogenesis

Syndromes

Treacher-Collins Syndrome (Mandibulofacial Dysostosis)

Hypoplasia of the midface

Associated with dental and ear abnormalities, microtia, micrognathia, hypoplastic malar bones, and low sideburns

Findings: lateral lid defects, absent lateral canthal tendon, absent medial lashes, antimongoloid slant, ectropion, poorly developed puncta and meibomian glands

Goldenhar's Syndrome (Oculoauriculovertebral Dysplasia)

Abnormalities of the 1st and 2nd brachial arches

Findings: limbal dermoids and dermolipomas; may have lower lid colobomas

Other findings: hypoplastic facial bones, pretragal auricular appendages, vertebral abnormalities; may have fistulas between the mouth and ear

Associated with Duane's syndrome

Hypertelorism

Findings: increased interpupillary distance due to increased distance between medial orbital walls

Associated with blepharophimosis, frontal meningoceles, encephaloceles, meningoencephaloceles, and fibrous dysplasia

Craniosynostoses

Premature closure of bony sutures; inhibits growth of the cranium perpendicular to the axis of the suture; growth can continue parallel to the suture

Findings: hypertelorism; proptosis can also occur

Plagiocephaly: premature closure of one-half of the coronal sutures

Skull develops normally on one side and is underdeveloped on the other side (resulting in a flattened face)

Other findings: midfacial hypoplasia, proptosis, telecanthus, V-pattern XT, oral and dental abnormalities, and respiratory problems

Crouzon's Syndrome (Craniofacial Dysostosis) (autosomal dominant [AD] or Sporadic)

Absence of forward development of the cranium and midface

Multiple combinations of suture closure can occur

Findings: proptosis, V-pattern exotropia, nystagmus, hypertelorism; shallow orbits; optic atrophy (in 25–50%; due to narrowing of optic canal, kinking or stretching of optic nerve)

Other findings: mental retardation, hypoplasia of maxilla, parrot's beak nose, high arched palate, external auditory canal atresia, anodonia

Apert's Syndrome (AD)

Crouzon's plus syndactyly

Anterior megalophthalmos

Associated with increased paternal age

Pfeiffer's Syndrome (AD)

Findings: hypertelorism and pointy head; may have shallow orbits, syndactyly, and short digits

Carpenter's Syndrome (autosomal recessive [AR])

Severe mental retardation

Involvement of sagittal, lambdoidal, and coronal sutures

Median Facial Cleft Syndrome

Findings: hypertelorism, exotropia

Other findings: medial cleft nose, lip, palate; widow's peak; cranium bifidum occultum

Waardenburg's Syndrome (AD)

Findings: lateral displacement of inner canthi/puncta, confluent eyebrows, heterochromia iridis, fundus hypopigmentation

Other findings: sensorineural deafness, white forelock

Hemifacial Microsomia

Findings: upper lid coloboma, strabismus

Other findings: facial asymmetry with microtia, macrostomia, mandibular anomalies, orbital dystopia, ear tags, vertebral anomalies

Hallermann-Streiff Syndrome

Sporadic

Findings: bilateral cataracts, glaucoma, microphakia, microcornea

Other findings: mandibular hypoplasia, beaked nose

Pierre Robin Sequence

Findings: retinal detachment, congenital glaucoma and/or cataracts, high myopia

Other findings: micrognathia, glossoptosis, cleft palate
Associated with Stickler's syndrome

Fetal Alcohol Syndrome

Findings: short palpebral fissures, telecanthus, epicanthal folds, comitant strabismus, optic disc anomalies; may have high myopia, anterior segment anomalies

Other findings: thin vermilion border of upper lip, variable mental retardation, small birth weight and height, cardiovascular and skeletal abnormalities

LID DISORDERS

Ablepharon

Absence of lids

Ankyloblepharon

Partial or complete fusion of lid margins; usually temporal, often bilateral

Often AD

Associated with craniofacial abnormalities

Can be secondary to thermal or chemical burns, inflammation, ocular cicatricial pemphigoid, Stevens-Johnson syndrome

Blepharophimosis

Horizontally and vertically shortened palpebral fissures with poor levator function

Absent lid crease

May be part of autosomal dominant syndrome (chromosome 3q) with ptosis, telecanthus, epicanthus inversus, lower lid ectropion, hypoplasia of nasal bridge and superior orbital rim, anteverted ears, hypertelorism

Treatment: surgical correction requires multiple procedures

Coloboma

Embryologic cleft involving lid margin; unilateral or bilateral; partial or full thickness

Ranges from notch to absence of entire lid

Upper lid: usually medial third, not associated with systemic abnormalities, usually full thickness

Lower lid: usually lateral third, associated with other abnormalities (Treacher-Collins, Goldenhar's syndromes), usually partial thickness
May have exposure keratitis

Treatment: method of surgical repair depends on size of defect (see section on Lid avulsion)

Congenital Blepharoptosis

Droopy eyelid; 75% unilateral; nonhereditary
Rarely causes amblyopia
Associated with blepharophimosis syndrome (AD)
Myogenic is most common

Etiology:
Myogenic:
   Dysgenesis of levator muscle
   Fibroadipose tissue in muscle belly
   Poor levator function, loss of lid crease, eyelid lag, sometimes lagophthalmos
Aponeurotic:
   Rare, possibly due to birth trauma
   Good eyelid excursion, high or indistinct lid crease

Neurogenic:
> Congenital CN 3 palsy
> Marcus Gunn jaw-winking (aberrant connections between motor division of CN 5 and levator muscle; jaw movements cause elevation of ptotic lid)

Congenital Horner's Syndrome

Ptosis, miosis, anhydrosis

May cause amblyopia

Treatment: surgical repair (levator resection), severe cases require frontalis sling

Congenital Ectropion

Eversion of eyelid margin due to vertical shortening of anterior lamella

Etiology: inclusion conjunctivitis, anterior lamella inflammation, Down's syndrome
Associated with blepharophimosis syndrome

Treatment: usually not required; otherwise, treat as the cicatricial form

Congenital Entropion

Inversion of eyelid margin

Etiology: lid retractor dysgenesis, tarsal plate defects, vertical shortening of posterior lamella

Usually involves lower eyelid

Treatment: may require surgical repair

Congenital Tarsal Kink

Upper eyelid bent back and open with complete fold of tarsal plate

May cause corneal abrasion and exposure keratopathy

Distichiasis

Partial or complete accessory row of eyelashes growing from or posterior to meibomian orifices

Due to improper differentiation of pilosebaceous units

Usually well tolerated, but trichiasis may develop

Treatment: lubrication, cryoepilation, surgical epilation

Epiblepharon

Pretarsal skin and orbicularis override the lid margin, causing a horizontal fold of tissue to push cilia vertically; no entropion

Most common among Asians

Usually occurs in lower lid and resolves spontaneously

Rarely requires surgery (excision of skin and muscle for significant trichiasis)

Epicanthus

Medial canthal vertical skin folds

Due to immature facial bones or redundant skin
Usually bilateral

Produces pseudoesotropia

Types:
Epicanthus tarsalis:
> Fold most prominent in upper eyelid
> Commonly associated with Asian eyelid
Epicanthus inversus:
> Fold most prominent in lower eyelid
> Associated with blepharophimosis syndrome
Epicanthus palpebralis:
> Fold is equally distributed in upper and lower eyelids
Epicanthus supraciliaris:
> Fold arises from eyebrow and extends to lacrimal sac

Euryblepharon

Horizontal widening of palpebral fissure due to inferior insertion of lateral canthal tendon

Associated with ectropion of lateral third of lid
Poor lid closure with exposure keratitis

Treatment: lubrication, may require surgical repair with resection of excess lid, lateral canthal tendon repositioning, and vertical eyelid lengthening

Microblepharon

Vertical shortening of lids

May have exposure keratitis

Telecanthus

Widened intercanthal distance due to long medial canthal tendons

Associated with fetal alcohol, Waardenburg's, and blepharophimosis syndromes

Treatment: surgery with transnasal wiring

LACRIMAL DISORDERS

Developmental Anomalies

Atresia of lacrimal puncta: ranges from thin membrane over punctal site to atresia of canaliculus

Supernumerary puncta: no treatment needed

Lacrimal fistula: usually located inferonasal to the medial canthus

Dacryocystocele

Cystic swelling of lacrimal sac accompanies obstruction of lacrimal drainage system above and below the sac

Presents at birth as bluish swelling inferior and nasal to medial canthus

Infection (dacryocystitis) develops if condition does not resolve spontaneously

Common organisms: *Haemophilus influenzae, S. pneumoniae, Staphylococcus, Klebsiella, Pseudomonas*

Treatment: digital massage, lacrimal probing, or surgical decompression (for dacryocystitis)

Nasolacrimal Duct Obstruction (NLDO)

Up to 5% of infants have obstruction of the NLD, usually due to membrane covering valve of Hasner

Most open spontaneously within 4–6 weeks of birth; ⅓ are bilateral

Findings: tearing, discharge; may develop dacryocystitis or conjunctivitis

Digital pressure over lacrimal sac producing mucoid reflux indicates obstruction of nasolacrimal duct

May have a dacryocystocele (dilated lacrimal sac), or amniotic fluid or mucus trapped in tear sac

Treatment: lacrimal sac massage, topical antibiotic, probing and irrigation by 13 months of age (95% cure rate); consider turbinate infracture and silicone intubation if probing unsuccessful; dacryocystorhinostomy (DCR) after multiple failures

CONJUNCTIVAL DISORDERS

Ocular Melanocytosis

Unilateral excessive pigment in uvea, sclera, and episclera

Increase in number of normal melanocytes

More common among Caucasians

Findings: slate grey appearance of sclera, darkened appearance of fundus

When associated with pigmentation of eyelid skin, called nevus of Ota (congenital oculodermal melanocytosis; more common among African Americans and Asians; malignant potential only in Caucasians)

Other findings: heterochromia iridis due to diffuse nevus of uvea; may develop glaucoma (due to melanocytes in trabecular meshwork), rarely uveal, orbital, or meningeal melanoma

Pathology: spindle-shaped pigment cells in subepithelial tissue

Conjunctivitis

Ophthalmia Neonatorum

Conjunctivitis within first month of life

Papillary conjunctivitis (no follicular reaction in neonate due to immaturity of immune system)

Etiology:

Chemical: caused by silver nitrate 1% solution (Crede's prophylaxis); occurs in first 24 hours, lasts 24 to 36 hours (therefore, prophylaxis is now with erythromycin or tetracycline ointment)
  FINDINGS: usually bilateral, bulbar injection with clear watery discharge
  No treatment necessary

Neisseria gonorrheae: days 1–2; can occur earlier with premature rupture of membranes
  FINDINGS: severe purulent discharge, chemosis, eyelid edema; can be hemorrhagic; may develop corneal ulceration or perforation
  DIAGNOSIS: Gram's stain (Gram-negative intracellular diplococci)
  TREATMENT: IV ceftriaxone × 7 days; bacitracin ointment topically
  High incidence of *Chlamydia* coinfection; therefore, also use oral erythromycin syrup and treat mother and sexual partners

Other bacteria: days 4–5; *Staphylococci, Streptococci, Haemophilus, Enterococci*
  TREATMENT: bacitracin, erythromycin, or gentamicin ointment; fortified antibiotics for *Pseudomonas*

HSV: days 5–14; type 2 in 70%
  FINDINGS: serous discharge, conjunctival injection, keratitis; may have vesicular lid lesions
  Can have systemic herpetic infection
  DIAGNOSIS: conjunctival scrapings with multinucleated giant cells; cultures take 5–7 days
  TREATMENT: Zirgan 5×/d or Viroptic q2h × 1 week; acyclovir 10 mg/kg IV tid × 10 days

Chlamydia (neonatal inclusion conjunctivitis): days 5–14; most common infectious cause of neonatal conjunctivitis
  FINDINGS: acute, mucopurulent, papillary (no follicles until 3 months of age); may have pseudomembranes
  Associated with pneumonitis, otitis, nasopharyngitis, gastritis
  DIAGNOSIS: intracytoplasmic inclusions on Giemsa stain
  TREATMENT: topical erythromycin, oral erythromycin syrup × 2–3 weeks (125 mg/kg/day qid) to prevent pneumonitis (onset 3–13 weeks later); treat mother and sexual partners with doxycycline 100 mg bid × 1 week (do not use in nursing mothers)
  Rule out concomitant *Gonococcus* infection

DDx: trauma, foreign body, corneal abrasion, congenital glaucoma, NLDO, dacryocystitis

Prophylaxis: tetracycline 1% or erythromycin 0.5% ointment at birth

Other Infections

Pediatric conjunctivitis is usually bacterial (50–80%) vs. adult infectious conjunctivitis, which is usually viral

Age dependent; more common in younger children (<3 years old)

Organisms: *H. influenzae* (50–65%), *S. pneumoniae* (20-30%), *Moraxella catarrhalis* (10%); rarely *Streptococcus pyogenes* or *S. aureus*

Findings: purulent discharge (80%), red eye (50%)

Other findings: otitis media (30% in <3 year olds; *H. influenzae*), preseptal cellulitis (>3 year olds with sinusitis, fever, and elevated WBCs; *S. pneumoniae*)

Diagnosis: culture refractory cases and neonates

Treatment: topical antibiotics; oral antibiotics (cefixime) for extraocular involvement (otitis media, sinusitis)

Vernal Keratoconjunctivitis

Form of seasonal (warm months), allergic conjunctivitis

Male > female (2:1); onset by age 10 years, lasts 2–10 years, usually resolves by puberty

Associated with atopic dermatitis (75%) or family history of atopy (66%)

Limbal vernal: more common among African Americans

Symptoms: intense itching, photophobia, pain

Findings: large upper tarsal papillae (cobblestones), minimal conjunctival hyperemia, Horner-Trantas' dots (elevated white accumulations of eosinophils at limbus), limbal follicles (gelatinous nodules at limbus), copious ropy mucus; may have pseudomembrane, keratitis, micropannus, shield ulcer (central oval epithelial defect with white fibrin coating); high levels of histamine and IgE in tears

Pathology: chronic papillary hypertrophy, epithelial hypertrophy then atrophy, conjunctiva contains many mast cells, eosinophils, and basophils

Treatment: topical allergy medication and steroids; consider topical ciclosporin (cyclosporine)

Ligneous

Rare, bilateral, pseudomembranous conjunctivitis in children; commonly young girls

Acute onset, chronic course

Etiology: appears to be exaggerated response to tissue injury following infection, surgery, or trauma

Findings: unilateral or bilateral highly vascularized, raised, friable lesion; with continued inflammation, a white, thickened avascular woody (ligneous) mass appears above the neovascular membrane, usually on palpebral conjunctiva; easily removed but bleeds; may recur

Process affects all mucous membranes (mouth, vagina, etc)

Pathology: acellular eosinophilic hyaline material (immunoglobulins, primarily IgG), granulation tissue, cellular infiltration (T cells, mast cells, eosinophils)

Treatment: complete excision (expect significant bleeding); any remaining portion of lesion results in rapid recurrence because retained lesion acts as physical barrier to topical medications; ENT evaluation before surgery to ensure respiratory tract not involved because many require general anesthesia

Postexcision: topical steroids every hour; hyaluronidase, acetylcysteine, and α-chymotrypsin every 4 hours; topical antibiotic; topical cyclosporine (ciclosporin) 2% (applied to surgical bed with sterile cotton-tipped applicator); oral prednisone (1mg/kg/day); daily débridement of any recurrence

Kawasaki's Disease (Mucocutaneous Lymph Node Syndrome)

Systemic childhood inflammatory disease/vasculitis with prominent mucocutaneous manifestations

Occurs in children <5 years old

More common among individuals of Japanese descent Epidemics suggest exposure to causal agent; siblings have 10∞ increased risk

More than 50% of familial cases occur within 10 days after onset of 1st case

Diagnostic criteria (requires 5 of 6): fever, bilateral conjunctivitis (90%), mild bilateral nongranulomatous uveitis (80%), rash, cervical lymphadenopathy, oral lesions (fissures, strawberry tongue), lesions of extremities (edema, erythema, desquamation)
Associated with polyarteritis

Treatment: aspirin; systemic steroids contraindicated (increased risk of coronary artery aneurysm)

Prognosis: 0.3% mortality

Complications: 15% develop coronary arteritis (can lead to coronary artery aneurysm or myocardial infarction)

Tumors

Epibulbar Osseous Choristoma

Hard mass, composed of mature bone

Usually located on bulbar conjunctiva (superotemporal fornix)

Does not enlarge

Not associated with other osteomas

No malignant potential

Treatment: observe or excise

Complex Choristoma

May contain cartilage, ectopic lacrimal gland tissue, smooth muscle, sweat glands, sebaceous glands, hair

Isolated or associated with linear nevus sebaceous syndrome

Ectopic Lacrimal Gland

Fleshy, vascularized tumor with raised translucent nodules

Usually extends into corneal stroma

Mild growth during puberty

Pathology: lacrimal gland parenchyma

Treatment: excision

CORNEAL DISORDERS

Anterior Megalophthalmos

Large anterior segment of eye

Associations: Marfan's syndrome, mucolipidosis type II, Apert's syndrome

Findings: high myopia and astigmatism; enlarged cornea, lens, iris, and ciliary ring; iris transillumination defects, lens dislocation, cataract

Congenital Corneal Staphyloma

Protuberant corneal opacity due to intrauterine keratitis

Findings: atrophic iris adheres to back of markedly thickened, scarred, and vascularized cornea; lens may be adherent to posterior cornea; cornea may perforate

Cornea Plana (AD or AR)

Mapped to chromosome 12q

Associations: sclerocornea, microcornea, and angle-closure glaucoma

Findings: flat cornea with curvature equaling that of sclera (usually 20–30 D), diffuse scarring and vascularization; may have coloboma, cataract, sclerocornea, shallow anterior chamber (AC), refractive error

Pathology: thickened epithelium, absent basement membrane, very thin Descemet's, anterior third of stroma is scarred and vascularized

Megalocornea

Horizontal diameter of cornea greater than 12 mm in newborn (>13 mm in adult)

Nonprogressive; most commonly X-linked (associated with anterior megalophthalmos), bilateral, 90% male; also AR

Associations: Marfan's syndrome, Alport's syndrome, Down's syndrome, dwarfism, craniosynostosis, facial hemiatrophy

Findings: large cornea; may have weak zonules, lens subluxation, hypoplastic iris, and ectopic pupil

Complications: ectopia lentis (enlarged limbal ring stretches the zonular fibers), glaucoma (due to angle abnormalities), cataract (PSC)

Microcornea

Corneal diameter less than 9 mm in newborn (<10 mm in adult)

Autosomal dominant or sporadic; unilateral or bilateral

Etiology: arrested corneal growth after 5th month of fetal development

Associations: dwarfism, Ehlers-Danlos syndrome

Findings: small cornea; often hyperopic (relatively flat corneas); may have cataract, coloboma, persistent hyperplastic primary vitreous (PHPV), microphakia; may develop angle-closure glaucoma or primary open-angle glaucoma (POAG)

DDx: nanophthalmos (small but structurally normal eye), anterior microphthalmos (small anterior segment), microphthalmos (small malformed eye)

Posterior Keratoconus

Discrete posterior corneal indentation with stromal haze and thinning

Female > male

Nonprogressive, usually central and unilateral

Anterior corneal surface is normal

Vision usually good; causes irregular astigmatism

Pathology: loss of stromal substance; Descemet's membrane may be thinned, but both it and endothelium are intact

Anterior Segment Dysgenesis (Mesodermal Dysgenesis Syndromes)

Bilateral, congenital, hereditary disorders affecting anterior segment structures

Axenfeld's anomaly: posterior embryotoxon (anteriorly displaced Schwalbe's line; found in 15% of normal individuals) with iris processes to scleral spur; 50% develop glaucoma; AD; mapped to chromosomes 4q25 (*RIEG1*), 13q14 (*RIEG2*), 6p25(*FOXC1*), 11p13 (*PAX6*)

Alagille's syndrome: Axenfeld's plus pigmentary retinopathy, corectopia, esotropia, and systemic abnormalities (absent deep tendon reflexes, abnormal facies, pulmonic valvular stenosis, peripheral arterial stenosis, biliary hypoplasia, and skeletal abnormalities); mapped to chromosome 20p12 *(JAG1)*; ERG and EOG are abnormal

Rieger's anomaly: Axenfeld's plus iris hypoplasia with holes; 50% develop glaucoma; mapped to chromosomes 4q25 *(RIEG1)*, 13q14 *(RIEG2)*, 6p25 *(FOXC1)*, and 11p13 *(PAX6)*

Rieger's syndrome: Rieger's anomaly plus mental retardation and systemic abnormalities (dental, craniofacial, genitourinary, and skeletal)

Peter's anomaly: central corneal leukoma (opacity due to defect in Descemet's membrane with absence of endothelium) with iris adhesions; lens involvement (cataract) may occur and 50% develop glaucoma; also associated with cardiac, craniofacial, and skeletal abnormalities; usually sporadic, bilateral (80%); AR or AD; mapped to chromosomes 11p13 *(PAX6)*, 4q25-q26 *(PTX2)*, 2p21-p22 *(CYP1B1)*, and 6p25 *(FOXC1)*

DDx: (Box 5-1)

Sclerocornea

Scleralized (white vascularized opacification) cornea; peripheral or entire

Nonprogressive; sporadic (50%) or hereditary (50%; AD or AR), mapped to chromosome 14; 90% bilateral

Corneoscleral limbus indistinct

Associations: persistent pupillary membrane, congenital glaucoma, cornea plana (80%)
Poor prognosis for corneal transplant

Descemet's Tear/Rupture

May be caused by forceps trauma (vertical or oblique) or glaucoma (horizontal or concentric to limbus; Haab's striae)

Acutely, edema occurs, scarring develops later
May cause astigmatism and amblyopia

Metabolic Disorders (Mucopolysaccharidoses, Mucolipidoses)

(see Table 5-4)

Congenital Hereditary Endothelial Dystrophy (CHED)

Rare, bilateral; mapped to chromosome 20p

Onset at or shortly after birth

Corneal clouding due to edema from defect of corneal endothelium and Descemet's membrane

Types:
CHED1 (AR): later onset (2nd year of life), pain, tearing, photophobia, no nystagmus, progressive

---

Box 5-1. DDx of congenital cloudy cornea: STUMPED

Sclerocornea

Tears in Descemet's membrane

Ulcers

Metabolic disease

Peter's anomaly

Edema (CHED)

Dermoids

Others: CHSD, rubella, posterior ulcer of von Hippel, posterior keratoconus, congenital corneal staphyloma

---

CHED2 (AR): more common, presents at birth, nystagmus, no pain or tearing, nonprogressive
No association with other systemic abnormalities

Findings: bilateral cloudy corneas, corneal edema

Pathology: thickened edematous stroma, massively thickened Descemet's membrane, atrophic or nonfunctioning endothelium

Congenital Hereditary Stromal Dystrophy (CHSD) (AD)

Rare, nonprogressive, diffuse opacification of superficial cornea

Findings: flaky, feathery appearance of anterior stroma, clear peripherally; no corneal edema
May cause strabismus, nystagmus, and amblyopia

Dermoid

Smooth, solid, yellow-white choristoma that may extend into corneal stroma to cover visual axis or cause astigmatism

No hereditary pattern; 25% bilateral

Types:
Conjunctival: (limbal) dermoid:
Straddles limbus, most commonly in inferotemporal quadrant
Isolated or associated with Goldenhar's syndrome (30%; includes accessory auricular appendages, aural fistulas, vertebral body abnormalities)
May cause astigmatism and amblyopia
Also associated with linear sebaceous nevus syndrome
Dermolipoma of the conjunctiva:
Usually located in superotemporal fornix; can extend deep into orbit
Consists of adipose and connective tissue
High surgical complication rate, with risk of marked ptosis, lateral rectus muscle paresis, and dry eye

Findings: dermoid, layer of lipid at leading edge in cornea; may cause proptosis, astigmatism, restricted motility, amblyopia

Pathology: thickened collagen fibers covered by skin-like epithelium; contains hair, sebaceous and sweat glands, and fat; lined by squamous epithelium

Treatment: observation; excision for cosmesis or if visual axis is blocked (*caution:* may be full thickness; granulomatous reaction if ruptures)

Other Causes of Corneal Opacity

Interstitial keratitis: congenital syphilis causes keratitis with edema followed by stromal vascularization ('salmon patch'), blood flow stops and 'ghost' vessels remain with corneal haze

Riley-day syndrome (familial dysautonomia; AR): autonomic nervous system dysfunction due to block of NE production; Eastern European Jews
  Findings: decreased corneal sensation, lack of tearing, poorly reactive pupils, light-near dissociation; may develop neurotrophic keratitis with risk of perforation
  Other findings: poor pain, temperature, and taste sensation; spinal curvature; increased sweating; constipation; hypotension
  Crisis (lasts 1–10 days): emotional lability, profuse sweating, postural hypotension, vomiting; treat with diazepam (Valium) and hydration
  Increased risk with general anesthesia: exquisite sensitivity to thiopental sodium (Pentothal) (hypotension, cardiac arrest)
  Diagnosis: high urinary homo-vanillic acid (HVA) and VMA, low hexamethylphosphorous triamide (HMPT)

Infections

Syphilis

Congenital: maternal transmission after 4th month of gestation (50% for primary or secondary syphilis, 30% for untreated or late syphilis)

Findings: interstitial keratitis (33%), ectopia lentis, Argyll-Robertson pupil, optic atrophy, panuveitis with various retinal pigmentary changes (usually salt and pepper or pseudo-RP)

Other findings:
  Early: stillbirth, failure to thrive, rhinitis ('snuffles'), osteochondritis, pneumonia, hepatosplenomegaly
  Late: Hutchinson's teeth (peg-shaped), mulberry molars, saber shins, frontal bossing, saddle nose, deafness (5%), tabes dorsalis

Hutchinson's triad: interstitial keratitis, Hutchinson's teeth, deafness
  Interstitial keratitis (IK): immune response to treponemal antigens
    Starts between ages of 5 and 20 years; triggered by minor corneal trauma

Bilateral with 2nd eye involvement at 1–2 months in 50%, 12 months in 75%
  3 STAGES:
    PROGRESSIVE: pain, photophobia, poor vision; blepharospasm, fine keratic precipitates (KP), perilimbal injection, diffuse or sectoral corneal haze (ground-glass appearance)
    FLORID: acute inflammatory response; salmon patch of Hutchinson (cornea appears pink due to deep vascularization)
    RETROGRESSIVE: vessels meet at center of cornea
  LATE FINDINGS: ghost vessels, Descemet's folds, guttata, secondary glaucoma (iris/angle damage)
  PATHOLOGY: stromal blood vessels just anterior to Descemet's
  TREATMENT: steroids (do not prevent involvement of fellow eye); systemic penicillin

DDx: acquired syphilis (IK usually sectoral and less severe), leprosy (superficial avascular keratitis, usually superotemporal quadrant; later, leprous pannus of blood vessels, beading of corneal nerves)

Herpes Simplex Virus (HSV)

Often an asymptomatic primary infection before age of 5 years; 3- to 5-day incubation period

Congenital: ocular involvement in 10% of disseminated cases

Findings: vesicular skin eruption, conjunctivitis, epithelial keratitis, stromal immune reaction, cataracts, necrotizing chorioretinitis

IRIS DISORDERS

Aniridia

Bilateral absence of iris, commonly a rudimentary iris stump exists

Incidence 1 in 100,000

Hereditary or sporadic; mapped to chromosome 11p13 (*PAX6*)

Types:
  AN1 (85%): AD, only eye involvement
  AN2 (13%): sporadic, associated with Wilms' tumor (Miller syndrome and WAGR [Wilms' tumor, aniridia, genitourinary abnormalities, and mental retardation])
  AN3 (2%): AR, associated with mental retardation and ataxia (Gillespie's syndrome)

Findings: visual acuity usually 20/100 or worse, foveal and optic nerve hypoplasia, nystagmus, photophobia, amblyopia, strabismus

May have cataracts (50–85%), glaucoma (30–50%), and corneal pannus

Treatment: consider cosmetic/painted contact lenses for photophobia; peripherally painted IOLs and PMMA rings have been used with cataract surgery but are not FDA approved

Coloboma

Iris sector defect due to incomplete closure of embryonic fissure; usually located inferonasal

May have other colobomas (lid, ciliary body, choroid, retina, and optic nerve)

Associated with trisomy 13, 18, and 22; chromosome 18 deletion; Klinefelter's syndrome, Turner's syndrome, CHARGE, basal cell nevus syndrome, Goldenhar's syndrome, Meckel's syndrome, Rubinstein-Taybi syndrome, linear sebaceous nevus syndrome

Treatment: consider surgical repair in symptomatic cases

Congenital Iris Ectropion

Ectropion uveae: ectropion of posterior pigment epithelium onto anterior surface of iris

Associated with neurofibromatosis, Prader-Willi syndrome

Congenital iris ectropion syndrome: unilateral congenital iris ectropion, high iris insertion, smooth cryptless iris surface, dysgenesis of angle, and glaucoma

Congenital Iris Hypoplasia

Thin iris stroma with transillumination of entire iris

Associated with albinism

Congenital Miosis

May be associated with other anterior segment abnormalities

Etiology: absence or malformation of dilator pupillae muscle or contracture of fibrous material on pupil margin from tunica vasculosa lentis remnant or neural crest cell abnormalities

Congenital Mydriasis

Etiology: iris sphincter trauma, pharmacologic, neurologic disease

Corectopia

Displacement of pupil

Isolated or associated with ectopia lentis et pupillae, Axenfeld-Rieger syndrome, iridocorneal endothelial syndrome, uveitis, or trauma

Dyscoria

Abnormally shaped pupil

Isolated or associated with posterior synechiae, Axenfeld-Rieger syndrome, ectopia lentis et pupillae

Persistent Pupillary Membrane

Remnants of anterior tunica vasculosa lentis that appear as fine iris strands

Common congenital ocular anomaly
Rarely visually significant

Type I: iris to iris, bridging pupil

Type II: iris to lens; may have associated anterior polar cataract

Primary Iris Cysts

Due to spontaneous separation of pigmented and nonpigmented epithelium

Occur anywhere between pupil and ciliary body
Miotics can cause cysts at pupillary border

Congenital stromal cysts occur in infants and young children from sequestration of epithelium during fetal development

Brushfield's Spots

Focal areas of iris stromal hyperplasia surrounded by relative hypoplasia

Appear as ring of peripheral, elevated, white-gray spots (10–20/eye)

Occur in 85% of Down syndrome patients

May be found in normal individuals (Kunkmann-Wolffian bodies)

Lisch Nodules

Neural crest hamartomas

Associated with neurofibromatosis type I

Number and frequency increase with age

Appear as tan nodules, usually in inferior iris

Juvenile Xanthogranuloma (JXG; Nevoxanthoendothelioma)

Histiocytic proliferation usually of skin

Yellow-orange nodules appear before 1 year of age

Orange because of vascularity (red) combined with high lipid content (yellow)

May involve iris (may cause spontaneous hyphema)

May involve muscles, salivary glands, stomach, and other internal organs

Rarely associated with an orbital granuloma (which causes proptosis)

Lesions often spontaneously regress by 5 years of age

Pathology: diffuse non-necrotizing proliferation of histiocytes with scattered touton giant cells (ring of nuclei separating a central eosinophilic cytoplasm from peripheral foamy [or clear] cytoplasm)

Treatment: iris lesions are treated with steroids, XRT, and excision

Medulloepithelioma (Diktyoma)

Primary neoplasm of ciliary body neuroectoderm (arises in nonpigmented epithelium); arises from primitive medullary epithelium that lines neural tube; can also arise in retina and ON

Occurs in both benign and malignant forms (locally invasive but limited metastatic potential)

May have heterotopic elements; no calcification

Unilateral, unifocal, usually arises before 6 years of age; no hereditary pattern

Types:
Nonteratoid or simple: pure proliferation of embryonic nonpigmented ciliary epithelium
Teratoid: contains heterotopic elements such as cartilage, brain tissue, and rhabdomyoblasts

Findings: decreased vision, pain, strabismus, leukocoria, iris mass, fleshy pink to white peripheral fundus tumor; rubeosis, hyphema, glaucoma, lens coloboma occurs in some congenital cases

Pathology: undifferentiated round to oval cells containing little cytoplasm, organized into ribbon-like structures that have distinct cellular polarity; lined on one side by thin basement membrane; stratified sheets of cells are capable of forming mucinous cysts that are clinically characteristic; Flexner-Wintersteiner and Homer-Wright rosettes can be seen; called **teratoid medulloepithelioma** when composed of cells from 2 different embryonic germ layers; may contain cartilage, brain tissue, and rhabdomyoblasts

Treatment: resection (iridocyclectomy) or enucleation (not radiosensitive)

Prognosis: good if no extraocular extension; rarely metastasizes

LENS DISORDERS

Congenital Anomalies

Mittendorf's dot: small white opacity on posterior lens capsule that represents a remnant of the posterior vascular capsule (tunica vasculosa lentis) where hyaloid artery is inserted

Chicken tracks (epicapsular star): brown or golden flecks on anterior lens capsule; remnant of anterior tunica vasculosa lentis

Lenticonus: cone-shaped lens deformity due to central bulge in area of thin capsule; causes irregular myopic astigmatism; 'oil-droplet' sign on retinoscopy; associated with cataract

Anterior: bilateral, male > female; associated with Alport's syndrome (anterior lenticonus, hereditary nephritis, and deafness)
Posterior: unilateral, sporadic, female > male, more common than anterior type, amblyopia common

Lens coloboma: focal flattening of lens edge due to absence of inferior zonules from ciliary body coloboma; not a true coloboma

Lentiglobus: generalized hemispherical deformity, very rare

Microphakia: small lens due to arrested development; associated with Lowe's syndrome

Microspherophakia: small, spherical lens, usually bilateral; zonules visible on pupillary dilation; iridodenesis; zonule rupture is common, pupillary block may occur especially with use of miotics (treat with cycloplegic to tighten zonules, flattening the lens and pulling it posteriorly)

Associated with Weill-Marchesani syndrome, hyperlysinemia, Lowe's syndrome, Alport's syndrome, congenital rubella, and Peter's anomaly
Treatment: cycloplegic (tightens zonules, flattening lens and pulling it posteriorly)

Congenital aphakia: rare, absence of lens

Ectopia Lentis

(see Ch. 10, Anterior Segment)

Congenital Cataracts

Characteristics:
Bilateral: usually AD; consider diabetes, galactosemia, or Lowe's syndrome; require metabolic workup and treatment by age 3 months, or irreversible nystagmus with poor visual acuity (≤20/200) occurs. Opacities greater than 3 mm can be visually significant. Surgery often performed on the better-seeing eye first: lensectomy, anterior vitrectomy, and contact lens fitting for infants; posterior capsulotomy is necessary due to significant postoperative inflammation, which causes posterior capsular opacification
Unilateral: generally not metabolic or genetic; therefore, laboratory testing is not needed. Usually local dysgenesis (PHPV, anterior polar or posterior lenticonus), often presents with leukocoria and strabismus. Requires treatment by 6–8 weeks of life

Types: classified by location or etiology
Polar (subcapsular cortex and capsule): anterior or posterior, sporadic, or AD
ANTERIOR: usually small, bilateral, symmetric, nonprogressive; good visual prognosis; 90% are idiopathic. Remnant of the hyaloid system. Associated with microphthalmos and anterior lenticonus

PATHOLOGY: fibrous plaque beneath folded anterior capsule secreted by irritated metaplastic epithelial cells

POSTERIOR: larger, usually stable, but may progress; more visually significant; AD (bilateral) or sporadic (unilateral); often with associated defect of posterior capsule

Associated with remnants of the tunica vasculosa lentis, posterior lenticonus, or lentiglobus

PATHOLOGY: posterior migration of lens epithelium

Sutural (AR): bilateral opacities of Y sutures; rarely affects vision. Occurs during development of fetal lens nucleus

Nuclear (usually AD): bilateral, opacification of embryonic/fetal nucleus; typically axial, dense, bilateral, and larger than 3 mm. Associated with small eye

Anterior pyramidal: congenital anterior subcapsular

Lamellar/zonular: bilateral, symmetric, appears like a sand dollar; circumscribed zone of opacity within lens, surrounding the nucleus. May be due to transient toxic exposure during embryogenesis (neonatal tetany); can be AD. Usually does not interfere with vision

Complete: no red reflex; unilateral or bilateral

Membranous: lens proteins resorb following trauma; anterior and posterior capsules fuse into a dense white membrane

Crystalline: rare, bilateral congenital cataract, with refractile, rhomboid crystals (containing tyrosine and cysteine) radiating outward from the center of the lens into the juvenile nucleus

Anterior axial embryonic: most common type of congenital/infantile cataract. White, clustered, punctate opacities near the Y sutures; not visually significant

Pulverulent (AR): central, translucent, ovoid, and cluster of dot-like opacities in the fetal nucleus

Coronary (AR): wreath of peripheral cortical opacities that encircle the nucleus in a radial fashion; smaller punctate bluish opacities within the nucleus. Associated with Down's syndrome

Etiology: 1/3 hereditary; 1/3 associated with systemic syndromes; 1/3 of unknown origin

Etiology of bilateral cataracts: Idiopathic (60%)

Intrauterine infection (3%): TORCH syndromes (Toxoplasmosis, Other infections (syphilis; also hepatitis B, Varicella-Zoster virus, HIV, parvovirus B19), Rubella, CMV, HSV) the alternate acronym is TORCHES (TOxoplasmosis, Rubella, CMV, HErpes simplex, Syphilis)

Associated with ocular disorders: Leber's congenital amaurosis, retinitis pigmentosa (RP), PHPV, retinopathy of prematurity (ROP), aniridia, Peter's anomaly, ectopia lentis, posterior lenticonus, uveitis, tumors (retinoblastoma, medulloepithelioma)

Metabolic: galactosemia, hypocalcemia, Lowe's syndrome, congenital hemolytic jaundice, hypoglycemia, mannosidosis, Alport's syndrome, Fabry's disease

Hereditary (30%, usually AD):

WITHOUT SYSTEMIC ABNORMALITIES: AD, AR, X-linked

WITH CHROMOSOMAL ABNORMALITIES: trisomy 18, trisomy 21 (Down's syndrome), Turner's syndrome, trisomy 13 (Patau's syndrome), 'cri-du-chat' syndrome

CRANIOFACIAL SYNDROMES: Crouzon's syndrome, Apert's syndrome, Hallermann-Streiff syndrome, Pierre Robin sequence

CNS ABNORMALITIES: Zellweger syndrome, Torsten-Sjögren syndrome, Marinesco-Sjögren syndrome, Lawrence-Moon-Biedl-Bardet syndrome, Norrie's disease, neurofibromatosis

SKIN ABNORMALITIES: Cockayne's syndrome, Rothmund-Thomson syndrome, Werner's syndrome, atopic dermatitis, ichthyosis, incontinentia pigmenti

Maternal drug ingestion/malnutrition

Trauma

Specific entities:

Galactosemia (AR): defect in 1 of 3 enzymes (galactose-1-P-uridyl transferase [most common], galactokinase, or uridine diphosphate [UDP] galactose-4-epimerase) causes inability to convert galactose into glucose; galactose is converted into galactitol, which serves as osmotic agent for influx of fluid

FINDINGS: oil-droplet cataract (reversible early on)

OTHER FINDINGS: mental retardation, hepatomegaly, jaundice, and malnutrition within 1st few weeks of life

TREATMENT: eliminate lactose from diet; fatal if untreated

Mannosidosis: α-mannosidase deficiency causes Hurler-like syndrome

FINDINGS: posterior spoke-like opacity; no corneal changes (unlike Hurler's)

OTHER FINDINGS: mental retardation, short stature, skeletal changes, hepatosplenomegaly

Fabry's disease: α-galactosidase A deficiency

FINDINGS: cornea verticillata; spoke-like cataract in 25%

OTHER FINDINGS: angiokeratomas, cardiovascular abnormalities, renal disorders, bouts of pain in digits

Hypocalcemia: either idiopathic or following surgery of parathyroid glands

Punctate iridescent opacities in anterior and posterior cortex

Lowe's (oculocerebrorenal) syndrome (X-linked): defect of amino acid metabolism; male > female

FINDINGS: congenital cataract (100%), usually bilateral; small, thin, discoid lens (microphakic) associated with retained lens nuclei; glaucoma (50%); congenital cataract and glaucoma are very rare

Female carriers have white, punctate cortical opacities and subcapsular plaque-like opacities

OTHER FINDINGS: renal tubular acidosis, aminoaciduria, renal rickets, mental retardation, muscular hypotonia, failure to thrive

Alport's syndrome (X-linked): triad of anterior lenticonus, deafness, and hemorrhagic nephropathy/renal failure

FINDINGS: conjunctival calcium crystals, corneal endothelial pigment, juvenile arcus, spherophakia, anterior polar cataract, retinal changes similar to retinitis pigmentosa or fundus albipunctatis, optic nerve drusen

Female carriers have lenticular changes

DIAGNOSIS: renal or skin biopsy (lack of α-5 type IV collagen in glomerular and epidermal basement membranes)

Hallermann-Streiff syndrome (mandibulo-oculofacial dysmorphia): hypoplasia of mandible with bird-like facies; one of the few syndromes with combined cataract and glaucoma

FINDINGS: microphakia, microcornea, glaucoma, and cataract (can develop within 1st few weeks of life); spontaneous rupture of lens capsule with absorption of lens proteins can occur; immune response to lens proteins resembles phacoanaphylactic uveitis

Intrauterine infections: usually occur early in first trimester because lens capsule is formed during week 5 of embryogenesis; rubella, HSV, mumps, toxoplasmosis, vaccinia, CMV

Hypoglycemia during pregnancy: congenital lenticular opacities; associated with optic atrophy, mental retardation

Down's syndrome: snowflake cataract, keratoconus

Diagnosis of bilateral cataracts: if AD pattern determined, no workup is necessary

Urinalysis: amino acids (Lowe's syndrome), reducing substance after milk feeding (galactosemia)

Blood tests: calcium (hypocalcemia/hyperparathyroidism), glucose (hypoglycemia), red blood cell galactokinase, TORCH titers

Karyotyping: trisomy 13 (Patau's syndrome), 18, and 21 (Down's syndrome); Turner's syndrome, 'cri-du-chat' syndrome

Bilateral audiograms: congenital rubella, Alport's syndrome

B-scan ultrasound: if no view of fundus

Etiology of unilateral cataracts:

Idiopathic (80%):

Ocular abnormalities (10%): PHPV, posterior lenticonus (90% unilateral), anterior segment dysgenesis, tumors (retinoblastoma, medulloepithelioma)

Trauma (9%):

Intrauterine infection: rubella; 33% unilateral

Diagnosis of unilateral cataracts: rule out trauma (child abuse), TORCH titers

DDx of leukocoria (white pupil): cataract, retinoblastoma, toxoplasmosis, toxocariasis, RD, ROP, PHPV, Coats' disease, coloboma, myelinated nerve fibers, retinal dysplasia, Norrie's disease, incontinentia pigmenti, retinoschisis, cyclitic membrane, medulloepithelioma

DDx of congenital cataracts and glaucoma: Lowe's syndrome, rubella, Hallermann-Streiff syndrome

Rubella: due to maternal infection late in the first trimester of pregnancy

FINDINGS (in 50%): cataract (usually bilateral, pearly white nuclear opacification; retention of lens nuclei in embryonic nucleus; virus remains viable in lens for years: viral shedding following cataract surgery can lead to intense and persistent AC inflammation), salt and pepper fundus (normal ERG), glaucoma (usually either cataract or glaucoma, rarely both), microphthalmos (15%), necrotizing iridocyclitis, corneal clouding

OTHER FINDINGS (especially during 1st trimester): cardiac defects (patent ductus arteriosis), deafness (infection of the organ of Corti [90%]), and mental retardation

Complications of surgery: chronic aphakic glaucoma (15%). Usually discovered 5–6 years after surgery; increased risk with trauma, microcornea, PHPV, preexisting anterior segment abnormalities, and retained lens material

Prognosis:

Good: lamellar cataracts (later onset and less risk of glaucoma)

Intermediate: nuclear cataracts

Poor: total cataracts (high incidence of microcornea, poor pupillary dilation, and increased risk of glaucoma). Microphthalmos, strabismus, nystagmus, and amblyopia; 90% of patients with visually significant congenital bilateral cataracts will develop nystagmus if not treated by 2 months of age; nystagmus and amblyopia may not resolve even after cataract surgery

GLAUCOMA

Childhood Glaucoma

Several types of glaucoma typically categorized by age of onset

Congenital (occurs in infants <3 months old; may be primary, secondary, or associated with a syndrome)

Infantile (between 3 months and 3 years of age)

Juvenile (between 3 and 35 years of age)

Types (Figure 5-6)

Primary Congenital Glaucoma

Etiology: mapped to chromosomes 1p36 (*GLC3B*), 2p21-p22 (*GLC3A, CYP1B1*); a mutation in the *CYP1B1* gene accounts for ~85% of congenital glaucoma. AR in 10%; affected parent has 5% chance of having a child with infantile glaucoma

Epidemiology: occurs in 1 of 12,500 births; 40% present at birth; 86% present during first year of life; 70% bilateral; 70% males

Primary infantile glaucoma (congenital glaucoma, trabeculodysgenesis)	
Secondary infantile glaucoma	
Associated with mesodermal neural crest dysgenesis	Iridocorneotrabeculodysgenesis • Rieger's anomaly or syndrome • Axenfeld's anomaly or syndrome • Peters' anomaly • systemic hypoplastic mesodermal dysgenesis (Marfan's syndrome) • systemic hyperplastic mesodermal dysgenesis (Weill–Marchesani syndrome)
	Iridotrabeculodysgenesis (aniridia)
Associated with phako-matoses and hamartomas	Neurofibromatosis (Von Recklinghausen's disease)
	Encephalotrigeminal angiomatosis (Sturge–Weber syndrome and variants, e.g. Klippel–Trénaunay–Weber syndrome)
	Angiomatosis retinae et cerebelli
	Oculodermal melanocytosis
Associated with metabolic disease	Oculocerebrorenal syndrome (Lowe's syndrome)
	Homocystinuria
Associated with inflammatory disease	Maternal rubella syndrome (congenital rubella)
	Herpes simplex iridocyclitis
Associated with mitotic disease	Juvenile xanthogranuloma (nevoxanthoendothelioma)
	Retinoblastoma
Associated with other congenital disease	Trisomy 13–15 syndrome (Patau's syndrome)
	Rubinstein–Taybi syndrome
	Persistent hyperplastic primary vitreous
	Congenital cataract • in phakic eyes • in aphakic eyes following surgery

Figure 5-6. Classification of the congenital and infantile glaucomas. (From Yanoff M, Duker JS [eds]: Ophthalmology, London, Mosby, 1999.)

Symptoms: tearing, photophobia, blepharospasm, eye rubbing. If younger than age 3 months, usually presents with corneal clouding or tearing; older than 3 years of age, usually asymptomatic with progressive myopia and insidious VF loss

Findings: IOP >21 mmHg; C/D ratio >0.3 (present in only 2.6% of normal infants; cupping is reversible in childhood); buphthalmos ('bull's-eye'; horizontal corneal diameter >13 mm; limbal ectasia; stretching of zonules can lead to lens subluxation; irreversible); corneal clouding/edema/Haab's striae (circumferential or horizontal Descemet's ruptures [vs oblique or vertical with forceps injury]; may result in chronic corneal edema, scarring, and astigmatism); myopia

Angle is of neural crest origin, as are facial bones, teeth, cartilage, and meninges; therefore, congenital glaucoma may be associated with malformation of these structures

Other ocular associations: microcornea, cornea plana, sclerocornea, Axenfeld's/Reiger's/Peter's anomaly (50%), aniridia (50–75% develop glaucoma by teens due to increased episcleral venous pressure, iris stump blocking TM, or angle malformation or agenesis), microspherophakia, nanophthalmos, PHPV, ROP, tumors (retinoblastoma [RB], JXG, medulloepithelioma), inflammation, trauma, steroid-induced

Associated syndromes: Lowe's syndrome (50%); Sturge-Weber syndrome (50%, especially if nevus flammeus involves upper lid, due to primary defect in angle and increased episcleral venous pressure); neurofibromatosis (25% if plexiform neurofibroma involves upper lid; may have hamartomatous infiltration of angle); congenital rubella (2–15%); also Marfan's syndrome, homocystinuria, Weill-Marchesani syndrome, Rubenstein-Taybi, Pierre Robin, nevus of Ota, trisomy 13 (Patau's), Hallermann-Streiff, Stickler's syndrome, mucopolysaccharidoses (Hurler's and Hunter's)

Diagnosis:

Examination under anesthesia (EUA): usually required for complete evaluation. Remember, ketamine and succinylcholine raise IOP, general anesthesia (halothane, thiopental, tranquilizers, and barbituates) lowers IOP. Best time for IOP measurement is just as patient goes under and is not too deep

Gonioscopy: landmarks are often poorly recognized due to 'Barkan's membrane' covering TM (but no histologic evidence of such a structure)

1. Open-angle with anterior iris insertion above scleral spur (usual configuration is flat iris insertion into trabecular meshwork; less commonly, concave insertion with plane of iris posterior to scleral spur and anterior iris sweeping upward and inserting into TM)
2. Thickening of TM
3. Peripheral iris stromal hypoplasia

Treatment: definitive treatment is surgical; medication is a temporizing measure

Goniotomy: perform in child <1½ years of age; TM incised under direct gonioscopic visualization; requires clear cornea; 77% success rate

Trabeculotomy (ab externo): if cornea hazy, if >1½ years old, or if goniotomy fails twice; Schlemm's canal is entered via an external incision, and the trabeculotome rotates into the AC and tears the TM; 77% success rate

If goniotomy and trabeculotomy fail, consider trabeculectomy with mitomycin C, drainage implant, cycloablation of CB

UVEITIS

Anterior Uveitis

DDx: JRA, trauma, infection, tumor, sympathetic ophthalmia, sarcoidosis, phacoantigenic

Juvenile Rheumatoid Arthritis (JRA)

Most common cause of uveitis in children: seronegative (RF–), ANA-positive, pauciarticular (<5 joints) arthritis in children <16 years old; mostly girls

Table 5-2. Classification of JRA

Type	Polyarticular RF-Negative	Polyarticular RF-Positive	Pauciarticular type I	Pauciarticular type II	Systemic (Still's disease)
Age	Any	Late childhood	Early childhood	Late childhood	Any
Sex	90% girls	80% girls	80% girls	90% boys	60% boys
RF	Negative	Positive	Negative	Negative	Negative
ANA	25%	75%	60%	Negative	Negative
HLA-B27	N/A	N/A	N/A	75%	N/A
Joints	Any	Any	Large joints (knee, elbow, ankle)	Large joints (hip, SI joints)	Any
Uveitis	Rare	No	30% Chronic	15% Acute	Rare
Other findings	Low-grade fever, delayed growth, anemia, malaise	Low-grade fever, anemia, malaise, rheumatoid nodules	Few	Few	High fever, rash, organomegaly, polyserositis

Types (Table 5-2)

Pauciarticular (<5 joints), early onset: 80% female; 30% with chronic iridocyclitis; 25% of all JRA; RF–; 60% ANA+

Pauciarticular, late onset: 90% male; 15% of all JRA; RF–; ANA–; 75% HLA-B27; 15% acute iridocyclitis

Polyarticular (<5 joints): 85% female; iridocyclitis rare; 40% of all JRA; 75% are RF–

Still's disease: throughout childhood; 60% male; small and large joints; iridocylitis rare; 20% of all JRA; RF–; ANA–; high fever, rash, organomegaly, polyserositis

Findings: chronic anterior uveitis (30%, usually bilateral; eyes are white and quiet even with active ocular inflammation [lots of flare]), glaucoma (20%), cataract (40%), band keratopathy (40%)

Other findings (30%): arthritis, fever, lymphadenopathy, maculopapular rash, myocarditis, hepatosplenomegaly

Treatment: topical steroids and cycloplegic; consider systemic steroids or sub-Tenon's steroid injection; treat complications. May require immunosuppressive agents, EDTA chelation for band keratopathy, treatment of secondary glaucoma, cataract surgery (eyes should be without AC reaction for at least 3 months; intraoperatively, anterior vitrectomy, synechialysis, removal of cyclitic membranes; no IOL; may be complicated by hypotony)

Intermediate Uveitis

Pars Planitis

(see Ch. 8, Uveitis)

Posterior Uveitis

DDx: toxoplasmosis, toxocariasis, presumed ocular histoplasmosis syndrome (POHS), HSV, syphilis, Lyme disease, sympathetic ophthalmia, masquerade syndromes (RB, leukemia, lymphoma, melanoma, JXG, intraocular foreign body, RD, RP, MS)

Toxoplasmosis

Due to infection with *Toxoplasma gondii*, usually congenital (maternal infection during gestation) 70% of women are seronegative

Primary retinal infection with coagulative necrosis and secondary granulomatous choroiditis with vitritis; intraretinal cysts cause recurrent disease

Most common cause of posterior uveitis (25%); 98% congenital

Most common cause of pediatric uveitis (50% of posterior uveitis in children)

Tachyzoite form is responsible for inflammation

Congenital infection: transplacental transmission of *T. gondii*

First-trimester infection: neonatal convulsions, intracerebral calcifications, retinitis

Later infection: may have retinitis only

Findings: inactive chorioretinal scar in posterior pole, often in macula (Figure 5-7); active focal white fluffy lesion ('headlight in fog' appearance) occurs adjacent to old scar with granulomatous uveitis and vitritis; may have white spots along arterioles (Kyrieleis' plaques); may have microphthalmia, nystagmus, strabismus

In AIDS: head CT may show ring-enhancing lesions; minimal AC reaction and vitritis because immunocompromised host is unable to mount normal immune response

Other findings:

Congenital toxoplasmosis: stillbirth, mental retardation, seizures, hydrocephalus, microcephaly, intracranial calcifications, hepatosplenomegaly, vomiting, diarrhea

Acquired toxoplasmosis: rash, meningoencephalitis, flu-like syndrome

Pathology: round *Toxoplasma* cysts (Figure 5-8); chronic granulomatous choroiditis

Diagnosis: ELISA or immunofluorescence assay (IFA) for *Toxoplasma* IgG or IgM

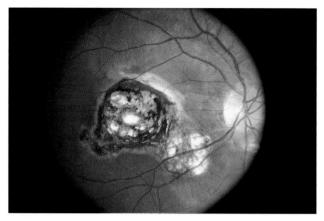

Figure 5-7. Congenital toxoplasmic retinitis. Note inactive satellite scars at the macula, the inferior juxtapapillary scar, and the temporal pallor of the disc. (From Khanna A, Goldstein DA, Tessler HH: Protozoal posterior uveitis. In Yanoff M, Duker JS [eds]: Ophthalmology, London, Mosby, 1999.)

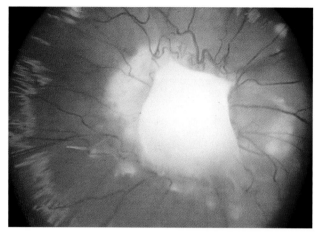

Figure 5-9. Typical toxocara granuloma located over the optic nerve. (In: Yanoff M, Duker JS [eds]: Ophthalmology (Ch. 173), London, Mosby, 1999.)

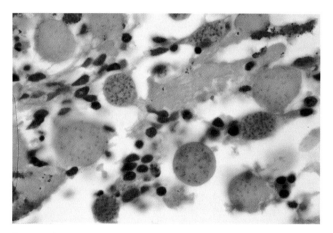

Figure 5-8. Viable and necrotic cysts of *Toxoplasma gondii* in the necrotic retina. (From Khanna A, Goldstein DA, Tessler HH: Protozoal posterior uveitis. In Yanoff M, Duker JS [eds]: Ophthalmology, London, Mosby, 1999.)

Table 5-3. Clinical presentations of toxocariasis

	Chronic endophthalmitis	Localized granuloma	Peripheral granuloma
Age range	2–9 years	6–14 years	6–40 years
Lesion	Exudation filling vitreous cavity, cyclitic membrane	Single localized granuloma in macula or peripapillary region	Peripheral granuloma with dense fibrotic strand, often to disc
Symptoms	Pain, photophobia, lacrimation, decreased vision, acute inflammation	Quiet eye, decreased vision, strabismus	Decreased vision, strabismus
Course	Often leads to destruction of globe	Nonprogressive	Nonprogressive

Treatment:

Indications: decreased vision; moderate to severe vitreous inflammation; lesions that threaten macula, papillomacular bundle, or optic nerve; small peripheral lesions may be observed (heal spontaneously)

Antibiotics: kill tachyzoites in retina during active retinitis, but do not affect cysts

CLINDAMYCIN: 300 mg qid (risk of pseudomembranous colitis)

SULFADIAZINE: 2 g loading, then 1 g qid

PYRIMETHAMINE (Daraprim): 75 mg loading, then 25 mg daily (bone marrow depression; prevent with use of folinic acid [leucovorin, citrovorum factor; 3-5 mg 2 times/week])

ALTERNATIVE: trimethoprim-sulfamethoxazole (Bactrim)

Steroids: systemic and periocular

Toxocariasis (Table 5-3)

Due to infection with 2nd-stage larval form of dog roundworm *Toxocara canis* (ocular larva migrans)

Acquired by ingestion of contaminated soil

Ocular larva migrans: usually unilateral, solitary lesion; does not complete life cycle (stool examination unnecessary), no other findings

Visceral larva migrans: fever, lymphadenopathy, hepatomegaly, pneumonitis, eosinophilia, no eye involvement

Findings: 3 clinical presentations depending on patient age (endophthalmitis, localized granuloma, or peripheral granuloma); vitreous abscess; dragging of macula temporally owing to peripheral lesion results in apparent XT; often presents with leukocoria; traction RD can occur (Figure 5-9)

Other findings: may affect lungs and liver

DDx: as for leukocoria

Diagnosis: AC tap for eosinophils; ELISA for *Toxocara* antibody titers; no ova/parasites in stool

Treatment: topical steroid and cycloplegic for active uveitis; vitrectomy, may require surgical repair of RD

METABOLIC DISORDERS

(Table 5-4 and Box 5-2)

Box 5-2. Ocular manifestations of childhood cerebral degenerations

Conjunctival telangiectasia: ataxia telangiectasia, Fabry's disease

Glaucoma: MPS I-Scheie, Zellweger's disease (rare)

Corneal opacity: MPS I, III, IV, VI; mucolipidoses III, IV; Fabry's disease, sialidosis with chondrodystrophy, Cockayne's disease, xeroderma pigmentosum, Zellweger's disease (occasionally), Wilson's disease (Kayser-Fleischer ring)

Lens opacity: Wilson's disease, galactosemia, Marinesco-Sjögren syndrome, Lowe's disease, cerebrocutaneous xanthomatosis, sialidosis, mannosidosis

Cherry red spot: Tay-Sachs disease, sialidosis, Niemann-Pick disease (50%), GM gangliosidosis (50%), Farber's disease, multiple sulfatase deficiency (metachromatic leukodystrophy variant)

Macular and pigmentary degeneration: ceroid lipofuscinosis, MPS 1-H, 1-S, II, III; mucolipidoses IV, Refsum's disease (phytanic acid lipidosis), Bassen-Kornzweig (abetalipoproteinemia), Kearns-Sayre syndrome

Optic atrophy: Krabbe's disease, metachromatic leukodystrophy, sphingolipidoses, adrenoleukodystrophy, Alexander's disease, spongy degeneration, Pelizaeus-Merzbacher disease, neuraxonal dystrophy, Alpers' disease, spinocerebellar degeneration, diseases with retinal pigmentary degeneration

Nystagmus: diseases with poor vision (searching nystagmus), Pelizaeus-Merzbacher disease, metachromatic leukodystrophy, Friedreich's ataxia, other spinocerebellar degenerations and cerebellar atrophies, neuraxonal dystrophy, ataxia telangiectasia, Leigh's syndrome, Marinesco-Sjögren syndrome, opsoclonus-myoclonus syndrome, Chédiak-Higashi disease

Ophthalmoplegia: Leigh's syndrome, Kearns-Sayre syndrome, Niemann-Pick variant with vertical ophthalmoplegia, Gaucher's disease, Bassen-Kornzweig syndrome, ataxia-telangiectasia, Tangier's disease

RETINAL DISORDERS

Persistent Hyperplastic Primary Vitreous (PHPV)

Unilateral microphthalmia with spectrum of findings from prominent hyaloid vessel remnant with large Mittendorf's dot and Bergmeister's papillae to angle-closure from fibrovascular invasion of lens through posterior lens capsule

Due to incomplete regression of tunica vasculosa lentis and primary vitreous

Sporadic, 90% unilateral

Findings: microphthalmia, vascularized retrolental plaque (may contain cartilage), elongated ciliary processes, prominent radial vessels on iris surface, shallow AC, iris vascularization; may have cataract, angle-closure glaucoma, vitreous hemorrhage, retinal detachment

DDx of intraocular cartilage: PHPV, medulloepithelioma, teratoma, trisomy 13

Treatment: observation, lensectomy with or without vitrectomy

Prognosis: depends on degree of amblyopia; visual prognosis variable after surgery, often depends on status of posterior segment

Coloboma

Yellow-white lesion with pigmented margins due to incomplete closure of embryonic fissure; usually located inferonasal

Retina is reduced to glial tissue; no RPE; may have colobomas of other ocular structures

Retinopathy of Prematurity (Retrolental Fibroplasia)

Vasoproliferative retinopathy occurring almost exclusively in premature infants; occasionally in full-term infants

Risk factors: low birth weight (<1.5 kg; if <1.25 kg, 65% develop some degree of ROP), early gestational age (<33 weeks), supplemental oxygen (>50 days; controversial), coexisting illness

Risk increases exponentially the more premature and the smaller the infant: <2000 g (4 pounds, 7 ounces), earlier than 36 weeks (at 36 weeks, nasal retina is completely vascularized; at 40 weeks, temporal retina is fully vascularized)

2 phases:
  Acute: abnormal vessels develop in association with fibrous proliferation; >85–90% spontaneously regress
  Chronic: retinal detachment, temporal displacement of macula, severe vision loss; occurs in 15%

Classification: (International Classification of ROP [ICROP])
  Zone:
  1. Posterior pole, area enclosed by 60° diameter circle centered on optic nerve
  2. Area between edge of zone 1 and circle centered on optic disc and tangent to nasal ora serrata
  3. Remaining crescent of temporal peripheral retina anterior to zone 2
  Extent: measured in clock hours of involvement
  Stage:
  1. Demarcation line between vascular and avascular retina (flat, white) (Figure 5-10)
  2. Ridge (elevated, pink/white) (Figure 5-11)
  3. Ridge with tufts of extraretinal blood vessels (popcorn) (Figures 5-12, 5-13)
  4. Subtotal retinal detachment (Figure 5-14)
     A. Extrafoveal
     B. Including fovea
  5. Total RD with funnel (open or closed)

Plus disease: engorged, tortuous vessels around disc, vitreous haze, and iris vascular congestion; progressive vascular incompetence throughout eye; poor prognostic sign

Threshold disease: (level at which 50% go blind without treatment) = stage 3 in zone 1 or 2 with Plus disease and at least 5 contiguous or 8 cumulative clock hours of involvement; usually develops at 27 weeks' postgestation (Figure 5-15)

Table 5-4. Metabolic diseases with eye findings

Disease	Enzyme deficiency	Inheritance	Findings	Other findings
Sphingolipidoses				
GM2 gangliosidoses				
Type I (Tay-Sachs disease)	Hexosaminidase A	Autosomal recessive	Cherry red spot, optic atrophy, blindness, nystagmus, ophthalmoplegia	Normal at birth, motor deterioration starts at 3–5 months of age, rapid after 10 months of age, Death by 2–3 years of age
Type I (Sandhoff's disease)	Hexosaminidase B	Autosomal recessive	Cherry red spot, optic atrophy, blindness	Death by 2–12 years of age
Type III (Bernheimer-Seitelberger disease)	Hexosaminidase A (partial)	Autosomal recessive	Optic atrophy, pigmentary retinopathy	Death by 15 years of age
GM1 gangliosidoses				
Type I (Landing disease)	β-Galactosidase A, B, and C	Autosomal recessive	Cherry red spots in 50%, optic atrophy, high myopia, blindness, subtle corneal clouding, nystagmus	Psychomotor delay present at birth with rapid neurologic deterioration and death by 2 years of age
Type II (Derry disease)	β-Galactosidase B and C	Autosomal recessive	RPE degeneration, possible optic atrophy, nystagmus, esotropia	Neurologic deterioration in 1st or 2nd year of life, seizures, death between 3 and 10 years of age
Mucopolysaccharidoses				
MPS type I-H (Hurler)	α-Iduronidase	Autosomal recessive	Corneal clouding, RPE degeneration, optic atrophy, glaucoma	Onset between 6 and 24 months of age, gargoyles facies, mental retardation, dwarfism, skeletal dysplasia
MPS type I-S (Scheie)	Iduronate sulfatase	X-linked recessive	RPE degeneration, optic atrophy	Coarse facial features, claw-like hands, aortic valve disease
MPS type II (Hunter)		Autosomal recessive	RPE degeneration, optic atrophy	Similar to 1-H, less skeletal deformity
MPS type III (Sanfilippo)	4 types: A, B, C, D Heparan N-sulfatase; N-acetyl D-glucosaminidase; acetyl-CoA-glucosaminidase- N,N-acetyltransferase;N-acetylglucosamine-6-sulfate sulfatase	Autosomal recessive	Corneal clouding, optic atrophy	Mild dysmorphism, progressive dementia
MPS type IV (Morquio)	2 types: A, B galactose-6-sulfatase; β-galactosidase	Autosomal recessive	Corneal clouding, RPE degeneration, optic atrophy	Short trunk, dwarfism, skeletal deformities, aortic valve disease, normal mental development
MPS type VI (Maroteaux-Lamy)	Arylsulfatase B	Autosomal recessive	Corneal clouding	Normal mental development, similar to 1-H
MPS type VII (Sly)	β-Glucuronidase	Autosomal recessive	Clear cornea	Onset after 4 years of age, similar to 1-H
MPS type VIII (Diferrante)	Glucosamine-S-sulfate sulfatase	Autosomal recessive		
Lipidoses				
Fabry's disease	α-Galactosidase A	X-linked recessive	Whorl-like corneal changes, granular opacities of lens, tortuosity of retinal and conjunctival vessels	Systemic ischemia and infarction (cerebrovascular, cardiac; skin)
Metachromatic leukodystrophy	Arylsulfatase A	Autosomal recessive	Nystagmus, cherry red spot, optic atrophy	Weakness, mental deterioration, developmental delay, may be infantile, juvenile, or adult onset
Krabbe's disease	Galactocerebrosidase	Autosomal recessive	Optic atrophy, blindness	Rapidly progressive and fatal, usually with infantile onset
Gaucher's disease	β-Galactosidase	Autosomal recessive	RPE degeneration, EOM abnormalities	Hepatosplenomegaly, bone complications, neurologic deterioration
Niemann-Pick disease	Sphingomyelinase	Autosomal recessive	Corneal opacities, cherry red spot, lens opacities	Severity of disease varies depending on type, loss of motor and cognitive skills, splenomegaly
Others				
Cystinosis	Defective transport of cystine	Autosomal recessive	Corneal crystals, secondary photophobia and blepharospasm, RPE degeneration	Infantile and late-onset forms; renal failure (Fanconi's syndrome), CNS damage
Galactosemia	Gal-1-UDP transferase	Autosomal recessive	Cataract (oil-drop)	Failure to thrive, hepatomegaly and liver dysfunction, developmental delay
Mannosidosis	α-Mannosidase	Autosomal recessive	Corneal clouding, lens opacification	Coarse features, hepatosplenomegaly, mental deterioration, hearing loss
Mucolipidoses II and III	Multiple lysosomal enzymes	Autosomal recessive	Corneal clouding	Coarse features, psychomotor retardation, organomegaly, cardiorespiratory problems
Refsum's disease	Phytanic acid oxidase	Autosomal recessive	Retinal degeneration, optic disc pallor, cataracts	Peripheral neuropathy, cerebellar ataxia, elevated CSF protein
Adrenoleukodystrophy	Peroxisomal disorder	X-linked, autosomal recessive	Optic atrophy, RPE degeneration, strabismus	CNS demyelination, adrenal insufficiency, high long-chain fatty acid levels
Homocystinuria	Cystathionine synthase	Autosomal recessive	Dislocated lenses, optic atrophy, glaucoma	Osteoporosis, thromboembolic disease, seizures

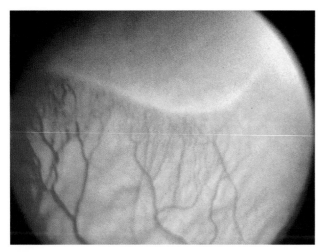

Figure 5-10. Stage 1 retinopathy of prematurity. The flat, white border between the avascular and vascular retina seen superiorly is called a demarcation line. (Reproduced from Earl A. Palmer, MD, and the Multicenter Trial of Cryotherapy for Retinopathy of Prematurity. From Yanoff M, Duker JS [eds]: Ophthalmology, London, Mosby, 1999.)

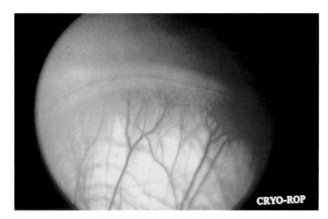

Figure 5-11. Stage 2 retinopathy of prematurity. The elevated mesenchymal ridge has height. Highly arborized blood vessels from the vascularized retina dive into the ridge. (Reproduced from Palmer EA, MD, and the Multicenter Trial of Cryotherapy for Retinopathy of Prematurity: In: Yanoff M, Duker JS [eds]: Ophthalmology, London, Mosby, 1999.)

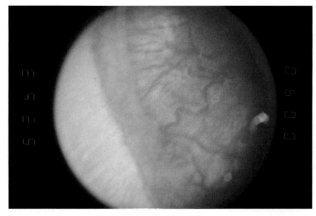

Figure 5-12. Stage 3 retinopathy of prematurity. Vessels on top of the ridge project into the vitreous cavity. The extraretinal proliferation carries with it a fibrovascular membrane. Note the opalescent avascular retina anterior to the ridge. (From Sears J, Capone A: Retinopathy of primaturity. In Yanoff M, Duker JS [eds]: Ophthalmology, London, Mosby, 1999.)

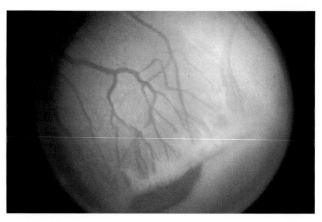

Figure 5-13. Stage 3 retinopathy of prematurity. Note finger-like projections of extraretinal vessels into the vitreous cavity. Hemorrhage on the ridge is not uncommon. (From Sears J, Capone A: Retinopathy of prematurity. In Yanoff M, Duker JS [eds]: Ophthalmology, London, Mosby, 1999.)

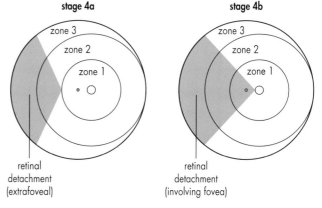

Figure 5-14. Stage 4a detachment spares the fovea. Stage 4b detachment involves the fovea. (From Sears J, Capone A: Retinopathy of prematurity. In Yanoff M, Duker JS [eds]: Ophthalmology, London, Mosby, 1999.)

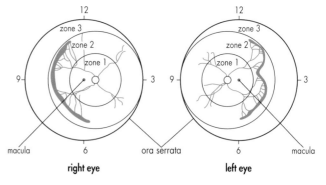

Figure 5-15. Definition of 'threshold' retinopathy of prematurity. (From Sears J, Capone A: Retinopathy of prematurity. In Yanoff M, Duker JS [eds]: Ophthalmology, London, Mosby, 1999.)

Aggressive posterior (AP) ROP or Rush disease: plus disease in zone 1 or posterior zone 2; rapidly progressive

Prethreshold:
1. Zone 1, any stage
2. Zone 2, stage 2+ or 3
3. Zone 2, stage 3+ for >5 clock hours

DDx of peripheral vascular changes and retinal dragging: FEVR, incontinentia pigmenti (Bloch-Sulzberger syndrome), X-linked retinoschisis

DDx of temporally dragged disc: FEVR, *Toxocara*, congenital falciform fold

Diagnosis: screen infants <1250 g, on supplemental oxygen during first 7 days of life, or <27 weeks' gestation

Treatment: observation, laser, cryo, surgery
Cryotherapy for ROP Study (Cryo-ROP): determined whether treatment for ROP would prevent poor outcomes (see below)

Treat with ablation of peripheral avascular retina: when patient reaches type 1 ROP, defined as:
Zone 1, any stage with Plus disease
Zone 1, stage 3
Zone 2, stage 2 or 3 with Plus disease
(Early Treatment of ROP Study [ETROP])

Indirect argon green or diode laser photocoagulation: 500 µm spots to entire avascular retina in zone 1 and peripheral zone 2 (at least as effective as cryotherapy; Laser-ROP study)

Cryotherapy: to entire avascular retina in zone 2, but not ridge (cryo-ROP study)

Serial exams: with type 2 ROP, defined as:
Zone 1, stage 1 or 2
Zone 2, stage 3

Surgery: vitrectomy with or without lensectomy, membrane peel, and possible scleral buckle for tractional retinal detachment (TRD) or rhegmatogenous retinal detachment (RRD) (cicatricial ROP, stages 4 and 5)

Prognosis: depends on extent of disease; most cases resolve spontaneously without visible residua
Some develop cicatricial changes: (retrolental fibroplasia)
GRADE I: myopia and peripheral glial scar (VA >20/40)
GRADE II: dragged retina, macular heterotopia (VA 20/50-20/200)
GRADE III: retinal fold (VA <20/200)
GRADE IV: partial retrolental membrane and RD (VA = HM or LP)
GRADE V: complete retrolental membrane and RD (VA = LP or NLP)

Complications:
Grade I-II: myopia (80%; due to forward displacement of lens–iris diaphragm), anisometropia, strabismus, amblyopia, macular heterotopia, pseudo-XT (change in angle κ due to macular dragging from peripheral cicatrization), increased risk of retinal tear or RD
Grade III-V: nystagmus, glaucoma, cataracts, heterochromia irides, rubeosis iridis, anterior uveitis, RD, band keratopathy, phthisis bulbi

MAJOR CLINICAL STUDY

Cryotherapy for ROP Study (Cryo-ROP)

Objective: to evaluate whether cryotherapy for ROP in preterm infants with birth weights <1251 g prevents unfavorable outcomes (posterior retinal fold, stage 4B or 5 retinal detachment, or visual acuity of 20/200 or worse)

Results:

The more posterior the zone and the greater the extent of stage 3+ ROP, the poorer is the outcome

All unfavorable fundus structural outcomes and almost all unfavorable visual acuity outcomes occurred in eyes with zone 1 or 2 ROP and >6 sectors of stage 3+ disease

Fewer unfavorable outcomes occurred in treated vs control eyes (44.4% vs 62.1% for visual acuity; 27.2% vs 47.9% for fundus status)

Retinal detachments remained stable in treated eyes (22%) but continued to occur in control eyes (from 38.6% at 5.5 years to 41.4% at 10 years)

After 10 years, treated eyes were much less likely than control eyes to be blind

Conclusions:

Cryotherapy preserves visual acuity in eyes with threshold disease

Initial examination: 4–6 weeks after birth or at 30 weeks' gestational age (whichever is later), then every 2 weeks until vessels reach zone 3

Prethreshold disease: examine every week until regression or threshold disease develops

Threshold disease: perform cryotherapy within 72 hours of diagnosis
Laser photocoagulation or cryotherapy to avascular retina, 90% regression rate
After 1 week, plus disease is usually less if treatment will work, fibrovascular proliferation often takes 2 weeks to begin regressing; consider retreatment if ROP is worse after 1 week; retreat untreated areas

Stage 4 disease: 60% reattachment rate with scleral buckle; 5% obtain useful vision

Stage 5 disease: vitrectomy (very poor success rate)

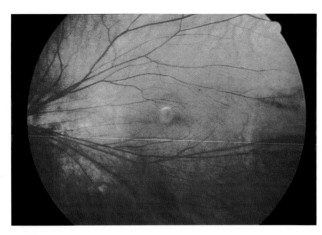

Figure 5-16. Fundus view of a patient who has familial exudative vitreoretinopathy. Note abnormally straightened retinal vasculature. (From Kimura AJ: Hereditary vitreoretinopathies. In Yanoff M, Duker JS [eds]: Ophthalmology, London, Mosby, 1999.)

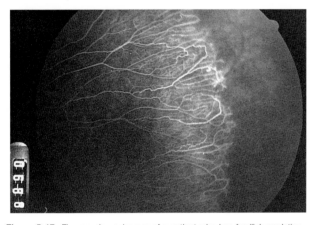

Figure 5-17. Fluorescein angiogram of a patient who has familial exudative vitreoretinopathy. (From Kimura AJ: Hereditary vitreoretinopathies. In Yanoff M, Duker JS [eds]: Ophthalmology, London, Mosby, 1999.)

Familial Exudative Vitreoretinopathy (FEVR) (AD or X-Linked Recessive)

Mapped to chromosome 11q13-q23 *(EVR1)*, 11p13-p12 *(EVR3)*

Most are unaware that they have this disorder

Rare, progressive developmental abnormality of peripheral retinal vasculature (especially temporally)

Findings: similar to ROP (Figures 5-16 and 5-17)
  Stage 1: avascular peripheral retina, white without pressure, vitreous bands, peripheral cystoid degeneration, microaneurysms, telangiectasia, straightened vessels, vascular engorgement; may have strabismus or nystagmus; most asymptomatic; may progress to stage 2
  Stage 2: fibrovascular proliferation with neovascularization, exudates, dragging of disc and macula, retinal folds and detachments; visual loss after 2nd–3rd decade of life rare unless progression to stage 3

Stage 3: cicatrization with rhegmatogenous retinal detachments (10–20%; usually in 3rd–4th decade of life), may develop proliferative vitreoretinopathy; prognosis poor

Treatment: prophylactic laser treatment to avascular retina (controversial); may require RD repair

Coats' Disease (Leber's Miliary Aneurysms)

Nonhereditary, proliferative exudative vascular disease

More common in males (10:1); bimodal distribution (peak in 1st decade and small peak in young adulthood [associated with hypercholesterolemia]) 90% unilateral; 50% progressive

Findings: usually presents with leukocoria and strabismus; telangiectatic blood vessels leak (with large amount of subretinal lipid in outer plexiform layer), noncalcified yellow subretinal lesions, exudative RD in 66% (especially in patients <4 years old), microaneurysms, capillary nonperfusion

Pathology: triad of retinal vascular anomalies, subretinal and intraretinal cholesterol deposits, and intraretinal PAS-positive deposits; loss of vascular endothelium and pericytes; gliotic retina over subretinal fluid with cholesterol clefts and hemosiderin-laden macrophages. Aspiration of subretinal exudates reveals cholesterol and pigment-laden macrophages

DDx: retinoblastoma, angiomatosis retinae (von Hippel-Lindau syndrome), PHPV

B-scan ultrasound: consider ruling out retinoblastoma

Fluorescein angiogram (FA): blood-fluid levels; saccular aneurysms ('light bulb' dilatations) of retinal arterioles and venules (Figure 5-18)

Treatment: cryo or laser to stop leaking blood vessels

Norrie's Disease (X-Linked Recessive)

Defect of retinal development

Findings: bilateral leukocoria (white, often hemorrhagic retrolental mass), retinal dysplasia, peripheral NV, hemorrhagic RD, and retinal necrosis

Other findings: deafness, mental retardation

Shaken Baby Syndrome

30–40% of children subjected to child abuse will have ophthalmic sequelae

Most common in children <3 years old

Findings: diffuse retinal hemorrhages, papilledema, vitreous hemorrhage, retinal tissue disruption (retinoschisis, retinal breaks, folds); may resemble CRVO, Terson's syndrome, or Purtscher's retinopathy

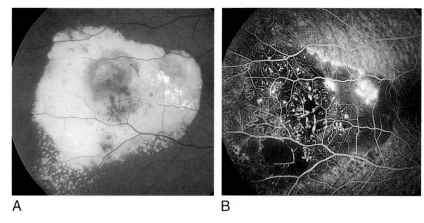

A   B

Figure 5-18. A, The classic fundus picture of Coats' disease with massive lipid exudation that causes an exudative retinal detachment. **B,** Fluorescein angiogram from the same patient with large telangiectatic vessels and numerous leaking aneurysms. (From Mittra RA, Mieler WF, Pollack JS: Retinal arterial macroaneurysms. In Yanoff M, Duker JS [eds]: Ophthalmology, London, Mosby, 1999.)

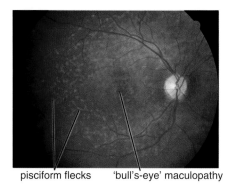

pisciform flecks   'bull's-eye' maculopathy

Figure 5-19. Stargardt's disease. (From Kaiser PK, Friedman NJ, Pineda II, R: Massachusetts Eye and Ear Infirmary Illustrated Manual of Ophthalmology, 2nd edn, Philadelphia, WB Saunders, 2004.)

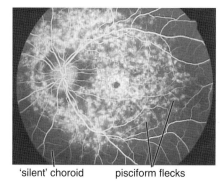

'silent' choroid   pisciform flecks

Figure 5-20. Fluorescein angiogram of Stargardt's disease demonstrating dark choroid and hyperfluorescent pisciform flecks. (From Kaiser PK, Friedman NJ, Pineda II, R: Massachusetts Eye and Ear Infirmary Illustrated Manual of Ophthalmology, 2nd edn, Philadelphia, WB Saunders, 2004.)

Associated with other injuries: subdural hematoma, subarachnoid hemorrhage, bruises, fracture of long bones or ribs

Prognosis: poor due to macular scarring, vitreous hemorrhage, RD

Inherited Retinal Diseases

Fundus Flavimaculatus (AR)

Mapped to chromosome 1p21-p13 *(ABCA4)*

Findings: bilateral pisciform, yellow-white flecks at level of RPE

Predominantly involves peripheral retina with macula involved to a lesser degree; flecks, then macular degeneration

Central vision preserved until macula involved

Pathology: lipofuscin deposits within hypertrophied RPE cells

ERG: degree of abnormality correlates with amount of fundus involvement

Stargardt's Disease

AR or less often AD; mapped to chromosomes 1p21-p22 *(STGD1)*, 4p *(STGD4)*, 6q14 *(STGD3)*

Juvenile macular degeneration with flecks

Most common hereditary macular dystrophy

Onset in first 2 decades of life with decreased vision

Symptoms: decreased vision, nyctalopia

Findings: bilateral pisciform, yellow-white flecks at level of RPE; change with time (new ones appear, others disappear); beaten-metal appearance of fundus; foveal atrophy; bull's-eye maculopathy; may have salt and pepper pigmentary changes of peripheral retina (Figure 5-19)

Pathology: RPE massively thickened by accumulation of lipofuscin

FA: dark choroid (85%) due to accumulation of lipofuscin in RPE; areas of hyperfluorescence do not directly correspond to flecks; pigmentary changes in macula appear as window defects (Figure 5-20)

ERG and EOG: normal or subnormal

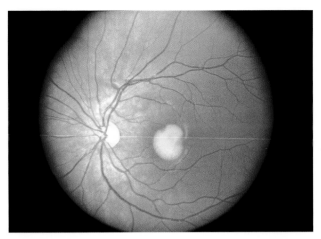

Figure 5-21. Best's disease. Vitelliform stage. (Courtesy of Ola Sandgren, University Hospital of Umea, Sweden. From Parnell JR, Small KW: Macular dystropies. In Yanoff M, Duker JS [eds]: Ophthalmology, London, Mosby, 1999.)

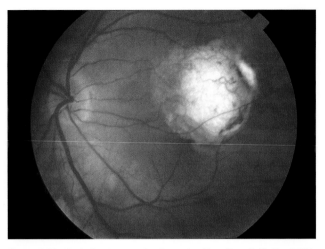

Figure 5-22. North Carolina macular dystrophy. (From Parnell JR, Small KW: Macular dystrophies. In Yanoff M, Duker JS [eds]: Ophthalmology, London, Mosby, 1999.)

Prognosis: 50% have at least 20/40 vision in one eye by age 19; only 22% have 20/40 vision by age 39; rapid progression to 20/200 – Counting fingers (CF)

Best's Disease (Vitelliform Dystrophy) (AD)

Variable penetrance; mapped to chromosome 11q13 (*VMD2* [bestrophin])

Second most common hereditary macular dystrophy

Progressive with onset in 1st decade of life

Macular dystrophy in which RPE is primarily affected; form of exudative central macular detachment in which pigmentation can occur in end stages with atrophic scarring and/or CNV

Associated with strabismus and hyperopia

Symptoms: none or mild decreased vision initially; later decreases to 20/50-20/100; better vision than expected by clinical appearance

Findings: progressive macular changes; can get CNV
  Previtelliform stage: small round submacular yellow dot
  Vitelliform stage: yellow-orange egg yolk/fried egg appearance; can be multiple; usually between ages 3 and 15 (Figure 5-21)
  Scrambled egg stage: irregular subretinal spots; vision usually still good
  Cyst stage
  Pseudohypopyon stage: RPE atrophy
  Round chorioretinal atrophy stage: atrophic scar; vision usually stabilizes at 20/100

DDx: central serous chorioretinopathy, RPED, toxoplasmosis, macular coloboma, solar retinopathy, old foveal hemorrhage, adult vitelliform macular dystrophy, syphilis

FA: blockage by egg yolk lesion; window defect when cyst ruptures

ERG: normal

EOG: abnormal (Arden ratio <1.6; also in carriers)

Dark adaptation: normal

Prognosis: good vision (20/30-20/100 range)

Familial Drusen (Doyne's Honeycomb Dystrophy) (AD)

Mapped to chromosome 2p16-p21 (*EFEMP1*)
Small yellow-white, round to oval deposits on Bruch's membrane; decreased vision after age 40

Complications: macular edema, hemorrhage, CNV

Maternal Inherited Diabetes and Deafness (MIDD)

Mitochondrial disease (maternal inheritance); point mutation at position 3243 of maternal mtDNA

Onset in 5th decade with ptosis, external ophthalmoplegia, ragged red fibers in extraocular muscles, chorioretinal atrophy, iris atrophy, pigmentary retinopathy (annular perifoveal RPE atrophy in macula or pattern-type dystrophy appearance)

VF: annular defect

FA: autofluorescence around dark pigment atrophy area

OCT: photoreceptor dropout

ERG: normal

North Carolina Macular Dystrophy (AD)

Mapped to chromosome 6q14-q16 *(MCDR1)*

Onset in 1st decade with drusen progressing to chorioretinal atrophy with staphyloma of macula (Figure 5-22)

May develop CNV

ERG, EOG, and dark adaptation: normal

Pseudoinflammatory Macular Dystrophy (Sorsby's) (AD)

Mapped to chromosome 22q12-q13 (SFD [*TIMP-3*])

Atrophy, edema, hemorrhage, and exudate

Decreased acuity and color vision occurs between ages 40 and 50

ERG and EOG: subnormal late

Dark adaptation: delayed

Pattern Dystrophies (Usually AD)

Group of diseases with central pigmentary disturbance, good central vision, normal ERG, abnormal EOG

May develop CNV

Sjögren's reticular: fishnet configuration; fishnet is hypofluorescent on FA

Butterfly: gray-yellow butterfly lesion with surrounding depigmentation; onset between ages 20 and 50 with slightly reduced vision; mapped to chromosome 6p21 (RDS [peripherin])

Adult vitelliform: onset between ages 30 and 50; early ring-like area of RPE clumping that develops into symmetric, solitary yellow macula lesions (like Best's egg yolk lesions but smaller [1/2 DD in central fovea] and do not break up); often have central area of pigment; CNV is more common than in Best's disease; normal EOG

Progressive Cone Dystrophy

Autosomal dominant or less often X-linked; mapped to chromosomes 6p21 (*COD3*), Xp21 (*COD1*) [*RPGR*]), Xq27 (*COD2*)

Progressive dysfunction of cones with normal rod function

Onset during first 3 decades of life with decreased vision, dyschromatopsia, photophobia

Symptoms: visual loss, photophobia (usually precede visible macular changes)

Findings: decreased vision (to 20/200), decreased color vision, central scotoma, nystagmus (25%), NFL loss, optic atrophy, macular degeneration (granular appearance early, then beaten-metal appearance); can have fine, golden subretinal deposits, bull's-eye maculopathy (Figure 5-23); can develop a pattern that mimics Stargardt's or fundus flavimaculatus

VF: normal

FA: may show window defects early

ERG: absent photopic, normal scotopic

EOG: normal

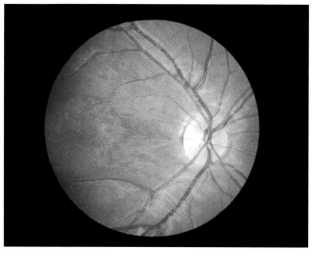

Figure 5-23. The 'bull's-eye' maculopathy in this 5-year-old male who has a cone–rod dystrophy is not found in all cases of this entity. (From Sieving PA: Retinis pigmentosa and related disorders. In Yanoff M, Duker JS [eds]: Ophthalmology, London, Mosby, 1999.)

Dark adaptation: rod phase only

Prognosis: poor vision (20/200 level) by 4th decade of life

Stationary Cone Disorders

Present at birth; nonprogressive

Complete rod monochromatism (congenital achromatopsia) (AR): mapped to chromosome 14 (*ACHM1*); absent or abnormal cones; nonprogressive
Findings: decreased vision (20/200 level), complete color blindness, photophobia, nystagmus, normal retinal examination
VF: central scotoma
Erg: normal scotopic, abnormal photopic

Blue cone monochromatism (X-linked recessive): have only blue-sensitive cones
Findings: decreased vision (20/40-20/200), photoaversion, nystagmus
ERG: absent cone response, normal rod response

Tapetoretinal Degeneration

Processes that involve the outer half of the retina (photoreceptor/RPE); RPE = tapetum nigran (black carpet)

Retinitis Pigmentosa (RP)

Group of progressive dystrophies caused by abnormal photoreceptor protein production

Most common hereditary degeneration, incidence 1:5000

RP type I (rod–cone):
Inheritance patterns:
AR (37%): most common form; may be due to defects in 2 RPE genes (which provide

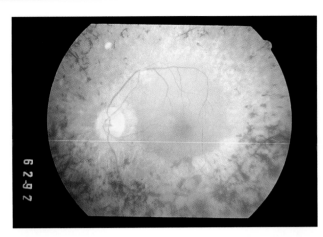

Figure 5-24. 'Typical' retinitis pigmentosa changes. (From Sieving PA: Retinis pigmentosa and related disorders. In Yanoff M, Duker JS [eds]: Ophthalmology, London, Mosby, 1999.)

instructions for vitamin A transport proteins): *RPE 65, CRALBP*

X-LINKED RECESSIVE (4%): rarest and most severe form; poor prognosis; vision <20/100 by 3rd decade of life; carriers may have fundus changes

AD (20%): least severe form, later onset; most likely to retain good vision

SPORADIC (30–50%)

Associations: keratoconus, macular cystoid degeneration, Coats' disease, optic disc drusen, astrocytic hamartoma of ON, myopia

Symptoms: nyctalopia, 'blue blindness,' decreased vision late

Findings: pigmentary retinal changes (bone spicules), attenuated arteries, waxy pallor of optic nerve (due to glial membrane formation over disc), retinal atrophy with increased visibility of choroidal vessels, vitreous cells, cataract; some forms can have prominent subretinal exudation (Coats'-like disease) (Figure 5-24)

Pathology: photoreceptor atrophy including outer nuclear layer; inner retina well preserved; RPE cells invade retina and surround retinal vessels (bone spicules)

VF: inferotemporal scotoma, enlarges to form ring/annular scotoma; constricted

ERG: early, increased rod threshold with normal cone response and decreased scotopic b-wave; late, nonrecordable; abnormalities precede retinal changes and visual complaints

EOG: abnormal

Dark adaptation: prolonged

RP carriers:

FUNDUS: bone spicules, salt and pepper changes, bronze sheen in macula

ERG: decreased scotopic amplitude and delayed cone B-wave implicit time in X-linked carriers

VITREOUS FLUOROPHOTOMETRY: abnormal in X-linked carriers

DDx of tunnel vision: glaucoma, functional, gyrate atrophy, vitamin A toxicity, occipital lobe stroke

DDx of nyctalopia: uncorrected myopia, vitamin A deficiency, zinc deficiency, choroideremia, gyrate atrophy, congenital stationary night blindness (CSNB), Goldman-Favre disease

DDx of salt and pepper fundus: rubella retinopathy, Leber's congenital amaurosis, carrier states (albinism, RP, choroideremia), syphilis, cystinosis, phenothiazine toxicity, pattern dystrophy, following resolution of an exudative RD

Macular complications: CME (no leakage on FA), epiretinal membrane, atrophy

RP type II (cone–rod): AD, AR, or X-linked

Findings: less pigment deposition; 50% are sine pigmento

ERG: cones more affected than rods

Treatment: low vision aids, dark glasses; vitamin A slows reduction of ERG (controversial)

Prognosis: poor

RP Variants

Treatable RP: Bassen-Kornzweig (abetalipoproteinemia), Refsum's (elevated phytanic acid), gyrate atrophy (elevated ornithine)

Leber's congenital amaurosis (AR): mapped to chromosomes 1p31 (*LCA2*), 14q11 (*RPGRIP1*), 17p13 (*LCA1,LCA4*), 19q13 (*CRX*)

Infantile form of RP; blind or severe visual impairment in infancy or early childhood; responsible for approximately 10% of childhood blindness

Associations: keratoconus, hyperopia, cataract, macular coloboma, mental retardation, deafness, seizures, renal and musculoskeletal abnormalities

Findings: decreased vision (HM-CF [hand movements–counting fingers]), nystagmus, hyperopia, poorly reactive pupils, range of fundus appearance from normal (most common) to variety of pigmentary changes (granular, fleck, salt and pepper, sheen, or atrophic)

OCULODIGITAL SIGN: child rubs eyes to elicit entopic stimulation of retina

Pathology: diffuse absence of photoreceptors

ERG: low or completely flat

Sector RP (AD or AR): retinal changes limited to focal area, usually inferonasal quadrant

VF: abnormal

ERG: abnormal; normal b-wave implicit time reflects nonprogression

Prognosis: good

Unilateral RP: very rare

Inverse RP: posterior pole affected (rather than midperiphery): bone spicules in macula, normal periphery

FA: dark choroid (probably a variant of Stargardt's)

Retinitis punctata albescens (AR): small white spots in midperiphery of retina, no bone spicules

RP sine pigmento: no retinal pigmentary changes

Pseudoretinitis pigmentosa: migration of RPE melanin into sensory retina leading to bone spicule pattern

Etiology: trauma, drug toxicity (chloroquine, chlorpromazine), infection/inflammation (syphilis, toxoplasmosis, measles, rubella), post-CVO, resolved exudative RD, ophthalmic artery occlusion

RP Syndromes

Usher's syndrome (AR): most common syndrome associated with RP; mapped to chromosome 1q41 (*USH2A*)

Findings: RP and deafness; ataxia, MR, low phosphate (rickets), muscle wasting 10–20% of RP patients are deaf; 5% of congenitally deaf individuals have Usher's type I

TYPE 1: night blindness (1st–2nd decade), profound deafness, unintelligible speech, ataxia

TYPE 2: night blindness (2nd–4th decade), partial deafness, intelligible speech, no ataxia

DDx of deafness and RP: Usher's, Hallgrenn's, Alstrom's, Laurence-Moon-Biedl-Bardet, and Cockayne's syndromes

Other eye syndromes associated with hearing loss: Cogan's (IK + hearing loss), Stickler's (vitreous changes, joint and orofacial abnormalities, hearing loss), Waardenburg-Klein (iris heterochromia, white forelock), Duane's (15% have hearing loss)

Refsum's disease (AR): deficiency of phytanic acid oxidase interferes with fatty acid metabolism

Phytanic acid accumulates in RPE cells, sensory retina deteriorates; onset in childhood

Mapped to chromosomes 7q21-q22 (*PEX1*), 10p15-p12 (*PNYH*)

Findings: atypical RP (often sine pigmento or starts in macula), cataracts, prominent corneal nerves

Other findings: ataxia, peripheral neuropathy, deafness, anosmia, ichthyosis, cardiac abnormalities, hypotonia, hepatomegaly, mental retardation

Diagnosis: increased serum copper and ceruloplasmin; increased CSF protein without pleocytosis

Treatment: dietary restriction of animal fats, milk products, leafy green vegetables

Bassen-Kornzweig syndrome (AR): hereditary abetalipoproteinemia; mapped to chromosome 4q24 (*MTP*)

Inability to transport and absorb lipids because apolipoprotein B is a major protein of chylomicrons; deficiency in fat-soluble vitamins (A, D, E, and K)

Findings: RP (usually without bone spicules); may have Bitot's spots on conjuctiva

Other findings: ataxic neuropathy, growth retardation, coagulopathy

Diagnosis: CBC, cholesterol (low), stool sample; elevated CSF protein; no apolipoprotein B-48 (low chylomicrons) or apolipoprotein B-100 (low LDL and VLDL)

Treatment: vitamin A and E supplements

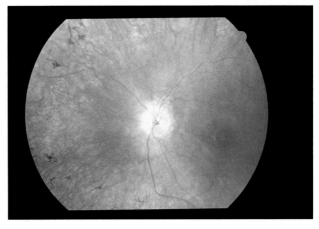

Figure 5-25. Bardet-Biedl syndrome with extensive peripheral retinal pigment epithelium and parafoveal retinal pigment epithelium atrophy. (From Sieving PA: Retinis pigmentosa and related disorders. In Yanoff M, Duker JS [eds]: Ophthalmology, London, Mosby, 1999.)

Other causes of treatable RP due to vitamin A deficiency: chronic pancreatitis, cirrhosis, bowel resection

Lawrence-Moon-Bardet-Biedl syndrome (AR): mapped to chromosomes 2q31 (*BBS5*), 3p13-p12 (*BBS3*), 11q13 (*BBS1*), 15q22-q23 (*BBS4*), 6q21 (*BBS2*), 20p12 (*BBS6*)

L-M and B-B: pigmentary retinopathy with flat ERG, mental retardation, hypogonadism, short stature

B-B: polydactyly and obesity (Figure 5-25)

L-M: spastic paraplegia

Spielmeyer-Vogt-Batten-Mayou syndrome: neuronal ceroid lipofuscinosis

Onset between 2 and 4 years of age in Jewish females

Findings: RP-like retinal degeneration with bull's-eye maculopathy

Other findings: seizures, progressive dementia, ataxia

Pathology: vacuolization of peripheral lymphocytes; metachromasia of skin fibroblasts in cell culture (carriers only)

Chronic progressive external ophthalmoplegia (CPEO): mitochondrial inheritance; 50% with positive family history

Findings: retinal degeneration (salt and pepper changes with normal retinal function; progresses to RP-like disease), ptosis, ophthalmoplegia, strabismus

Other findings: facial weakness, dysphagia, small stature, limb girdle myopathy, cardiac conduction defects (Kearns-Sayre syndrome)

Olivopontocerebellar atrophy: retinal degeneration; tremors, ataxia, dysarthria

Alstrom's disease: mapped to chromosome 2p13 (*ALMS1*)

RP with profound visual loss in 1st decade of life; diabetes, obesity, deafness, renal failure, baldness, acanthosis nigricans, hypogenitalism

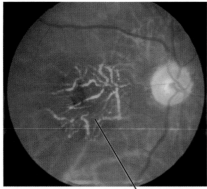

central areolar choroidal dystrophy

Figure 5-26. Central geographic atrophy in a patient with central areolar choroidal dystrophy. (From Kaiser PK, Friedman NJ, Pineda II, R: Massachusetts Eye and Ear Infirmary Illustrated Manual of Ophthalmology, 2nd edn, Philadelphia, WB Saunders, 2004.)

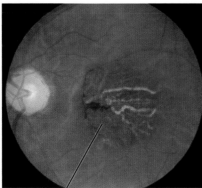

central areolar choroidal dystrophy

Figure 5-27. Left eye of same patient as shown in Figure 5-26 demonstrating similar central geographic atrophy. (From Kaiser PK, Friedman NJ, Pineda II, R: Massachusetts Eye and Ear Infirmary Illustrated Manual of Ophthalmology, 2nd edn, Philadelphia, WB Saunders, 2004.)

Cockayne's syndrome: RP with profound visual loss by 2nd decade of life; dwarfism, deafness, mental retardation, premature aging, psychosis, intracranial calcifications

Neuronal ceroid lipofuscinosis (Batten's disease): juvenile or adult onset of seizures, dementia, ataxia, mental retardation

Central Areolar Choroidal Dystrophy (AD)

Mapped to chromosome 6p (*RDS* [peripherin]), 17p13 (*CACD*)

Decreased vision in 4th decade

Findings: RPE mottling in macula progressing to geographic atrophy (choroidal vessels visible) (Figures 5-26, 5-27)

FA: window defect of central lesion

ERG: normal or subnormal

EOG, dark adaptation: normal

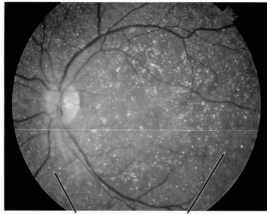

Bietti's crystalline retinopathy

Figure 5-28. Bietti's crystalline retinopathy. (From Kaiser PK, Friedman NJ, Pineda II, R: Massachusetts Eye and Ear Infirmary Illustrated Manual of Ophthalmology, 2nd edn, Philadelphia, WB Saunders, 2004.)

Bietti's Crystalline Retinopathy (AR)

Decreased vision in 5th decade

Findings: yellow-white refractile spots throughout fundus, geographic atrophy; may have crystals in peripheral corneal stroma (Figure 5-28)

FA: crystals hyperfluoresce, window defects and areas of blockage

ERG: reduced

Congenital Stationary Night Blindness (CSNB)

Poor night vision (nyctalopia)

Group of nonprogressive rod disorders classified by fundus appearance

Findings: normal vision, VF, and color vision; may show paradoxical pupillary dilation to light; no Purkinje shift (always most sensitive to 550 nm)

ERG: scotopic and photopic implicit times are identical; decreased scotopic ERG; photopic ERG almost normal

Normal fundus:
Nougaret type (AD): no rod function; mapped to chromosome 3p21 (*GNAT1*)
Riggs type (AR): some rod function
Schubert-Bornschein type (X-linked or AR): some or no rod function, myopia

Abnormal fundus:
Fundus albipunctatus (AR): mapped to chromosome 12q13-q14
  FINDINGS: midperipheral deep yellow-white spots spare macula (Figure 5-29)
  ERG: normalization of scotopic after 4–8 hours of dark adaptation
  ALPORT'S SYNDROME (AD): kidney failure, deafness, anterior lenticonus with anterior polar cataract;

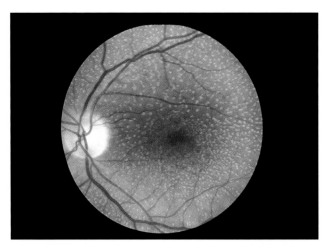

Figure 5-29. Fundus albipunctatus. This posterior pole and beyond show multiple small, discrete, round, white dots that spare the fovea. (From Noble KG: Congenital stationary night blindness. In Yanoff M, Duker JS [eds]: Ophthalmology, London, Mosby, 1999.)

may have retinal appearance similar to fundus albipunctatus

Oguchi's disease: mapped to chromosomes 2q37 (*Oguchi 1, Arrestin, SAG*), 13q34 (*Oguchi 2 [RHOK]*)

    MIZUO-NAKAMURA PHENOMENON: golden-brown fundus (yellow/gray sheen) in light-adapted state, normal-colored fundus in dark-adapted state (takes about 12 hours) (Figure 5-30)

    ERG: absent b-wave; only scotopic a-wave

Kandori's flecked retina (AR): yellow-white spots scattered in equatorial region; spares macula

Choroideremia (X-Linked Recessive)

Mapped to chromosome Xq21

Progressive disorder of choriocapillaris; considered a form of rod–cone degeneration

Onset during late childhood with nyctalopia, photophobia, constricted visual fields in affected males

Findings:
early – degeneration of RPE and choriocapillaris in periphery (scalloped RPE atrophy); late – absence of RPE and choriocapillaris except in macula (Figure 5-31) Female carriers have salt and pepper fundus

Pathology: defect in choroidal vasculature

ERG: markedly reduced; undetectable late

Gyrate Atrophy (AR)

Mapped to chromosome 10q26

Deficiency of ornithine aminotransferase; elevated ornithine levels (10–20× normal), low lysine levels; chorioretinal dystrophy itself is not due to high ornithine levels

Progressive retinal degeneration; starts peripherally and spreads toward posterior pole

Onset by 2nd decade of life with decreased vision, nyctalopia, and constricted visual fields

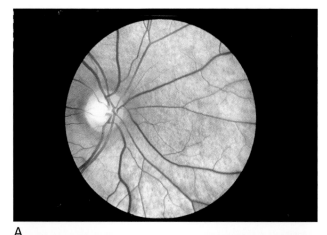

A

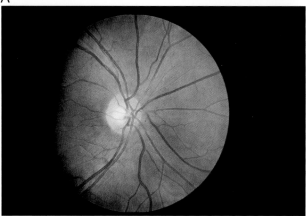

B

Figure 5-30. Oguchi's disease. **A,** The yellowish metallic sheen is apparent nasal to the optic disc. **B,** After 3 hours of dark. (From Noble KG: Congenital stationary night blindness. In Yanoff M, Duker JS [eds]: Ophthalmology, London, Mosby, 1999.)

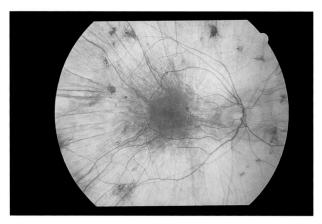

Figure 5-31. Fundus changes in the right eye from a patient with late-stage choroideremia. (From Grover S, Fishman GA: Choroidal dystrophies. In Yanoff M, Duker JS [eds]: Ophthalmology, London, Mosby, 1999.)

Findings: scalloped areas of absent choriocapillaris and RPE in periphery with abrupt transition between normal and atrophic areas (Figure 5-32); eventually lose choriocapillaris and medium-sized choroidal vessels; myopia (90%), cataracts, vitreous degeneration, CME

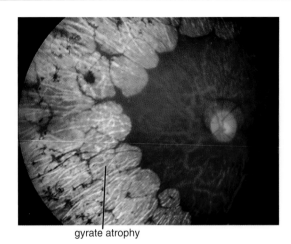

gyrate atrophy

Figure 5-32. Gyrate atrophy. (From Kaiser PK, Friedman NJ, Pineda II, R: Massachusetts Eye and Ear Infirmary Illustrated Manual of Ophthalmology, 2nd edn, Philadelphia, WB Saunders, 2004.)

Other findings: seizures, structural changes in muscle and hair fibers

Diagnosis: blood tests (increased ornithine, decreased lysine), urinalysis (increased ornithine)
 Carrier: decreased levels of ornithine ketoacid transaminase

ERG and ECG: abnormal

Dark adaptation: prolonged

Treatment: restrict arginine and protein in diet; consider vitamin B_6 supplementation (pyridoxine; reduces ornithine)

Metabolic Diseases

Mucopolysaccharidoses (AR Except Hunter [X-Linked Recessive])

Accumulation of acid mucopolysaccharides due to lysosomal enzyme defects

Syndromes in which heparin sulfate accumulates are associated with pigmentary retinopathy

Findings: may have corneal clouding (stromal; progressive), retinopathy (RPE degeneration), and/or optic atrophy (see Table 5-4)
 Corneal clouding and retinopathy: Hurler (type Ia), Scheie (type Ib), Maroteaux-Lamy (type VI)
 Retinopathy only: Hunter (type II), Sanfilippo (type III)
 Corneal clouding only: Morquio (type IV), Sly (type VII)
 No corneal clouding or retinopathy: Sly (type VII)

Sphingolipidoses (AR)

Accumulation of sphingolipids due to lysosomal enzyme defects

Sphingolipids accumulate in retinal ganglion cells; result in cherry red spot (macula has highest concentration of ganglion cells) (see Table 5-4)

Cherry red spot: Tay-Sachs, Sandhoff's, Neimann-Pick, and Gaucher's disease
 Tay-Sachs: most common; hexosaminodase A deficiency; death by 3 years of age; cherry red spot and mental retardation
 Sandhoff's: similar to Tay-Sachs; extensive visceral involvement
 Niemann-Pick: cherry red spot, macular halo, optic atrophy; hepatosplenomegaly, infiltration of lungs, foam cells in bone marrow, no mental retardation

DDx of cherry red spot: CRAO, commotio retinae, macular hole, macular hemorrhage, ocular ischemic syndrome, subacute sclerosing panencephalitis, quinine toxicity, methanol toxicity

No cherry red spot: Fabry's and Krabbe's diseases
 Fabry's (X-linked dominant): α-galactosidase A deficiency; accumulation of trihexosylceramide in smooth muscle of blood vessels
 FINDINGS: cornea verticillata (whorl-like opacities in basal epithelium), tortuous conjunctival and retinal vessels, cataracts (posterior lenticular spoke-like changes); manifest in heterozygous females (carriers) and 90% of affected males
 OTHER FINDINGS: paresthesias in extremities, cutaneous telangiectases, angiokeratomas, poor temperature regulation, abdominal pain, anemia, renal failure, hypertension; vascular anomalies of heart, kidney, and brain; renal failure is leading cause of death
 DIAGNOSIS: failure to detect α-galactosidase in tears

Cystinosis

Mapped to chromosome 17p13

Amino acid disorder; lysosomes cannot excrete cystine

Findings: iridescent fusiform cystine crystals in conjunctiva, cornea, iris, lens, and retina; photophobia
 Infantile form (nephropathic form) (AR): Fanconi's syndrome: polyuria, growth retardation, rickets, progressive renal failure, salt and pepper fundus changes (but no visual disturbance); the only form with retinopathy; most die before puberty
 Adolescent form (AR): less severe nephropathy than in Fanconi's syndrome
 Adult form: benign; no renal problems; deposits limited to anterior segment

Treatment: cysteamine (systemically for renal disease, topically for corneal crystals)

Long-Chain 3-Hydroxyacyl-CoA Dehydrogenase Deficiency (LCHAD Deficiency)

Disorder of mitochondrial fatty acid beta-oxidation due to mutation of guanine to cytosine at position 1528

Findings: normal fundus at birth, followed by RPE pigment dispersion; eventually develop chorioretinal atrophy and occlusion of choroidal vessels; deterioration of central vision; may have posterior staphylomas, developmental cataracts, progressive myopia

Treatment: low-fat, high-carbohydrate diet with carnitine supplementation

Prognosis: usually fatal by 2 years of age (hepatic or cardiorespiratory failure) unless dietary treatment is started

Vitreoretinal Dystrophies

Vitreous abnormalities associated with schisis cavity at level of NFL and ganglion cell layer

Juvenile Retinoschisis (X-Linked Recessive)

Mapped to chromosome Xp22 (*XLRS1* [retinoschisin])

Males; bilateral; present at birth; progresses rapidly during first 5 years of life; stable by age 20

Cleavage of retina at NFL (in senile retinoschisis, cleavage is at outer plexiform layer)

Findings:
  Foveal retinoschisis (only abnormality in 50%): pathognomonic; earliest change is radial, spoke-like ILM folds centered on fovea because of dehiscence of NFL; appears like CME. Later, cystoid structure appears in fovea with round microcysts in perifoveal area and marked pigmentary degeneration; bullous schisis cavities develop; retinal vessels are only remaining structure within inner layer and may bleed causing vitreous hemorrhage
  Marked sclerosis/sheathing of blood vessels with appearance of vitreous veils
  Vitreous cells (30%)
  True retinoschisis (NFL) in periphery in 50% (usually inferotemporal); does not extend to ora
  Vitreous syneresis
  Hyperopia
  Reduced vision (20/50-20/100 level)
Carriers have normal retinal appearance and function

VF: absolute scotoma

FA: microcysts with no leakage

ERG: normal a-wave until late, reduced b-wave (especially scotopic) in proportion to amount of retinoschisis, markedly reduced oscillatory potentials

EOG: normal

Complications: RD and VH (uncommon)

Goldmann-Favre Disease (AR)

Mapped to chromosome 15q23 (*PNR*)

Rare, vitreotapetoretinal degeneration with nyctalopia and constricted visual fields (like RP + juvenile retinoschisis)

Findings: decreased vision, nyctalopia, optically empty vitreous with strands and veils, bilateral central and peripheral retinoschisis, attenuated retinal vessels, peripheral bone–spicule retinal pigmentary changes, lattice degeneration, optic disc pallor, cataracts

ERG: markedly reduced

EOG: abnormal (distinguishes from juvenile retinoschisis)

Treatment: may require retinal surgery for retinal tears or detachments

Vitreoretinal Degenerations

Wagner Syndrome (AD)

Mapped to chromosomes 5q13-q14 (*WGN1*), 12q13 (*COL2A1*)

Findings: optically empty vitreous (abnormal vitreous structure; vitreous liquefaction and fibrillar condensation result in a clear vitreous space with membranes, veils, and strands), no RD, equatorial and perivascular pigmented lattice-like changes, peripheral vessel sheathing, RPE atrophy, cataract (wedge and fleck opacities between ages 20 and 40), moderate myopia, optic atrophy

ERG: may be abnormal

Treatment: cataract extraction; genetic counseling

Jansen Syndrome (AD)

Wagner syndrome + RD

Stickler's Syndrome (AD)

Mapped to chromosomes 1p21 (*COL11A1*), 6p21 (*COL11A2*), 12q13 (*COL2A1*)

Progressive arthro-ophthalmopathy; Wagner-like ocular changes with severe myopia and marfinoid habitus

Findings: optically empty vitreous, lattice degeneration, RD (50%), optic atrophy, cataract, glaucoma, high degree of myopia (Figure 5-33)

Other findings: orofacial abnormalities (Pierre Robin anomaly: midfacial flattening and cleft palate), marfinoid

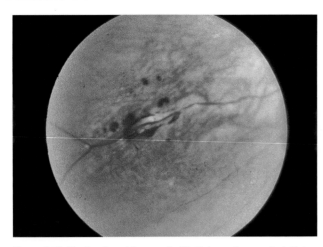

Figure 5-33. Fundus view of the eye of a Stickler's syndrome patient. Note the radial perivascular pigmentary changes. (From Kimura AJ: Hereditary vitreoretinopathies. In Yanoff M, Duker JS (eds) Ophthalmology, London, Mosby, 1999.)

habitus, hearing loss, mitral valve prolapse, joint abnormalities (hyperextensibility, enlargement, arthritis)

ERG: decreased b wave

Hereditary Arthro-Ophthalmopathy (Weill-Marchesani-Like Variety)

Similar to Stickler's but short stature with stubby hands and feet; increased risk of ectopia lentis

Snowflake Degeneration (AD)

Very rare, progressive vitreoretinal degeneration

Manifests after 25 years of age

Findings: optically empty vitreous; associated with peripheral NV, increased risk of RD, early cataracts
  Stage 1: Extensive white without pressure
  Stage 2: Snowflakes (white dots in superficial retina) within white without pressure
  Stage 3: Sheathing of retinal vessels and early peripheral pigmentation
  Stage 4: Disappearance of retinal vessels in periphery and increased retinal pigmentation

ERG: decreased scotopic b-wave amplitude

EOG: normal

Dark adaptation: elevated rod threshold later in disease

Miscellaneous Retinal Disorders

Albinism

Albinoidism: only minimal reduction in vision; no nystagmus

Albinism: AR or less frequently AD disorder characterized by decreased melanin and congenitally subnormal vision (foveal hypoplasia and nystagmus)
  Oculocutaneous: lack of pigmentation of skin, hair, and eyes
    TYROSINASE-NEGATIVE (no pigmentation):
      Defect in chromosome 11
      FINDINGS: decreased vision, iris transillumination, foveal hypoplasia, hypopigmented fundus, nystagmus, photophobia, high myopia, strabismus
      OTHER FINDINGS: hypopigmentation of skin and hair (white hair, pink skin)
    TYROSINASE-POSITIVE (some pigmentation):
      Defect in chromosome 15 (paternal = Prader-Willi syndrome; maternal = Angelman's syndrome)
      Ocular and systemic characteristics less severe
    POTENTIALLY LETHAL VARIANTS:
      CHÉDIAK-HIGASHI SYNDROME: large melanosomes on skin biopsy, reticuloendothelial dysfunction with pancytopenia, recurrent infections, and malignancies (leukemia, lymphoma)
      HERMANSKY-PUDLAK SYNDROME: clotting disorder due to abnormal platelets, commonly of Puerto Rican descent
  Ocular: abnormal melanogenesis limited to eye (decreased number of melanosomes)
    X-LINKED RECESSIVE: iris transillumination less prominent, female carriers with variable retinal pigmentation (mosaic pattern)
      Giant melanosomes in skin, normal pigmentation of skin
      Associated with deafness
    AUTOSOMAL RECESSIVE: both males and females affected
  ERG and EOG: supranormal

Aicardi's Syndrome (X-Linked Dominant)

Only females, lethal in males
Lacunar defects in RPE

Findings: widespread depigmented round chorioretinal lesions, ON head coloboma, microphthalmos

Other findings: infantile spasms, severe mental retardation, agenesis of corpus collosum

Colorblindness (Tables 5-5 and 5-6)

Incidence up to 13% of population

Red-green disorders are X-linked recessive (male preponderance); men and women can have tritan disorders (AD)

Table 5-5. Incidences of color vision abnormalities	
Deuteranomaly	5% (XR)
Deuteranopia	1% (XR)
Protonanomaly	1% (XR)
Protonanopia	1% (XR)
Tritanomaly	0.0001% (AD)
Tritanopia	0.001% (AD)

Congenital color vision defect is typically red-green; acquired color vision defect is typically blue-yellow

Table 5-6. Comparison of dyschromatopsias

Congenital dyschromatopsia	Acquired dyschromatopsia
Deuteranomalous trichromats are most common (5% of male population)	
Red-green axis	Blue-yellow axis
Males > females	Females = males
Nonprogressive	May be slowly progressive
Bilateral and symmetric	Unilateral or nonsymmetric
Normal eye examination	Associated with abnormality on eye examination
X-linked recessive	No heritability
Deep blue is perceived as purple	Deep blue is perceived as gray

Color vision defects do not cause decreased vision, except for red and blue cone monochromatism

Normal individuals are trichromats: 3 types of cones (red, green, blue); 92% of population

Prot = Red; Deuter = Green; Trit = Blue (Greek for 1st, 2nd, 3rd; order in which these deficits were described)

Anopia = absent; Anomaly = abnormal; An = unspecified

Anomalous trichromatism: all 3 cones present but in abnormal proportions; can distinguish fully saturated colors but has difficulty distinguishing colors of low saturation

According to which pigment is abnormal, the disorders are called:
Protanomaly: abnormal level of red pigment
Deuteranomaly: abnormal level of green pigment
Tritanomaly: abnormal level of blue pigment

Congenital dichromatism: substantial lack of one type of color cone
Protanopia: red cones contain chlorolabe (green pigment)
Deuteranopia: green cones contain erythrolabe (red pigment)
Tritanopia: defect of blue cones
2 forms of congenital dyschromatopsia associated with low vision:
Rod monochromatism (AR): cones are absent, therefore complete achromatopsia; poor vision and nystagmus in infants
ERG: normal under scotopic conditions; reduced during photopic conditions
Blue cone monochromatism (X-linked recessive): nystagmus, decreased vision, photophobia, myopia

Tritan color defect and slightly subnormal vision: consider Kjer's dominant optic atrophy

Diagnosis: color vision testing
Farnsworth-Munsell 100 hue test: consists of 85 hue caps contained in 4 separate racks with 2 end caps fixed; patient arranges caps between fixed ends in order of hue; tests for both red-green and blue-yellow defects
Farnsworth's panel D-15: derived from 100-hue test, but uses only 15 caps
City university test: derived from 100-hue test, but uses 10 charts with a central color and 4 peripheral colors; select outer color that matches central color
Pseudoisochromatic plates: Ishihara plates (for protanopes and deuteranopes; detect only red-green defects), and Hardy-Rand-Ritter (HRR) polychromatic plates (test for both red-green and blue-yellow defects)

Kollner's rule: errors made by persons with optic nerve disease tend to resemble those made by protans and deutans (red and green), whereas errors made by individuals with retinal disease resemble those made by tritans (blue)

Retinal Tumors

Congenital Hypertrophy of the RPE (CHRPE)

Usually unilateral, congenital, asymptomatic

Findings: flat, well-circumscribed black lesion with surrounding halo; larger lesions often contain depigmented lacunae (choroid visible through lacunae); multiple patches with sector distribution called 'bear tracks' (Figures 5-34 to 5-36)

Pathology: melanosomes in RPE cells are larger and more spherical than normal; densely packed round melanocytes and increased thickness of RPE; focal areas of RPE loss (lacunae)

Atypical multifocal bilateral variant: occurs in 75% of patients with familial adenomatous polyposis (FAP: AD, mapped to chromosome 5q; high incidence of multiple adenomas of colon and rectum; eventually undergo malignant transformation.. Gardner's syndrome [variant of FAP]: combination of colonic polyps and extracolonic manifestations [osteomas, dermoid tumors])

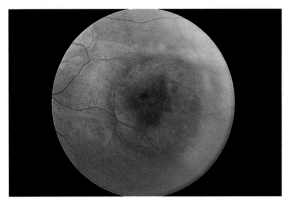

Figure 5-34. Typical congenital hypertrophy of retinal pigment epithelium. (From Augsburger JJ, Bolling JJ: Hypertrophy of retinal pigment epithelium. In Yanoff M, Duker JS [eds]: Ophthalmology, London, Mosby, 1999.)

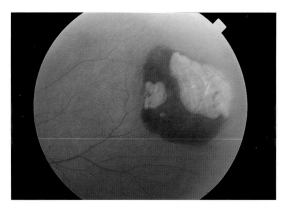

Figure 5-35. Congenital hypertrophy of retinal pigment epithelium with prominent depigmented lacunae. (From Augsburger JJ, Bolling JJ: Hypertrophy of retinal pigment epithelium. In Yanoff M, Duker JS [eds]: Ophthalmology, London, Mosby, 1999.)

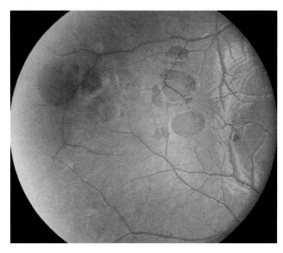

Figure 5-36. Congenital hypertrophy of retinal pigment epithelium (grouped by pigmentation of retina). (From Augsburger JJ, Bolling JJ: Hypertrophy of retinal pigment epithelium. In Yanoff M, Duker JS [eds]: Ophthalmology, 2nd edn, St Louis, Mosby, 2004.)

DDx: (Box 5-3)

> **Box 5-3.** Differential diagnosis of congenital hypertrophy of the retinal pigment epithelium. (From Augsburger JJ, Bolling JJ: Hypertrophy of retinal pigment epithelium. In Yanoff M, Duker JS [eds]: Ophthalmology, London, Mosby, 1999.)
>
> Reactive hyperplasia of retinal pigment epithelium
>
> Massive gliosis of retina
>
> Combined hamartoma of retina
>
> Melanotic choroidal nevus or melanoma
>
> Bilateral diffuse uveal melanocytic proliferation associated with systemic carcinoma syndrome
>
> Adenoma or adenocarcinoma of retinal pigment epithelium
>
> Metastatic melanoma to retina

Table 5-7. Chances of having a baby with retinoblastoma

Offspring of	NEGATIVE FH		POSITIVE FH	
	Unilateral (%)	Bilateral (%)	Unilateral (%)	Bilateral (%)
Parents with an affected child	1	6	40	40
Affected patient	8	40	40	40
Normal sibling of affected patient	1	<1	7	7

Retinoblastoma (RB)

Most common intraocular malignancy in children

Incidence 1 in 20,000

No sex or race predilection

90% diagnosed by 5 years of age; fatal in 2–4 years if untreated

30% bilateral, 30% multifocal

Genetics: (Table 5-7)
Mapped to chromosome 13q14, must have gene defect on both chromosomes

94% sporadic (75% somatic, 25% germinal mutation); 6% autosomal dominant

40% heritable, 80% penetrance

Most occur sporadically in infants with no family history; bilateral cases are usually familial (risk that additional offspring will have retinoblastoma is 40%)

75% are caused by mutation (inactivation of both RB genes) in a single retinal cell; these tumors are unilateral and unifocal; the chance of inactivation of both RB genes is very small
  Parents with 1 affected child: 6% risk of producing more affected children
  Parents with 2 or more affected children: 40% risk (because only 80% penetrance)
  Retinoblastoma survivor with hereditary form: 50% chance of transferring to children (but children have only 40% chance of manifesting a tumor)

Presentation: leukocoria (60%), strabismus (22%), decreased vision (5%)

Findings: yellow-white retinal mass, rubeosis, pseudohypopyon, hyphema, angle-closure glaucoma, uveitis

Types:
  Endophytic: arises from inner retina and grows toward vitreous; can simulate endophthalmitis; can have pseudohypopyon (Figure 5-37)

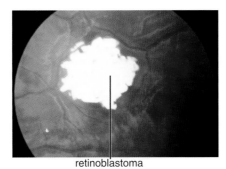

retinoblastoma

Figure 5-37. Retinoblastoma demonstrating discrete round tumor. (From Kaiser PK, Friedman NJ, Pineda II, R: Massachusetts Eye and Ear Infirmary Illustrated Manual of Ophthalmology, 2nd edn, Philadelphia, WB Saunders, 2004.)

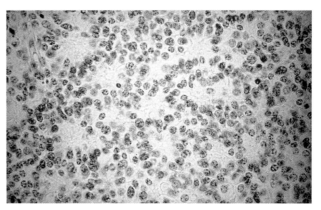

Figure 5-38. Homer-Wright rosettes. (From Augsburger JJ, Bornfeld M, Giblin ME: Retinoblastoma. In Yanoff M, Duker JS [eds]: Ophthalmology, London, Mosby, 1999.)

Exophytic: arises from outer retina and grows toward choroid causing solid RD; can extend through sclera; can simulate Coats' disease or traumatic RD

Tumor necrosis when outgrows blood supply, then calcification (seen on CT and ultrasound); may develop NV glaucoma (17%); no macular tumors after 1.5 months of age

ON involvement: present in 29% of enucleated eyes
Risk for ON invasion: exophytic tumors >15 mm, and eyes that have secondary glaucoma

Second tumors: commonly present around age 17; osteogenic sarcoma of femur (most common), malignant melanoma of eye or orbit, leiomyosarcoma of eye or orbit, lymphoma, leukemia, rhabdomyosarcoma, medulloblastoma

Trilateral retinoblastoma: bilateral RB with a pinealoblastoma or parasellar neuroblastoma; occurs in 3% of children with unilateral RB and 8% with bilateral RB; 95% have a positive family history and/or other tumors; spontaneous regression occurs with subsequent necrosis and phthisis

Pathology: rosettes are histologic markers for tumor differentiation
In order of increasing differentiation:
Homer-Wright rosette: no lumen; nuclei surround tangle of neural filaments; reflects low-grade neuroblastic differentiation; can be found in other types of neuroblastic tumors (adrenal neuroblastoma, medulloblastoma) (Figure 5-38)
Flexner-Wintersteiner rosette: ring of single row of columnar cells around central lumen; cells have eosinophilic cytoplasm and peripheral nuclei; photoreceptors contain cilia with a 9 + 0 pattern; represent early retinal differentiation; attempt of outer photoreceptor production; special stains show hyaluronidase-resistant acid mucopolysaccharides in lumen; also present in medulloepitheliomas (Figure 5-39)

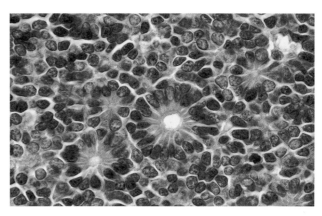

Figure 5-39. Flexner-Wintersteiner rosettes. (From Augsburger JJ, Bornfeld M, Giblin ME: Retinoblastoma. In Yanoff M, Duker JS [eds]: Ophthalmology, London, Mosby, 1999.)

Fleurettes: bouquet of pink bulbous neoplastic photoreceptor inner segments; highest degree of differentiation in retinoblastoma; found in relatively eosinophilic areas of tumor (photoreceptor differentiation)
Pseudorosettes: circumferential arrangements of viable tumor cells surrounding a central vessel
Cells have round, spindle-shaped hyperchromatic nuclei and very little cytoplasm; high mitotic activity; as tumor grows, outgrows blood supply creating necrosis with areas of calcification (80%)
H&E stain:
BLUE AREAS: represent viable tumor; differentiated cells that have basophilic nuclei and little cytoplasm
PINK AREAS: represent necrotic tumor; lose basophilic nuclei and appear eosinophilic (pink)
PURPLE AREAS: represent calcified tumor; occur in necrotic areas; calcium stains purple (Figure 5-40)

DDx: (DDx of leukocoria): cataract, retrolental mass (PHPV, ROP, Norrie's disease, RD), tumor (choroidal metastases, retinal astrocytoma), exudates (FEVR, Coats' disease, Eales' disease), change in retinal pigment (incontinentia pigmenti, high myopia, myelinated nerve

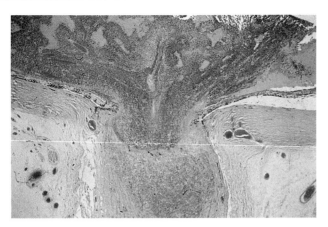

Figure 5-40. RB demonstrating necrosis and optic nerve invasion. (From Yanoff M, Fine BS: Ocular Pathology, 5th edn. Mosby, Philadelphia, 2002.)

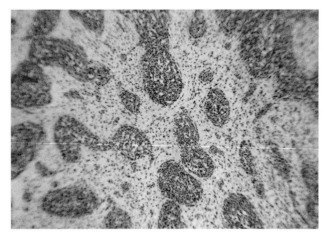

Figure 5-41. Leukemic infiltrate in optic nerve. (From Yanoff M, Fine BS: Ocular Pathology, 5th edn. Mosby, Philadelphia, 2002.)

fiber, retinal dysplasia, choroideremia, coloboma), infections (toxoplasmosis, toxocariasis, endophthalmitis)

Diagnosis:

LDH levels: ratio of aqueous:plasma LDH >1.0

Ultrasound: acoustic solidity and high internal reflectivity; calcium appears as dense echoes

FA: early hyperfluorescence with late leakage of lesions

CT scan: calcification; look for pineal tumor with CT or MRI, and for ON involvement

Metastatic workup: bone scan, bone marrow aspirate, LP (cytology)

Treatment:

Enucleation: all blind and painful eyes; affected eye in most unilateral cases; worse eye in most asymmetric cases; both eyes in many symmetric cases; excise at least 10 mm of ON to prevent spread

External beam radiation: salvageable eyes with vitreous seeding or large tumor; most eyes with multifocal tumors; eyes that have failed coagulation therapy; RB is very radiosensitive; used to treat most 2nd tumors

Episcleral plaque radiation: salvageable eyes with single medium-sized tumor that does not involve ON or macula, even with localized vitreous seeding

Photocoagulation/cryotherapy: occasional eyes with one or a few small tumors, not involving ON or macula

Prognosis: 90–95% of children with retinoblastoma survive (same with either growth pattern); 3% spontaneously regress

Metastases: most commonly to CNS along ON; 50% are to bone

Familial RB: location related to age, earliest in macula, later in periphery; 2nd eye tumor develops up to 44 months later; 45% mortality by age 35 (vs 19% long-term survival for all patients with RB by age 35); multiple primary tumors in an eye does not worsen prognosis

Increased risk of 2nd unrelated malignancy in 25% of children with heritable retinoblastoma

Poor prognostic signs: ON invasion, uveal invasion, extrascleral extension, multifocal tumors (represent seeding); delay in diagnosis, degree of differentiation

Bilateral involvement does not worsen prognosis; prognosis depends on status of tumor in worst eye; degree of necrosis and calcification does not influence prognosis

Reese-Ellsworth classification: predicts visual prognosis (not survival) in eyes treated by methods other than enucleation

Retinocytoma/Retinoma

Benign tumor with same appearance and genetics as RB

Pathology: numerous fleurettes among cells with varying degrees of photoreceptor differentiation

Differentiation from RB: more cytoplasm, more evenly dispersed nuclear chromatin, no mitoses, calcification may be present, and necrosis is usually absent in retinocytoma

13q Deletion Syndrome

Associated with retinoblastoma, microcephaly, hypertelorism, microphthalmos, ptosis, and epicanthus

Leukemia

Most common malignancy of childhood

Usually affects choroid with retinal hemorrhages; usually unilateral

Symptoms: blurred vision, floaters

Findings (Figures 5-41 and 5-42): cellular infiltration of vitreous; infiltrative lesions of retina, optic nerve, or uvea; multiple hemorrhages, Roth spots, cotton wool spots (CWS); heterochromia irides, pseudohypopyon, spontaneous hyphema, uveitic glaucoma, cataract

Optic nerve infiltration causes loss of vision and papilledema

Orbital infiltration (rare) causes proptosis, lid swelling, ecchymosis (1-2% of patients)

Treatment: emergent XRT for ON infiltration; patient is more susceptible to developing radiation optic neuropathy when chemotherapy is used concurrently

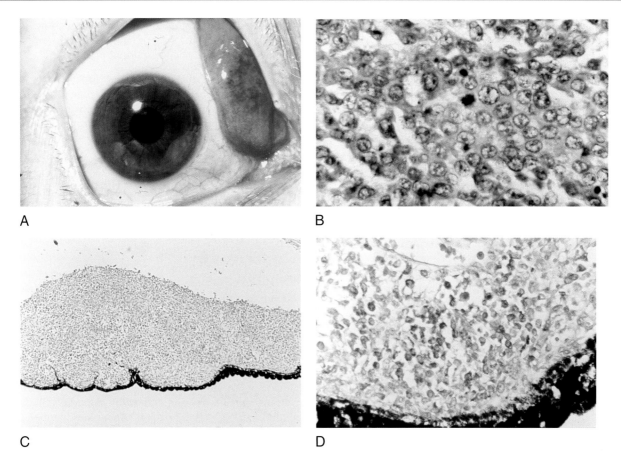

Figure 5-42. Acute leukemia. **A,** A patient presented with a large infiltrate of leukemic cells positioned nasally within the conjunctiva of the right eye, giving this characteristic clinical picture. These lesions look similar to those caused by benign lymphoid hyperplasia, lymphoma, or amyloidosis. **B,** A biopsy of the lesion shows primitive blastic leukocytes. **C,** In another case, the iris is infiltrated by leukemic cells. A special stain (Lader stain) shows that some of the cells stain red, better seen when viewed under increased magnification in **D.** This red positiveness is characteristic of myelogenous leukemic cells. (From Augsburger JJ, Tsiaras WG: Lymphoma and leukemia. In Yanoff M, Duker JS [eds]: Ophthalmology, London, Mosby, 1999.)

Prognosis: poor; high mortality; can be rapidly fatal if untreated

PHAKOMATOSES

Group of disorders (neurocutaneous syndromes) characterized by ocular and systemic hamartomas. Most are AD with variable penetrance except Sturge-Weber and Wyburn-Mason (no hereditary pattern) and ataxia-telangiectasia (AR) (Table 5-8)

Table 5-8. Genetics of the phakomatoses

Disorder	Chromosome
Neurofibromatosis:	
Type 1	17
Type 2	22
Sturge-Weber	None
von Hippel-Lindau	3
Tuberous sclerosis	9
Ataxia-telangiectasia	11
Wyburn-Mason	None

Treatment: often requires CT scans and medical consultations; may require treatment of elevated IOP

Neurofibromatosis (AD)

Variable expressivity

Disorder of Schwann cells and melanocytes with hamartomas of nervous system, skin, and eye

Types:

NF-1 (von Recklinghausen's syndrome): mapped to chromosome 17q11 (neurofibromin), 50% due to new mutation; 80% penetrance

More common form (prevalence 1 in 3000 to 5000)

  CRITERIA (2 or more of the following):

    6 or more café au lait spots >5 mm in diameter in prepubescent or >15 mm in postpubescent individuals

    2 or more neurofibromas or 1 plexiform neurofibroma

    Freckling of intertriginous areas

    Optic nerve glioma

    2 or more Lisch nodules

Osseous lesion (sphenoid bone dysplasia, thinning of long bone cortex)

First-degree relative with NF-1

FINDINGS: plexiform neurofibroma (plexus of abnormal markedly enlarged nerves; occur in 25%; 10% involve face, often upper eyelid or orbit; 'bag of worms' appearance and S-shaped upper lid; congenital glaucoma in ipsilateral eye in up to 50%), fibroma molluscum, plexiform neurofibroma of conjunctiva, prominent corneal nerves, Lisch nodules (glial/melanocytic iris hamartomas), diffuse uveal thickening due to excess melanocytes and neurons (similar to ocular melanocytosis), ectropion uveae, retinal astrocytic hamartoma (less likely to be calcified than in tuberous sclerosis), increased incidence of myelinated nerve fibers and choroidal nevi (33%), ON glioma (juvenile pilocytic astrocytoma in >30%; may cause visual loss, hypothalamic dysfunction or hydrocephalus; neuroimaging shows fusiform enlargement of nerve with kinking; if have glioma, 25% have NF), meningioma, orbital plexiform neurofibroma, schwannoma, absence of sphenoid wing (pulsating exophthalmos)

OTHER FINDINGS: café au lait spots, intertriginous (axillary) freckling, cutaneous peripheral nerve sheath tumors

NF-2: mapped to chromosome 22q

Prevalence 1 in 50,000

CRITERIA:

Bilateral cerebellar–pontine angle tumors (acoustic neuromas; cause hearing loss, ataxia, headache)

First-degree relative with NF-2 and either a unilateral acoustic neuroma or 2 of the following: meningioma, schwannoma, neurofibroma, glioma, posterior subcapsular cataract

May have pheochromocytoma and other malignant tumors

No Lisch nodules

Encephalotrigeminal Angiomatosis (Sturge-Weber Syndrome)

Nonhereditary
No racial or sex predilection

Facial hemangioma: nevus flammeus (port wine stain) limited to first 2 divisions of CN 5; 5–10% bilateral

Findings: dilated tortuous vessels of the conjunctiva and episclera, congenital or juvenile glaucoma (25% risk, especially if upper lid is involved), heterochromia irides (due to angiomas of iris), angiomas of episclera and CB, diffuse cavernous choroidal hemangioma ('tomato-ketchup' fundus [50%]), peripheral retinal AV malformations, may get RD or severe RPE alterations (pseudo-RP)

Mechanism of glaucoma: neovascular, increased episcleral venous pressure, immature angle structures

Other findings: leptomeningeal vascular malformations (ipsilateral to port wine stain), central calcifications, mental retardation, seizures, pheochromocytoma

Klippel-Trénaunay-Weber: variant of Sturge-Weber with cutaneous nevus flammeus, hemangiomas, varicosities, intracranial angiomas, and hemihypertrophy of limbs

Findings (uncommon): congenital glaucoma, conjunctival telangiectasia; can have AV malformation similar to Wyburn-Mason

Angiomatosis Retinae (Von Hippel–Lindau Disease) (AD)

Incomplete penetrance; mapped to chromosome 3p26-p25 (*VHL*)

Prevalence 1 in 100,000

50% bilateral

Hamartomas of eye, brain (cerebellum), kidney/adrenal gland

(Note: disease has 3 names, 3 locations for tumors, and defect on chromosome 3)

Findings: retinal angioma (hemangioma or hemangioblastoma; round orange-red mass fed by dilated tortuous retinal artery and drained by engorged vein; may be multifocal as well as bilateral; often in midperiphery, may be near disc; leaks heavily causing serous RD and/or macular edema; treat with yellow dye laser if enlarges)

Other findings: 25% of retinal capillary hemangiomas associated with CNS tumor (hemangioblastoma of cerebellum [60%]; pons, medulla, and/or spinal cord is less common); visceral lesions (cysts and tumors of kidney, pancreas, liver, adrenal glands, including renal cell carcinoma [25%], pheochromocytoma [5%])

Von Hippel disease: only ocular involvement

Treatment: observation, cryotherapy, or laser photocoagulation

Tuberous Sclerosis (Bourneville's Disease) (AD or Sporadic)

Mapped to chromosomes 9q34 (*TSC1* [hamartin]), 16p13 (*TSC2* [tuberin])

Prevalence 1 in 10,000 to 100,000

Triad of adenoma sebaceum, mental retardation, and epilepsy

Findings: astrocytic hamartoma of the retina (flat or mulberry-shaped with calcifications; usually in posterior pole; consists of nerve fibers and undifferentiated glial cells; occurs in 50%; bilateral in 15%), astrocytic hamartoma of the ON ('giant drusen'; benign)

Other findings:

Cutaneous: facial angiofibroma (adenoma sebaceum; vascularized red papules in butterfly distribution, not present at birth, become visible between ages 2 and 5), ash leaf spots (hypopigmented spots that fluoresce under Wood's light, considered pathognomonic), shagreen patches (25%; areas of fibromatous infiltration, usually on trunk), periungual fibromas, may have café au lait spots

CNS: subependymal hamartomas (calcify, forming 'brain stones' with root-like appearance; concentrated in periventricular area), mental retardation (60%), seizures (80%), cerebral calcification

Other: cardiac rhabdomyoma, spontaneous pneumothorax (from pleural cyst), renal angiomyolipomas, pheochromocytoma

Early mortality

Ataxia-Telangiectasia (Louis-Bar Syndrome) (AR)

Mapped to chromosome 11q22 (*ATM*)

Prevalence 1 in 40,000

Findings: prominent dilated conjunctival vessels, impaired convergence, nystagmus, oculomotor apraxia

Other findings: cutaneous telangiectasia in butterfly distribution during 1st decade of life, mental retardation, cerebellar ataxia (due to cerebellar atrophy), thymic hypoplasia with defective T-cell function and IgA deficiency with increased risk of infections, malignancy (leukemia/lymphoma)

Racemose Hemangiomatosis (Wyburn-Mason Syndrome)

Nonhereditary, usually unilateral

Findings: racemose hemangioma of retina (arteriovenous malformation with markedly dilated and tortuous shunt vessels); may have intraocular hemorrhage or glaucoma

Other findings: arteriovenous malformations in brain (may cause seizures, paresis, mental changes, VF defects), orbit and facial bones; may have small facial hemangiomas

Others

Retinal Cavernous Hemangioma

Cluster of intraretinal aneurysms filled with venous blood

Appears as 'cluster of grapes'

Vitreous hemorrhage is rare

May be associated with cutaneous and CNS hemangiomas

FA: fluid levels without leakage within lesions

Incontinentia Pigmenti (Bloch-Sulzberger Syndrome) (X-Linked Dominant)

Occurs exclusively in females (lethal in males)

Findings: proliferative retinal vasculopathy (resembles ROP); may have retinal detachment and retrolental membrane (Figure 5-43)

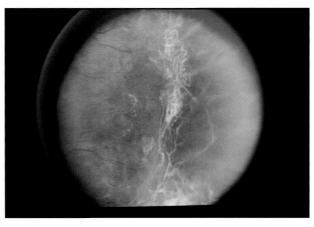

Figure 5-43. Incontinentia pigmenti. The peripheral retina of a patient who has incontinentia pigmenti demonstrates somewhat elevated vessels with vessel walls. A majority of these vessels show nonperfusion. The more posterior retina was perfused, and the anterior retina was ischemic. (From Ebroom DA, Jampol JM: Proliferation retinopathies. In Yanoff M, Duker JS [eds]: Ophthalmology, London, Mosby, 1999.)

Other findings:

Skin lesions:
STAGE 1 (at birth): erythematous macules, papules, and bullae on trunk and extremities (intraepithelial vesicles containing eosinophils)

STAGE 2 (2 months of age): vesicles are replaced by verrucous lesions

STAGE 3 (3-6 months of age): lesions take form of pigmented whorls on trunk

STAGE 4: skin is atrophic with hypopigmented patches

Hair abnormalities: alopecia

CNS abnormalities: microcephaly, hydrocephalus, seizures, mental deficiency

Dental abnormalities: missing and cone-shaped teeth

Treatment: photocoagulation (variable results)

OPTIC NERVE DISORDERS

Aplasia

Complete absence of optic nerve; very rare; may occur with anencephaly or major cerebral maldevelopment

Hypoplasia

Variable visual compromise

Etiology unclear

No sex predilection

Associations: aniridia, Goldenhar's syndrome, midline anomalies, endocrine abnormalities, congenital intracranial tumors (craniopharyngioma, optic glioma), maternal diabetes or drug ingestion during pregnancy (alcohol, LSD, quinine, dilantin)

Findings: double ring sign (thin ring of pigment surrounding nerve tissue; halo of retina and RPE partially covering lamina cribrosa), strabismus, amblyopia, nystagmus, positive RAPD, VF defects

Other findings: CNS abnormalities (45%), growth retardation, endocrine abnormalities

De Morsier's syndrome (septo-optic dysplasia): bilateral ON hypoplasia, septum pellucidum abnormality, pituitary and hypothalamus deficiency; associated with agenesis of the corpus callosum; may have chiasmal developmental anomalies with VF defects; at risk for sudden death

Treatment: brain MRI, endocrine workup

Coloboma

Due to incomplete closure of embryonic fissure; usually located inferonasal

Unilateral or bilateral

Variable visual acuity and visual field defects

Associated with other ocular colobomas

Findings: large anomalous discs, deep excavation with abnormal vascular pattern (ranges from complete chorioretinal coloboma to involvement of proximal portion of embryonic fissure causing only optic nerve deformity); may resemble physiologic cupping if mild

Morning Glory Disc

Probably represents a dysplastic coloboma

Generally unilateral

Female > male (2 : 1)

Often seen with high myopia

May be associated with cranial defects or other ocular anomalies

Findings: cup filled with glial tissue surrounded by pigment ring, adjacent retinal folds common; also described as funnel-shaped, enlarged, excavated disc with central white connective tissue; vessels radiate in spoke-like fashion; usually poor vision; may develop peripapillary RD

Optic Pit

Gray-white depression in optic disc usually in inferotemporal area

85% unilateral

Associated with peripapillary RPE disturbances

May develop serous retinal detachment extending from pit (40%)

Tilted Disc

Findings (any of the following may occur, alone or in combination): apparent tilting (usually inferiorly with superior pole of disc elevated), scleral crescent, situs inversus arteriosus (vessels emerge temporally from optic nerve [rather than nasally] and course nasally before sweeping temporally), myopia and/or astigmatism, reduced visual acuity, visual field defects (usually bitemporal and do not respect vertical midline)

Myelinated Nerve Fibers

Myelination begins at lateral geniculate body and usually ceases at lamina cribrosa; however, some retinal fibers may acquire myelin sheath during first month of life

More common in males

Unilateral or bilateral (20%)

Vision generally good unless macula involved

Findings: superficial white flame-shaped patches with feathery margins; usually peripapillary; can be extensive

Relative or absolute scotoma corresponds to area of myelination

Persistence of Hyaloid System

Common; ranges from tuft of glial tissue on disc (Bergmeister's papillae) to patent artery extending from disc to lens

Megalopapilla

Enlarged optic disc

Peripapillary Staphyloma

Posterior bulging of sclera in which optic disc occupies bottom of bulge

Optic Nerve Drusen

Superficial or buried hyaline bodies in prelaminar portion of optic nerve

Sporadic or AD; 75% bilateral

Incidence 0.3–1% clinically; 2% histopathologically

More common in Caucasians; no sex predilection

Associations: angioid streaks, retinitis pigmentosa, Alagille's syndrome (familial intrahepatic cholestasis, posterior embryotoxin, bilateral optic disc drusen [80%])

Findings: disc margins may show irregular outline, bumpy nodular chunky appearance to nerve head (pseudopapilledema); VF defects (especially with deep drusen; enlarged blind spot, arcuate scotoma, sectoral scotoma); may have transient visual obscurations, positive RAPD (unilateral ON drusen); often calcify with age

Pathology: hyaline bodies that become calcified; stain positively for amino acids, calcium, acid mucopolysaccharides, and hemosiderin; stain negatively for amyloid

Diagnosis: B-scan ultrasound, CT scan, autofluorescence

Complications: rarely visual loss due to axonal compression, AION, CNV, subretinal or vitreous hemorrhage, vascular occlusion

Melanocytoma (Magnocellular Nevus of the Optic Disc)

Deeply pigmented tumor with feathery border located over ON

Derived from uveal dendritic melanocytes

May have choroidal and NFL involvement

15% show minimal enlargement over 5 years

Findings: VF defect; may have positive RAPD (even with good vision)

Pathology: benign, plump, round polyhedral melanocytes

Malignant transformation very rare

Hereditary Optic Neuropathy

Kjer's syndrome (AD): dominant optic neuropathy; most common form of heritable optic atrophy; mapped to chromosome 3q28 (*OPA1*); insidious onset between ages of 4 and 8; bilateral and symmetric; decreased vision (20/40-20/200), blue–yellow dyschromatopsia, temporal wedge of disc pallor

Behr's syndrome (AR): infantile optic neuropathy; onset before age 10, male > female, nonprogressive; moderate to severe decreased vision, nystagmus, diffuse optic atrophy; ataxia, spasticity, hypotonia, mental retardation

Wolfram syndrome (AR): onset between ages of 5 and 21; slowly progressive; decreased vision (<20/400), diffuse optic atrophy; DIDMOAD (Diabetes Insipidus, Diabetes Mellitus, Optic Atrophy, Deafness), ataxia, seizures, mental retardation

Leber's hereditary optic neuropathy

(LHON): maternal mitochondrial DNA; point mutations in mitochondrial gene for NADH subunit 4 (position 11778 [most common], 3460, 14484); male > female (9:1); maternal transmission to all sons (50% affected) and all daughters (15% of daughters affected, 85% are carriers); onset between ages of 15 and 30; subacute sequential bilateral vision loss (≤20/200) over days; tobacco or alcohol can trigger decompensation

Findings: disc hyperemia, peripapillary telangiectatic vessels (do not leak fluorescein, also found in 60% of asymptomatic family members), tortuous vessels, peripapillary NFL edema, late optic disc pallor; may have cardiac conduction abnormalities

DDx: acquired optic neuropathies: compressive (tumors [craniopharyngioma, optic nerve/chiasmal gliomas],

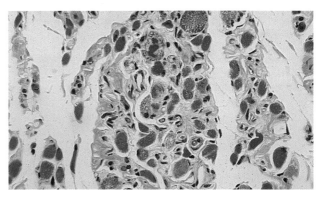

Figure 5-44. MELAS syndrome demonstrating degenerated EOM with trichome stain shows 'ragged red' fibers. (Case presented by Dr. R. Folberg to the meeting of the Verhoeff Society, 1993, and reported by Rummett V, Folberg R, Ionasescu V et al: Ocular pathology of MELAS syndrome with mitochondrial DNA nucleotide 3243 point mutation. Ophthalmology, 100:1757-66, 1993.)

hydrocephalus), toxic (anoxia at birth or in neonatal period), traumatic, infiltrative (leukemia, metabolic storage diseases)

Treatment: no treatment; genetic counseling

Mitochondrial Diseases

Maternal inheritance; children of both sexes affected; only female offspring can pass on

Findings: optic atrophy, CPEO, pigmentary retinopathy, retrochiasmal visual loss

Disorders:

Maternal inherited diabetes and deafness (MIDD): see earlier

Leber's hereditary optic neuropathy (LHON): see earlier

Kearns-Sayre syndrome: onset before age 20

   FINDINGS: chronic progressive external ophthalmoplegia with ptosis, pigmentary retinopathy (salt and pepper, bone spicules, and/or RPE atrophy), mild visual loss (50%)

   OTHER FINDINGS: neck and limb weakness, cardiac conduction defects (arrhythmias, heart block, cardiomyopathy), cerebellar ataxia

   PATHOLOGY: 'ragged red' fibers (contain degenerated mitochondria) on muscle biopsy

   EKG: heart block

   CSF: elevated protein

MELAS: Mitochondrial Encephalopathy, Lactic Acidosis, and Stroke-like episodes

Onset before age 15; point mutations (3242, 3271) or deletions

   FINDINGS: retrochiasmal visual loss; recurrent attacks of headache, vomiting, seizures; transient focal neurologic deficits (hemiplegia, hemianopia/cortical blindness), CPEO, optic neuropathy; pigmentary retinopathy, dementia, hearing loss, short stature, muscle weakness

   PATHOLOGY: 'ragged red' fibers on muscle biopsy, abnormal mitochondria in blood vessels (Figure 5-44)

DIAGNOSIS:
Elevated serum and CSF lactate
CT SCAN: basal ganglia calcification
MRI: posterior cortex lesions, spare deep white matter; can resolve
MERRF: Myoclonus, Epilepsy, and Ragged Red Fibers
FINDINGS: encephalopathy with myoclonus, seizures, ataxia, spasticity, dementia; may have dysarthria, optic neuropathy, nystagmus, short stature, hearing loss
PATHOLOGY: 'ragged red' fibers on muscle biopsy (Gomori trichrome stain)

Strabismus

ANATOMY AND PHYSIOLOGY

Subconjunctival Fascia (Figure 5-45)

Tenon's capsule:
Anterior: fuses with conjunctiva just behind limbus
Posterior: separates orbital fat from muscles and globe

Intermuscular septum: extension of Tenon's, connects muscles

Check ligaments: connect muscles to overlying Tenon's and inserts on orbital walls to support globe

Lockwood's ligament: fusion of sheaths of inferior rectus and inferior oblique; attaches to medial and lateral retinaculi and supports globe

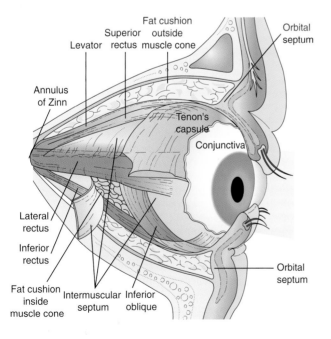

Figure 5-45. Muscle cone. (From Campolattaro BN, Wang FM: Anatomy and physiology of the extraocular muscles and surrounding tissues. In Yanoff M, Duker JS [eds]: Ophthalmology, 2nd edn. Mosby, St Louis.) 2004.)

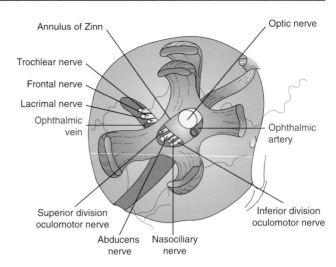

Figure 5-46. The annulus of Zinn and surrounding structures. (From Campolattaro BN, Wang FM: Anatomy and physiology of the extraocular muscles and surrounding tissues. In Yanoff M, Duker JS [eds]: Ophthalmology, 2nd edn, St Louis, Mosby, 2004.)

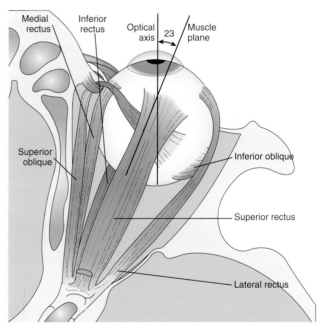

Figure 5-47. The extrinsic mucles of the right eyeball in the primary position, seen from above. The muscles are shown as partially transparent. From Campolattaro BN, Wang FM: Anatomy and physiology of the extraocular muscles and surrounding tissues. In Yanoff M, Duker JS [eds]: Ophthalmology, 2nd edn, St Louis, Mosby, 2004.)

Extraocular Muscles (Table 5-9, Figures 5-46 to 5-48)

All rectus muscles have 2 accompanying ciliary arteries except lateral rectus, which has 1

Spiral of Tillaux: Continuous curve that passes through insertions of rectus muscles; the temporal aspect of vertical muscles lies farther from limbus than the nasal aspect (Figure 5-49)

Table 5-9. Extraocular muscles

Muscle	Muscle length (mm)	Tendon length (mm)	Arc of contact (mm)	Anatomic insertion from limbus	Action from primary position	Origin	Innervation
Medial rectus (MR)	40	4.5	7	5.5 mm	Adduction	Annulus of Zinn	CN 3, (inferior division)
Lateral rectus (LR)	40	7	12	6.9 mm	Abduction	Annulus of Zinn	CN 6
Superiorrectus (SR)	40	6	6.5	7.7 mm	1. Elevation 2. Intorsion 3. Adduction	Annulus of Zinn	CN 3, (superior division)
Inferior rectus (IR)	40	7	6.5	6.5 mm	1. Depression 2. Extorsion 3. Adduction	Annulus of Zinn	CN 3, (inferior division)
Superior oblique (SO)	32	26	7-8	Posterior to equator insuperotemporal quadrant	1. Intorsion 2. Depression 3. Abduction	Orbital apex above annulus of Zinn	CN 4
Inferior oblique (IO)	37	1	15	Posterior to equator ininferotemporal quadrant	1. Extorsion 2. Elevation 3. Abduction	Behind lacrimal fossa	CN 3, (inferior division)
Levator palpebrae	40	14-20	—	Septa of pretarsal orbicularis and anterior surface of tarsus	Lid elevation	Orbital apex above annulus of Zinn	CN 3, (superior division)

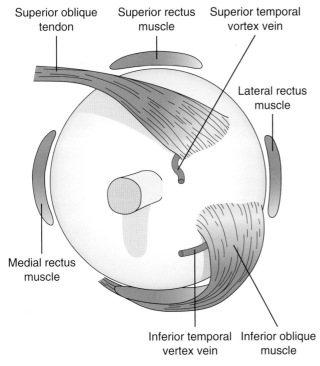

Figure 5-48. Posterior view of the eye with Tenon's capsule removed. (From Campolattaro BN, Wang FM: Anatomy and physiology of the extraocular muscles and surrounding tissues. In Yanoff M, Duker JS [eds]: Ophthalmology, 2nd edn, St Louis, Mosby, 2004.)

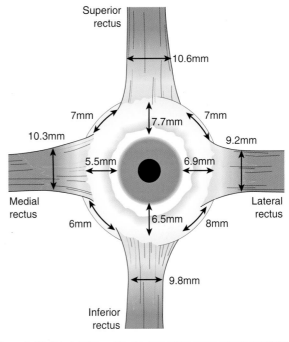

Figure 5-49. Spiral of Tillaux. The structure of the rectus muscle insertions. (From Campolattaro BN, Wang FM: Anatomy and physiology of the extraocular muscles and surrounding tissues. In Yanoff M, Duker JS [eds]: Ophthalmology, 2nd edn, St Louis, Mosby, 2004.)

Medial rectus (MR):
1. Pure adductor
2. Closest to limbus
3. Hardest to find if slipped because no fascial attachment to an oblique muscle

Lateral rectus (LR):
1. Pure abductor
2. Easiest exposure
3. Connected to inferior oblique

Superior rectus (SR):
1. Elevates, adducts, and incyclotorts
2. Inserts 23° temporal to visual axis in primary position; pure elevator only in 23° abduction

3. Fascial connections: SO, upper eyelid elevators. Therefore, SR recession may cause lid retraction, and resection may cause fissure narrowing
4. Passes over superior oblique

Inferior rectus (IR):

1. Depresses, abducts, and excyclotorts
2. Inserts 23° temporal to visual axis in primary position; pure depressor only in 23° abduction
3. Fascial connections: IO, lower eyelid retractors (Lockwood's ligament). Therefore, IR recession may cause lid retraction, and resection may cause fissure narrowing

Superior oblique (SO):

1. Incyclotorts, abducts, and depresses
2. Inserts 51° to visual axis; pure depressor only in 51° adduction
3. Passes inferior to SR
4. Arises from orbital apex above annulus of Zinn (lesser wing of sphenoid)

Inferior oblique (IO):

1. Excyclotorts, abducts, and elevates
2. Inserts 51° to visual axis; pure elevator only in 51° adduction
3. Passes inferior to IR
4. Originates from periosteum of maxillary bone
5. Inserts near macula
6. Avoid inferotemporal vortex vein during surgery
7. The inferior division of CN 3 up to the inferior oblique carries parasympathetic supply to iris constrictor; injury to these fibers results in mydriasis

Pediatric Eye Examination

Visual development:

At birth: blinking response to bright light
At 7 days: vestibulo-ocular response
At 2 months: fixation well developed
At 6 months: VER acuity at adult level
At 2 years: Snellen acuity at adult level
At 7 years: stereoacuity at adult level
Hyperopia (average of 2 D) increases during first year of life; 50% have >1 D with-the-rule astigmatism; decreases after 7 years of age

Vision testing:

Infancy: optokinetic (OKN) response, forced preferential looking (Teller acuity cards), visual evoked response (VER)
Older children: Allen pictures, HOTV, tumbling E, Snellen acuity

Sensory Testing

Binocular vision:

Horopter: the set of object points imaged on corresponding retinal points
Panum's fusional space: region around horopter in which binocular vision exists (Figure 5-50)

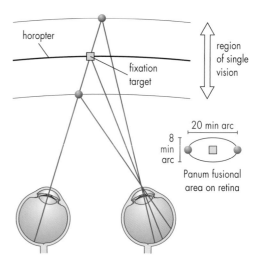

Figure 5-50. Panum's fusional area. The left eye fixates a square target, and a search object visible only to the right eye is moved before and behind this target. The ellipse of retinal area, for which typical dimensions are given for the parafoveal area, is the projection of Panum's fusional area. Diplopia is not perceived for 2 targets within this area. (From Diamond GR: Sensory status in strabismus. In Yanoff M, Duker JS [eds]: Ophthalmology, London, Mosby, 1999.)

Table 5-10. Normal fusional amplitudes (prism diopters [Δ])

Testing Distance	Convergence (Δ)	Divergence (Δ)	Vertical (Δ)
6 m	14	6	2.5
25 cm	38	16	2.6

Types of binocularity:

SIMULTANEOUS PERCEPTION: ability to see 2 images, 1 on each retina (super-imposed, not blended)
FUSION: simultaneous perception of 2 similar images blended as 1 (Table 5-10)
STEREOPSIS: perception of 2 slightly dissimilar images blended as 1 with appreciation of depth
  STEREOACUITY: occurs when retinal disparity is too small to cause diplopia, but too great to allow superimposition of fusion of the 2 visual directions. Normal is 20–50 seconds of arc
  TITMUS STEREOTEST: readily available, monocular clues present. Determines normal retinal correspondence (NRC) in binocular patient.
Example: Fly = 3000 arc seconds; animals = 400, 200, 100 arc seconds; circles = 800 – 40 arc seconds
RANDOM DOT STEREOGRAMS: monocular clues absent but more difficult for children to understand

Sensory phenomena associated with strabismus:

Diplopia: simultaneous perception of similar images falling on noncorresponding retinal points
Visual confusion: simultaneous perception of dissimilar images falling on corresponding retinal points

Sensory adaptations to diplopia and visual confusion:

Suppression (scotoma): image from 1 eye is inhibited or does not reach consciousness (Figure 5-51)

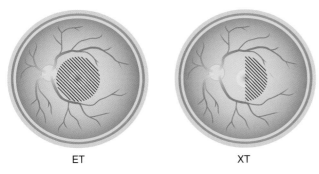

ET   XT

Figure 5-51. Suppression scotomas for esotropia (ET) and exotropia (XT).

Esotropic left eye with ARC and suppression or with monofixation syndrome, fixing with right eye

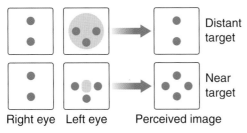

Right eye   Left eye   Perceived image

Esotropic right eye with ARC and suppression or with monofixation syndrome, fixing with left eye

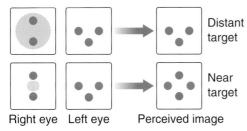

Right eye   Left eye   Perceived image

Figure 5-52. Possible Worth 4 Dot percepts in binocular patients. Note the similar distant responses in patients who have esotropia with abnormal retinal correspondence (ARC) and suppression and in those who have monofixation syndrome. Patients who have exotropia with ARC and suppression give the same responses, but the suppression scotoma is larger and shaped somewhat differently. The red lens is over the right eye, and the green lens is over the left eye. (From Diamond GR: Sensory status in strabismus. In Yanoff M, Duker JS [eds]: Ophthalmology, 2nd edn, St Louis, Mosby, 2004.)

CENTRAL: adaptation to avoid confusion
PERIPHERAL: adaptation to avoid diplopia
OBLIGATORY: present all the time
FACULTATIVE: present only when eyes are deviated
TESTS:
  WORTH 4 DOT: with red lens over 1 eye and green lens over other eye, patient views red, green, and white lights. Green light is visible to eye under green lens, red light visible to eye under red lens, and white light visible to both eyes. Determines binocularity (Figures 5-52, 5-53). May be used to define the size and location of a suppression scotoma in patients with strabismus. Performed at distance (central fusion) and at near (peripheral fusion)

Any strabismus in patient fixing right eye

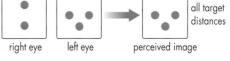

right eye   left eye   perceived image   all target distances

Any strabismus in patient fixing left eye

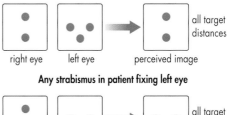

right eye   left eye   perceived image   all target distances

Figure 5-53. Possible Worth 4 Dot responses in patients who do not have binocularity. The red lens is over the right eye, and the green lens is over the left eye. (From Diamond GR: Sensory status in strabismus. In Yanoff M, Duker JS [eds]: Ophthalmology, London, Mosby, 1999.)

Results:
  Suppression: 2 red or 3 green lights seen
  Fusion: 4 lights seen
  Diplopia: 5 lights seen
4-PRISM DIOPTER BASE-OUT PRISM TEST: for small suppression scotomas. 4-prism diopter (Δ) prism placed base-out over 1 eye; if suppression scotoma is present, eye will not move
HORROR FUSIONIS: intractable diplopia with absence of central suppression
Abnormal retinal correspondence (ARC): (see following)
Monofixation syndrome: binocular sensory state in patients with small angle strabismus (<8 Δ; microtropia)
  CHARACTERISTICS: central scotoma and peripheral fusion present with binocular viewing
  Usually ET, may appear XT or orthophoric
  Amblyopia common, usually mild
  Stereoacuity reduced
  Central or eccentric fixation
  Typically occurs when preexisting strabismus is controlled nonoperatively or after surgery, but may occur in nonstrabismic patients, also from macular lesions and anisometropia
  Decompensation occurs when the deviation changes from a latent to a manifest one
  DIAGNOSIS: 4 Δ base-out prism test (used to shift image outside scotoma to cause eye movement). In normal patient, when prism is placed in front of 1 eye, eyes turn and then refixate
  In monofixation syndrome, when prism is placed in front of normal eye, there is no refixation movement, and when prism is placed in front of eye with scotoma, there is no initial eye turn

Retinal correspondence: the ability of the sensory system to appreciate the perceived direction of the fovea and other retinal elements in each eye relative to each other
  Corresponding retinal points: 2 retinal points (1 in each eye) that, when stimulated simultaneously, result in the subjective sensation that the stimulating target comes from the same direction in space. If diplopia occurs, then the 2 points are noncorresponding

Normal retinal correspondence: corresponding areas of the retina that have identical relationships to the fovea of each eye

CHARACTERISTICS: occurs in straight eyes under binocular conditions

Occurs in eyes in which the objective and subjective angles of strabismus are the same; measured with amblyoscope (patient superimposes dissimilar targets)

OBJECTIVE ANGLE: measured angle

SUBJECTIVE ANGLE: the amount of prism required to superimpose the images or promote fusion

Other dissimilar target tests: Lancaster red-green test and Hess screen; require NRC; used to measure paretic strabismus

Abnormal retinal correspondence (ARC): corresponding areas of the retina that have dissimilar relationships to their respective foveas. Sensory adaptation eliminates peripheral diplopia and confusion by permitting fusion of similar images projecting onto noncorresponding retinal areas

CHARACTERISTICS: change in visual direction of retinal points

Manifests only during binocular viewing

Objective and subjective angles are not equal

Sensory adaptation of immature visual system to strabismus

Prevents diplopia

Accompanied by scotoma

No fusional amplitudes and no stereopsis

Fovea in deviating eye and fovea in fixing eye do not have the same visual direction

Fovea of fixing eye shares common visual direction with peripheral area of the nonfixing eye

HARMONIOUS ARC: subjective angle is zero

UNHARMONIOUS ARC: subjective angle is greater than zero but less than objective angle

TESTS FOR ARC:

AFTERIMAGE TEST: label fovea of each eye with a linear light afterimage (vertical image for deviating eye and horizontal image for fixing eye). Each eye is stimulated individually (monocular), then patient draws perceived afterimages (Figure 5-54):

NRC: cross with central gap

ET with ARC: afterimages crossed

XT with ARC: afterimages uncrossed

BAGOLINI LENSES: glasses have no dioptric power but have narrow striations running at 45° and 135°. With glasses on, patient fixes on a light and draws perceived image. Allows determination of strabismus as well as retinal correspondence. Break in line is proportional to size of suppression scotoma (Figure 5-55)

RED GLASS TEST: with red glass in front of deviating eye, patient fixes on light; angular deviation can be measured with a Maddox rod to determine retinal correspondence

ET: uncrossed images

XT: crossed images

Harmonious ARC: patient sees pink light

AMBLYOSCOPE: device with which patient views 2 dissimilar targets and attempts to superimpose them

NRC: objective and subjective angles of strabismus are equal

Harmonious ARC: subjective angle equals zero (arms of amblyoscope are parallel)

Unharmonious ARC: subjective angle is between zero and objective angle

Amblyopia

Unilateral or bilateral reduction of visual acuity that cannot be attributed directly to any structural abnormality of the eye or visual system. Due to disuse of fovea

Characteristics: prevalence 2–4%; preventable or reversible with appropriately timed intervention

Types:

Strabismic: crowding phenomenon (letters or symbols are more difficult to recognize if closely surrounded

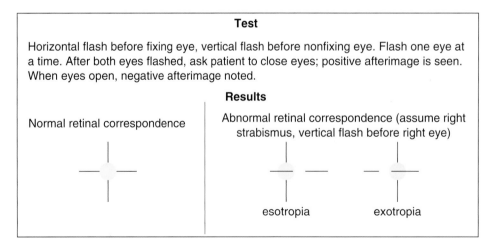

Test
Horizontal flash before fixing eye, vertical flash before nonfixing eye. Flash one eye at a time. After both eyes flashed, ask patient to close eyes; positive afterimage is seen. When eyes open, negative afterimage noted.

Results

Normal retinal correspondence

Abnormal retinal correspondence (assume right strabismus, vertical flash before right eye)

esotropia   exotropia

Figure 5-54. Afterimage test percepts, central fixation. Shown are those possible in patients who have central fixation and binocular vision. (From Diamond GR: Sensory status in strabismus. In Yanoff M, Duker JS [eds]: Ophthalmology, 2nd edn, St Louis, Mosby, 2004.)

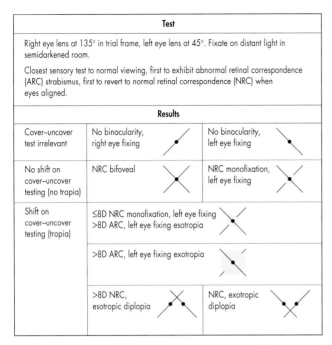

Test
Right eye lens at 135° in trial frame, left eye lens at 45°. Fixate on distant light in semidarkened room.
Closest sensory test to normal viewing, first to exhibit abnormal retinal correspondence (ARC) strabismus, first to revert to normal retinal correspondence (NRC) when eyes aligned.

Figure 5-55. Possible Bagolini lens percepts, central fixation. (From Diamond GR: Sensory status in strabismus. In Yanoff M, Duker JS [eds]: Ophthalmology, London, Mosby, 1999.)

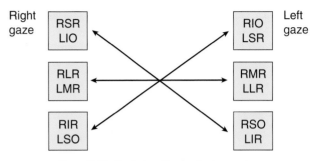

Table 5-11. Agonists, synergists, and antagonists

Agonist	Synergists	Antagonists
Medial rectus (MR)	SR, IR	LR, SO, IO
Lateral rectus (LR)	SO, IO	MR, SR, IR
Superior rectus (SR)	IO, MR	IR, SO
Inferior rectus (IR)	SO, MR	SR, IO
Superior oblique (SO)	IR, LR	IO, SR
Inferior oblique (IO)	SR, LR	SO, IR

Figure 5-56. Cardinal positions and yoke muscles.

by similar forms; therefore, visual acuity may substantially improve with isolate letters); neutral density filters do not reduce acuity as much in the amblyopic eye as in the normal eye

Refractive: high ametropia (hyperopia of +5 D, myopia of −8 D, astigmatism of 2.5 D) or anisometropia (1 D for hyperopia, 3 D for myopia, 1.5 D for astigmatism)

Deprivation: media opacity, ptosis, occlusion

Diagnosis: reduced visual acuity that cannot be entirely explained by physical abnormalities

Treatment: treat amblyopia before strabismus surgery (eliminate any obstacle to vision, remove significant congenital lens opacity by 2 months of age). Force use of poorer eye by limiting use of better eye (full-time occlusion, part-time occlusion, optical degradation of better eye, atropinization of better eye). Full-time occlusion for 1 week per year of age at most prior to reexamination; continue until no further improvement. Re-evaluate until 10 years of age

Prognosis: good for strabismic, poor for deprivation

Motor Testing

Ductions: monocular rotations of eye

Versions: conjugate binocular eye movements

Vergence: disconjugate binocular eye movement

Agonist: primary muscle moving eye in given direction (Table 5-11)

Synergist: secondary muscle that acts with agonist to move eye in given direction

Antagonist: muscle that acts to move eye in opposite direction as agonist

Yoke muscles: 2 muscles, 1 in each eye, that act to move respective eyes into a cardinal position

Cardinal positions: 6 positions of gaze in which 1 muscle of the eye is the prime mover (Figure 5-56)

Midline positions: straight up and straight down from primary position

Hering's law (equal innervation): equal and simultaneous innervation to synergistic muscles; amount of innervation to eyes is determined by the fixating eye; therefore, the amount of deviation depends on which eye is fixating:

Primary deviation (paralytic strabismus): deviation measured with normal eye fixing

Secondary deviation (paralytic strabismus): deviation measured with paretic eye fixing; larger than primary deviation

Hering's law also explains the term 'inhibitional paresis of the contralateral antagonist'

This is the incorrect impression that a muscle in the normal eye is responsible for the ocular misalignment and may occur in an SO palsy when the paretic eye fixes (e.g. in SO palsy, less innervation is required by the antagonist [IO], and therefore less innervation is directed to the yoke [contralateral SR]). The contralateral antagonist is actually the antagonist of the yoke of the paretic muscle

Sherrington's law (reciprocal innervation): innervation to ipsilateral antagonist decreases as innervation to the agonist increases

Angle Kappa (κ): angle between visual axis and anatomic axis (pupillary axis) of eye (Figure 5-57)

Positive-angle (κ): temporal position of fovea relative to pupillary axis; causes slight temporal rotation of globe to keep image in focus; light reflex appears nasal. May cause a pseudoexotropia or increase the apparent degree of an XT, and lessen or mask an ET

Example: ROP, *Toxocara*

Negative-angle κ: nasal position of fovea relative to pupillary axis; causes slight nasal rotation of globe to keep image in focus; light reflex appears temporal.

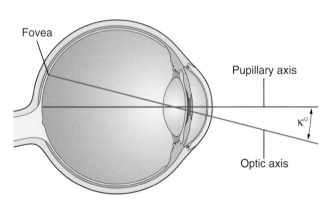

Fovea

Pupillary axis

κ°

Optic axis

Figure 5-57. The angle κ. This is the displacement in degrees of the pupillary axis from the optic axis. The positive-angle κ provides the illusion of exotropia in the left eye. (From Diamond GR: Sensory status in strabismus. In Yanoff M, Duker JS [eds]: Ophthalmology, 2nd edn, St Louis, Mosby, 2004.)

May cause a pseudoesotropia or increase the apparent degree of an ET, and lessen or mask an XT

Eccentric fixation: consistent use of a nonfoveal region of retina for monocular viewing in an amblyopic eye; a monocular phenomenon

Detecting deviations:

Corneal light reflex: if equal, no manifest deviation (tropia) but may have latent deviation (phoria); if unequal, tropia is present

Monocular cover–uncover test: tests for phoria or tropia by detecting movement of eyes when 1 eye is covered and then uncovered (Figure 5-58)

Measuring deviations:

Modified Krimsky's method: place prism over fixating eye to center the corneal light reflex over the pupil; place over deviating eye in incomitant or paralytic deviations (Figure 5-59)

Hirschberg's method: estimate each millimeter of decentration of corneal light reflex from the center of the pupil (1 mm equals 7° or 15 Δ of deviation) (Figure 5-60)

Simultaneous prism cover test or cover–uncover test: measures tropia

Alternate cover testing: measures tropia and phoria

Measurements are affected by corrective lenses: minus (concave lenses; myopia) measures more, and plus (convex lenses; hyperopia) measures less, due to the prismatic effect of the lenses. Difference = 2.5% × D

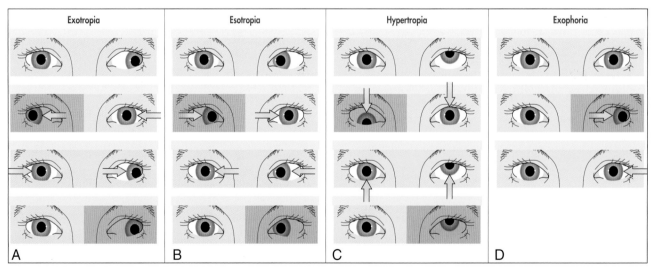

Exotropia	Esotropia	Hypertropia	Exophoria

A B C D

Figure 5-58. Cover test for tropias and phorias. **A,** For exotropia, covering the right eye drives inward movement of the left eye to take up fixation; uncovering the right eye shows recovery of fixation by the right eye and leftward movement of both eyes; covering the left eye discloses no shift of the preferred right eye. **B,** For esotropia, covering the right eye drives outward movement of the left eye to take up fixation; uncovering the right eye shows recovery of fixation by the right eye and rightward movement of both eyes; covering the left eye discloses no shift of the preferred right eye. **C,** For hypertropia, covering the right eye drives downward movement of the left eye to take up fixation; uncovering the right eye shows recovery of fixation by the right eye and upward movement of both eyes; covering the left eye shows no shift of the preferred right eye. **D,** For exophoria, the left eye deviates outward behind a cover and returns to primary position when the cover is removed. An immediate inward movement denotes a phoria, a delayed inward movement denotes an intermittent exotropia. (From Diamond G, Eggers H: Strabismus and Pediatric Ophthalmology, London, Mosby, 1993.)

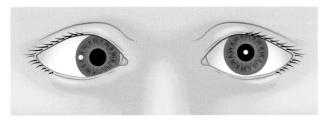

A

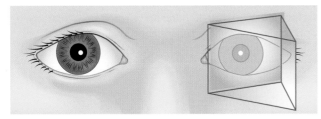

B

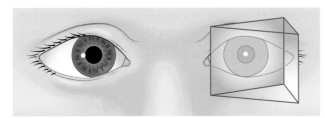

C

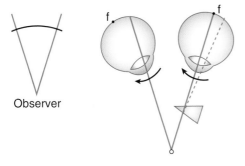

Observer

D

Figure 5-59. Modified Krimsky's method of estimating deviation. (From von Noorden GK: Von Noorden-Maumenee's Atlas of Stabismus, 3rd edn, St Louis, Mosby, 1977.)

Other tests:

Double Maddox rod test: measures torsion
Parks-Bielschowsky 3-step test: identifies cyclovertical palsy
1. Which eye has hyperdeviation?
   Identify weak depressors in higher eye (IR, SO) and elevators in lower eye (IO, SR)
2. Is hyperdeviation greater in right or left gaze?
   Identify muscles that act in direction as hyperdeviation increases
   Right gaze: SR and IR of right eye, IO and SO of left eye
   Left gaze: IO and SO of right eye, SR and IR of left eye
3. Is hyperdeviation greater with right or left head tilt?

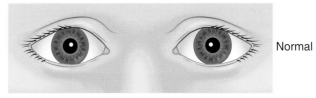

Normal

A

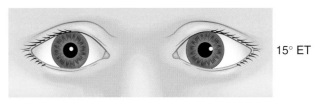

15° ET

B

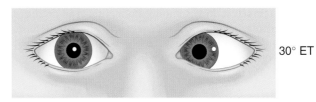

30° ET

C

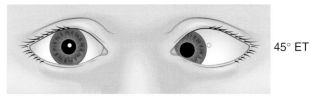

45° ET

D

Figure 5-60. Hirschberg's method of estimating deviation. (From von Noorden GK: Von Noorden-Maumenee's Atlas of Stabismus, 3rd edn, St Louis, Mosby, 1977.)

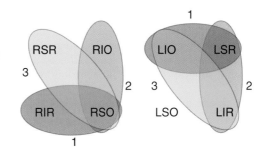

Figure 5-61. Parks-Bielschowsky 3-step test for RSO palsy.

Identify torting muscles that act in direction as hyperdeviation increases
Right head tilt:
  Intorsion of right eye (SR and SO)
  Extorsion of left eye (IO and IR)
Left head tilt is reversed
(Remember: **s**upinate–**s**uperiors **i**ntort)
Circle involved muscles at each step described previously. Muscle with 3 circles is the one with palsy
Example: RSO palsy (Figure 5-61)

143

Forced duction test: determines deviation due to muscle restriction

Forced generation test: measures muscle strength

NYSTAGMUS

Oscillation of eyes

Childhood forms are most commonly congenital, latent, sensory, and spasmus nutans

Congenital

Benign disorder of eye movement calibration system (between sensory and motor systems)

Characteristics: long-standing, horizontal in all positions, may have rotary component, increases intensity with fixation, null point, no oscillopsia, may have head posture, dampened by convergence (better near than distance vision), exponentially increasing velocity of slow phase, OKN reversal in 60%, strabismus in 33%, similar monocular and binocular vision (20/20–20/70), absent during sleeping, latent nystagmus can be present (cover 1 eye, nystagmus converts to jerk away from covered eye), may develop head oscillations at 3 months of age, wide-swinging eye movements; at 1 year, small pendular movements; at 2 years, jerk nystagmus with null zone, discover convergence dampens nystagmus and may develop nystagmus blockage syndrome

Waveform: exponentially increasing velocity of slow phase

Associations: albinism, aniridia, Leber's congenital amaurosis, ON hypoplasia, congenital cataracts, achromatopsia

Treatment: base-out prisms in glasses dampen nystagmus by forcing patient to converge (only fusional convergence [overcoming exophoria] diminishes the nystagmus; therefore, minus lenses that stimulate accommodative convergence do not dampen nystagmus); if head posture >50% of time, surgical correction (Kestenbaum procedure)

Distinguish congenital nystagmus from latent nystagmus:

Cover 1 eye: latent nystagmus worsens

Reversal of normal OKN response: congenital nystagmus

Dampens with convergence: congenital nystagmus

Examine slow-phase velocity: increases (congenital), decreases (latent)

Latent

Jerk nystagmus during monocular viewing away from covered eye

Associated with congenital esotropia and DVD

Pure form is rare

Etiology: abnormal cortical binocularity, proprioceptive imbalance, defective egocentric localization

Characteristics: cover 1 eye and uncovered eye develops nystagmus, fast phase to side of fixing eye; long-standing; normal OKN response; nulls with adduction; normal vision when both eyes open, vision decreases when each eye is tested separately; may have strabismus, especially infantile esotropia, DVD (50%)

Waveform: exponentially decreasing velocity of slow phase

Alexander's rule: intensity increases when looking toward fast phase and decreases when looking toward slow phase (i.e. adduction nulls; therefore, no head posture)

Treatment: surgery for strabismus or head turn

Sensory

Pendular nystagmus due to visual loss; more common than congenital nystagmus

Etiology: aniridia, albinism, rod monochromatism (achromatopsia), CSNB, optic nerve coloboma, cataracts, optic nerve hypoplasia, Leber's congenital amaurosis, bilateral macular coloboma

Spasmus Nutans

Benign form of nystagmus consisting of fine, rapid, often monocular or markedly asymmetric eye movements

Diagnosis of exclusion

Onset during first year of life with spontaneous resolution by age 3 years

Triad of findings: eye movements, head nodding/bobbing, torticollis (diagnosis can be made in absence of head nodding)

Waveform: high frequency, low amplitude, pendular, asymmetric (dissociated form of nystagmus)

DDx: chiasmal glioma, subacute necrotizing encephalomyopathy

Neuroimaging: rule out tumor

Acquired Nystagmus

(see Ch. 4, Neuro-ophthalmology)

OCULAR ALIGNMENT

Horizontal Deviations

At birth, $\frac{1}{3}$ of babies are orthophoric and $\frac{2}{3}$ are slightly XT

Orthophoria: normal alignment; eyes are straight; no latent or manifest deviation

Comitant: deviation is equal in all positions of gaze

Incomitant: deviation varies in different positions of gaze (paralytic or restrictive etiologies)

Esodeviations: latent or manifest convergence of the visual axes

Most common deviation (50–75%)

Types:

PSEUDOESOTROPIA: patient is orthophoric but has appearance of esotropia. Due to broad nasal bridge, prominent medial epicanthal folds, or negative-angle κ

ESOPHORIA (E): latent deviation controlled by fusional mechanisms; may manifest under certain conditions (fatigue, illness, stress, or tests that dissociate eyes [alternate cover test])

INTERMITTENT ESOTROPIA (E(T)): deviation that is sometimes latent and sometimes manifest; partially controlled by fusional mechanisms

ESOTROPIA (ET): manifest deviation (Box 5-4)

Exodeviations: latent or manifest divergence of the visual axes

Less common than ET

Account for 25% of strabismus in children

In neonates, up to 60% have a constant, transient exodeviation

Most common form is intermittent exotropia

Types:

PSEUDOEXOTROPIA: patient is orthophoric but has appearance of exotropia. Due to positive- angle κ without other abnormalities, macular heterotopia

---

Box 5-4. Classification of esotropia

Infantile

Classic congenital

Early-onset accommodative

Duane's syndrome type I

Abducens paralysis from birth trauma

Nystagmus blockage syndrome

Möbius' syndrome

Acquired

Accommodative

Refractive

Nonrefractive

Mixed (partially accommodative and partially basic)

Decompensated

Nonaccommodative

Stress-induced acquired

Cyclic

Acute comitant

Sensory deprivation

Divergence insufficiency

Divergence paralysis

Spasm of near synkinetic reflex

Restrictive (thyroid-related, medial orbital wall fracture, overresected MR)

Lateral rectus weakness (CN 6 palsy, iatrogenic/surgical [slipped, detached, overrecessed LR])

(temporally dragged macula [PHPV, ROP, toxocariasis] with large angle κ), wide interpupillary distance

EXOPHORIA (X): latent deviation; detected by alternate cover testing; may be related to asthenopia

INTERMITTENT EXOTROPIA (X(T)): deviation that is sometimes latent and sometimes manifest; partially controlled by fusional mechanisms

EXOTROPIA (XT): manifest deviation

BASIC: exodeviation equal at distance and near

DIVERGENCE EXCESS: exodeviation greater at distance than near by at least 10 Δ

Types:

Simulated (pseudodivergence excess): enhanced fusional convergence at near related to accommodation 30-minute patch test: binocular fusional impulses suspended and exodeviation becomes equal at distance and near. If near deviation increases to close to distance deviation with +3.00 lenses, then high AC/A ratio exists

True: after 30-minute patch test, still has divergence excess at distance

CONVERGENCE INSUFFICIENCY: near exotropia is greater than distance exotropia

Congenital Esotropia

1–2% of all strabismus

Equal sex distribution

Present by 6 months of age

Family history of strabismus is common

Increased frequency in cerebral palsy or hydrocephalus

Findings: deviation usually ≥30 Δ, low amounts of hyperopia, often cross fixation with equal visual acuity in each eye, rarely develop normal binocular vision (even with surgery)

Associations:

Dissociated vertical deviation (DVD) in 70%

Overaction of inferior obliques in 70%

Involved eye elevates with adduction

Onset usually in second year of life; greatest occurrence between ages 3 and 7

Treat with IO weakening procedure

Latent nystagmus

Congenital, conjugate, horizontal jerk nystagmus that occurs under monocular conditions

When 1 eye is occluded, nystagmus develops in both eyes with fast phase toward the fixing eye and slow phase toward the occluded eye

MANIFEST LATENT NYSTAGMUS: nystagmus present when both eyes are open

Because of induced nystagmus in the uncovered eye with latent nystagmus, binocular visual acuity is better than when each eye is tested individually

NYSTAGMUS BLOCKAGE SYNDROME: overaccommodation to dampen nystagmus results in ET at near (usually large). Can differentiate from essential infantile esotropia (EIE) with manifest latent nystagmus because nystagmus does not increase with occlusion of 1 eye. Nystagmus dampens in convergence or adduction and increases in primary or lateral gaze. Adduction continues even when 1 eye is occluded, and head turn occurs toward the uncovered eye when the fellow eye is occluded. With adduction effort, the pupil constricts, demonstrating that accommodative mechanisms are present. May treat with large (6 mm+) bimedial resections using a Faden suture

Asymmetry of the monocular, optokinetic motion–processing response
  Nasal to temporal smooth pursuit less well developed than temporal to nasal pursuit
  Can establish congenital nature of ET in an older patient
  Asymmetry also seen in healthy newborns and disappears by 6 months of age

Diagnosis: demonstrate potential for full abduction with vestibular ocular reflex and doll's head maneuver to rule out congenital CN 6 palsy
  Look for synkinetic lid or eye movements with attempted horizontal gaze to rule out Duane's syndrome
  Rule out accommodative component with glasses if older than age 1 or phospholine iodide 0.125%

Treatment:
  Nonsurgical: correct amblyopia before surgery; cross fixation suggests equal visual acuity of both eyes
  Early surgery (as early as 6 months): potential for sensory binocular fusion; aim for alignment within 10 Δ of orthophoria
    PROCEDURES:
      Bilateral medial rectus recession
      Recess medial rectus muscle and resect lateral rectus muscle of 1 eye
      Associated surgery of inferior obliques if overaction present
      3 or 4 muscle surgeries for large deviation

Accommodative Esotropia

Onset 6 months to 7 years

May be intermittent at onset

Often, positive family history

Associated with amblyopia (generally from anisometropia)

May be precipitated by trauma or illness

Types: (Table 5-12)

Accommodative convergence to accommodation
(AC/A) ratio: normally between 3:1 and 5:1 prism diopters per diopter of accommodation
  High AC/A ratio: usually present when near deviation exceeds distance deviation by >10 to 15 Δ
  Calculation (2 methods):
    HETEROPHORIA METHOD:
      $AC/A = IPD + [(N - D)/Diopt]$
      IPD = interpupillary distance (cm)
      N = near deviation
      D = distance deviation
      Diopt = accommodative demand at fixation distance
    Example: near deviation = 35 Δ; distance deviation =10 Δ; accommodative demand = 20 cm (5 D); IPD = 60 mm (6 cm). Therefore, AC/A = 6 + [(35 − 10)/5] = 11:1
    LENS GRADIENT METHOD: $AC/A = (WL - NL)/D$
      WL = deviation with lens in front of eye
      NL = deviation without lens in front of eye
      D = dioptric power of lens used
    Example: near deviation with a +1.00 lens is 50 Δ and without a lens is 35 Δ. Therefore, AC/A = (50 −35)/1.00 =15:1

Natural history: hyperopia may decrease with age, AC/A ratio may normalize, and fusional divergence can improve; may begin to reduce strength of glasses and bifocals slowly as child gets older

Treatment: correct refractive error and treat amblyopia; consider surgery for residual component
  Satisfactory: residual esotropia <10 Δ; peripheral fusion and expansion of fusional amplitudes possible

Table 5-12. Types of accommodative esotropia

Type	Characteristics	Treatment
Refractive accommodative (normal AC/A ratio)	• Esotropia at distance and near within 10 Δ	• Full cycloplegic refraction
	• High hyperopia (range +3.00 to +10.00, average = +4.00)	• Treat amblyopia
Nonrefractive accommodative (high AC/A ratio)	• Lower amount of hyperopia (average = +2.25)	• Consider bifocal when esotropia at near exceeds distance by 10 Δ (executive type)
	• Esotropia greater at near than at distance (may resolve with age)	• Consider miotics (phospholine iodide 0.125%)
	• Esotropia reduced at near with plus lens	• Surgery if needed for residual esotropia
Mixed mechanism	• Partially accommodative	• Full cycloplegic refraction
	• Angle of deviation reduced but not eliminated with spectacles	• Surgery for nonaccommodative component
Decompensated accommodative	• Residual esotropia after correction with full cycloplegic refraction	• Full cycloplegic refraction
	• Occurs more commonly with high AC/A ratio	• Surgery

Unsatisfactory: try atropine with glasses or long-acting cholinesterase inhibitors; recheck refraction for increased or latent hyperopia

Echothiophate (phospholine iodide) causes accommodation that removes convergence with accommodative effort

Nonaccommodative, Acquired ET

Stress-induced acquired ET: breakdown of fusional divergence that occurs after illness, emotional trauma, or injury; requires surgery

Cyclic ET: intermittent, usually present every other day (48-hour cycle) and becomes constant with time

Findings: V-pattern ET is common; amblyopia can develop; on days when ET is not present, normal binocular visual acuity with good stereovision

Treatment: prescribe full hyperopic correction; may also require surgery if glasses do not fully correct deviation; phenobarbital and amphetamines can alter the frequency of the cycles

Sensory ET: due to loss of vision (sensory deprivation) in 1 or both eyes, usually during childhood (age <6); identify and treat obstruction to vision

Divergence insufficiency: ET greater at distance than near; fusional divergence is reduced

Treat with base-out prisms (to correct diplopia) or surgery

Rule out divergence paralysis (associated with pontine tumors, head trauma, or other neurologic abnormalities; may mimic bilateral CN 6 paralysis)

Spasm of near synkinetic reflex (ciliary spasm):

Intermittent episodes of sustained convergence with accommodative spasm and miosis

Findings: headache, blurred distance visual acuity (recent onset of myopia is present in history [pseudomyopia]), abnormally close near point, and fluctuating visual acuity; variable angle of deviation; monocular abduction is normal; large difference between manifest and cycloplegic refraction

Treatment: cycloplegia may break spasm; on postcycloplegic refraction push plus

Incomitant ET:

Etiology:

MR restriction: thyroid, orbital wall fractures, or excessively resected MR muscle

Slipped muscle following strabismus surgery

Neurogenic: CN 6 palsy (spontaneous or due to intracranial lesions [33%], infections, or birth trauma)

Myasthenia gravis

Consecutive esotropia: follows surgery for exotropia; rule out slipped muscle

Prism Adaptation Test: prisms are used to help patients obtain binocular fusion while awaiting surgical alignment of the eyes. Used to preoperatively predict which patients will develop residual esotropia after surgery. Patients who respond with increasing deviation are given stronger prism until orthophoria is obtained. The largest angle is the target for surgical correction

Intermittent Exotropia

Most common form of XT

Onset varies from infancy to age 4 years

May be progressive

Often have reflex closure of 1 eye in bright light

Suppression only when eyes are deviated (facultative suppression)

Amblyopia is uncommon

Natural history:

Phase 1: X(T) at distance and straight at near

Present when fatigued

May see double

Most maintain excellent stereovision

Phase 2: X(T) becomes more constant at distance with X(T) at near

Suppression increases

Phase 3: XT at distance and near

Often no diplopia because of suppression

Most common cause of a constant XT

Treatment: treat amblyopia, alternate occlusion therapy, induce accommodative convergence by prescribing overminus spectacles (also for consecutive exotropia), prism therapy with base-in prisms, fusional convergence training (progressive base-out prism to induce convergence)

Surgery for increased tropic phase, poor recovery of fusion once tropic, increasing ease of dissociation, XT greater than 50% of time at home

PROCEDURES:

Bilateral lateral rectus recession

Recess lateral rectus and resect medial rectus of 1 eye

3 of 4 muscle surgeries for large deviation

Congenital Exotropia

Rare

May be primary (otherwise healthy patients) or secondary (from ocular or systemic abnormalities)

Usually large angle of deviation (average >35 Δ)

Amblyopia is uncommon; similar refractive error to general population

Most resolve by age 6 months; if not, consider surgery

Associations: DVD and oblique muscle overaction; orbital or skull defects, neurologic disease, or other ocular, genetic, or systemic conditions

Convergence Insufficiency

Exophoria greater at near than at distance (not exotropic at near)

Reduced near point of convergence and amplitudes of convergence

Female > male

Common in teenagers and young adults

Associations: can be exacerbated by fatigue, drugs, uveitis, or Adie's tonic pupil; may also follow head trauma. Also associated with systemic illnesses, or as a conversion reaction

Findings: asthenopia, diplopia; may have reduced amplitude of accommodation and remote near point of accommodation

Treatment: observation; orthoptic exercises to improve fusional amplitudes, base-out prisms; rarely surgery (medial rectus resection)

Convergence Paralysis Secondary to Intracranial Lesion

Normal adduction and accommodation

XT and diplopia on attempted near fixation

Associations: Parinaud's syndrome

Treatment: base-in prisms or occlusion of 1 eye to relieve diplopia

Sensory Exotropia

Due to loss of vision or long-standing poor vision in 1 eye

Children age <6 with unilateral vision loss may develop ET or XT; adults usually develop XT

Angle of deviation may be variable and usually increases with time

Consecutive Exotropia

Follows previous strabismus surgery for esotropia

Vertical Deviations

Dissociated Vertical Deviation (DVD; DHD [Dissociated Horizontal Deviation]; DTD [Dissociated Torsional Deviation])

Intermittent deviation of nonfixing eye consisting of upward excursion, extorsion, excyclotorsion, abduction, or lateral deviation

Exact etiology unknown but associated with early disruption of binocular development

Usually asymptomatic because of poor fusion and suppression

Often asymmetric

Does not obey Hering's law (fellow eye does not exhibit refixation movement in opposite direction)

Occurs with eye occlusion or visual inattention

May be latent or manifest

Usually presents before 12 months of age

Usually more marked when patient is fatigued, daydreaming, under stress, or sick

Associations: nystagmus (latent or manifest latent), inferior oblique overaction, often occurs in patients with history of congenital ET; isolated in 40% of patients

Findings: slow movement of eye in the characteristic direction, amount of deviation variable (accurate measurements difficult to obtain), dissociated deviation occurs in all directions of gaze

Diagnosis:
Bielschowsky's phenomenon: occurs in 50% of patients with DVD
Elevated eye will drift downward when light in fixing eye is reduced
Conversely, increased illumination in an eye with DVD will cause it to drift up
Red lens phenomenon: place red lens over either eye while patient fixates on light source
Red image is always seen below the white image
In patients with a true hypertropia, the red image is seen above or below the primary image, depending on whether the red filter is placed in front of the hyperdeviated or hypodeviated eye

Treatment:
Increase fusional mechanisms: give optimal spectacle correction; switch fixation to nonpreferred eye
Surgery:
INDICATIONS: increasing size or frequency of manifest DVD, abnormal head position
PROCEDURES:
SR recession
IR resection
IO weakening or anterior transposition (in patients with IOOA and DVD)
CAUTIONS: perform bilateral surgery (unilateral surgery often reveals occult contralateral DVD); often recurs or persists after surgery

Inferior Oblique Overaction (IOOA)

Occurs in 2/3 of patients with congenital ET

Usually bilateral and asymmetric

Early surgery for ET is important for development of binocular vision but does not reduce incidence of IO dysfunction

May be primary (due to paralysis of the antagonist [SO]) or secondary

Findings: when fixing eye is abducted, adducting eye is elevated; when fixing eye is adducted, abducted eye is depressed; V-pattern deviation; primary position extorsion of fundus on indirect ophthalmoscopy

Treatment: IO weakening procedure (recession, myectomy, anteriorization)

Inferior Oblique Palsy

Rare

Usually idiopathic but may follow orbital trauma, viral illness, or other neurologic problems

May be bilateral

Findings: eye is hypotropic when fixing with normal eye, hypertropia of normal eye when fixing with involved eye, deviation worsens with gaze into field of action of involved inferior oblique, deviation is worse with head tilt opposite of paretic eye, poor elevation in adduction, normal forced duction (distinguishes from Brown's syndrome), A pattern

Treatment:
With associated SO overaction: SO weakening procedure. If hyperdeviation develops in downgaze, then weaken contralateral IR
IO palsy with hypotropia in primary gaze and no SO overaction: IR recession (2.5 Δ per mm of recession)

Superior Oblique Overaction

Less common than IO overaction or DVD

Findings: A pattern; associated with depression on attempted adduction if fixing with uninvolved eye; may have associated horizontal deviation

Treatment: weaken overacting SO with tenotomy (uncontrolled) or silicone spacer (controlled)

Superior Oblique Palsy

Most common isolated cyclovertical muscle palsy

Congenital (75%): large fusional amplitudes (as much as 15 Δ or more)
SO tendon often long or floppy; sometimes absent
Long-standing CN 4 palsy results in ocular torticollis, which can lead to facial asymmetry
Examine old photographs to determine duration of head tilt
Can mimic a double elevator palsy (if fixation preference is for the affected eye, the contralateral SR muscle can appear to underact [inhibitional palsy of the contralateral antagonist] and the contralateral IR can undergo contracture, leading to double elevator palsy)

Acquired: often due to trauma (long course of 4th nerve makes it especially vulnerable)
Findings: diplopia (vertical, horizontal, or torsional). In long-standing cases of SO palsy, comitance develops and the deviation becomes more difficult to localize (hypertropia can be present in all fields of gaze)

Bilateral: objective torsion is often >10° of excyclotorsion (measure with double Maddox rod), often have inferior oblique overaction with V-pattern ET and chin-down head posture, alternate hypertropia with head tilt

Diagnosis: Parks-Bielschowsky 3-step test (i.e. right superior oblique palsy produces right hypertropia in primary gaze, worsens in left gaze and in right head tilt)

Treatment: surgery
Indications: significant head tilt, large hypertropia in primary gaze, diplopia
Procedures:
If deviation in primary gaze is ≤15 Δ, operate on 1 muscle; if deviation >15 Δ, operate on 2 or more muscles
With IO overaction, weaken ipsilateral IO (corrects approximately 15 Δ of vertical deviation)
If hyperdeviation is >15 Δ in primary gaze, strengthen ipsilateral IR or weaken contralateral SR
With no inferior oblique overaction, consider weakening ipsilateral SR or recessing contralateral IR; SO tuck may also be considered if there is laxity of the tendon
Knapp classification for treatment of superior oblique palsy offers guidance
General principle is to match the fields of greatest deviation to the muscles that work most in those fields to guide surgical approach
Check traction test in operating room to assess laxity of superior oblique tendon
Torsional symptoms: most people can tolerate 7° of torsion
Consider Harada-Ito procedure: lateral transposition of anterior portion of SO tendon; corrects excyclotorsion only; no effect on vertical deviation or fusion

Inferior Rectus Palsy

Due to trauma to CN 3 or IR

May occur at time of injury or repair of an orbital fracture

May resolve with time

Double Elevator Palsy (Monocular Elevation Deficiency)

Sporadic, unilateral defect of upgaze associated with ipsilateral ptosis

There are 2 elevators of the eye: the SR (provides most of elevation) and the IO

May be supranuclear (may not involve both elevators)

May be congenital or acquired (cerebrovascular disease, tumor, or infection)

Types:
IR restriction: unilateral fibrosis syndrome
Positive forced ductions to elevation
Positive force generation (no muscle paralysis)
Normal saccades of SR
Elevator weakness: (SR and IO)
Free forced ductions to elevation
Reduced force generation (muscle paralysis)
Reduced velocities of upgaze movements

Combination: IR restriction plus weak elevators
    Positive forced ductions to elevation
    Reduced force generation (muscle paralysis)
    Reduced velocities of upgaze movements

Findings: unilateral limitation of upgaze above midline with accompanying ptosis in both adduction and abduction, variable head position (normal or chin-up), hypotropia increases on upgaze, fixing with involved eye causes large secondary hypotropia in nonparetic eye

Treatment: surgery
Indications: chin-up head position, large vertical deviation in primary position, poor fusion in primary position
Procedures:
    DOUBLE ELEVATOR PALSY WITH TIGHT IR: IR recession
    DOUBLE ELEVATOR PALSY WITH SR WEAKNESS: Knapp procedure (elevation and transposition of MR and LR to the side of SR)
    DOUBLE ELEVATOR PALSY WITH PTOSIS: correct strabismus then residual ptosis

Brown's Syndrome (SO Tendon Sheath Syndrome)

Inability to elevate the eye in adduction, both actively and passively on forced duction testing

May be congenital or acquired (traumatic, inflammatory, iatrogenic [following SO tuck, glaucoma drainage implant, scleral buckle])

Findings: limitation of elevation in adduction, less elevation deficiency in midline, minimal or no elevation deficiency in abduction, V-pattern divergence in upgaze, restricted forced ductions, minimal or no superior oblique overaction; may have 'clicking' (suggests a trochlear problem), anomalous head posture or hypotropia in primary position

Treatment:
Observation: spontaneous improvement may occur
Surgery:
    INDICATIONS: abnormal head position, large hypotropia in primary position, constant deviation causing amblyopia and threatening binocularity
    PROCEDURE: superior weakening procedure (SO tenectomy, tenotomy, or silicone spacer)
    COMPLICATION: SO palsy

A and V Patterns

Change in horizontal deviation as eyes move between upgaze and downgaze

Up to 50% of all strabismus has an associated A or V pattern

May present as compensatory head posture (chin-up or chin-down) in child with binocular function

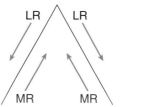 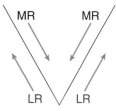

Figure 5-62. Direction of muscle transposition for A and V patterns.

A pattern: increasing convergence or decreasing divergence in upgaze, increasing divergence in downgaze

Clinically significant when eyes diverge >10 Δ from upgaze to downgaze

V pattern: increasing convergence or decreasing divergence in downgaze, increasing divergence in upgaze

Clinically significant when eyes converge >15 Δ from upgaze to downgaze

Etiology: oblique muscle dysfunction (obliques are abductors, IO overaction creates a V pattern), horizontal rectus muscle dysfunction, vertical rectus muscle dysfunction, structural factors (e.g. craniosynostosis is associated with a V pattern, abnormal insertions of rectus muscles, absence of SO tendon)

Diagnosis: measure deviation in primary position, then with eyes directed 25° in upgaze and downgaze

Treatment: surgery
Indications: abnormal head position; to improve motor alignment
Procedures:
    If no oblique muscle overaction is present, vertical transposition of horizontal muscles (Figure 5-62)
    Corrects about 15 Δ of the A and V patterns, muscles are transposed ½ to 1 tendon width up or down, transposition is in the direction of the desired weakening
    Mnemonic: MALE (Medial rectus to Apex of pattern; Lateral rectus to the Empty space)
    If oblique muscle overaction present, oblique muscle weakening
        IO WEAKENING: corrects ≥15 Δ of eso shift in upgaze, with no effect on horizontal alignment in primary gaze
        BILATERAL SO TENOTOMIES: corrects up to 30–40 Δ of eso shift in downgaze; torsional symptoms may occur in patients with good fusion

SPECIAL FORMS OF STRABISMUS

Duane's Retraction Syndrome

Usually sporadic, may be inherited

Cocontraction of medial and lateral rectus muscles causes retraction of the globe with secondary narrowing of the palpebral fissure

Vertical deviations may be present with characteristic upshoot or downshoot (leash phenomenon)

Bilateral in 15–20%

Head turn common (for fusion)

Etiology: abnormal innervation of lateral rectus by a branch of CN 3; electromyography shows decreased firing of lateral rectus during abduction and paradoxical innervation of the lateral rectus during adduction
   Exact etiology unclear, proposed mechanisms include hypoplasia of 6th nerve nucleus, midbrain pathology, fibrosis of lateral rectus

Types:
   Type 1: (most common): limitation of abduction, retraction and narrowing of palpebral fissures in adduction; appears esotropic
   Type 2: limitation of adduction; appears exotropic
   Type 3: limitation of abduction and adduction

Associations: deafness, crocodile tears, syndromes (Goldenhar's syndrome, Klippel-Feil syndrome, Wildervanck's syndrome [Duane's syndrome associated with Klippel-Feil], thalidomide toxicity, fetal alcohol syndrome, cat-eye syndrome)

Treatment: correct any refractive error, treat amblyopia
   Surgery
      INDICATIONS: abnormal head position or deviation in primary gaze
      PROCEDURES:
         For esotropia: recession of medial rectus muscle
         For globe retraction: simultaneous lateral rectus recession
         For upshoot or downshoot: splitting of lateral rectus or Faden procedure
         Avoid muscle resection (increases globe retraction, upshoots and downshoots)

Möbius' Syndrome

CN 6 and 7 palsies

Due to aplasia of involved brain stem nuclei

Associations: congenital facial diplegia (mask facies); combined CN 6, 7, 9, and 12 palsies; gaze palsy (PPRF involvement); chest, limb, tongue defects

Findings: esotropia with limitation of abduction, exposure keratitis from poor lid closure

Congenital Fibrosis Syndrome

Group of congenital anomalies characterized by variable amounts of restriction of extraocular muscles and replacement of the muscles with fibrous tissue

Nonprogressive

1 or more muscles may be involved

Positive forced duction testing

Types:
   Generalized fibrosis:
      Most severe
      Usually autosomal dominant, may be recessive
      All extraocular muscles involved, including levator (with ptosis)
   Congenital fibrosis of inferior rectus:
      Sporadic or familial
      Levator may be involved
   Strabismus fixus:
      Severe esotropia
      Horizontal rectus muscles involved (usually MR, occasionally LR)
   Vertical retraction syndrome:
      SR fibrosis (inability to depress eye)
   Congenital unilateral fibrosis:
      Enophthalmos and ptosis
      Fibrosis of all muscles, including levator

Chronic Progressive External Ophthalmoplegia (CPEO)

Sporadic or maternal inheritance (mitochondrial DNA)

May present at any age

Associations:
   Kearns-Sayre syndrome: triad of CPEO, retinal pigmentary changes, and cardiomyopathy
   Bassen-Kornzweig syndrome: (abetalipoproteinemia): retinal pigmentary changes similar to RP, diarrhea, ataxia, and other neurologic signs
   Refsum's disease: RP-like syndrome with elevated phytanic acid levels
   Oculopharyngeal dystrophy (AR): difficulty in swallowing
   Cardiac conduction defects

Findings: severe ptosis with complete ophthalmoplegia, absent Bell's phenomenon, no restrictions on forced ductions, large angle strabismus (often exotropia)

Orbital Floor Fracture

Findings: ecchymosis, diplopia in some or all positions of gaze immediately after injury, paresthesia or hypesthesia in distribution of infraorbital nerve, entrapment of inferior rectus muscle or inferior oblique muscle; may have associated ocular damage, may have associated wall fractures (e.g. medial wall with medial rectus entrapment)

Diagnosis: forced duction testing, orbital imaging

Treatment: observation (usually 5 to 10 days until edema and hematoma resolve, then reevaluate), surgery

Following Surgery

Commonly after cataract, scleral buckle, and glaucoma drainage implant procedures

May be transient and resolve spontaneously

Horizontal, vertical, or torsional

Etiology:

Mechanical: adhesions, mass effect (implant or buckle)

Motor: trauma, ischemia, slipped or disinserted muscle, toxicity (local anesthetic; most commonly IR fibrosis with hypotropia in primary gaze that worsens in abduction; positive forced ductions)

Sensory: fusion breakdown, anisometropia, aniseikonia, image distortion

Treatment: observation, prism spectacles, surgery

Other Forms of Strabismus

Myasthenia gravis, thyroid-related ophthalmopathy, CN 3 palsy, skew deviation

STRABISMUS SURGERY

Indications: establish binocularity, improve fusion, improve symptoms or appearance

Anesthesia:

Topical: may consider for recession procedures

Retrobulbar: use shorter-acting anesthetic for adjustable sutures

General: for children; consider in adults undergoing bilateral surgery

Incisions:

Fornix: in superior or inferior cul-de-sac on bulbar conjunctiva

Limbal: conjunctival/Tenon's flap at limbus

Swan: over the muscle (causes more scarring)

Weakening Procedures

Recession: most common technique used to weaken rectus muscles by moving muscle posteriorly; also used to weaken inferior oblique

Myotomy (cutting across muscle) **or myectomy** (excising a portion of muscle): used to weaken inferior oblique

Denervation and extirpation: used to weaken inferior oblique by ablating all muscle within Tenon's capsule

Tenotomy (cutting across tendon) **or tenectomy** (excising a portion of tendon): most commonly used to weaken superior oblique

Posterior fixation suture (Faden procedure): suture placed 11–18 mm from insertion through belly of muscle and sclera to weaken muscle only in its field of action; decreases mechanical advantage of muscle acting on globe; often combined with recession

Strengthening Procedures

Resection: used to strengthen rectus muscles by excising portion of muscle and reattaching muscle at its insertion site

Advancement (moving muscle forward): often used for muscles previously recessed, also in Harada-Ito procedure

Tuck: technique used to strengthen superior oblique by shortening the tendon (may produce iatrogenic Brown's syndrome)

Other Techniques

Adjustable suture: slipknot or noose suture to enable muscle adjustment postoperatively under topical anesthesia

Transposition: moving muscle out of original plane of action; used in cases of paralysis, double elevator palsy, or A and V patterns

Harada-Ito procedure: anterior temporal displacement of anterior half of superior oblique tendon; used to correct excyclotorsion

Kestenbaum procedure: bilateral resection/recession to dampen nystagmus in patients with nystagmus and head turn; eyes are surgically moved toward direction of head turn

Botulinum toxin (Botox): interferes with release of acetylcholine to paralyze muscle into which it is injected. When an extraocular muscle is paralyzed by Botox, the antagonist contracts to change the alignment of the eyes

Used in cases of paralytic strabismus to prevent contracture of muscles or postoperative residual strabismus, and when surgery is inappropriate

General Principles

Needles: use spatulated needles (cutting surface on the side) to decrease risk of perforation (sclera is thinnest just posterior to insertion of rectus muscles [0.3 mm])

Vertical deviations: in general, surgery should be performed on muscles whose field of action is in same field as the vertical deviation (e.g. left hypertropia that is greatest down and to patient's right might be addressed by either weakening right inferior rectus or strengthening left superior oblique)

Horizontal incomitancy: can be treated by adjusting amount of surgery performed on each muscle (i.e. if exotropia increases from right gaze to primary gaze to left gaze, consider larger recession on left lateral rectus to have a greater effect on exotropia to left [in field of action of that muscle])

Distance–near disparity: perform surgery on lateral rectus muscles if exodeviation is greater at distance than at near. Perform surgery on medial rectus muscles if esodeviation is greater at near than at distance

Complications of Strabismus Surgery

Residual strabismus (most common): alignment in postoperative period can change owing to poor fusion, poor vision, altered accommodation, and contracture of scar tissue

Scleral perforation: usually creates only a chorioretinal scar but can also lead to vitreous hemorrhage, retinal tear, retinal detachment, or endophthalmitis. If suspected during surgery, perform indirect ophthalmoscopy to determine whether a perforation is present; consider retinal laser treatment, cryotherapy, or observation

Infection: uncommon; includes endophthalmitis, cellulitis, and subconjunctival abscess

Foreign body granuloma: may develop weeks after surgery, often at suture site. Localized, elevated, slightly hyperemic, tender mass, usually <1 cm; may require surgical excision

Conjunctival inclusion cyst: may occur when conjunctiva is buried during closure of incision. Appears days to weeks later as noninflamed, transluscent mass under conjunctiva. May resolve spontaneously or require excision if symptomatic

Conjunctival scarring: can occur with orbital fat encroaching under bulbar conjunctiva because of inadvertent openings through Tenon's capsule

Fat adherence syndrome: violation of Tenon's capsule with prolapsed orbital fat into sub-Tenon's space can lead to fibrofatty scar. May have positive traction test and restricted motility

Delle: thin, dehydrated area of cornea caused by elevated limbal conjunctiva that prevents adequate corneal lubrication during blinking

Anterior segment ischemia: most blood to anterior segment supplied by anterior ciliary arteries that travel in rectus muscles. Usually occurs with surgery on 3 or more muscles. Corneal edema and anterior uveitis are present. Treat with topical steroids

Diplopia: Change in eyelid position: most commonly with surgery of vertical rectus muscles

Lost or slipped muscle: when only the capsule is sutured to insertion site, muscle can slip back; prevented with locking bites during suturing

Oculocardiac reflex: slowing of heart rate with traction on extraocular muscles

Malignant hyperthermia: acute metabolic disorder that may be fatal if diagnosis or treatment is delayed. Triggered by inhalation agents and succinylcholine. Signs include tachycardia, unstable BP, arrhythmias, increased temperature, muscle rigidity, cyanosis, dark urine

REVIEW QUESTIONS (Answers start on page 361)

1. The approximate age of onset for accommodative ET is closest to
   a. 1 year old
   b. 3 years old
   c. 5 years old
   d. 7 years old

2. A 15-year-old girl with strabismus is examined, and the following measurements are recorded: distance deviation of 10 Δ, near deviation of 35 Δ at 20 cm, and interpupillary distance of 60 mm. Her AC/A ratio is
   a. 11 : 1
   b. 10 : 1
   c. 5 : 1
   d. 3 : 1

3. Duane's syndrome is thought to be due to a developmental abnormality of the
   a. trochlear nucleus
   b. motor endplate
   c. oculomotor nucleus
   d. abducens nucleus

4. The most helpful test in a patient with aniridia is
   a. EKG
   b. abdominal ultrasound
   c. chest X-ray
   d. CBC

5. The best test for an infant with a normal fundus and searching eye movements is
   a. VER
   b. ERG
   c. EOG
   d. OKN

6. The most common congenital infection is
   a. toxoplasmosis
   b. HSV
   c. CMV
   d. rubella

7. ARC is most likely to develop in a child with
   a. congenital esotropia
   b. amblyopia and suppression
   c. alternating exotropia
   d. small-angle esotropia

8. Which of the following most accurately reflects what a patient with harmonious ARC reports when the angle of anomaly is equal to the objective angle?
   a. fusion
   b. crossed diplopia
   c. simultaneous macular perception
   d. uncrossed diplopia

9. The inferior oblique muscle is weakened most by which procedure?
   a. disinsertion
   b. recession
   c. myotomy
   d. anteriorization

10. The test that gives the best dissociation is
    a. Maddox rod
    b. Worth 4 Dot
    c. Bagolini glasses
    d. Red glass

11. The 3-step test shows a left hypertropia in primary position that worsens on right gaze and with left head tilt. The best surgical procedure is
    a. RIR resection
    b. RSO tuck
    c. LIR recession
    d. LIO weakening

12. In the treatment of a superior oblique palsy, Knapp recommended all of the following except
    a. SO plication
    b. recession of the contralateral IR
    c. IO weakening
    d. resection of the contralateral SR

13. The best results of cryotherapy for ROP occur for treatment of disease in which location?
    a. zone 1
    b. anterior zone 2
    c. posterior zone 2
    d. zone 3

14. Characteristics of congenital ET include all of the following except
    a. dissociated vertical deviation
    b. cross fixation
    c. amblyopia
    d. inferior oblique overaction

15. The contalateral antagonist of the right superior rectus
    a. passes under another muscle
    b. causes incyclotorsion when paretic
    c. adducts the eye
    d. is innervated by the inferior division of CN 3

16. With respect to Panum's area, physiologic diplopia occurs at what point?
    a. on the horopter
    b. within Panum's area
    c. in front of Panum's area
    d. none of the above

17. The best treatment of an A-pattern ET with muscle transposition is
    a. MR resection with upward transposition
    b. LR resection with upward transposition
    c. MR recession with downward transposition
    d. LR resection with downward transposition

18. A superior rectus Faden suture is used for the treatment of which condition?
    a. Duane's syndrome
    b. dissociated vertical deviation
    c. Brown's syndrome
    d. double elevator palsy

19. Which medication should be administered to a child who develops trismus under general anesthesia?
    a. atropine
    b. edrophonium chloride (Tensilon)
    c. lidocaine
    d. dantrolene

20. Congenital superior oblique palsy is characterized by all of the following except
    a. excyclotorsion <10°
    b. head tilt
    c. facial asymmetry
    d. <10 D of vertical vergence amplitudes

21. Which of the following statements regarding monofixation syndrome is false?
    a. there is no diplopia with the 4 Δ base-out prism test
    b. fusion with the Worth 4 Dot test is absent at distance
    c. fusional vergence amplitudes are absent
    d. titmus test for fly is normal

22. Iridocyclitis is most commonly associated with which form of JRA?
    a. Still's disease
    b. polyarticular
    c. spondyloarthropathy
    d. pauciarticular

23. Congenital rubella is most commonly associated with
    a. retinal pigment epitheliopathy
    b. cataracts
    c. glaucoma
    d. strabismus

24. The most common cause of proptosis in a child is
    a. idiopathic orbital inflammation
    b. orbital cellulitis
    c. cavernous hemangioma
    d. Graves' disease

25. Which form of rhabdomyosarcoma has the worst prognosis?
    a. botryoid
    b. pleomorphic
    c. alveolar
    d. embryonal

26. Which of the following conditions is the least common cause of childhood proptosis?
    a. cavernous hemangioma
    b. rhabdomyosarcoma
    c. lymphangioma
    d. mucocele

27. A child with retinoblastoma is born to healthy parents with no family history of RB. The chance of RB occurring in a second child is approximately
    a. 5%
    b. 25%
    c. 40%
    d. 50%

28. The best chronologic age to examine a baby for ROP is
    a. 28 weeks
    b. 32 weeks
    c. 36 weeks
    d. 40 weeks

29. All of the following are associated with trisomy 13 except
    a. anophthalmos
    b. retinal dysplasia
    c. epiblepharon
    d. intraocular cartilage

30. Paradoxical pupillary response does not occur in
    a. achromatopsia
    b. CSNB
    c. Leber's congenital amaurosis
    d. albinism
31. An infant with bilateral cataracts is diagnosed with galactosemia. Which enzyme is most likely to be defective?
    a. galactokinase
    b. galactose-1-P-uridyl transferase
    c. galactose-6-sulfatase
    d. UDP galactose-4-epimerase
32. All of the following are associated with optic nerve drusen except
    a. peripapillary hemorrhage
    b. inferior nasal visual field loss
    c. increased risk of intracranial tumors
    d. autosomal dominant inheritance
33. The etiology of torticollis and intermittent, fine, rapid, pendular nystagmus of the right eye in a 10-month-old baby is most likely
    a. metastatic neuroblastoma
    b. posterior fossa tumor
    c. optic nerve meningioma
    d. none of the above
34. The most common malignant tumor of the orbit in a 6-year-old boy is
    a. neuroblastoma
    b. rhabdomyosarcoma
    c. optic nerve glioma
    d. lymphosarcoma
35. Retinitis pigmentosa and deafness occur in all of the following disorders except
    a. Usher's syndrome
    b. Alstrom's syndrome
    c. Refsum's disease
    d. Cockayne's syndrome
36. Which of the following agents is most likely to increase IOP during an EUA (examination under anesthesia)?
    a. halothane
    b. chloral hydrate
    c. thiopental
    d. ketamine
37. α-galactosidase A deficiency is associated with
    a. cornea verticillata
    b. corneal clouding
    c. corneal vascularization
    d. no corneal changes
38. Congenital cataracts and glaucoma may occur in all of the following disorders except
    a. Hallerman-Streiff syndrome
    b. Alport's syndrome
    c. rubella
    d. Lowe's syndrome
39. RPE degeneration and optic atrophy are found in all of the following mucopolysaccharidoses except
    a. MPS type I
    b. MPS type II
    c. MPS type III
    d. MPS type IV
40. Which vitamin is not deficient in a patient with abetalipoproteinemia (Bassen-Kornzweig syndrome)?
    a. A
    b. C
    c. D
    d. E
41. Hearing loss is not found in
    a. Cogan's syndrome
    b. Refsum's disease
    c. Duane's syndrome
    d. Stickler's syndrome
42. Pheochromocytoma may occur in all of the following phakomatoses except
    a. Louis-Bar syndrome
    b. von Hippel-Lindau disease
    c. Sturge-Weber syndrome
    d. Bourneville's disease
43. Maternal ingestion of LSD is most likely to result in which congenital optic nerve disorder
    a. coloboma
    b. optic pit
    c. hypoplasia
    d. morning glory disc
44. A patient with strabismus wearing −6 D glasses is measured with prism and cover test. Compared with the actual amount of deviation, the measurement would find
    a. more esotropia and less exotropia
    b. more esotropia and more exotropia
    c. less esotropia and more exotropia
    d. less esotropia and less exotropia
45. Prism glasses are least helpful for treating
    a. incomitant esotropia
    b. divergence insufficiency
    c. sensory esotropia
    d. intermittent exotropia
46. A 4-year-old boy has bilateral lateral rectus recessions for exotropia. Two days after surgery he has an esotropia measuring 50 Δ. The most appropriate treatment is
    a. atropinization
    b. prism glasses
    c. alternate patching
    d. surgery
47. The most common cause of a vitreous hemorrhage in a child is
    a. ROP
    b. shaken baby syndrome
    c. FEVR
    d. Coat's disease
48. A 5-year-old girl with 20/20 vision OD and 20/50 vision OS is diagnosed with an anterior polar cataract OS. The most appropriate treatment is
    a. start occlusion therapy
    b. observe and reexamine in 6 months
    c. perform cataract surgery and use aphakic contact lens
    d. perform cataract surgery with lens implant
49. Chronic iritis in a child is most commonly caused by
    a. JRA
    b. trauma
    c. sarcoidosis
    d. Lyme disease

50. All are features of ataxia-telangiectasia except
    a. sinopulmonary infections
    b. thymic hyperplasia
    c. IgA deficiency
    d. autosomal recessive inheritance
51. All of the following vitreoretinal disorders are inherited in an autosomal dominant pattern except
    a. familial exudative vitreoretinopathy
    b. Wagner's syndrome
    c. Stickler's syndrome
    d. Goldmann-Favre disease
52. The most common location for an iris coloboma is
    a. superotemporal
    b. superonasal
    c. inferotemporal
    d. inferonasal
53. Von Hippel-Lindau disease has been mapped to which chromosome?
    a. 3
    b. 9
    c. 11
    d. 17
54. Which X-linked disorder is not associated with an ocular abnormality in the female carrier?
    a. choroideremia
    b. albinism
    c. juvenile retinoschisis
    d. retinitis pigmentosa

55. Which tumor is not associated with von Hippel-Lindau disease?
    a. hepatocellular carcinoma
    b. pheochromocytoma
    c. renal cell carcinoma
    d. cerebellar hemangioblastoma

SUGGESTED READINGS

American Academy of Ophthalmology: Pediatric Ophthalmology and Strabismus, vol 6. San Francisco, AAO, 2012.

Burian HM, von Noorden GK: Binocular Vision and Ocular Motility: Theory and Treatment of Strabismus. St Louis, Mosby, 1974

Del Monte MA, Archer SM: Atlas of Pediatric Ophthalmology and Strabismus Surgery. Philadelphia, Butterworth-Heinemann, 1991.

Nelson LB, Olitsky SE: Harley's Pediatric Ophthalmology, 5th edn. Philadelphia, Lippincott Williams & Wilkins, 2005.

Nelson LB, Catalano RA: Atlas of Ocular Motility. Philadelphia, WB Saunders, 1997.

Von Noorden GK: Atlas of Strabismus, 4th edn. St Louis, Mosby, 1983.

Von Noorden GK, Campos EC: Binocular Vision and Ocular Motility: Theory and Treatment of Strabismus, 6th edn. St Louis, Mosby, 2002.

6

Orbit / Lids / Adnexa

ANATOMY
IMAGING
ORBITAL DISORDERS
EYELID DISORDERS
NASOLACRIMAL SYSTEM DISORDERS
ORBITAL SURGERY

ANATOMY

Dimensions

Orbit: pear-shaped (widest diameter is 1 cm posterior to orbital rim); 40 mm wide, 35 mm high, 45 mm deep, volume = 30 cc (Table 6-1)

Optic nerve: orbital length = 25–30 mm; length from globe to optic foramen = 18 mm; width = 1.5 mm in globe, 3.5 mm posterior to lamina cribrosa (due to myelin), 5.0 mm with the addition of the optic nerve sheath (see Figure 4-2)

Proptosis: measure with Hertel exophthalmometer (Table 6-2)

Apertures

(Figures 6-1 to 6-3)

Superior orbital fissure:
Separates greater and lesser sphenoid wings
Between roof and lateral wall
Transmits: CN 3, 4, V_1, and 6, superior ophthalmic vein, and sympathetic fibers to iris dilator

Optic canal (orbital foramen):
Within lesser wing of sphenoid: 10 mm long
Enlarged with ON glioma
Transmits: Optic nerve (CN 2), ophthalmic artery, and sympathetic nerves to ocular and orbital blood vessels

Inferior orbital fissure:
Bordered medially by maxillary bone, anteriorly by zygomatic bone, and laterally by greater wing of sphenoid
Transmits: CN V_2, zygomatic nerve, inferior ophthalmic vein, venous communication between ophthalmic vein and pterygoid plexus, sphenopalatine ganglion branches

Nasolacrimal canal:
Runs from lacrimal sac fossa to inferior meatus under the inferior turbinate
Contains the nasolacrimal duct
Lateral wall = maxillary bone
Medial wall = lacrimal bone and inferior turbinate

Zygomaticofacial and zygomaticotemporal canals:
Transmit: vessels and branches of the zygomatic nerve through the lateral wall to cheek and temporal fossa

Ethmoidal foramina:
Transmit: anterior and posterior ethmoid arteries
Potential route for spread of infectious sinusitis

Frontosphenoidal foramina:
Transmit: anastomosis between the middle meningeal and lacrimal arteries, which provides collateral blood supply to the orbit

Foramen ovale:
Transmits: CN V_3

Foramen rotundum:
Transmits: CN V_2

Foramen lacerum:
Transmits: internal carotid artery

Vascular Supply to Eye

(Figures 6-4 to 6-6)

Ophthalmic artery: 1st branch of internal carotid within skull
Central retinal artery:
Enters optic nerve 13 mm posterior to globe
Supplies blood to inner ⅔ of retina

Table 6-1. Osteology

Orbit	Bones	Related structures/miscellaneous
Roof	Sphenoid (lesser wing)	Lacrimal gland fossa
	Frontal	Trochlea
		Supraorbital notch (medial)
Lateral wall	Sphenoid (greater wing)	Lateral orbital tubercle of Whitnall
	Zygomatic	Strongest orbital wall
		Lateral orbital rim at equator of globe
Floor	Maxilla	Contains infraorbital nerve and canal
	Palatine	Forms roof of maxillary sinus
	Zygomatic	
Medial wall	Sphenoid	Lacrimal sac fossa
	Maxilla	Adjacent to ethmoid and sphenoid sinuses
	Ethmoid	Posterior ethmoidal foramen
	Lacrimal	Weakest orbital wall

Table 6-2. Hertel exophthalmometry measurements

	Mean (mm)	Upper Limit of Normal (mm)
Caucasian male	16.5	21.7
Caucasian female	15.4	20
African American male	18.5	24.7
African American female	17.8	23.0

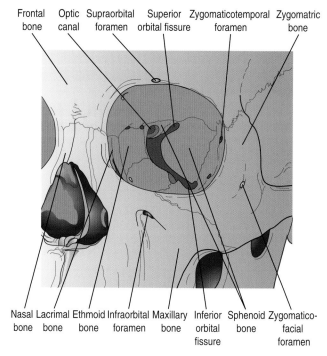

Figure 6-1. Bony anatomy of the orbit in frontal view. (From Dutton JJ: Atlas of Clinical and Surgical Orbital Anatomy, Philadelphia, WB Saunders, 1994.)

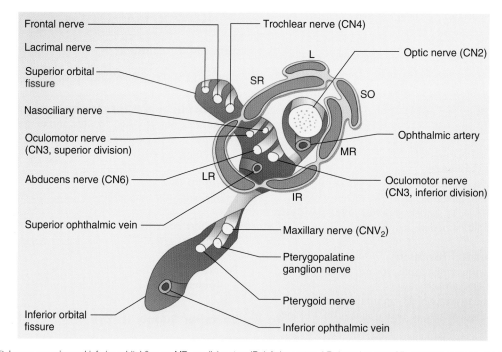

Figure 6-2. Orbital apex, superior and inferior orbital fissure. MR, medial rectus; IR, inferior rectus; LR, lateral rectus; SR, superior rectus; L, levator; SO, superior oblique. Note that the trochlear nerve lies outside the muscle cone.

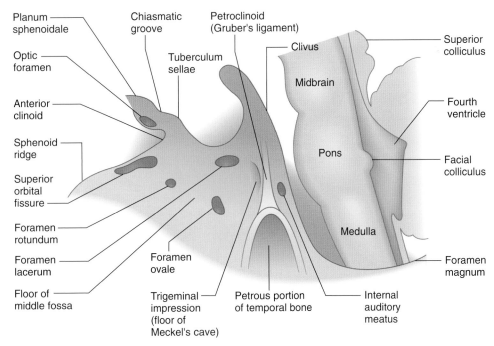

Figure 6-3. Schematic representation of the landmarks, temporal view. (From Bajandas FJ, Kline BK: Neuro-Ophthalmology Review Manual, Thorofare, NJ, Slack, 1988.)

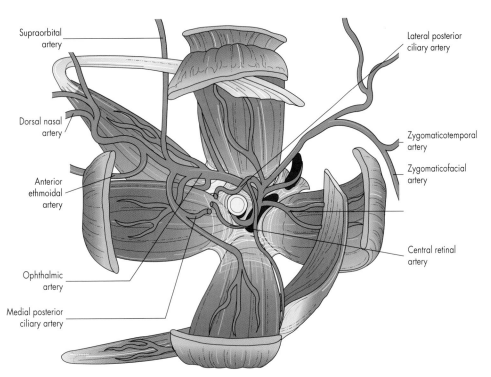

Figure 6-4. Arterial supply to the orbit, in coronal view. (From Dutton JJ: Atlas of Clinical and Surgical Orbital Anatomy, Philadelphia, WB Saunders, 1994.)

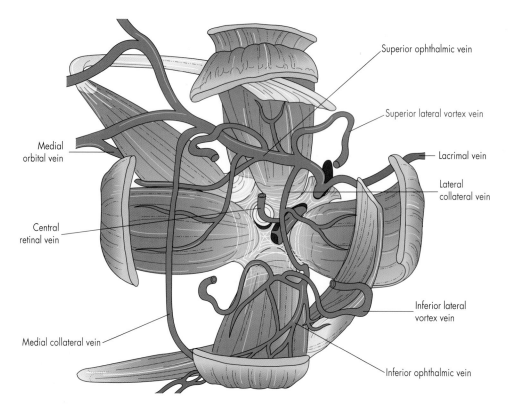

Figure 6-5. Orbital veins. Venous drainage from the orbit, in coronal view. (From Dutton JJ: Atlas of Clinical and Surgical Orbital Anatomy, Philadelphia, WB Saunders, 1994.)

Posterior ciliary arteries:
  Long posterior ciliary arteries supply anterior segment
  Short posterior ciliary arteries supply choroid
  Optic nerve head is primarily supplied by blood from the vascular **circle of Zinn-Haller** (collection of anastomotic arteries arising from the short posterior ciliary arteries)

Venous system: Orbital veins do not have valves
  Vortex veins:
    4–8 per eye; 1–2 per quadrant
    Exit posterior to the equator
    Drain choroid and merge into the superior or inferior ophthalmic veins
  Superior ophthalmic vein:
    Exits via superior orbital fissure into the cavernous sinus
    2 superior vortex veins
  Inferior ophthalmic vein:
    Exits via inferior orbital fissure
    2 inferior vortex veins
  Central retinal vein:
    Joins superior or inferior ophthalmic vein
    Leaves nerve 10 mm behind globe

Innervation of Eye

Sensory innervation provided by ophthalmic and maxillary division of trigeminal nerve (CN 5) (Figure 6-7)

Ophthalmic division (V_1):

  Nasociliary nerve:
    Enters orbit within the annulus of Zinn

    Short ciliary nerves pass through ciliary ganglion
    Long ciliary nerves supply iris, cornea, and ciliary muscle
  Frontal nerve:
    Enters orbit above annulus of Zinn
    Divides into supraorbital nerve and supratrochlear nerve
    Innervates medial canthus, upper lid, and forehead
  Lacrimal nerve:
    Enters orbit above annulus of Zinn
    Innervates upper eyelid and lacrimal gland

Maxillary nerve (V_2):

  Passes through foramen rotundum, then passes through inferior orbital fissure
  Divides into infraorbital nerve, zygomatic nerve, and superior alveolar nerve

Parasympathetic innervation:

  Controls accommodation, pupillary constriction, and lacrimal gland stimulation
  Enters eye as short posterior ciliary nerves after synapsing in the ciliary ganglion

Sympathetic innervation:

  Controls pupillary dilation, vasoconstriction, smooth muscle function of eyelids and orbit, and hidrosis
  Dysfunction: Horner's syndrome (ptosis, miosis, anhidrosis, and vasodilation)
  Nerve fibers follow arterial supply as well as long ciliary nerves

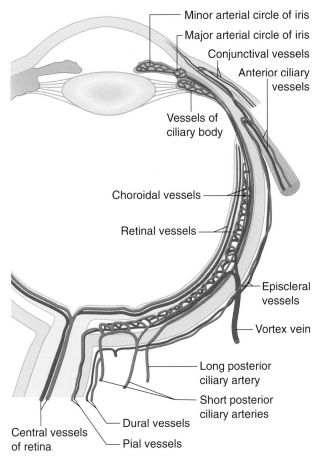

Figure 6-6. Vascular supply to the eye. All arterial branches originate with the ophthalmic artery. Venous drainage is through the cavernous sinus and the pterygoid plexus.

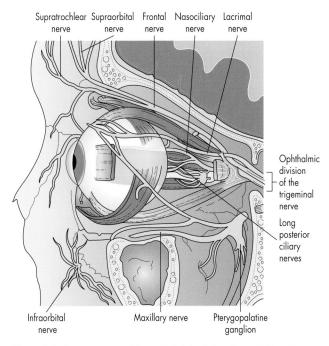

Figure 6-7. Sensory nerves of the orbit, in lateral view. (From Dutton JJ: Atlas of Clinical and Surgical Orbital Anatomy, Philadelphia, WB Saunders, 1994.)

Sinuses

(Figure 6-8)

Frontal:
Not radiographically visible before age 6
Drains into anterior portion of the middle meatus

Ethmoid:
Multiple thin-walled cavities
First sinus to aerate
Anterior and middle air cells drain into the middle meatus
Posterior air cells drain into the superior meatus
Ethmoidal sinusitis is the most common source of infection that leads to orbital cellulitis

Sphenoid:
Rudimentary at birth
Reaches full size after puberty
Optic canal is superior and lateral to sphenoid sinus
Drains into sphenoethmoid recess of each nasal fossa

Maxillary:
Largest sinus
Roof contains the infraorbital nerve
Drains into middle meatus

Soft Tissues

(Figure 6-9)

Periorbita:
Periosteum is attached firmly at the orbital rim and suture lines
Arcus marginalis: fusion of periosteum and orbital septum at orbital rim
Fuses with the dura covering the optic nerve

Annulus of Zinn:
Fibrous tissue ring arising from periorbita that surrounds the optic canal
Origin of the 4 recti muscles
Fuses with dura covering ON at apex

Adipose tissue:
Surrounds most of orbital contents; divided by fine fibrous septa
Preaponeurotic fat pads: lie immediately posterior to orbital septum
2 FAT PADS IN UPPER LID: anterior to levator aponeurosis; nasal pad smaller and paler than central pad; with aging, nasal pad moves anteriorly and may cause bulging of upper nasal orbit
3 FAT PADS IN LOWER LID: anterior to capsulopalpebral fascia; inferior oblique muscle separates the nasal and middle pads; lateral pad is small and more inferior

Lacrimal gland:
2 lobes: orbital (larger) and palpebral, separated by levator aponeurosis

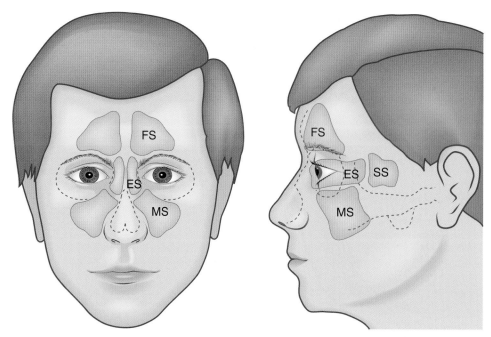

Figure 6-8. Relationship of the orbits to the paranasal sinuses: FS, frontal sinus, ES, ethmoid sinus; MS, maxillary sinus; SS, sphenoid sinus. (Reprinted with permission from Slamovits TL: Basic and Clinical Science Course, Section 7: Orbit, Eyelids and Lacrimal System. American Academy of Ophthalmology, San Francisco, 1993.)

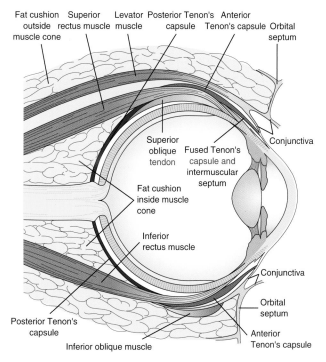

Figure 6-9. Sagittal section of orbital tissues through the vertical recti. (Adapted from Parks MM: Extraocular muscles. In Duane TD Clinical Ophthalmology, Philadelphia, Harper and Row, 1982.)

Ducts from both lobes pass though the palpebral lobe and empty into the superior fornix

Innervation: secretomotor from superior salivatory nucleus via CN 7; sensory from CN 5; sympathetic from superior cervical ganglion via deep petrosal nerve, pterygopalatine ganglion, and zygomatic nerve

Blood supply: lacrimal artery

Accessory lacrimal glands: glands of Wolfring located in tarsus and glands of Krause located in the conjunctival fornices (10% of production)

Eyelid

Lamellae of upper eyelid: (Figure 6-10)

Anterior: skin, orbicularis

Posterior: tarsus, levator aponeurosis, Müller's muscle, palpebral conjunctiva

Skin:

Thinnest skin of the body, no subcutaneous fat layer

Upper eyelid crease approximates attachments of the levator aponeurosis to the pretarsal orbicularis and skin

Histology of epidermis:

BASILAR LAYER (stratum basalis): cuboidal cells with scant cytoplasm; responsible for generating superficial layers

PRICKLE CELL LAYER: multiple layers of cells with abundant cytoplasm attached to each other by desmosomes

GRANULAR CELL LAYER (stratum granulosum): cells contain granular material that stains blue with H&E

KERATIN LAYER: superficial, acellular keratin devoid of nuclei; stains pink with H&E

Orbicularis oculi: (Figure 6-11)

Main protractor of the eyelid; acts as lacrimal pump; innervated by CN 7

3 anatomic parts: palpebral portion (pretarsal and preseptal) involved with involuntary blinking; orbital portion involved with voluntary, forced lid closure

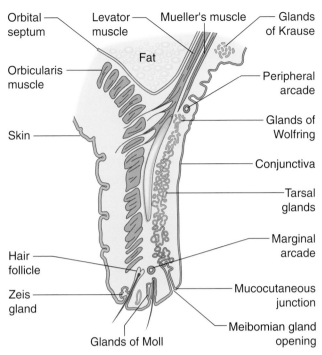

Figure 6-10. Cross section of upper eyelid. Note position of cilia, tarsal gland orifices, and mucocutaneous junction. (Reprinted with permission from Grand MG: Basic and Clinical Science Course, Section 2: Fundamentals and Principles of Ophthalmology. American Academy of Ophthalmology, San Francisco, 1993.)

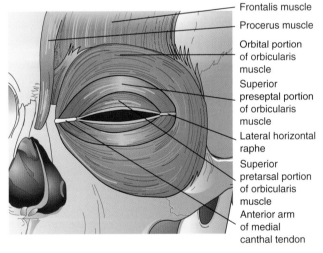

Figure 6-11. The orbicularis and frontalis muscles. (From Dutton JJ: Atlas of Clinical and Surgical Orbital Anatomy, Philadelphia, WB Saunders, 1994.)

PRETARSAL: overlies tarsus, originates from lateral orbital tubercle, forms muscle of Riolan (seen as gray line at lid margin)
SUPERFICIAL HEAD: medially inserts into anterior lacrimal crest, contributes to medial canthal tendon, laterally inserts into zygomatic bone
DEEP HEAD: medially inserts into posterior lacrimal crest, called Horner's muscle, surrounds canaliculi facilitating tear drainage, laterally inserts into lateral orbital tubercle, contributes to lateral canthal tendon

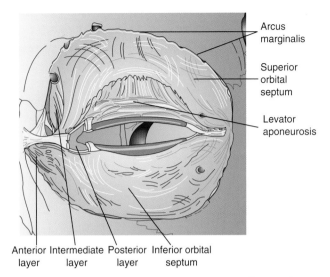

Figure 6-12. The orbital septum. (From Dutton JJ: Atlas of Clinical and Surgical Orbital Anatomy, Philadelphia, WB Saunders, 1994.)

PRESEPTAL: overlies orbital septum
Originates from anterior limb of the medial canthal tendon, and from posterior lacrimal crest and lacrimal sac fascia
Forms lateral palpebral raphe overlying the lateral orbital rim
ORBITAL: lies beneath skin
Thickest portion of orbicularis
Inserts at medial canthal tendon
Interdigitates with the frontalis muscle superiorly at eyebrow

Other muscles of forehead and eyebrow:
Frontalis: moves scalp anteriorly and posteriorly; raises eyebrows; innervated by CN 7
Corrugator: pulls medial eyebrow inferiorly and medially producing vertical glabellar wrinkle; originates from nasal process of frontal bone; inserts laterally into subcutaneous tissue; innervated by CN 7
Procerus: pulls forehead and medial eyebrow inferiorly producing horizontal lines in nose; interdigitates with inferior edge of frontalis; innervated by CN 7

Orbital septum: (Figure 6-12)
Dense fibrous sheath that acts as barrier between the orbit and eyelid; stops spread of infection
Originates from periosteum of the superior and inferior orbital rims
Inserts into levator aponeurosis superiorly (2–5 mm above superior tarsal border in non-Asians) and into lower eyelid retractors inferiorly (capsulopalpebral fascia just below inferior tarsal border)
Medially inserts into lacrimal crest
Structures posterior to the septum: palpebral lobe of lacrimal gland, lateral canthal tendon, trochlea of superior oblique muscle
In Asians, orbital septum fuses with levator aponeurosis between the eyelid margin and the superior border of the tarsus

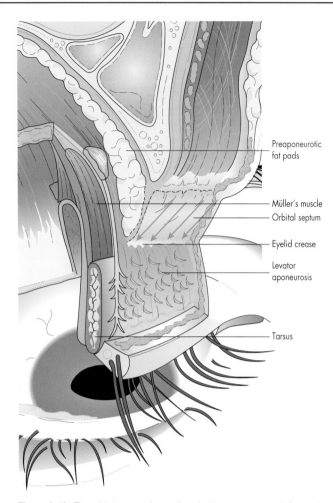

Figure 6-13. The orbital septum inserts into the levator aponeurosis *(arrows)*. The preaponeurotic fat pads are located posterior to the septum. In downgaze, the lid crease becomes attenuated (weakened), and in a normal young eyelid, the fold is absent. (From Zide BW, Jelks BW: Surgical Anatomy of the Orbit. New York, Raven Press, 1985.)

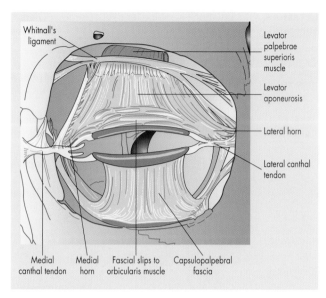

Figure 6-14. The levator aponeurosis, and the medial and lateral canthal tendons. (From Dutton JJ: Atlas of Clinical and Surgical Orbital Anatomy, Philadelphia, WB Saunders, 1994.)

Whitnall's ligament (superior transverse ligament):
    condensation of levator muscle sheath
    Visible as horizontal white line 10 mm above superior
        edge of tarsus
    Arises from the sheath of anterior portion of levator
        muscle
    Medially attaches to trochlea
    Laterally forms septa through stroma of lacrimal gland
        and attaches to inner aspect of lateral orbital wall
        at the frontozygomatic suture (10 mm above
        orbital tubercle [Whitnall's tubercle]) and at the
        orbital tubercle
    Acts to change direction of pull of levator and serves
        as check ligament to prevent excessive lid elevation
Müller's muscle (superior tarsal muscle):
    Posterior to levator aponeurosis
    Sympathetic innervation
    Originates from undersurface of levator approximately
        at level of Whitnall's ligament
    Inserts into upper border of tarsus
    12–15 mm long; raises eyelid 2 mm
    Peripheral arterial arcade found between aponeurosis
        and Müller's muscle

Lower eyelid retractors: (Figure 6-15)
Capsulopalpebral fascia: analogous to levator aponeurosis
    Originates from inferior rectus muscle sheath, divides
        as it encircles inferior oblique muscle, and then
        joins to form Lockwood's ligament
    Fuses with septum and inserts into inferior tarsus
Lockwood's suspensory ligament: analogous to Whitnall's
    ligament
    Arises posteriorly from fibrous attachments to inferior
        side of the IR muscle and continues anteriorly as
        capsulopalpebral fascia
    Medial and lateral horns attach to retinacula forming
        a suspensory hammock for the globe

Upper eyelid retractors: (Figure 6-13)
Levator palpebrae:
    Originates from lesser wing of sphenoid above
        annulus of Zinn
    Innervated by CN 3
    MUSCULAR PORTION: 40 mm
    APONEUROTIC PORTION: 14–20 mm and has lateral
        and medial extensions (horns) (Figure 6-14)
        LATERAL HORN:
            Inserts onto lateral orbital tubercle
            Divides lacrimal gland into orbital and
               palpebral portions
        MEDIAL HORN:
            Inserts onto posterior lacrimal crest
            More delicate and weaker than lateral horn
            Anterior portion inserts into septa between
               pretarsal orbicularis muscle bundles
            Posterior portion inserts onto anterior surface of
               lower half of tarsus; forms eyelid crease
            Disinsertion of aponeurosis results in loss of
               eyelid crease

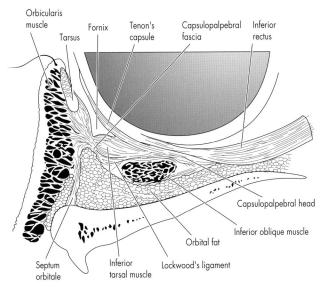

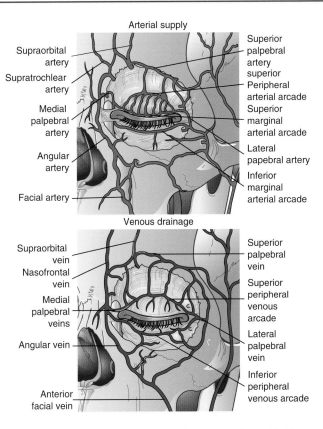

Figure 6-15. Anatomy of the lower eyelid retractors. (Adapted from Hawes MJ, Dortzbach RK: The microscopic anatomy of the lower eyelid retractors, Arch Ophthalmol 100:1313-1318, 1982.)

Inferior tarsal muscle: analogous to Müller's muscle
Sympathetic innervation
Arises from capsulopalpebral fascia

Tarsus:
Dense connective tissue plate in each eyelid; not cartilage
Contains meibomian glands
29 mm long and 1 mm thick; tapered at ends
Rigid attachments to periosteum medially and laterally
Superior tarsal plate: 10 mm in height
Inferior tarsal plate: 4 mm in height

Medial canthal tendon:
Fusion of tendinous insertions of pretarsal and preseptal
orbicularis muscles
Attaches to tarsal plates
Anterior limb: attaches to frontal process of maxillary
bone and serves as origin of superficial head of
pretarsal orbicularis; passes in front of lacrimal sac
and attaches to anterior lacrimal crest
Posterior limb: attaches to posterior lacrimal crest; passes
behind lacrimal sac. More important than anterior
limb for normal medial canthal appearance and
function (maintaining apposition of lids to globe)

Lateral canthal tendon:
Broad band of connective tissue from lateral borders of
upper and lower tarsal plates
Inserts onto lateral orbital tubercle of Whitnall; 3 mm
superior to medial canthal tendon insertion

Eyelid margin: 3 distinguishing landmarks
Lash line: 2–3 rows of lashes; 100 in upper lid, 50 in
lower lid; 10-week growth, 5-month resting phase
Gray line: border of pretarsal orbicularis (muscle of
Riolan); junction of anterior and posterior lamellae;
vascular watershed
Meibomian gland orifices: 30 in upper lid, 20 in lower lid

Figure 6-16. Arterial supply to, and venous drainage from, the eyelids. (From Dutton JJ: Atlas of Clinical and Surgical Orbital Anatomy, Philadelphia, WB Saunders, 1994.)

Vascular supply: (Figure 6-16)
Upper lid: internal carotid artery → ophthalmic artery →
superior marginal arcade (deep to orbicularis and
anterior surface of tarsus)
Lower lid: external carotid artery → facial artery →
angular artery → inferior marginal arcade
Angular artery is 6–8 mm medial to medial canthus,
posterior to orbicularis, 5 mm anterior to
lacrimal sac
Peripheral and marginal arcades allow for anastomosis
between the ICA and ECA
Venous drainage:
PRETARSAL: angular vein medially, superficial
temporal vein temporally
POST-TARSAL: orbital vein, anterior facial vein, and
pterygoid plexus

Innervation:
Sensory: CN V$_1$ (upper lid), CN V$_2$ (lower lid)
Motor: CN 3, CN 7, sympathetics

Lymphatic drainage:
Submandibular nodes: drain medial ⅓ of upper lid,
medial ⅔ of lower lid
Preauricular nodes: drain lateral ⅔ of upper lid, lateral
⅓ of lower lid
No lymphatic vessels or nodes are found within
the orbit
Lymphatic vessels are found in the conjunctiva

Table 6-3. Glands of the eyelids

Gland	Location	Type	Function	Pathology
Lacrimal	Superotemporal orbit	Eccrine	Reflex tear (aqueous) secretion	Dacryoadenitis Tumors
Accessory lacrimal: Krause Wolfring	Fornix Just above tarsus	Eccrine	Basal tear (aqueous) secretion	Sjögren's syndrome GVH disease Rare tumors (BMT)
Meibomian	Within tarsus	Holocrine	Lipid secretion Retards tear evaporation	Chalazion Sebaceous carcinoma
Zeis	Near lid margin Caruncle Associated with cilia	Holocrine	Lipid secretion Lubricates cilia	External hordeolum Sebaceous carcinoma
Moll	Near lid margin	Apocrine	Modified sweat glands Lubricates cilia	Ductal cyst Apocrine carcinoma
Sweat		Eccrine	Electrolyte balance	Ductal cyst Syringoma Sweat gland carcinoma
Goblet cells	Conjunctiva Plica Caruncle	Holocrine	Mucin secretion Enhances corneal wetting	Dry eye

Glands of the eyelids: (Table 6-3)

Eccrine: secretion by simple exocytosis

Holocrine: secretion by release of entire cellular contents (disruption of cell)

Apocrine: secretion by pinching or budding off of a portion of cellular cytoplasm

Nasolacrimal System

(Figure 6-17)

Puncta:

Upper and lower; 6 mm from medial canthus, lower is slightly more temporal

Slightly inverted against globe

Open into ampulla (2 mm long) oriented perpendicular to eyelid margin

Canaliculi:

10 mm long (2 mm vertical segment [ampulla] and 8 mm horizontal portion parallel to lid margin)

Combine to form single common canaliculus in 90% of individuals

Valve of Rosenmüller prevents reflux from lacrimal sac into canaliculi

Nasolacrimal sac:

10 mm long, occupies the lacrimal fossa

Lies between anterior and posterior crura of the medial canthal tendon, anterior to orbital septum

Lateral to middle meatus of nose

Nasolacrimal duct:

15 mm long

Passes inferiorly, posteriorly, and laterally within canal formed by maxillary and lacrimal bones

Extends into inferior meatus, which opens under inferior turbinate (2.5 cm posterior to naris)

Partially covered by valve of Hasner

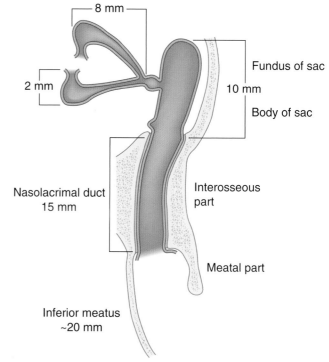

Figure 6-17. Excretory lacrimal system. (From Grand MG: Basic and Clinical Science Course, Section 2, Fundamentals and Principles of Ophthalmology, San Francisco, American Academy of Ophthalmology, 1993.)

Lacrimal pump:

Lids close: pretarsal orbicularis contracts, compresses ampulla, shortens canaliculus; punctum moves medially; lacrimal sac expands, creates negative pressure, draws fluid from canaliculus into sac

Lids open: muscles relax, lacrimal sac collapses, tears forced into nose, punctum moves laterally, tears enter canaliculus

IMAGING

Ultrasound

Optimal sound wave frequency is 10 MHz

Higher frequencies give better resolution; lower frequencies provide better penetration (Table 6-4)

Table 6-4. Ultrasound characteristics of lesions	
Good sound transmission	**Poor sound transmission**
Cavernous hemangioma	Metastatic cancer
Lymphangioma	Orbital pseudotumor
Mucocele	Glioma
Dermoid	Neurofibroma
High Reflectivity	**Low Reflectivity**
Neurofibroma	Metastatic cancer
Fresh hemorrhage	Orbital pseudotumor
Hemangioma	Cyst
Thyroid eye disease	Mucocele
	Varix
	Dermoid
	Lymphoma

MRI

Strong magnetic field results in alignment of nuclei of atoms with odd numbers of protons or neutrons

Radiofrequency pulse disturbs the alignment by energizing protons or neutrons

When pulse terminates, protons return to previous alignment and emit absorbed energy as radiofrequency signal, generating an image

Can provide axial, coronal, and sagittal views

Relaxation times:

Longitudinal relaxation time (T1): time required for net bulk magnetization to realign itself along original axis
   Blood, orbital fat, melanin, and mucus appear bright
   Acute hemorrhage, vitreous, optic nerve sheath, and extraocular muscles appear dark
   Most orbital tumors are hypointense to fat on T1-weighted images
   EXCEPTIONS: mucinous lesions (orbital dermoid cyst, mucocele), lipoma, liposarcoma, melanoma, subacute hemorrhage
   Gadolinium: bright white on T1-weighted images
   Must perform fat suppression on T1-weighted images when gadolinium is used
   Fat suppression renders orbital fat hypointense and permits better visualization of optic nerve and extraocular muscles
Transverse relaxation time (T2): mean relaxation time
   Based on interaction of hydrogen nuclei within a given tissue
   Provides more information about pathologic processes
   Helps differentiate melanotic lesions from hemorrhagic process
   Vitreous is bright on T2-weighted images
   Blood and fat appear dark

Demyelinating plaques of MS are best seen with T2-weighted images (hyperintense foci, usually in periventricular white matter)

Advantages: better for soft tissues and posterior fossa, sagittal sections, no artifacts from bone or teeth, no ionizing radiation

Disadvantages: poor bony detail, longer imaging time, more expensive, certain contraindications

Contraindications: patients with retained metallic foreign body, pacemaker, aneurysm clip

CT Scan

Use with orbital trauma to detect foreign body or calcification, or for evaluation of orbital soft tissue lesion with suspicion of bony erosion

Bone and metal appear bright

Advantages: better bony detail and for acute hemorrhage, sinuses, and trauma; shorter imaging time; less expensive

Disadvantages: poor posterior fossa detail; no sagittal sections, ionizing radiation
(Table 6-5)

Table 6-5. CT and MRI characteristics of lesions	
Most common orbital lesions with well-circumscribed appearance on CT and MRI	**Most common orbital lesions with Ill-defined appearance on CT and MRI**
Children:	**Children:**
Dermoid cyst	Capillary hemangioma
Lymphangioma	Orbital pseudotumor
Rhabdomyosarcoma	Plexiform neurofibroma
ON glioma	Leukemic infiltrate
	Eosinophilic granuloma
Adults:	**Adults:**
Cavernous hemangioma	Orbital pseudotumor
Neurofibroma	Metastasis
Neurilemmoma	Leukemic infiltrate
Fibrous histiocytoma	Primary malignant tumor
(Lymphoproliferative disorders)	Lymphoproliferative disorders

Radiographs

Specific views can be helpful, especially when CT is unavailable or to quickly rule out a metallic foreign body

Plain film radiography also detects sinus pathology, calcification, hyperostosis, and lytic lesions

Canthomeatal line: radiographic baseline of skull (line between lateral canthal angle and tragus of ear)

Waters view: occipitomental; head extended until canthomeatal line lies at 37° to the central beam; best view of orbital roof and floor

Caldwell view: posteroanterior view with central beam tilted 25° toward feet; best view of superior and lateral orbital rim, medial wall, and ethmoid and frontal sinuses

Lateral view: best for evaluation of sella turcica

Submental vertex view: basal or Hirtz view with head tilted back until canthomeatal line is perpendicular to central beam; best view of sphenoid and ethmoid sinuses, nasal cavities, and zygomatic arch

Oblique (×2) views: PA view with central beam tilted 32° toward feet and 37° from perpendicular; best views of optic foramina

ORBITAL DISORDERS

Congenital and Developmental Anomalies

(See Ch. 5, Pediatrics/Strabismus)

Trauma

Orbital Contusion

Bruising from blunt trauma

Pain, decreased vision

Often have associated lid, orbit, and ocular injuries

Treatment: ice compresses, systemic NSAIDs

Orbital Fractures

Fractures of orbital bones, often associated with ocular or intracranial injuries
  Orbital floor (blow-out): Maxillary bone
  Posterior medial floor is weakest area
  Findings: may have enophthalmos, diplopia, infraorbital
    hypesthesia, orbit or lid emphysema, and medial
    wall fracture
  Complications: orbital contents may become entrapped in
    maxillary sinus with resultant restriction of ocular
    motility, diplopia, and globe ptosis

Medial wall:
  Maxillary, lacrimal, and ethmoid bones
  Findings: may have depressed nasal bridge, telecanthus,
    floor fracture
  Complications: epistaxis from injury of anterior
    ethmoidal artery, CSF rhinorrhea, lacrimal drainage
    injury, orbit or lid emphysema

Orbital apex:
  Can involve optic canal and superior orbital fissure
  Complications: CSF rhinorrhea, carotid-cavernous
    fistula

Orbital roof:
  Uncommon
  May affect frontal sinus, cribriform plate, and brain
  Complications: CSF rhinorrhea, pneumocephalus

Zygomatic (tripod):
  Fracture of zygoma at 3 sites (zygomaticomaxillary
    suture, zygomaticofrontal suture, and zygomatic arch)
    and orbital floor
  Findings: discontinuity of orbital rim, flattening of malar
    eminence, enophthalmos, infraorbital hypesthesia,
    trismus, orbit or lid emphysema, downward
    displacement of lateral canthus

LeFort (I, II, III):
  I: low transverse fracture of maxillary bone above teeth;
    no orbital involvement
  II: pyramidal fracture of nasal, lacrimal, and maxillary
    bones; involves medial orbital floors
  III: craniofacial dysjunction; involves orbital floor, lateral
    and medial walls; may involve optic canal
  CT scan: identify and localize fracture and coexisting
    injuries

Treatment:
  Systemic steroids and antibiotics
  Surgical repair depends on type, location, and severity
    of fracture and associated findings

Intraorbital Foreign Bodies

Commonly associated with intraocular and/or optic nerve injury

Inert material can be well tolerated and may be observed

Copper and organic material are poorly tolerated and must be removed

Often asymptomatic, but may have pain or decreased vision

CT scan (MRI is contraindicated for metallic foreign bodies)

Treatment: systemic antibiotics, tetanus booster, consider surgical removal

Orbital (Retrobulbar) Hemorrhage

Compartment syndrome due to bleeding in orbit with globe and nerve compression

Ocular emergency

Findings: pain, decreased vision, subconjunctival hemorrhage, proptosis, restriction of ocular motility, increased IOP, tense orbit

Treatment: lateral canthotomy and cantholysis

Degeneration

Atrophia Bulbi

Progressive degeneration and decompensation of globe following severe injury

3 stages: atrophia bulbi without shrinkage, atrophia bulbi with shrinkage, atrophia bulbi with disorganization (phthisis bulbi)

Increased risk of intraocular malignancy

Annual B scan to rule out malignancy

Findings: cataract, retinal detachment, hypotony, corneal edema, globe shrinkage, intraocular hemorrhage, inflammation, calcification, and disorganization

Treatment: topical steroid and cycloplegic for pain; consider retrobulbar alcohol injection or enucleation for severe pain

Infections

Bacterial

Preseptal cellulitis, orbital cellulitis (see Ch. 5, Pediatrics/Strabismus)

Fungal

Most commonly *Phycomycetes*

Mucormycosis:

Most common and virulent fungal orbital disease

Non-septated, large, branching hyphae, with invasion of blood vessels, thrombosis, and necrosis

Black eschar may be visible in nose or palate

Intracranial spread is hematogenous via ophthalmic artery

Risk factors: diabetes mellitus (70%), immunosuppression (18%), renal disease (5%), leukemia (3%)

Findings: painful orbital apex syndrome, proptosis, ptosis, ophthalmoplegia, decreased vision, corneal anesthesia; may develop retinal vascular occlusions; stains with H&E

Treatment: requires immediate and emergent management

Surgical débridement, IV amphotericin B; control underlying illness

Complications: intracranial involvement, death

Aspergillosis: Septated branching hyphae

Disseminated form: occurs in immunosuppressed hosts; widespread necrotizing angiitis, thrombosis, endophthalmitis

Local form: sclerosing granulomatous infiltrative mass that originates in the sinus; proptosis, periorbital pain, visual loss

Treatment: surgical débridement, amphotericin B, flucytosine, rifampin (IV and oral)

Viral

Dengue fever:

Flavivirus

75% with ocular soreness and pain on eye movement

Parasitic

Trichinosis:

Trichinella spiralis

Larvae from ingestion of raw meat migrate to muscle and brain and become encysted

Associated with fever, myalgia, diarrhea, eosinophilia, and periorbital edema

Cysticercosis:

Taenia solium

Larvae penetrate intestinal wall, enter bloodstream, and migrate to eyes, lungs, brain, muscle, and connective tissue; becomes encysted

Inflammation

Idiopathic Orbital Inflammation (Orbital Pseudotumor)

Idiopathic inflammatory disease of orbital tissues

Findings: acute orbital pain, lid erythema and edema, lacrimal gland enlargement, restricted eye movements, proptosis, diplopia, increased IOP; may have impaired vision from optic nerve involvement

Adults: usually unilateral; bilateral cases need workup for systemic vasculitis and lymphoproliferative disorders

Children: bilateral in 33%; commonly have headache, fever, vomiting, and lethargy; may have associated papillitis or iritis; work up usually not needed (see Ch. 5, Pediatrics/Strabismus)

Pathology: enlargement of extraocular muscles and tendons; patchy infiltrate of lymphocytes, plasma cells, and eosinophils

DDx: thyroid-related ophthalmopathy, orbital cellulitis, tumor, vasculitis, trauma, AV fistula, cavernous sinus thrombosis, CN palsy

Diagnosis:

Lab tests: eosinophilia, elevated ESR, positive ANA, CSF pleocytosis

CT scan: enlargement of extraocular muscles and tendons, ring sign (contrast enhanced sclera), enlarged lacrimal gland

B-scan ultrasound: may show acoustically hollow area corresponding to edematous Tenon's capsule

Treatment: systemic NSAIDs, systemic steroids (60–120 mg oral prednisone, taper slowly over months); consider radiation if unresponsive to steroids, perform biopsy first; chemotherapy (cyclophosphamide)

Orbital myositis: localized to extraocular muscles

MR and LR most commonly involved (33% each), IR 10%

Findings: diplopia, pain, proptosis, ptosis, conjunctival injection, and chemosis

Complications: fibrosis with strabismus

Tolosa-Hunt syndrome: localized to superior orbital fissure, optic canal, and cavernous sinus

Findings: painful ophthalmoplegia, decreased vision

Sclerosing orbital pseudotumor: fibrosis of orbit and lacrimal gland

Insidious onset

More steroid resistant

Pain is less common, and eye is often white and quiet

Associated with retroperitoneal fibrosis

A-scan ultrasound: low reflectivity (seen with both orbital pseudotumor and lymphoma)

Thyroid-Related Ophthalmopathy

Autoimmune disease with spectrum of ocular manifestations

Most common cause of unilateral or bilateral proptosis in adults

Most common cause of acquired diplopia in adults

Women affected 8–10× more often than men

Patient can be hyperthyroid (90%), euthyroid (5–10%), or hypothyroid (1%); most commonly associated with Graves' disease; increased incidence in Graves' patients who smoke (7× more likely)

Associated with myasthenia gravis (in 5% of patients with Graves' disease)

Usually asymptomatic

Findings: eyelid retraction (90%), proptosis (63%), restrictive myopathy with diplopia; overaction of levator (secondary to restrictive myopathy of inferior rectus muscle); pseudoretraction (secondary to proptosis); lagophthalmos; lid lag on downgaze (von Graefe's sign); dry eye (due to corneal exposure and infiltration of lacrimal glands); conjunctival injection and chemosis; corneal exposure (from combination of eyelid retraction, proptosis, and lagophthalmos); increased IOP on upgaze; choroidal folds or disc hyperemia; compressive optic neuropathy (<5%) with decreased acuity and color vision, RAPD, and VF defect

Werner Classification of Eye Findings in Graves' Disease (**NO SPECS**):
  No signs or symptoms
  Only signs
  Soft tissue involvement (signs and symptoms)
  Proptosis
  Extraocular muscle involvement
  Corneal involvement
  Sight loss (optic nerve compression)

Pathology: enlargement of extraocular muscles; patchy infiltrates of lymphocytes, monocytes, mast cells, and fibroblasts; fibroblasts produce mucopolysaccharides, which leads to increased water content of muscles; inflammation spares tendons (Figure 6-18)

CT scan: enlargement of extraocular muscles sparing tendons; inferior rectus > medial rectus > superior rectus > lateral rectus > obliques (IMSLO)

Treatment: control underlying thyroid abnormality; ocular lubrication; consider lid taping or tarsorrhaphy; systemic steroids; radiation (effects take 2–4 weeks)
  Surgery:
    ORBITAL DECOMPRESSION: perform before strabismus surgery; 2, 3, or 4 walls; 80% will experience postoperative diplopia

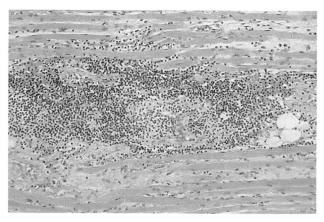

Figure 6-18. Thyroid-related ophthalmopathy demonstrating thickened extraocular muscles with inflammatory cell infiltrate and fluid. (Courtesy of Dr. RC Eagle, Jr. Reported in Hufnagel TJ, Hickey WF, Cobbs WH et al: Immunohistochemical and ultrastructural studies on the exenterated orbital tissues of a patient with Graves' disease, Ophthalmology 91:1411-9, 1984.)

    STRABISMUS SURGERY: perform before lid surgery
      INDICATIONS: diplopia, abnormal head position, large-angle strabismus
      Strabismus must be stable for at least 6 months
      Avoid if anterior inflammatory signs present
      Recession of affected muscles is mainstay of treatment, avoid resections (can exacerbate restrictions already present)
      Vertical muscle surgery can affect eyelid position (recession of inferior rectus can cause increased lid retraction due to connection of IR to lower lid retractors; recession of IR can decrease upper lid retraction in that the SR now has to work less against the tight IR [thus, the associated levator muscle is less stimulated, causing less eyelid retraction])
      Beware late slippage of inferior rectus
      Consider adjustable sutures
    LID SURGERY: eyelid retraction repair; perform after orbital decompression and strabismus surgery

Sarcoidosis

(See Ch. 8, Uveitis)

Chronic, idiopathic, multisystem, granulomatous disease primarily affecting lung, skin, eye

More common among young African Americans

Findings: bilateral panuveitis, corneal abnormalities (thickening of Descemet's membrane, calcific band keratopathy, nummular keratitis, and deep stromal vacuolation), pars planitis, chorioretinitis, optic nerve involvement, orbital apex syndrome, ptosis, conjunctival nodules, dacryoadenitis; most frequently involves lacrimal gland

Pathology: noncaseating granulomas and Langhans' giant cells

Diagnosis: chest X-ray (CXR), purified protein derivative (PPD) and controls, angiotensin-converting enzyme (ACE), serum lysozyme, gallium scan, pulmonary function tests

Treatment: systemic steroids, chemotherapy; treat ocular complications

Wegener's Granulomatosis

Systemic disease of necrotizing vasculitis and granulomatous inflammation involving sinuses, respiratory system, kidneys, and orbit

Findings: painful proptosis, reduced ocular motility, chemosis, scleritis (25%), keratitis, optic nerve edema, nasolacrimal duct obstruction

Pathology: triad of vasculitis, granulomatous inflammation, and tissue necrosis

Diagnosis: antineutrophil cytoplasmic antibodies (ANCA) (positive in 67%)

Treatment: systemic steroids, immunosuppressive therapy

Complications: fatal if untreated

Vascular Abnormalities

Varix

(See Ch. 5, Pediatrics/Strabismus)

AV Fistula

Direct or indirect communication between previously normal carotid artery and venous structures of the cavernous sinus

Direct carotid-cavernous sinus fistula: high flow; associated with head trauma, especially basal skull fracture; due to spontaneous rupture of aneurysm
> *Findings:* dilated corkscrew scleral/episcleral vessels, conjunctival injection and chemosis, elevated IOP on involved side, proptosis (may be pulsatile), orbital bruit that may be abolished by ipsilateral carotid compression, dilated tortuous retinal veins; may develop ischemic maculopathy or retinal artery occlusion, enlarged cup-to-disc ratio, ophthalmoplegia (often CN 6), anterior segment ischemia, blood in Schlemm's canal
> *CT/MRI scan:* dilated superior ophthalmic vein
> *Treatment* (for severely affected patients): embolization, surgical ligation

Dural-sinus fistula: low-flow communication between meningeal branches of carotid artery and dural walls of cavernous sinus; often asymptomatic; associated with hypertension, atherosclerosis, and connective tissue diseases; may close spontaneously; need MRI/MRA

Tumors

(Table 6-6)

Hamartomas: growth arising from tissue normally found at that site (e.g., nevus, neurofibroma, neurilemmoma,

schwannomma, glioma, hemangioma, hemangiopericytoma, lymphangioma, trichoepithelioma)

Choristomas: growth arising from tissue not normally found at that site (e.g., dermoid cyst, dermatolipoma, ectopic lacrimal gland)

Cystic Tumors

(See Ch. 5, Pediatrics/Strabismus)

Vascular Tumors

Lymphangioma

(See Ch. 5, Pediatrics/Strabismus)

Capillary Hemangioma

(See Ch. 5, Pediatrics/Strabismus)

Cavernous Hemangioma

Most common benign orbital tumor in adults (usually middle-aged women)

Findings: slowly progressive proptosis; may induce hyperopia, may also have retinal striae, IOP elevation, strabismus, or optic nerve compression

Growth may accelerate during pregnancy

Pathology: encapsulated lesion composed of blood-filled cavernous spaces, lined by endothelial cells (Figure 6-19)

CT scan: well-demarcated, encapsulated, intraconal mass

MRI: hypointense to fat on T1-weighted images, hyperintense to fat and equivalent to vitreous on T2-weighted images

A-scan ultrasound: high internal reflectivity

Treatment: observation, surgical excision

Hemangiopericytoma

Rare tumor of abnormal pericytes surrounding blood vessels
Occurs in middle-aged adults
More common in women

Table 6-6. Common orbital tumors	
In Children (see Chapter 5, Pediatrics/Strabismus)	**In Adults**
90% are benign; 10% are malignant	Mucocele
Rhabdomyosarcoma (most common primary orbital malignancy)	Cavernous hemangioma
Capillary hemangioma (most common benign orbital tumor)	Meningioma
Lymphangioma	Fibrous histiocytoma
Neuroblastoma (most common metastatic orbital tumor)	Neurilemmoma
Dermoid (most common orbital mass)	Pleomorphic adenoma (BMT)
Teratoma	Lymphoid tumors
ON glioma	Metastatic tumors
Granulocytic sarcoma ('chloroma')	
Burkitt's lymphoma	
Histiocytic tumors	

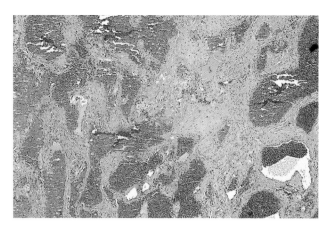

Figure 6-19. Cavernous hemangioma demonstrating large, blood-filled spaces and fibrous septa. (Case presented by Dr. WC Frayer to the meeting of the Verhoeff Society, 1989. From Yanoff M, Fine BS: Ocular Pathology, 5th edn, St Louis, Mosby, 2002.)

Often located in superior orbit

Can metastasize to lung, bone, liver

Findings: slowly progressive proptosis, pain, decreased vision, diplopia

CT scan: well-circumscribed, encapsulated mass

A-scan ultrasound: low to medium internal reflectivity

Treatment: complete surgical excision because it may metastasize

Neural Tumors

Optic Nerve Glioma

(See Ch. 5, Pediatrics/Strabismus)

Neurofibroma

(See Ch. 5, Pediatrics/Strabismus)

Neurilemmoma (Schwannoma)

Encapsulated tumor consisting of benign proliferation of Schwann cells

No malignant potential

Occurs in middle-aged individuals

Lesion can be painful due to perineural spread and compression of nerve

Usually located in the superior orbit causing gradual proptosis and globe dystopia

Schwannomas can grow along any peripheral or cranial nerve, most commonly CN 8 (acoustic neuroma)

Rarely associated with neurofibromatosis

Pathology: stains with S-100
  Antoni A: spindle cells arranged in interlacing cords, whorls, or palisades; contains Verocay bodies (collections of cells resembling sensory corpuscles) (Figure 6-20)
  Antoni B: loose, myxoid; stellate cells with a mucoid stroma (Figure 6-21)

CT scan: well-circumscribed, fusiform mass

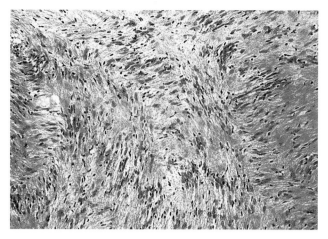

Figure 6-20. Antoni A pattern demonstrating palisading spindle cells with Verocray bodies (areas that appear acellular). (From Yanoff M, Fine BS: Ocular Pathology, 5th edn, St Louis, Mosby, 2002.)

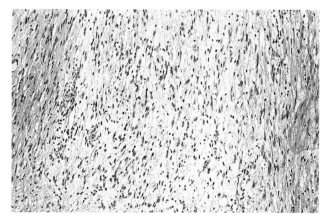

Figure 6-21. Antoni B pattern demonstrating necrosis with inflammatory cells. (From Yanoff M, Fine BS: Ocular Pathology, 5th edn, St Louis, Mosby, 2002.)

Treatment: complete surgical excision; can recur after complete surgical removal

Meningioma

Optic nerve sheath meningioma:
  More common in women
  Accounts for 33% of all primary optic nerve tumors
  Increased incidence in neurofibromatosis
  Arises from arachnoid cells in the meninges
  Findings: decreased visual acuity and color vision, visual field loss, proptosis, disc edema or pallor, optociliary shunt vessels
  Spencer's triad: optociliary shunts, optic atrophy, optic nerve meningioma
  Pathology: sheets of cells or whorls; psammoma bodies (calcified) in the center of whorls
  CT scan: tubular enlargement of optic nerve that enhances with gadolinium; optic foramen enlargement
  Treatment: observation, surgical excision to prevent involvement of optic nerve or chiasm

Sphenoid wing meningioma:
  Most common tumor to spread to orbit from intracranial space

Findings: temporal fullness, proptosis, lid edema
CT scan: hyperostosis and calcifications
Treatment: observation, surgical excision

Rhabdomyosarcoma

(See Ch. 5, Pediatrics/Strabismus.)

Lymphoid Tumors

Spectrum of disorders characterized by abnormal proliferation of lymphoid tissue

20% of all orbital tumors; 90% are non-Hodgkins B-cell lymphoma

Usually occur in adults 50–70 years old; rare in children

Conjunctival or lacrimal gland lesions

Cause painless proptosis

Tissue biopsy with immunohistochemical studies required for diagnosis

All lymphoid lesions of orbit must have a workup for systemic lymphoma, including CBC with differential, serum protein electrophoresis (SPEP), physical examination for lymphadenopathy, CT of thoracic and abdominal viscera, and bone scan

Perform every 6 months for 2 years

Bone marrow biopsy (better than bone marrow aspirate)

Monoclonal proliferations do not all progress to systemic disease; some polyclonal proliferations do progress

Benign Reactive Lymphoid Hyperplasia

Findings: bilateral painless lacrimal gland enlargement, limitation of ocular motility, visual disturbances

Pathology: mature lymphocytes with reactive germinal centers; T cells, 60–80% with scattered polyclonal B cells; high degree of endothelial cell proliferation

Atypical Lymphoid Hyperplasia

Low-grade lymphoma, no mitotic activity

Pathology: follicles and polymorphous response consistent with benign process

40% develop systemic disease within 5 years

Orbital Lymphoma

Orbital lymphoma occurs primarily in adults and usually involves superior orbit (only Burkitt's occurs in children); increased risk of systemic disease

Findings: limitation of ocular motility, painless lacrimal gland swelling, conjunctival salmon patches, visual changes; 17% bilateral

Pathology: atypical immature lymphocytes with mitoses; diffuse or follicular growth; monoclonal B-cell proliferations 60–90% with scattered or reactive T cells; involves reticuloendothelial system, including retroperitoneal lymph nodes (Figure 6-22)

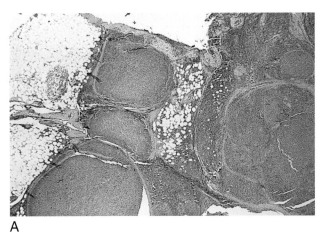

A

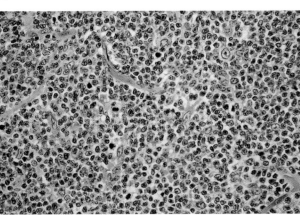

B

Figure 6-22. **A,** Nodular lymphoid infiltrate. **B,** Higher magnification shows uniform lymphocyte infiltrate with mitotic figures. (From Yanoff M, Scheie HG: Malignant lymphoma of the orbit – difficulties in diagnosis, Surv Ophthalmol 12:133-140, 1967.)

CT scan: putty-like molding of tumor; orbital tissues not displaced

Treatment: radiotherapy for localized orbital disease, chemotherapy for systemic involvement

Prognosis: location appears more important than histopathology for determining systemic involvement: lymphoma of eyelids (67% have systemic involvement) > orbit (35%) > conjunctiva (20%)

Malignant lymphoma: 60% risk of systemic lymphoma

Plasmacytoma

Tumor composed of plasma cells

Pathology: plasmacytoid lymphocytes, immunoblasts, mature plasma cells

DDx: Waldenström's macroglobulinemia, multiple myeloma, lymphoma with immunoglobulin production

Granulocytic Sarcoma ('Chloroma')

(See Ch. 5, Pediatrics/Strabismus)

Burkitt's Lymphoma

(See Ch. 5, Pediatrics/Strabismus)

Systemic Lymphoma and Waldenström's Macroglobulinemia

Solid infiltrating tumor with putty-like molding of tumor to pre-existing structures

Pathology: Dutcher bodies (intranuclear PAS-positive inclusions of immunoglobulin)

Fibro-osseous Tumors

Fibrous Dysplasia

(see Chapter 5, Pediatrics/Strabismus)

Ossifying Fibroma

Variant of fibrous dysplasia

Occurs in second and third decades of life

More common in women

Well-circumscribed, slow-growing, monostotic lesion

Pathology: vascular stroma containing lamellar bone with a rim of osteoid and osteoblasts

Osteoma

Dense bony lesions originating in the frontal and ethmoid sinus

Well-circumscribed, slow-growing mass

Symptoms secondary to sinus obstruction and intracranial or intraorbital extension

Pathology: lamellar bone with variable amounts of fibrous stroma

Fibrous Histiocytoma

Firm orbital mass composed of fibroblasts and histiocytes

Usually benign (malignant in 10%)

Distinguished from hemangiopericytoma only on biopsy

Most common mesenchymal orbital lesion of adults

Pathology: storiform (cartwheel or spiral), nebular pattern of tumor cells (fibroblasts); both fibrous histiocytoma and hemangiopericytoma are spindle cell tumors, and they can be difficult to differentiate (Figure 6-23)

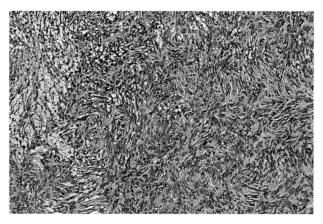

Figure 6-23. Histiocytes *(on left)* and fibrous *(on right,* with storiform [matted] appearance) components. (From Jones WD 3rd, Yanoff M, Katowitz JA: Recurrent facial fibrous histiocytoma, Br J Plast Surg 32:46-51, 1979.)

CT scan: well-circumscribed mass anywhere in the orbit (upper nasal most common)

Treatment: surgical excision; moderate risk of recurrence

Histiocytosis X

(Langerhans' cell histiocytosis) (see Ch. 5, Pediatrics/Strabismus)

Juvenile Xanthogranuloma

(JXG; nevoxanthoendothelioma) (see Ch. 5, Pediatrics/Strabismus)

Epithelial Lacrimal Gland Tumors

50% of lacrimal gland lesions are inflammatory and lymphoproliferative; contour around the globe

50% of lacrimal gland tumors are of epithelial origin

50% of epithelial tumors are benign pleomorphic adenomas

50% of malignant tumors are adenoid cystic carcinomas

Pleomorphic Adenoma (Benign Mixed Tumor)

Most common epithelial tumor of the lacrimal gland

Occurs in 4th–5th decade of life

More common in men

Slow onset (6–12 months)

Firm mass in lacrimal fossa with painless proptosis; globe often displaced medially and downward

Progressive expansile growth may indent bone of lacrimal fossa

Tumor growth stimulates periosteum to deposit a thin layer of new bone (cortication)

Pathology: proliferation of epithelial cells into a double layer, forming lumina with ductal and secretory elements; ductal inner cells secrete mucus; outer stromal cells give rise to fibrous stroma and osteoid and cartilaginous metaplasia, pseudoencapsulated with surface bosselations (Figure 6-24)

CT scan: well-circumscribed but may have nodular configuration

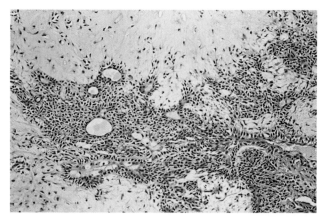

Figure 6-24. BMT demonstrating ductal structures in a myxoid stroma. (From Yanoff M, Fine BS: Ocular Pathology, 5th edn, St Louis, Mosby, 2002.)

Treatment: complete en bloc excision without biopsy; incomplete excision may result in recurrence and malignant transformation into pleomorphic adenocarcinoma

Pleomorphic Adenocarcinoma (Malignant Mixed Tumor)

Long history of mass in lacrimal fossa

Occurs in elderly individuals

Findings: rapid, progressive, painful proptosis

Pathology: similar to benign mixed tumor but with foci of malignant change

Treatment: radical orbitectomy and bone removal

Adenoid Cystic Carcinoma

Most common malignant tumor of the lacrimal gland

Highly malignant

Presents in 4th decade of life

Rapidly progressive proptosis, pain and paresthesia due to perineural invasion and bony destruction

Pathology: small, benign-appearing cells arranged in nests, tubules, or in a 'Swiss-cheese' (cribriform) pattern (Figure 6-25)

CT scan: poorly circumscribed mass, bony destruction, calcifications

Treatment: removal of any bone that is involved, exenteration, adjunctive radiation and chemotherapy

Prognosis: poor; survival rate of 20–70%

Sinus Tumors

Sinus Mucocele

Cystic, slowly expanding sinus lesion

Entrapment of mucus in aerated space due to obstruction of sinus ostia

Exerts pressure on surrounding bony structures

May become infected (mucopyocele)

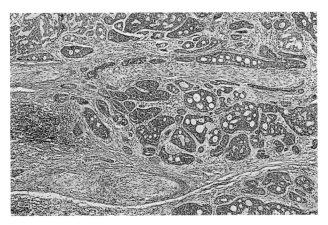

Figure 6-25. Adenoid cystic carcinoma demonstrating characteristic 'Swiss-cheese' appearance. (From Yanoff M, Fine BS: Ocular Pathology, 5th edn, St Louis, Mosby, 2002.)

Causes of ostial obstruction: inflammation with scarring, congenital narrowing of ostia, trauma, osteomas, polyps, septal deviation, mucus retention cysts

Associated with cystic fibrosis

Must rule out encephalocele and meningocele
  Findings:
  Frontoethmoid sinus (most common location): outward and downward displacement of globe, fullness in superonasal and medial canthal regions, above the medial canthal tendon
  Sphenoid and posterior ethmoid sinus: visual symptoms, retrobulbar pain; may have cranial nerve palsies; 50% have nasal symptoms
  Maxillary sinus (rare): upward displacement of globe, erosion of orbital floor may cause enophthalmos

CT scan: homogeneous opacified cyst with bowing of sinus wall and attenuation/erosion of bone

MRI: highly variable signal intensities

Treatment: surgical excision with IV antibiotics; reestablish normal drainage; obliteration of sinus (only if frontal)

Sinus Carcinoma

Usually squamous cell

Most commonly from maxillary sinus

No early signs except for sinusitis

Late findings: nonaxial proptosis, epiphora, epistaxis, infraorbital anesthesia

Metastatic Tumors

In contrast to adults, pediatric tumors metastasize to the orbit more frequently than to the uvea

Orbital metastases produce rapid painful proptosis with restricted ocular motility

Neuroblastoma

(See Ch. 5, Pediatrics/Strabismus)

Leukemia

(See Ch. 5, Pediatrics/Strabismus)

Ewing's Sarcoma

(See Ch. 5, Pediatrics/Strabismus)

Breast Carcinoma

Most common primary source of orbital metastasis in women

May occur many years after primary diagnosis

May elicit a fibrous response and cause enophthalmos and ophthalmoplegia

May respond to hormonal manipulation

Lung Carcinoma

Most common primary source of orbital metastasis in men

Very aggressive

Prostate Carcinoma

May present similarly to acute pseudotumor

Less aggressive than lung carcinoma

EYELID DISORDERS

Congenital Anomalies

(See Ch. 5, Pediatrics/Strabismus)

Trauma

Lid Laceration

Partial- or full-thickness cut in eyelid that may involve the lid margin, canthus, or canaliculus

Treatment: antibiotics, tetanus booster; surgical repair; technique depends on severity and location of injury

Lid Avulsion

Complete or partial tearing of eyelid with or without tissue loss

Treatment: technique of repair depends on severity and location of injury
  Small defect (<25%): direct closure
  Moderate defect (25–50%): Tenzel's flap
  Large defect (>50%): bridge flap reconstruction (Cutler-Beard [for upper lid] or Hughes' [for lower lid] procedure with flap advancement)

Inflammation

Hordeolum

Obstruction and infection of Zeiss (external hordeolum, stye) or meibomian (internal hordeolum, chalazion) glands

Painful erythematous eyelid swelling

Accumulation of secretions causes acute inflammatory response

Lipogranuloma formation (chalazion) often evolves from internal hordeolum

Pathology: epithelioid and giant cells surrounding empty lipid vacuoles, zonal granulomatous inflammation (zonal lipogranuloma) (Figure 6-26)

Treatment: warm compresses, topical antibiotic ointment, lid scrubs (for associated blepharitis); if no response, consider local steroid injection, or incision and curettage

Blepharitis

Inflammation of lid margin

Anterior lid margin disease: seborrheic or staph blepharitis

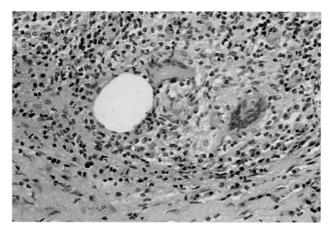

Figure 6-26. Chalazion demonstrating epithelioid and giant cells surrounding clear areas that contained lipid. (From Yanoff M, Fine BS: Ocular Pathology, 5th edn, St Louis, Mosby, 2002.)

Posterior lid margin disease: meibomitis

Angular blepharitis: associated with *Moraxella*

Symptoms: burning, itching, redness, tearing

Findings: lid thickening, crusting, scurf, collarettes, inspissated meibomian glands, foamy tears, lash loss, redness

Associated with dry eye, acne rosacea, and chalazia

Treatment: lid scrubs, topical antibiotic ointment, lubrication (for associated dry eye), oral supplements (omega-3 fatty acids); consider oral tetracycline/doxycycline, topical azithromycin, topical steroid

Acne Rosacea

Idiopathic, chronic skin disorder affecting sebaceous glands of face (including meibomian glands)

Type IV hypersensitivity may play a role

Common between ages 40 and 60 years

Ocular involvement in >50%

Findings: chronic blepharitis, meibomitis, lid margin telangiectasia, conjunctival injection, abnormal tear film (foam, mucin particles, excess oil), decreased tear breakup time, meibomian gland plugging, recurrent chalazions; may develop keratitis with peripheral corneal infiltrates, vascularization, scarring, thinning, ulceration, and rarely perforation

Other findings: acne-like skin changes, telangiectatic vessels, papules, and rhinophyma

Pathology: granulomatous inflammation

Treatment: warm compresses and lid scrubs, oral doxycycline or erythromycin, oral flaxseed oil and omega-3 fatty acids, topical azithromycin, lubrication (for associated dry eye); topical metronidazole to facial skin; consider topical steroid

Contact Dermatitis

Inflammation of lid skin due to exogenous irritant or allergic hypersensitivity reaction

Symptoms: red, swollen, itchy periorbital skin

Findings: erythematous, scaling lesions; may have vesicles or weeping areas

Treatment: eliminate inciting agent; use mild steroid cream or tropical tacrolimus 0.1% (Protopic)

Infections

Molluscum Contagiosum

Shiny, white-yellow papule with central umbilication Infection by poxvirus

Spread by direct contact; consider HIV in healthy adult

Usually asymptomatic

Can cause follicular conjunctivitis and punctate keratitis

Pathology: lobular acanthosis, large basophilic poxviral intracytoplasmic inclusions composed of nucleic acids from DNA virus (Figure 6-27)

Treatment: surgical excision, cryo, incision and curettage

Phthiriasis Palpebrum/Pediculosis

Lice infection of lashes

Spread by direct contact, usually sexually transmitted

Produces blepharoconjunctivitis

Findings: follicles, injection, small white eggs (nits) and lice attached to lashes

Treatment: remove nits and lice, topical ointment to suffocate lice, delousing creams and shampoo

Verruca Vulgaris (Papilloma)

Pink, pedunculated or sessile mass

Associated with papillomavirus (HPV)

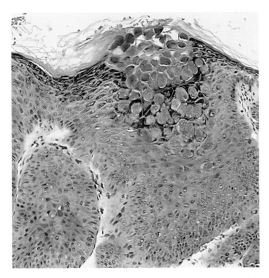

Figure 6-27. Intracytoplasmic, eosinophilic molluscum bodies in epidermis; they become larger and more basophilic near the surface. (Courtesy of Dr. WC Frayer. From Skin and lacrimal drainage system. In Yanoff M, Fine BS: Ocular Pathology, 5th edn, St Louis, Mosby, 2002.)

Usually asymptomatic

Often multiple and resolve spontaneously

Herpes Infection

Herpes simplex virus (HSV):

Primary infection causes vesicular dermatitis

May be associated with follicular conjunctivitis and keratitis

Treatment: antibiotic ointment to skin lesions, topical antiviral if eye involved

Varicella zoster virus (VZV):

Vesicular dermatitis with ulceration, crusting, and scarring

Reactivation of latent infection along distribution of trigeminal nerve (most often 5_1)

Dermatomal distribution, does not cross midline

May have constitutional symptoms and ocular involvement

Treatment: antibiotic ointment to skin lesions, (see Ch. 7, Cornea/External Disease for ocular involvement)

Leprosy

Organism is acid-fast bacillus *Mycobacterium leprae*

Tuberculoid and lepromatous leprosy can affect lids

Findings: loss of lashes, trichiasis, ectropion, and exposure keratitis

Treatment: systemic antibiotics (dapsone, rifampin)

Malposition and Other Disorders

Blepharospasm

Bilateral, intermittent, involuntary contractions of orbicularis and facial muscles causing uncontrolled blinking; may cause functional blindness

Etiology unknown but may be due to abnormality of basal ganglia

Usually occurs in 5th–7th decade of life; female > male (3:1); associated with Parkinson's disease

Absent during sleep

Meige's syndrome: essential blepharospasm with facial grimacing

DDx: secondary blepharospasm (due to ocular irritation), hemifacial spasm (usually unilateral, due to compression of CN 7, can be caused by cerebellopontine angle [CPA] tumor, present during sleep), myokymia, Tourette's syndrome, trigeminal neuralgia, basal ganglia disease, tardive dyskinesia

Consider CT/MRI scan to rule out posterior fossa lesion

Treatment: Botox (botulinum toxin type A) injections, surgery (excision of lid protractors or differential section of CN 7), medications (tetrabenazine, lithium, carbidopa, clonazepam)

Botox: derived from *Clostridium botulinum,* freeze-dried solution; subcutaneous injection, no more than 200 units/month

> **MECHANISM:** blocks neuromuscular conduction by binding to receptors on nerve terminals and stops release of ACh by disrupting calcium metabolism; does not cross blood–brain barrier
>
> **INDICATIONS:** blepharospasm (effective in 90%, lasts 3 months), hemifacial spasm (lasts 4 months), strabismus (lasts 1–8 weeks)
>
> **ADVERSE EFFECTS** (no systemic toxicity): exposure keratopathy, ptosis, diplopia, flaccid lower lid ectropion

Blepharochalasis

Idiopathic inflammatory edema of the eyelids

Familial, most often in young women

Recurrent attacks of transient, painless eyelid edema resulting in atrophy, wrinkling, and redundancy of eyelid skin

May develop ptosis and herniation of orbital lacrimal gland

Dermatochalasis

Redundancy of eyelid skin with orbital fat prolapse due to involutional changes

Blepharoptosis (Acquired)

Eyelid malposition characterized by drooping upper eyelid

Myogenic: uncommon; due to local or systemic muscular disease (e.g., myotonic dystrophy, chronic progressive external ophthalmoplegia, myasthenia gravis)

> Treat underlying condition; usually requires frontalis sling

Involutional (aponeurotic): most common form of ptosis; disinsertion of levator aponeurosis due to aging or chronic inflammation; may be exacerbated by eye surgery or trauma

> High eyelid crease with good levator function; ptotic lid in all positions of gaze (no lid lag on downgaze as in congenital cases); may have thinning of eyelid above tarsal plate

Neurogenic: due to CN 3 palsy, aberrant regeneration of CN 3 (Marcus Gunn jaw-winking ptosis), Horner's syndrome, multiple sclerosis, ophthalmoplegic migraine

> *Treatment for Horner's:* shorten Müller's muscle (Putterman [conjunctival-Müller's muscle resection]) or Fasanella-Servat [tarsoconjunctival resection] procedure)

Mechanical: due to mass effect of orbital or eyelid tumors, dermatochalasis, blepharochalasis, cicatrix

Traumatic: due to trauma to levator aponeurosis; may have lagophthalmos from cicatricial changes

> May improve spontaneously, therefore observe for 6 months

Examination:

> *Palpebral fissure height* (PF): normally 10–11 mm in primary gaze

Marginal reflex distance (MRD): distance between corneal light reflex and upper lid margin in primary gaze; normally 4 mm

Levator function (LF): distance of upper lid excursion while frontalis is immobilized; normal >12 mm, fair if 6–11 mm, poor if <5 mm

2.5% phenylephrine test: activates sympathetic fibers of Müller's muscle; resulting lid elevation simulates position after Müller's muscle resection

DDx: pseudoptosis (nanophthalmos, microphthalmos, phthisis bulbi, hypotropia, dermatochalasis, enophthalmos, contralateral eyelid retraction or proptosis)

Treatment: eyelid crutches, levator aponeurosis advancement, levator muscle resection, Müller's muscle resection, frontalis suspension with autogenous fascia lata, banked fascia lata, or synthetic materials

Surgical complications: overcorrection or under-correction, lid lag, lagophthalmos, exposure keratopathy

Eyelid Retraction

Upper eyelid at or above superior limbus

Lower eyelid exposing sclera

DDx: thyroid-related ophthalmopathy (most common, lateral upper eyelid more retracted than medial eyelid, fibrous contraction of eyelid retractors), orbital pseudotumor (idiopathic orbital inflammation [IOI]), pharmacologic (phenylephrine, α-agonists, cocaine), resection of superior rectus, overcorrection of ptosis, contralateral ptosis (Hering's law)

Treatment: lubrication; surgical repair (levator aponeurosis recession, levator myotomy, spacer insertion, full-thickness skin graft for lower eyelid, hard palate grafts for lower eyelid)

Ectropion

Eversion of eyelid margin; may cause keratinization and hypertrophy of conjunctiva

Symptoms: tearing, foreign body sensation, redness

Involutional: most common cause of ectropion; often in lower eyelid

> *Etiology:* horizontal laxity, disinsertion of lower eyelid retractors
>
> *Diagnosis:* snap-back test
>
> *Treatment:* horizontal eyelid shortening, lateral canthoplasty, repair of lower eyelid retractors

Paralytic: occurs after CN 7 palsy

> Frequent complaints of tearing from chronic reflex secretion
>
> *Treatment:* lubrication, taping of temporal lower eyelid, moisture chamber goggles, lateral tarsorrhaphy, horizontal tightening procedure, hard palate mucosal

graft for lower eyelid elevation, gold weight implantation to aid in closure of upper eyelid

Cicatricial: shortening of anterior lamella
Etiology: burns, trauma, tumor, infection, chronic inflammation causing secondary anterior lamellar contraction (acne rosacea, atopic dermatitis, eczema, herpes zoster dermatitis, scleroderma, epidermolysis bullosa, porphyria, xeroderma pigmentosum)
Treatment: revision and relaxation of cicatrix, horizontal tightening procedure, may require vertical lengthening with full-thickness graft

Mechanical:
Etiology: tumors of eyelid, herniated orbital fat, poorly fitted spectacles, chronic edema
Treat underlying condition

Entropion

Inversion of eyelid margin

Lower eyelid entropion usually involutional

Upper eyelid entropion usually cicatricial

Symptoms: tearing, foreign body sensation, redness

Congenital: very rare; due to epiblepharon or tarsal kink (see Ch. 5, Pediatrics / Strabismus)
Usually does not require treatment

Spastic: associated with ocular inflammation, trauma, and prolonged patching
Squeezing of eyelids causes inward rolling of eyelid margin; ocular surface irritation perpetuates cycle
Treatment: taping of eyelid, cautery, Botox injection, Quickert suture

Involutional:
Etiology: canthal tendon laxity (horizontal lid laxity, diagnose with snap-back test), eyelid retractor dehiscence (vertical lid laxity), overriding preseptal orbicularis muscle, involutional enophthalmos
Treatment: Quickert suture, horizontal lid-shortening procedure (Bick, lateral tarsal strip, marginal wedge resection), vertical lid-shortening procedure (Jones, Hotz, Wies marginal rotation), retractor advancement, excision of preseptal orbicularis

Cicatricial: shortening of posterior lamella
Etiology: ocular cicatricial pemphigoid, Stevens-Johnson syndrome, trachoma, herpes zoster dermatitis, surgery, trauma, chemical burns, miotics
Digital pressure on inferior border of tarsus corrects eyelid position in involutional entropion but not cicatricial entropion
Treatment: lubrication, avoid surgery during acute phase of autoimmune disease, remove lashes in contact with cornea, use tarsal fracture operation, apply tarsoconjunctival grafts or hard palate mucosal grafts to replace scarred tarsus; may require symblepharon ring and amniotic membrane graft to prevent recurrent scarring

Trichiasis

Misdirection of eyelashes and contact with ocular surface

May be associated with posterior lamellar scarring

Associated with distichiasis, entropion, OCP, Stevens-Johnson syndrome, chronic blepharitis, chemical burns

Symptoms: tearing, foreign body sensation, redness

Treatment: lubrication, epilation, electrolysis, cryodestruction with double-freeze/thaw technique, argon laser, full-thickness wedge resection

Floppy Eyelid Syndrome

Easily everted upper eyelids

Chronic papillary conjunctivitis due to lid autoeversion during sleep with resultant mechanical irritation from bed sheets

Associated with obesity, keratoconus, eyelid rubbing, and sleep apnea

Treatment: lubrication, tape/patch/shield lids during sleep; consider horizontal eyelid tightening

Madarosis

Loss of eyelashes and/or eyebrows due to local or systemic disorders

DDx: eyelid neoplasms, chronic blepharitis, trauma, burns, trichotillomania, alopecia, seborrheic dermatitis, chemotherapy agents, malnutrition, lupus, leprosy

Poliosis / Vitiligo

Premature whitening of the eyelashes / eyebrows (poliosis) or skin (vitiligo) due to local systemic disorders

Associated with Vogt-Koyanagi-Harada syndrome, sympathetic ophthalmia, Waardenburg syndrome, tuberous sclerosis, radiation, and dermatitis

Eyelid Tumors

Benign Epithelial Tumors
Squamous Papilloma

Keratinized epidermal fronds with fibrovascular cores

Most common benign lesion of eyelid

Associated with papovavirus (HPV) infection

May be sessile or pedunculated

Pathology: papillary configuration, proliferating fibrovascular tissue covered by hyperplastic prickle cell layer of the epidermis, hyperkeratosis and parakeratosis may be present, vacuolated cells containing virus particles may be seen in the upper squamous layer (Figure 6-28)

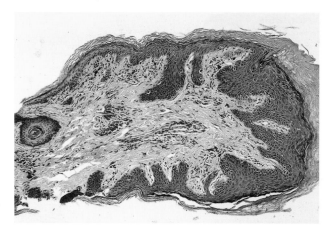

Figure 6-28. Squamous papilloma demonstrating acanthosis and hyperkeratosis. (From Yanoff M, Fine BS: Ocular Pathology, 5th edn, St Louis, Mosby, 2002.)

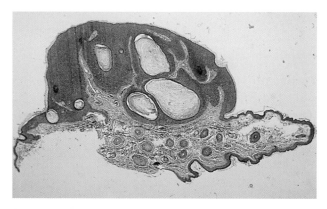

Figure 6-29. Seborrheic keratosis appears as blue lesion above skin surface with blue basaloid cells and keratin cysts. (From Yanoff M, Fine BS: Ocular Pathology, 5th edn, St Louis, Mosby, 2002.)

Treatment: surgical excision, cryo or laser ablation

Seborrheic Keratosis

Papillomatous proliferation of suprabasalar (prickle) cells

Pigmented keratin crust with greasy 'stuck-on' appearance

Occurs in elderly

Pathology: acanthosis, hyperkeratosis, parakeratosis, and squamous eddies may be present (Figure 6-29)

Inverted Follicular Keratosis

Nodular or verrucous lesion

Looks like a cutaneous horn

Inflamed seborrheic keratosis

Pathology: acanthosis, squamous and basal cell proliferation

Cysts

Epithelial lined chambers filled with debris

Epidermal Inclusion Cyst (Epidermoid Cyst)

Single-lumen, round or oval lesion lined by keratinized, stratified squamous epithelium (epidermis) and filled with cheesy keratin debris

Occurs after a fragment of epidermis is carried into the subepithelium by trauma

Trapped but viable epithelium proliferates and produces keratin

Rupture can cause a foreign body granulomatous reaction

Dermoid Cyst

Lined by keratinized squamous epithelium and dermal appendages such as hair shafts and sebaceous glands

Contains keratin, cilia, and sebum

Often congenital; most common orbital tumor in children

Can be found in eyelid or orbit

Hydrocystoma (Sudiforous Cyst)

Multilocular, branching lumen that appears empty or contains serous fluid
Lined by a double row of cuboidal epithelium (resembling sweat duct)

Most are eccrine hydrocystomas (can be apocrine if arising from the glands of Moll)

Occur most commonly at eyelid margin or lateral canthus

Sebaceous Gland Tumors

Congenital Sebaceous Gland Hyperplasia

Proliferation of normal sebaceous glands

20% degenerate into basal cell carcinoma

Acquired Sebaceous Gland Hyperplasia

Multiple well-circumscribed yellow nodules

Lobules of mature sebaceous glands around a dilated duct

Muir-Torre syndrome

multiple sebaceous neoplasms, keratoacanthomas, and visceral tumors (especially GI)

Sweat Gland Tumors

Syringoma

Waxy, yellow nodules on lower lid

Usually occur in young women

Benign proliferation of eccrine ductal structures

Hydrocystoma

Translucent, bluish cyst

Arises from eccrine or apocrine glands

Tumors of Hair Follicle Origin

Trichoepithelioma

Firm, skin-colored nodule

More common in women

Usually occurs on forehead, eyelids, nasolabial fold, and upper lip

Pathology: basaloid cells surrounding a keratin center

Multiple lesions: Brooke's tumor (AD)

Trichofolliculoma

A keratin-filled dilated cystic hair follicle, surrounded by immature hair follicles

Appears as a small umbilicated nodule usually with central white hairs

Tricholemmoma

Small crusty lesion with rough ulcerated surface

Usually occurs on face

Arises from glycogen-rich clear cells of the outer hair sheath

May resemble basal, squamous, or sebaceous cell carcinoma

Cowden's disease (AD): multiple facial tricholemmomas; marker for breast (40%) or thyroid cancer

Pilomatrixoma ('Calcifying Epithelioma of Malherbe')

Solitary, firm, deep nodule with overlying normal, pink, or bluish skin

Freely movable subcutaneous pink-purple nodule

Most common cystic lesion of childhood

In young adult, arises from hair matrix of upper lid or brow

Occurs on the eyelid, face, neck, or arms

Can range from 5 to 30 mm in diameter

May resemble an epidermal cyst

Associated with myotonic dystrophy and Gardner's syndrome

Precancerous Lesions

Actinic Keratosis

Most common precancerous lesion

Related to sun exposure

Occurs in middle-aged individuals

Scaly, white, flat-topped lesion with surrounding erythema

Common on face, eyelid, and scalp

May be single or multiple

12% evolve into squamous cell carcinoma (less aggressive than if it arises de novo); 25% spontaneously resolve

May also evolve into basal cell carcinoma

Pathology: elastotic degeneration in the dermis, overlying hyperkeratosis, focal parakeratosis, clefts in dyskeratotic areas (Figure 6-30)

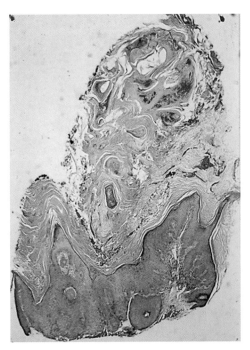

Figure 6-30. Actinic keratosis appears as pink papillomatous lesion with marked hyperkeratosis and acanthosis about skin surface. (From Yanoff M, Fine BS: Ocular Pathology, 5th edn, St Louis, Mosby, 2002.)

Treatment: surgical excision, cryo or freezing with liquid nitrogen

Nevus

Congenital or acquired hamartoma

Can be flat, but is usually elevated and pigmented

Arises from neural crest cells

Pigmentation and size tend to increase during puberty

With time, nevi tend to move deeper, migrating into the dermis

Contains benign-appearing dermal melanocytes

Malignant transformation is rare

Classified by location

Junctional nevus: occurs at epidermal/dermal junction; flat
  Greatest malignant potential

Compound nevus: both intradermal and junctional components (Figure 6-31); slightly elevated or papillomatous, often pigmented
  Junctional component gives malignant potential

Intradermal nevus: most common, most benign; can be papillomatous, dome-shaped, or pedunculated
  Slightly pigmented or amelanotic; hair shafts indicate intradermal variety

Kissing nevus: congenital; involves both upper and lower lids, secondary to fusion of lids during embryonic development

Spindle cell nevus: compound nevus of childhood; bizarre cellular components

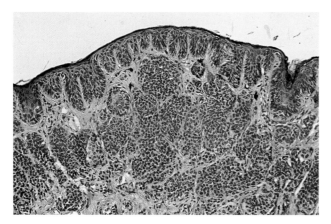

Figure 6-31. Compound nevus with cells at junction and in dermis. (From Yanoff M, Fine BS: Ocular Pathology, 5th edn, St Louis, Mosby, 2002.)

No malignant potential

Giant hairy nevus of the face and scalp: congenital; thickened eyelids can cause amblyopia

Nevus of Ota (Oculodermal Melanocytosis)

(See Ch. 5, Pediatrics/Strabismus.)

Lentigo Maligna (Melanotic Freckle of Hutchinson)

Acquired cutaneous pigmentation

Often periocular

Occurs in middle-aged or older individuals

Conjunctival pigmentation may be noted

No episcleral pigmentation

Melanoma arises in approximately 30%

Cutaneous counterpart of primary acquired melanosis (PAM) of the conjunctiva

Xeroderma Pigmentosa (AR)

Defect in DNA repair (UV light endonuclease)

Freckles and scaling at early age

Susceptible to a variety of malignant tumors (basal cell carcinoma, squamous cell carcinoma, malignant melanoma, sarcoma)

3% incidence of skin malignant melanoma

Malignant Epithelial Tumors

Risk factors: increased age, sun exposure, fair skin, previous history of skin cancer, positive family history

Characteristics: irregularity, induration, and altered lid anatomy

Basal Cell Carcinoma (BCC)

Most common malignancy of the eyelid (90%)

40 times more common than squamous cell carcinoma

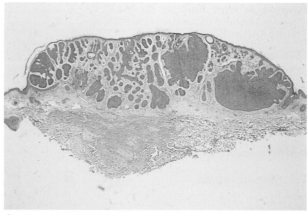

A

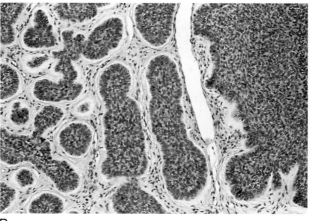

B

Figure 6-32. A, BCC appears as blue nests of basal cells proliferating over pale pink desmoplasia (dermal fibroblast proliferation). **B,** Basal cell nests with peripheral palisading and mitotic figures. (Courtesy of HG Scheie. From Yanoff M, Fine BS: Ocular Pathology, 5th edn, St Louis, Mosby, 2002.)

Develops on sun-exposed skin in elderly patients; smoking is also a risk

Location (in order of frequency): lower lid (50–60%), medial canthus (20–30%), upper lid (15%), outer canthus (5%)

Poorest prognosis when found in medial canthus because tumor often extends deeper and can involve lacrimal drainage system

Morbidity and mortality occur from local invasion of skull and CNS

Rarely metastasizes

Pathology: blue basaloid tumor cells arranged in nests and cords (H&E stain), peripheral palisading commonly seen (Figure 6-32)

Nodular basal cell carcinoma: most common form; firm, raised, pearly, discrete mass, often with telangiectases over tumor margin; if center is ulcerated, called a rodent ulcer

Morpheaform basal cell carcinoma: less common, but much more aggressive; firm, flat lesion with indistinct borders; penetrates into dermis, pagetoid spread can occur;

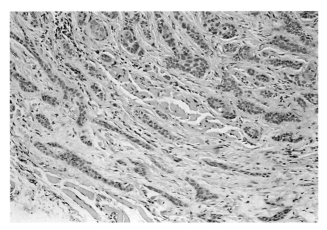

Figure 6-33. Morpheaform type demonstrating thin cords of basal cells. (From Yanoff M, Fine BS: Ocular Pathology, 5th edn, St Louis, Mosby, 2002.)

tumor cells may line up in single cell layer ('Indian-file' pattern) (Figure 6-33)

Treatment: excisional biopsy, wide excision with frozen section, Mohs' micrographic surgery, may require supplemental cryotherapy or radiation therapy, exenteration for orbital extension

Squamous Cell Carcinoma (SCC)

Flat, keratinized, ulcerated, erythematous plaque

Can arise de novo or from preexisting actinic keratosis

May spread by direct extension or may metastasize via local lymphatics or hematogenously

May be associated with HIV and HPV infection

More aggressive than basal cell carcinoma

Usually occurs on lower eyelid

Pathology: pink dyskeratotic cells forming keratin pearls (H&E stain), cord-like infiltrating strands into the dermis containing atypical anaplastic cells (Figure 6-34)

Treatment: excisional biopsy, wide excision with frozen section, Mohs' micrographic surgery, may require supplemental cryotherapy or radiation therapy, exenteration for orbital extension

Keratoacanthoma

Dome-shaped squamous lesion

Rapid onset (4–8 weeks); occurs in elderly

Central keratin-filled crater and elevated rolled edges; clinically resembles basal cell carcinoma

Previously considered a form of pseudoepitheliomatous hyperplasia, now classified as a squamous carcinoma

Spontaneous involution

May cause permanent damage to lid margin and madarosis (loss of lashes)

Pathology: acanthotic, hyperkeratotic, dyskeratotic epithelium and inflammatory cells (Figure 6-35)

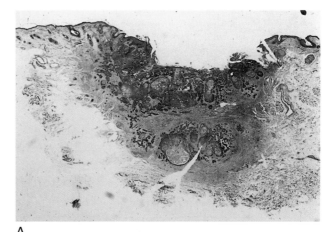

A

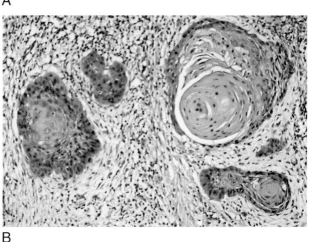

B

Figure 6-34. SCC demonstrating **A**, pink epithelial cells invading dermis with overlying ulceration. **B**, squamous cells in dermis making keratin. (From Yanoff M, Fine BS: Ocular Pathology, 5th edn, St Louis, Mosby, 2002.)

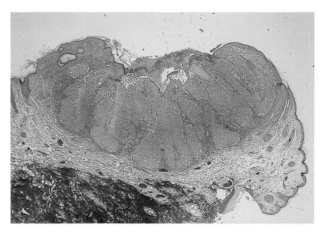

Figure 6-35. Keratoacanthoma appears as cup-shaped lesion with central keratin core above skin surface. (From Yanoff M, Fine BS: Ocular Pathology, 5th edn, St Louis, Mosby, 2002.)

Treatment: observation, surgical excision, local steroid injection

Sebaceous Adenocarcinoma

Orange-yellow nodule

Second most common malignancy of the eyelid (after BCC)

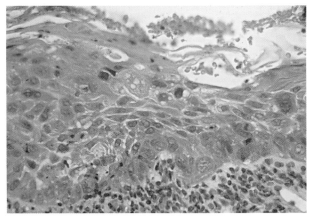

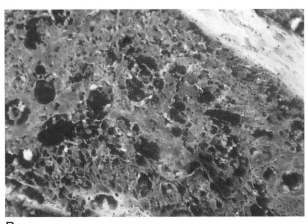

Figure 6-36. Sebaceous adenocarcinoma **A,** Large, foamy tumor cells in epidermis demonstrating pagetoid spread. **B,** Oil-red-O stains fat in cells. (From Yanoff M, Fine BS: Ocular Pathology, 5th edn, St Louis, Mosby, 2002.)

Occurs in the elderly (6th–7th decade of life)

Arises from meibomian glands, glands of Zeis, and glands of caruncle

Upper lid more commonly involved (greater number of meibomian glands)

Can masquerade and be misdiagnosed as a recurrent chalazion or chronic blepharitis

Often associated with madarosis

Highly malignant and lethal tumor; regional lymph node and hematogenous metastasis; 5-year mortality rate = 30%

Pathology: lobules of anaplastic cells with foamy, lipid-laden, vacuolated cytoplasm, large hyperchromic nuclei, skip areas and pagetoid invasion (spread of tumor into conjunctival epithelium), positive lipid stains (oil-red-O stain) (Figure 6-36)

Treatment: wide excision with frozen section and conjunctival map biopsy, exenteration for orbital extension or pagetoid spread, radiotherapy for palliation

Muir-Torre syndrome: multiple sebaceous neoplasms, keratoacanthomas, and visceral tumors (especially GI)

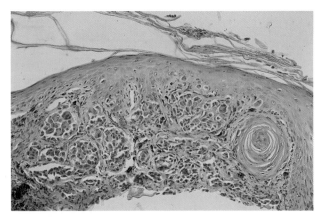

Figure 6-37. Malignant melanoma. (From Yanoff M, Fine BS: Ocular Pathology, 5th edn, St Louis, Mosby, 2002.)

Malignant Melanoma (MM) (Figure 6-37)

<1% of all eyelid cancers

Lentigo maligna melanoma (Hutchinson's malignant freckle) (10%): occurs in sun-exposed areas of elderly patients; arises from lentigo maligna (see Precancerous lesions)

Findings: flat, pigmented macule with irregular borders
Pathology: fascicles of spindle-shaped cells
10% metastasize; 5 year survival = 90%

Superficial spreading melanoma (80%): occurs in sun exposed and non-exposed skin (this form is not directly related to sun exposure) of younger individuals

Initial horizontal growth phase before invading deeper
Findings: spreading macule with irregular outline, variable pigmentation, invasive phase marked by papules and nodules
Pathology: pagetoid nests in all levels of epidermis
5-year survival = 69%

Nodular melanoma (10%): most common type of melanoma in the eyelid; usually occurs in 5th decade of life, more common in men (2:1); always palpable

More aggressive, with early vertical invasion; 5-year survival = 44%
20% of nodular and 50% of superficial spreading arises from nevi

Signs of transformation: change in color, change in shape or size, unduration, ulceration, bleeding

Treatment: wide surgical excision, lymph node dissection if microscopic evidence of lymphatic or vascular involvement

Prognosis: depends on depth of vertical invasion; <0.75 mm indicates favorable prognosis

Neurogenic Tumors

Neurofibroma

(See Ch. 5, Pediatrics/Strabismus)

Nodular form (fibroma molluscum): usually not associated with neurofibromatosis (NF)

Plexiform form: associated with NF; produces S-shaped lid deformity

Pathology: combined proliferation of axons, Schwann cells, and endoneural fibroblasts

Treatment: observation or resection

Neurilemmoma (Schwannoma)

(See Orbit section)

Solitary eyelid nodule composed of Schwann cells

Usually located near medial canthus

Usually not associated with NF

Pathology: proliferation of Schwann cells

Treatment: local excision

Merkel Cell Tumor

Rare, vascular, red-blue, sausage-shaped lesion

Rapid growth from Merkel cells (mechanical receptors for touch; amine precursor uptake and decarboxylation [APUD] system)

Usually occurs in upper lid

Occurs in older individuals

Metastasis and death in 30% of patients

Treatment: wide excision with immunohistochemical stains, lymph node dissection, radiation therapy

Vascular Tumors

Lymphangioma

(See Ch. 5, Pediatrics/Strabismus)

Capillary Hemangioma

(See Ch. 5, Pediatrics/Strabismus)

Cavernous Hemangioma

Appears as a port wine stain (nevus flammeus)

Associated with Sturge-Weber syndrome

Grows with the patient; does not involute

Pathology: dilated capillaries without endothelial cell proliferation

Kaposi's Sarcoma

Malignant soft tissue sarcoma (solitary or multiple)

More common in immunocompromised patients and those of Mediterranean descent

May involve orbit

Nontender, violaceous nodules and plaques

May cause lid distortion with edema and entropion

Treatment: complete surgical excision, also responsive to radiotherapy and chemotherapy

Other Lesions

Xanthelasma

Soft, flat or slightly elevated yellow plaques

More common on the medial aspect of the eyelids

$\frac{2}{3}$ of patients have normal serum lipids

Can occur in hyperlipid syndromes such as familial hypercholesterolemia, juvenile xanthogranuloma, histiocytosis X

Associated with **Erdheim-Chester disease** (lipoid granulomatosis): multisystem disease with lipogranuloma formation in the liver, heart, kidneys, lungs, and bones
　　Findings: proptosis and xanthelasma-like lesions
　　Pathology: histiocytes and Touton giant cells

Pathology: aggregates of lipid-containing macrophages (foam cells) with surrounding inflammation

Treatment: observation; may recur after excision

Sarcoidosis

(See Orbit section)

Slightly elevated, umbilicated papules

Noncaseating granulomas

Amyloidosis

Confluent, yellow, waxy papules

May hemorrhage with minor trauma

Lid lesions are associated with systemic involvement

Pathology: heterogeneous group of substances that stains with Congo red

Necrobiotic Xanthogranuloma

Zonal granuloma with necrobiotic center

Associated with JXG, monoclonal gammopathies, and plasma cell dyscrasias

Pathology: Touton giant cells and xanthoma cells

Mycosis Fungoides

Cutaneous T-cell lymphoma

Pathology: Lutzner cells and Pautrier abscesses

NASOLACRIMAL SYSTEM DISORDERS

Obstructions

Congenital tearing: (see Ch. 5, Pediatrics/Strabismus)
　　Must rule out congenital glaucoma; also consider corneal trauma, trichiasis, and superficial foreign body

Acquired tearing:

Etiology: primary idiopathic hypersecretion, ocular surface irritation with reflex tearing, outflow obstruction

Diagnosis:

> **DYE DISAPPEARANCE TEST:** instill fluorescein in inferior fornix of both eyes, wait 5 minutes, then evaluate for asymmetric clearance of dye from tear meniscus
>
> **JONES I TEST:** perform dye disappearance test, then attempt to recover fluorescein in inferior nasal meatus with cotton-tipped applicator; abnormal result (no fluorescein) occurs in 33% of normal individuals
>
> **JONES II TEST:** perform Jones I test, then irrigate saline into nasolacrimal system; dye recovery from nose indicates functional occlusion of nasolacrimal duct; clear saline recovery indicates canalicular occlusion or nonfunctioning lacrimal pump
>
> **DACRYOSCINTOGRAM:** instillation of technetium 99, physiologic test
>
> **DACRYOCYSTOGRAM:** injection of Lipiodol (Ethiodol; radiopaque) outlines drainage system
>
> **PROBING AND IRRIGATION**

Punctal Obstruction

Etiology: senile, cicatrizing (ocular cicatricial pemphigoid, Stevens-Johnson syndrome), trauma, tumor, drug-induced

Treatment: dilation, punctoplasty, reapposition of puncta

Canalicular Obstruction

Etiology: trauma, toxic medications (antivirals, strong miotics, epinephrine), infections (HSV, EBV, trachoma), dacryolith, inflammation (ocular cicatricial pemphigoid, Stevens-Johnson syndrome), allergy, radiation, tumor, canaliculitis

Treatment:

> Repair of canalicular system (in trauma)
>
> *Partial obstruction:* Crawford tubes or Viers rods
>
> *Obstruction within 8 mm of punctum:* Jones tubes
>
> *Obstruction >8 mm from punctum:* dacryocystorhinostomy (DCR) with O'Donoghue tubes

Nasolacrimal Duct Obstruction

Congenital: (see Chapter 5, Pediatrics/Strabismus)

Acquired:

Etiology: involutional stenosis (most common cause, more common in women [2:1], inflammatory infiltrates compress nasolacrimal duct), trauma, chronic sinus disease, nasal polyps, dacryocystitis, granulomatous disease (e.g. sarcoidosis, Wegener's granulomatosis)

Treatment: silicone intubation, DCR

Lacrimal Sac Obstruction

Etiology: trauma, acute or chronic dacryocystitis

Treatment: DCR

Infections

Canaliculitis

Infection of canaliculus, usually chronic

Organisms: *Actinomyces israelii* is most common (filamentous Gram-positive rod). Also, *Candida albicans, Aspergillus, Nocardia asteroides,* HSV, and VZV

More commonly occurs in middle-aged women

Symptoms: tearing, redness, pain, discharge

Findings: erythematous, dilated, tender, pouting punctum; expressible discharge, recurrent conjunctivitis; may have bloody tears

Grating sensation with probing

Often find sulfur granules

Treatment: warm compresses, probing and irrigation with penicillin, canalicular curettage, incision and débridement

Dacryocystitis

Infection of nasolacrimal sac

Organisms: *Staphylococcus, Streptococcus, Pseudomonas, H. influenzae* (young children), *Klebsiella, Actinomyces, Candida*

Findings:

Acute: edema, erythema, and distention below the medial canthal tendon; may result in mucocele formation, chronic conjunctivitis, or orbital cellulitis

Chronic: distended lacrimal sac, minimal inflammation

Treatment: warm compresses, topical and systemic antibiotics, incision and drainage if abscess present, avoid irrigation and probing during acute infection, DCR after acute inflammation subsides

Dacryoadenitis

Acute or chronic inflammation of lacrimal gland

Etiology:

Acute: infection (*Staphylococcus, N. gonorrheae,* mumps, Epstein-Barr virus [EBV], VZV)

Chronic: inflammation or infection (IOI, sarcoidosis, Mikulicz's syndrome, lymphoid lesions, syphilis, TB)

Symptoms: swelling, redness; may have pain, tearing, discharge with acute infection

Findings: enlarged lacrimal gland; may have tenderness, fever, preauricular lymphadenopathy, globe dystopia, restricted ocular motility

Diagnosis: CT scan; consider culture, laboratory tests (serologies), and biopsy

Treatment: may require systemic antibiotics, incision and drainage, or excision

Table 6-7. DDx of common disorders

Epithelial Eyelid Lesions
Slow-growing:
  Squamous cell papilloma
  Actinic keratosis
  Seborrheic keratosis
  Basal cell carcinoma
  Squamous cell carcinoma
Fast-growing:
  Molluscum contagiosum
  Keratoacanthoma

Subepithelial Eyelid Lesions
Cystic
  Cyst of Moll
  Cyst of Zeiss
  Sebaceous cyst
Solid
  Meibomian cyst
  Hordeolum
  Chalazion
  Xanthelasma
  Sebaceous adenocarcinoma

Pseudoproptosis
High myopia (axial myopia)
Contralateral enophthalmos
Shallow orbits (Crouzon's, Apert's syndrome)
Buphthalmos
Contralateral ptosis
Upper lid retraction

Infantile Proptosis
Capillary hemangioma (most common)
Orbital cellulitis
Dermoid
Encephalocele
Histiocytosis X
Leukemia
Retinoblastoma
Craniofacial disorders

Childhood Proptosis
Orbital cellulitis (most common)
Capillary hemangioma
Dermoid cyst
Inflammatory pseudotumor
Lymphangioma
Metastatic neuroblastoma
Granulocytic sarcoma
Orbital extension of retinoblastoma
Optic nerve glioma
Rhabdomyosarcoma
Lymphoma/leukemia
Meningioma
Neurofibromatosis
Spheno-orbital encephalocele
Optic nerve glioma
Plexiform neurofibroma in the orbit

Adult Proptosis
Thyroid-related ophthalmopathy (50%)
Hemangioma
Orbital pseudotumor

Bilateral Proptosis
Thyroid-related ophthalmopathy (most common)
Orbital pseudotumor
Wegener's granulomatosis
Orbital lymphoma
Metastatic tumor
Chloroma
Metastatic neuroblastoma
Crouzon's disease
Cavernous sinus thrombosis
Acromegaly
Histiocytosis X
Multiple myeloma

Pigmented Eyelid Lesions
Nevus
Pigmented basal cell carcinoma
Lentigo maligna (Hutchinson's freckle)
Malignant melanoma
Oculodermal melanocytosis (nevus of Ota)

Enlarged Extraocular Muscles on CT Scan
Thyroid-related ophthalmopathy (muscle tendons spared)
Orbital pseudotumor (muscle tendons involved)
Metastatic cancer
Lymphoma
Infection
Carotid-cavernous sinus fistula
Acromegaly
Amyloid
Nodular fasciitis
Fibrous histiocytoma
Tenon's cyst
Wegener's granulomatosis

Enhancing Lesions with Contrast
Cavernous hemangioma
Neurilemmoma
Fibrous histiocytoma
Hemangiopericytoma

Lacrimal Gland Inflammation/Swelling
Mumps
Glandular fever
Suppurative adenitis
Extension of conjunctivitis
Tuberculosis
Sarcoidosis
Malignant lymphoma
Lacrimal gland tumor
Thyroid-related ophthalmopathy
Orbital pseudotumor

Unilateral Periorbital Inflammation
Ruptured dermoid cyst
Rhabdomyosarcoma
Orbital pseudotumor
Leukemia
Eosinophilic granuloma
Infantile cortical hyperostosis

Enophthalmos
Orbital floor fracture
Metastatic tumors with sclerosis (breast carcinoma)

Painless Proptosis
Cavernous hemangioma
Optic nerve tumor
Neurofibroma
Neurilemmoma
Benign lacrimal gland tumors
Rhabdomyosarcoma
Fibrous histiocytoma
Lymphoma
Osteoma

Painful Proptosis
Orbital pseudotumor
Posterior scleritis
Dacryoadenitis
Orbital hemorrhage
Malignant lacrimal gland tumor
Nasopharyngeal carcinoma
Lymphangioma
Orbital abscess
Wegener's granulomatosis
Primary orbital tumors
Hemangioma
Lacrimal gland tumors
Optic nerve meningioma or glioma
Rhabdomyosarcoma

Tumors of the Lacrimal Sac

Rare; secondary to dacryocystitis

Findings: painless mass located above medial canthal tendon, tearing, may have bloody tears; bleeding with probing

Must be differentiated from dacryocystitis

Dacryocystogram outlines tumor

Squamous papilloma: most common primary lacrimal sac tumor

Squamous cell carcinoma: most common primary malignant lacrimal sac tumor

Lymphoma: second most common primary malignant lacrimal sac tumor

Lacrimal sac can be invaded by other malignant tumors of eyelids and conjunctiva

ORBITAL SURGERY

Evisceration

Removal of intraocular contents leaving the sclera intact

Indications: blind painful eye, process not involving sclera

Complications: implant extrusion due to epithelial downgrowth and poor closure

Enucleation

Removal of entire globe and portion of optic nerve

Implant material: PMMA, silicone, hydroxyapatite

Integrated implant: painted prosthesis fits into implant

Indications: blind painful eye, intraocular malignancy, after severe trauma to avoid sympathetic ophthalmia

Exenteration

Removal of all orbital contents

Indications: adenoid cystic carcinoma, mucormycosis, orbital extension of sebaceous cell, basal cell, malignant melanoma, and squamous cell carcinomas

Dacryocystorhinostomy (DCR)

Creation of passage between lacrimal sac and nasal cavity

Osteotomy is made by removing the lacrimal sac fossa and superior nasal wall of NLD at level of middle turbinate; bony window should measure 15 mm × 15 mm

Indications: focal distal canalicular obstructions and NLDOs

Complications: failure due to obstruction at common canaliculus or at bony ostomy site

1. The most common causative organism of canaliculitis is
   a. *Candida albicans*
   b. HSV
   c. *Actinomyces israelii*
   d. *Nocardia asteroides*
2. Sequelae of a CN 7 palsy may include all of the following except
   a. filaments
   b. ptosis
   c. decreased vision
   d. dry eye
3. Which procedure is the best treatment option for the repair of a large upper eyelid defect?
   a. Cutler-Beard
   b. Bick
   c. Hughes
   d. Fasanella-Servat
4. The extraocular muscle with the largest arc of contact is the
   a. LR
   b. IO
   c. MR
   d. SO
5. The risk of systemic involvement is highest for an ocular lymphoid tumor in which location?
   a. orbit
   b. eyelid
   c. conjunctiva
   d. bilateral orbit
6. The rectus muscle with the shortest tendon of insertion is the
   a. IR
   b. SR
   c. MR
   d. LR
7. Which of the following bones does not make up the medial orbital wall?
   a. lacrimal
   b. maxilla
   c. sphenoid
   d. palatine
8. Which of the following clinical features is least commonly associated with a tripod fracture?
   a. restriction of the inferior rectus
   b. flattening of the malar eminence
   c. hypesthesia
   d. displacement of the lateral canthus
9. A carotid-cavernous fistula can be differentiated from a dural-sinus fistula by all of the following characteristics except
   a. proptosis
   b. afferent pupillary defect
   c. bruit
   d. CN 6 palsy
10. Basal cell carcinoma is least likely to occur at which site?
    a. upper eyelid
    b. medial canthus

c. lower eyelid

d. lateral canthus

11. All of the following are sites of attachment of the limbs of the medial canthal tendon except
    a. frontal process of the maxillary bone
    b. anterior lacrimal crest
    c. orbital process of the frontal bone
    d. posterior lacrimal crest

12. Which muscle is most commonly responsible for vertical diplopia after 4-lid blepharoplasty?
    a. superior oblique
    b. inferior oblique
    c. superior rectus
    d. inferior rectus

13. Congenital and involutional ptosis can be distinguished by all of the following except
    a. degree of levator function
    b. presence of lid crease
    c. width of palpebral fissure
    d. presence of jaw wink

14. Congenital obstruction of the lacrimal drainage system usually occurs at the
    a. valve of Rosenmüller
    b. common canaliculus
    c. lacrimal sac
    d. valve of Hasner

15. What is the correct order of structures that would be encountered when the upper eyelid is penetrated 14 mm above the lid margin?
    a. preseptal orbicularis muscle, orbital septum, levator aponeurosis, Müller's muscle
    b. preseptal orbicularis muscle, orbital septum, levator muscle
    c. pretarsal orbicularis muscle, levator muscle, conjunctiva
    d. pretarsal orbicularis muscle, levator aponeurosis, orbital septum, fat

16. What is the best treatment option for a child who develops recurrent proptosis after upper respiratory infections?
    a. observation
    b. XRT
    c. chemotherapy
    d. surgery

17. All of the following are features of mucormycosis except
    a. internal ophthalmoplegia
    b. ipsilateral CN 7 palsy
    c. diplopia
    d. involvement of the first branch of the trigeminal nerve

18. All of the following are associated with blepharophimosis except
    a. trisomy 18
    b. ectropion
    c. AR inheritance
    d. wide intercanthal distance

19. Which of the following is the most important test to perform in a patient with a capillary hemangioma?
    a. ECHO
    b. hearing test

c. EKG

d. bleeding time

20. For entropion repair, the lateral tarsal strip is sutured
    a. below and anterior to the rim
    b. below and posterior to the rim
    c. above and anterior to the rim
    d. above and posterior to the rim

21. Staged surgery for a patient with severe thyroid-related ophthalmopathy is best done in what order?
    a. decompression, strabismus, lid repair
    b. strabismus, decompression, lid repair
    c. lid repair, decompression, strabismus
    d. decompression, lid repair, strabismus

22. Which of the following best explains why when a ptotic lid is lifted, the contralateral lid falls?
    a. inhibition of Müller's muscle
    b. Sherrington's law
    c. relaxation of the frontalis muscle
    d. Hering's law

23. Which study is most helpful in the evaluation of a patient with opsoclonus?
    a. EKG
    b. MRI
    c. ERG
    d. angiogram

24. What is the most appropriate treatment for a benign mixed tumor of the lacrimal gland?
    a. radiation
    b. excision
    c. observation
    d. biopsy

25. What is the most appropriate treatment for a biopsy-positive basal cell carcinoma of the lower eyelid?
    a. cryotherapy to the cancer and margins
    b. local antimetabolite treatment
    c. radiation with 2500 rads to the lesion and margins
    d. excision with frozen section control of the margins

26. CT enhancement is most associated with which lesion?
    a. rhabdomyosarcoma
    b. glioma
    c. lymphangioma
    d. meningioma

27. Which of the following factors is least likely to contribute to the development of entropion?
    a. preseptal orbicularis override
    b. horizontal lid laxity
    c. posterior lamella foreshortening
    d. capsulopalpebral fascia disinsertion

28. A 24-year-old woman presents after blunt trauma to the left orbit with enophthalmos and restriction of upgaze. Which plain film radiographic view would be most helpful?
    a. Caldwell view
    b. lateral view
    c. Waters view
    d. axial view

29. All of the following may cause enophthalmos except
    a. breast carcinoma
    b. lymphoma
    c. orbital floor fracture
    d. phthisis bulbi

30. All of the following nerves pass through the superior orbital fissure except
    a. CN 3
    b. CN 4
    c. CN V_2
    d. CN 6
31. Blepharospasm is associated with
    a. myotonic dystrophy
    b. syphilis
    c. vertebrobasilar insufficiency
    d. Parkinson's disease
32. The anatomic boundaries of the superior orbital fissure are
    a. the greater wing of the sphenoid and the zygoma
    b. the greater and lesser wings of the sphenoid
    c. the lesser wing of the sphenoid and the maxilla
    d. the lesser wing of the sphenoid and the zygoma
33. Which of the following is most likely to exacerbate the symptoms of thyroid-related ophthalmopathy?
    a. alcohol
    b. cigarettes
    c. aspirin
    d. caffeine
34. A 44-year-old woman develops a left lower eyelid ectropion following a severe facial burn. The most appropriate procedure includes
    a. horizontal tightening
    b. vertical shortening
    c. repair of lower eyelid retractors
    d. levator myotomy
35. All of the following are methods of treating spastic entropion except
    a. eyelid taping
    b. Botox injection
    c. Wies marginal rotation
    d. Quickert suture
36. The most common complication of a hydroxyapatite orbital implant is
    a. implant migration
    b. infection
    c. orbital hemorrhage
    d. conjunctival erosion
37. Which collagen vascular disease is associated with malignancy?
    a. dermatomyositis
    b. scleroderma
    c. Wegener's granulomatosis
    d. systemic lupus erythematosus
38. Oral antibiotics are indicated for
    a. canaliculitis
    b. dacryocystitis
    c. dacryoadenitis
    d. nasolacrimal duct obstruction
39. The levator muscle inserts onto all of the following structures except
    a. tarsus
    b. lateral orbital tubercle
    c. posterior lacrimal crest
    d. trochlea
40. When performing a DCR, the osteum is created at the level of the
    a. superior turbinate
    b. middle turbinate
    c. inferior turbinate
    d. none of the above

SUGGESTED READINGS

American Academy of Ophthalmology: Orbit, Eyelids and Lacrimal System, vol 7. San Francisco, AAO, 2012.

Bosniak SL: Principles and Practice of Ophthalmic Plastic and Reconstructive Surgery. Philadelphia, WB Saunders, 1996.

Collin JRO: Manual of Systematic Eyelid Surgery, 3rd edn. Philadelphia, Butterworth-Heinemann, 2002.

Dutton JS: Atlas of Clinical and Surgical Orbital Anatomy, 2nd edn. Philadelphia, Saunders, 2011.

Levine MR: Manual of Oculoplastic Surgery, 4th edn. Thorofare, SLACK, 2010.

Chen and Kahn: Color Atlas of Cosmetic Oculofacial Surgery, 2nd edn. Elsevier, 2009.

Fagien S: Putterman's Cosmetic Oculoplastic Surgery, 4th edn. Philadelphia, Saunders, 2007.

Rootman J: Diseases of the Orbit, 2nd edn. Philadelphia, Lippincott Williams and Wilkins, 2002.

Smith BC, Nesi FA, Cantarella VH, et al: Smith's Ophthalmic Plastic and Reconstructive Surgery, 2nd edn. St Louis, Mosby, 1998.

7

Cornea / External Disease

ANATOMY / PHYSIOLOGY
CONJUNCTIVAL DISORDERS
CORNEAL DISORDERS
SCLERAL DISORDERS
SURGERY

ANATOMY / PHYSIOLOGY

Conjunctiva

Nonkeratinized stratified columnar epithelium with goblet cells (most numerous in fornices) underlying loose stromal tissue (substantia propria)

Palpebral conjunctiva: firmly adherent to tarsus

Bulbar conjunctiva: loosely adherent to globe except at limbus where it fuses with Tenon's capsule

Plica semilunaris: narrow fold of medial bulbar conjunctiva near caruncle; rudimentary structure analogous to nictitating membrane in certain animals

Caruncle: tissue at medial canthus intermediate between conjunctiva and skin; contains accessory dermal appendages

Precorneal Tear Film

Layers:
  Lipid: outer layer; reduces evaporation; cholesterol and lipids; produced by meibomian, Zeis', and Moll's glands
  Aqueous: middle layer; provides oxygen to epithelium; 98% water, 2% protein, pH = 7.2; osmolarity ~ 302 mOsm/L; produced by lacrimal and accessory lacrimal glands (Krause's and Wolfring's), basal secretion rate = 2 μL/min; lysozyme (antibacterial enzyme) constitutes 30% of total protein in tear film; also, lactoferrin, IgA and IgG (not IgD), electrolytes, oxygen
  Mucin: inner layer; reduces surface tension and allows aqueous tear film to be spread evenly; helps structure the tear film; glycoproteins; 3 types: secreted mucins

(MUC4 and MUC7) produced by lacrimal gland, gel-forming mucins (MUC5-AC) produced by conjunctival goblet cells (glands of Manz and crypts of Henle, primarily in fornix), and membrane associated mucins (MUC1 and MUC16) that protect the ocular surface; 2–3 mL/day

Cornea (Figure 7-1)
Average measurements:
  Diameter: vertical = 11.5 mm, horizontal = 12.5 mm; at birth, horizontal diameter = 9.5–10.5, reaches adult size by age 2
  Thickness: central = 550 μm, peripheral = 1.0 mm; typically, inferotemporal paracentral cornea is thinnest, superior paracentral cornea is thickest
  Radius of curvature: 7.8 mm anteriorly; 6.2–6.8 mm posteriorly (peripheral cornea is flatter)
  Power: anterior surface = +49 D, posterior surface = −6D, total = 43 D (75% of total power of eye)
  Refractive index: 1.36

Epithelium: 50 μm thick (5% of corneal thickness); hydrophobic (hydrophilic molecules penetrate poorly)
  Smooth refractive surface; protects against infection
  Aerobic metabolism (accounts for 70% of ATP production)
  Oxygen is obtained via diffusion from the tear film when the eye is open and from the lid vasculature when the eye is closed; also, small amount from the aqueous
  Regenerates from limbal stem cells (turnover = 6–7 days)
  Approximately 4–6 cells thick centrally and 7–10 cells thick at limbus
  Layers:
    TOP: 3–4 layers of squamous cells (uppermost are apical cells)

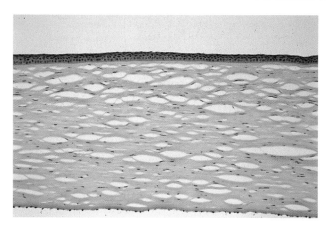

Figure 7-1. Normal cornea. (From Yanoff M, Fine BS: Ocular Pathology, 5th edn, St Louis, Mosby, 2002.)

MIDDLE: 1–3 layers of wing cells (flattened polygonal shape)

DEEP: 1 layer of basal cells

Cells:

APICAL CELLS: secrete proteins that form the glycocalyx extending from epithelial surface into mucin layer of tear film

WING CELLS: tightly packed, linked by desmosomes; form protective barrier

BASAL CELLS: anchor epithelium to stroma by hemidesmosomes; secrete basement membrane

NERVE CELLS: epithelium contains sensory nerve endings

Pathology:

CORNEAL EPITHELIAL EDEMA:

INTRACELLULAR: due to epithelial hypoxia and nutritional compromise; associated with contact lens use; fine, frosted-glass appearance (Sattler's veil)

INTERCELLULAR: due to elevated IOP; causes microcystic edema and epithelial bullae

CORNEAL FILAMENTS: composed of mucus and desquamated epithelial cells; due to increased mucus production and abnormal epithelial turnover

Basal lamina: scaffold for epithelium; adjacent to Bowman's membrane; composed of type IV collagen secreted by basal epithelium (use PAS stain)

2 layers: lamina lucida and lamina densa

Basal epithelium is secured by hemidesmosomes; adheres to stroma by anchoring fibrils

Bowman's membrane: 10 μm thick; type I collagen enmeshed in GAG matrix, rich in fibronectin, acellular; formed from secretion from both basal epithelial cells and stromal keratocytes

Not a true basement membrane

Heals with scarring; does not regenerate

Stroma: 480 μm thick centrally, 900 μm peripherally; 78% water by weight

Type I, IV, V collagen in mucopolysaccharide matrix

Collagen lamellae: 250 sheets composed of parallel small-diameter (20-30 nm) fibrils

Glycosaminoglycans: maintain lamellar spacing, contain water

Keratan sulfate:

Cells: keratocytes (produce tropocollagen; in wound repair, tropocollagen is different, resulting in nonparallel collagen fibrils and opacity), Langerhans' cells, pigmented melanocytes, lymphocytes, macrophages, histiocytes

Matrix metalloproteinases (MMP): family of enzymes that break down components of the extracellular matrix; help maintain the normal corneal structure; play a critical role in restructuring the cornea after injury

MMP-1 (collagenase-1): breaks down collagen types I, II, and III

MMP-2 (gelatinase A): breaks down collagen types IV, V, and VII, as well as gelatins and fibronectin

MMP-3 (stomalysin): breaks down proteoglycans and fibronectins

MMP-9 (gelatinase B): breaks down collagen types IV, V, and VII, as well as gelatins and fibronectin.

MMP-1, 2, and 3 are made by the stroma; MMP-9 is made by the epithelium; only MMP-2 is found in healthy cornea, the others are found only after injury

Pathology: during processing, stromal lamellae separate forming clefts (artifact); if these are absent, suggests corneal edema (lamellae are same thickness, but space between fills with fluid)

Descemet's membrane: 3 (birth) to 12 μm (adults) thick; PAS-positive basement membrane

Anchors endothelium to stroma

Type IV collagen secreted by endothelial cells

Layers:

FETAL BANDED LAYER: anterior layer (closer to stroma), striated pattern; organized collagen lamellae (like stroma); no change with age (3 μm)

ADULT NONBANDED LAYER: posterior layer (closer to endothelium), no striations; nonorganized; thickens with age (2–10 μm)

Regenerates after damage as long as endothelium is intact

Pathology:

BREAKS: edges tend to coil or roll into a scroll shape (Haab's striae, forceps injury, hydrops) (Figure 7-2)

FOCAL THICKENING: Fuchs' dystrophy, iridocorneal touch, vitreocorneal touch, guttata (Figure 7-3)

Endothelium: 4–6 μm thick

Monolayer of interdigitating hexagonal cells joined by tight junctions

Transports nutrients into cornea, pumps fluid out of cornea

Rich in mitochondria; metabolizes carbohydrates at 5–6 times the rate of epithelium

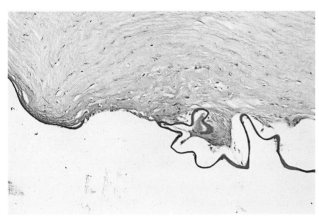

Figure 7-2. Hydrops demonstrating corneal edema (thickening) with breaks in Descemet's membrane. (From Yanoff M, Fine BS: Ocular Pathology, 5th edn, St Louis, Mosby, 2002.)

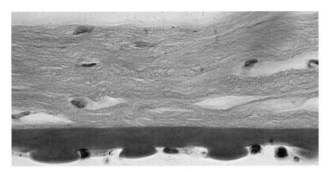

Figure 7-3. PAS stain demonstrating guttata as wart-like excrescences of Descemet's membrane. (From Yanoff M, Fine BS: Ocular Pathology, 5th edn, St Louis, Mosby, 2002.)

Functions:
1. Barrier between stroma and anterior chamber
2. Keeps cornea dehydrated and clear 1 million cells at birth (~3800 endothelial cells/mm^2); loss of approximately 50% with aging; adjacent cells stretch to fill gaps (no regeneration), insufficient pump when <500 cells/mm^2

Morphology: at least 60% of cells should be hexagonal; less than this represents unhealthy cornea

Pathology:

PLEOMORPHISM: variation in cell shape

POLYMEGATHISM: variation in cell size

Responses to stress (large, unusually shaped cells); surgery, contact lens wear, certain drugs may cause an osmotic challenge or inhibition of the Na$^+$/K$^+$ pump causing stromal edema

Example: diabetes (buildup of sorbitol in endothelial cells with hyperglycemia); contact lens (inhibits Na$^+$/K$^+$ pump and cells swell); earliest endothelial change (endothelial bleb response) occurs within minutes of insertion of a thick, soft or rigid contact lens (resolves rapidly after lens removal or slowly after 30 minutes of lens wear)

SCHWALBE'S LINE: termination of corneal endothelium (junction between endothelium and trabecular meshwork)

POSTERIOR EMBRYOTOXIN: thickening and anterior displacement of Schwalbe's line

Innervation: Innervation to cornea occurs via CN V$_1$
Approximately 70–80 branches of long posterior ciliary nerves enter peripheral cornea after myelin sheath is lost 1–2 mm before limbus

Stains:
Fluorescein: stains epithelial defects; negative staining occurs in areas of epithelial irregularity
PATTERN GIVES CLUE TO ETIOLOGY:
INTERPALPEBRAL: dry eye
HORIZONTAL BAND ACROSS INFERIOR ⅓ OF CORNEA: lagophthalmos/exposure
SUPERIOR PUNCTATE: SLK, floppy eyelid syndrome
CENTRAL PUNCTATE: focal epithelial keratitis (Thygeson's SPK, epidemic keratoconjunctivitis [EKC], molluscum)
INFERIOR PUNCTATE: blepharitis
PERILIMBAL (360°): soft contact lens wear
Rose bengal: stains tissue deficient of albumin and mucin, including devitalized cells
Lissamine green: devitalized cells, CIN; more comfortable than rose bengal

Special techniques:
Pachymetry: measures corneal thickness
Keratometry: measures corneal curvature (only 2 points 3 mm apart in paracentral region)
Topography: measures curvature of entire cornea

Limbus

Area 1–2 mm wide at which cornea and sclera meet; contains corneal epithelial stem cells, goblet cells, lymphoid cells, Langerhans' cells, mast cells (see Ch. 10, Anterior Segment)

Sclera

White fibrous layer composed of collagen and elastin

Thickness: 0.66 mm at muscle insertion, 0.33 mm beneath recti, 1.0 mm posteriorly

3 layers (ill defined): episclera, sclera proper, and lamina fusca

CONJUNCTIVAL DISORDERS

Inflammation

Follicles

Gray-white round elevations with avascular center and vessels at periphery

Well-circumscribed focus of lymphoid hypertrophy (lymphocytes with a germinal center) due to reactive hyperplasia

Generally most prominent in inferior fornix (except in trachoma)

Papillae

Small to large elevations with central vascular tuft and pale avascular valleys

Epithelial proliferation, hypertrophy, and infoldings; hyperplasia of vascular stroma with chronic inflammatory cells

Usually upper eyelid

Nonspecific reaction to conjunctival inflammation (edema and leakage of fluid from vessels)

Subepithelial substantia propria of tarsal and limbal conjunctivae contains fibrous tissue septa that interconnect to form polygonal lobules with a central vascular bundle

Giant papillae: >1 mm in diameter

Chemosis

Conjunctival edema; may be caused by allergy or infection, can occur after eyelid surgery or be idiopathic

Phlyctenule

Usually unilateral; more common in children

Etiology: type IV hypersensitivity reaction to *Staphylococci*, coccidioidomycosis, *Candida*, HSV, lymphogranuloma venereum (LGV), TB

Findings: round, elevated, focal, sterile infiltrate on bulbar conjunctiva, limbus, or cornea; overlying epithelium breaks down (stains with fluorescein); may have corneal vascularization

Pathology: infiltration of lymphocytes; atypical ulceration; fibrosis

Treatment: topical steroids and antibiotic

Symblepharon

Adhesion between conjunctival surfaces (palpebral and bulbar)
Due to inflammation, trauma, or surgery
Bilateral in ocular cicatricial pemphigoid and Stevens-Johnson syndrome

Degenerations

Amyloidosis

Yellow-salmon, subepithelial, interpalpebral plaque in primary localized disease
Systemic amyloidosis is not associated with conjunctival amyloid but is associated with amyloid of lid

Pathology: acellular eosinophilic material that stains with Congo red, thioflavin T, metachromatic with crystal violet, apple-green birefringence and dichroism with polarization microscopy

Concretions (Lithiasis)

Small, round, yellow-white deposits in palpebral conjunctiva
May contain calcium
May erode through conjunctiva and abrade ocular surface causing foreign body sensation
  Treatment: remove with needle if erodes through conjunctiva

Conjunctivochalasis

Redundant, loose, nonedematous inferior bulbar conjunctiva interposed between globe and lower eyelid
Due to elastoid degeneration, possible mechanical factor from dry eye or blepharitis (lid rubbing, dry conjunctiva)

Symptoms: tearing (interference with tear meniscus and lacrimal drainage), irritation

Treatment: treat underlying dry eye; consider short course of topical steroids or conjunctival resection

Pingueculum

Small nodule composed of abnormal subepithelial collagen; may calcify
Located at limbus, nasal more common than temporal; does not involve cornea
Caused by actinic (UV light) exposure

Pathology: elastoid degeneration (basophilic degeneration of collagen)

Pingueculitis: inflamed pingueculum due to dryness and irritation
  Treatment: lubrication, short course of topical steroids

Pterygium

Interpalpebral, wing-shaped, fibrovascular tissue that invades cornea
Associated with actinic exposure

Findings: Stocker's line (corneal iron line at head of pterygium); may induce astigmatism with flattening in meridian of pterygium; may decrease vision if crosses visual axis

Pathology: elastoid degeneration with destruction of Bowman's membrane; may have epithelial dysplasia; in recurrences after excision may have fibrotic response not elastoid degeneration

Treatment: observation or surgical excision
  High recurrence rate with primary excision (50% within 4 months, 95% within 1 year)
  Decreased risk of recurrence with amniotic membrane, conjunctival autograft, or mitomycin application at surgery

Deposits

Exogenous

Argyrosis, mascara, adenochrome (topical epinephrine is metabolized to melanin)

Endogenous

Addison's disease, Nelson's syndrome, alkaptonuria (AR, absence of homogentisic acid oxidase)

Biopsy: for cystinosis or oxalosis, fix in 50% alcohol so crystals do not dissolve; if urate suspected, use absolute alcohol

Conjunctival Telangiectasia

Associated with Louis-Barr syndrome (ataxia telangiectasia), Osler-Weber-Rendu (hereditary telangiectasia), Sturge-Weber syndrome, diabetes, sickle cell disease, Fabry's disease, increased orbital pressure (C-C fistula), blood-filled lymphatic tissue, irradiation

Allergy

Type I hypersensitivity reaction: airborne allergens (pollen, mold, dander) cross link IgE receptors on mast cells causing degranulation with release of histamine, eosinophil chemotactic factors, platelet-activating factor, major basic protein, and prostaglandin D_2

Symptoms: itching (H_1 receptors), hyperemia (H_2 receptors)

Conjunctival scraping: abundant eosinophils (normally, there are very few)

Treatment: topical antihistamine (emedastine [Emadine], levocabastine [Livostin]), mast cell stabilizer (pemirolast [Alamast], nedocromil [Alocril], lodoxamide [Alomide], cromolyn sodium [Crolom]), antihistamine/mast cell stabilizer combination (azelastine [Optivar], olopatadine [Patanol, Pataday], ketotifen [Zaditor, Alaway], epinastine [Elestat], bepotastine [Bepreve], alcaftadine [Lastacaft]), NSAID (ketorolac [Acular]), steroid, artificial tears, cold compresses

Allergic Conjunctivitis

20% of the US population has allergies
90% of patients with systemic allergies will have ocular symptoms
Most commonly seasonal or perennial allergic conjunctivitis
Associated with allergic rhinitis

Symptoms: itching, tearing, redness

Findings: lid swelling, conjunctival injection, chemosis

Giant Papillary Conjunctivitis

Etiology: allergic reaction to material coating a foreign body (e.g. contact lens [CL], exposed suture, ocular prosthesis); true giant papillae also occur in vernal and atopic keratoconjunctivitis
Atopic individuals are at higher risk

Symptoms: itching, tearing, mucus discharge, CL discomfort, then intolerance

Findings: giant papillae (>1.0 mm) on upper palpebral conjunctiva

Treatment: removal of inciting factor (e.g. CL, suture), topical allergy medication; symptoms resolve months before the giant papillae resolve; avoid thimerosal

Atopic Keratoconjunctivitis (AKC)

Atopy: hereditary allergic hypersensitivity (10–20% of population)
Types I < IV hypersensitivity reactions
Onset usually between ages 30 and 50 years
Clinical diagnosis (atopic skin disease [eczema], hay fever, asthma)

Eczema (atopic dermatitis): 3% of population; AKC in 15–40% of those with atopic dermatitis

Symptoms: itching, burning, photophobia, tearing, blurred vision

Findings: atopic dermatitis of eyelids (may have blepharitis, madarosis [loss of lashes], punctal ectropion), papillary conjunctivitis (small or medium-sized papillae in inferior fornix); may develop symblepharon, corneal vascularization, and scarring
Associated with keratoconus (10%), subcapsular cataracts (Maltese cross pattern), bilateral HSV keratitis, pellucid marginal degeneration

Pathology: mast cell infiltration of conjunctival epithelium

Treatment: topical allergy medication; consider systemic antihistamine, cyclosporine (up to 5 mg/kg/day)

Vernal Keratoconjunctivitis (VKC)

(See Ch. 5, Pediatrics/Strabismus)

Toxic Keratoconjunctivitis

Etiology: direct contact of medication or chemical substance with ocular surface

Findings: conjunctival injection, follicles, papillae, keratitis (SPK, occasionally pseudodendrite)

Superior Limbic Keratoconjunctivitis (SLK)

Recurrent inflammation of superior bulbar and palpebral conjunctiva; unknown etiology

Associated with CL wear and thyroid dysfunction (50%)

Female preponderance (70%), onset usually between ages 30 and 55 years

Recurrent episodes; lasts 1–10 years, eventually resolves permanently

70% bilateral; symptoms worse than signs

Symptoms: foreign body sensation, burning, photophobia, blurred vision

Findings: conjunctival injection, thickening, redundancy of superior bulbar conjunctiva with fine punctate staining (rose bengal), velvety papillary hypertrophy of upper palpebral conjunctiva, micropannus, filamentary keratitis (50%), decreased Schirmer's test (25%)

Pathology: thickening and keratinization of superior bulbar conjunctiva with loss of goblet cells

Conjunctival scraping: neutrophils, lymphocytes, plasma cells

Treatment: variety of options, usually requires scarring of superior bulbar conjunctiva
> Steroids of little use
> Pressure patch
> Large-diameter bandage contact lens
> Mechanical scraping of affected area may provide temporary relief
> Topical silver nitrate solution 0.5–1.0% to produce chemical burn, can retreat for recurrence (never use silver nitrate stick)
> Thermocauterization of upper bulbar conjunctiva
> Recession or resection of upper bulbar conjunctiva

Conjunctivitis Associated with Systemic Diseases

Mucocutaneous disorders: Stevens-Johnson syndrome, ocular cicatricial pemphigoid (OCP), bullous pemphigoid, pemphigus, epidermolysis bullosa, dermatitis herpetiformis, arthropathies (Reiter's syndrome, psoriatic arthritis), infections (Parinaud's oculoglandular syndrome, Kawasaki's disease), Wegener's granulomatosis

Infectious Conjunctivitis

May be hyperacute, acute, or chronic
Usually viral in adults and bacterial in children

Findings: papillae, follicles, conjunctival injection, chemosis, discharge; may have preauricular lymphadenopathy, lid swelling, membranes, keratitis, corneal infiltrates, AC reaction
> *Subepithelial infiltrates* (SEI): collections of inflammatory cells (mostly lymphocytes) at level of Bowman's membrane and anterior stroma
>> Typically occur 2 weeks after onset of EKC, can last months

Thought to be immunologic response to viral antigens trapped in stroma
May cause decreased vision, glare, and photophobia
DDx: hypoxia (contact lens overwear), infectious keratitis, EKC, Thygeson's SPK, hypersensitivity (staph marginal keratitis), medication (postsurgical topical NSAID without concomitant topical steroid), corneal graft rejection, Reis-Bucklers' dystrophy, Cogan's dystrophy
TREATMENT: topical steroids (SEIs fade but may return if steroids abruptly discontinued)
Subconjunctival hemorrhages: hemorrhagic conjunctivitis
ETIOLOGY: coxsackie A24, Picorna (enterovirus 70), EKC (adenovirus types 8 and 19)
True membrane: fibrin exudation, inflammatory cells, and invasion by vessels; firmly adherent to epithelium, bleeding occurs when peeled (diphtheria, *gonococcus*, β-hemolytic *streptococcus*, Stevens-Johnson syndrome)
Pseudomembrane: less adherent fibrin exudate (HSV, EKC, pharyngoconjunctival fever [PCF], bacterial, chlamydial, VKC, chemical burn, OCP, foreign body, ligneous, Kawasaki's disease, GVH disease)

DDx of conjunctivitis with preauricular lymphadenopathy: EKC, HSV, *Gonococcus*, *Chlamydia*, Parinaud's oculoglandular syndrome, Newcastle's disease

DDx of acute follicular conjunctivitis: EKC, PCF, chlamydial, primary HSV, medicamentosa (antivirals, atropine, Propine, apraclonidine [Iopidine], brimonidine [Alphagan], neomycin), viral lid infections (verruca, molluscum), Newcastle's disease, acute hemorrhagic (enteroviral) conjunctivitis

DDx of chronic follicular conjunctivitis (>4 weeks): chlamydial, medicamentosa, viral lid lesion, HSV, psittacosis, Lyme disease, Parinaud's oculoglandular syndrome, chronic fiber granuloma (nylon in fornix), type I hypersensitivity (atopic), molluscum, trachoma

Viral

Adenovirus

Most common; double-stranded DNA; primary infection provides lifelong immunity; 51 stereotypes, 1/3 associated with ocular infection

Findings: initially diffuse epithelial keratitis with normal vision; later, focal epithelial keratitis, coalescence of fine spots that become subepithelial infiltrates

Epidemic keratoconjunctivitis (EKC): adenovirus types 8, 19 and 37; bilateral in 75% to 90%
> *Findings:* preauricular lymphadenopathy, follicular conjunctivitis, lid swelling, watery discharge, pseudomembrane, subconjunctival hemorrhage, conjunctival scarring (symblepharon), SEIs; rarely, corneal edema, AC reaction, hypopyon; pharyngitis and rhinitis in 50%; can cause corneal ulceration
> *Treatment:* steroids are useful primarily with a true membrane or vision worse than 20/40 from SEIs

Pharyngoconjunctival fever (PCF): adenovirus types 3, 4, 5 and 7; young children; spread by respiratory secretions

Findings: fever, pharyngitis, follicular conjunctivitis; may have punctate keratitis, rarely SEIs

Newcastle's Disease

Unilateral follicular conjunctivitis, pneumonitis, preauricular lymphadenopathy

Occurs in poultry handlers; self-limited, lasts 1 week

Etiology: RNA virus; causes fatal disease in turkeys and other birds

Measles

Conjunctivitis, epithelial keratitis (associated with vitamin A xerosis)

Molluscum Contagiosum:

Chronic follicular conjunctivitis associated with elevated umbilicated lid lesions

Due to release of toxic viral products

Treatment: excision of lesions or cryosurgery

Bacterial

Hyperacute (<24 hours)

Copious purulent discharge, marked conjunctival injection and chemosis

Neisseria gonorrheae: preauricular lymphadenopathy, corneal infiltrates; can penetrate intact corneal epithelium; can perforate within 48 hours

Diagnosis: Gram's stain (Gram-negative intracellular diplococci)

Treatment: systemic ceftriaxone (1g IM if no corneal involvement; 1g IV or IM qd × 5 days with corneal involvement); topical antibiotic (fluoroquinolone or bacitracin); erythromycin or doxycycline × 1 week (to cover concurrent *Chlamydia* infection)

Acute (hours to days)

Purulent discharge, not as severe as hyperacute

Streptococcus pneumoniae, Staphylococcus, Haemophilus influenzae, Pseudomonas

Treatment: topical antibiotic (Polytrim, tobramycin, azithromycin, or fluoroquinolone); add systemic antibiotic for *H. influenzae*

Chronic

Staphylococcus, Moraxella (chronic angular blepharoconjunctivitis), occasionally Gram-negative rods

Diagnosis: culture

Treatment: topical antibiotic (Polytrim)

Chlamydial

Inclusion Conjunctivitis (TRIC – Trachoma Inclusion Conjunctivitis)

Chlamydia trachomatis serovars D to K

Chronic, follicular conjunctivitis

Associated with urethritis (5%)

Findings: bulbar follicles, subepithelial infiltrates, no membranes

Treatment: doxycycline, also need to treat sexual partners

Trachoma

Bilateral keratoconjunctivitis; leading cause of preventable blindness

Chlamydia trachomatis serovars A to C

Findings (progressive): bilateral infection of upper tarsal and superior bulbar conjunctiva, papillary reaction, conjunctival follicles, repeated infections, conjunctival scarring (Arlt's line), tarsal shortening, entropion, trichiasis, corneal abrasion, superior corneal pannus, corneal scarring, cicatrized limbal follicles (Herbert's pits)

Classification:
World Heath Organization:
- **TF = TRACHOMATOUS INFLAMMATION** (follicular): >5 follicles larger than 0.5 mm on upper tarsus
- **TI = TRACHOMATOUS INFLAMMATION** (intense): inflammatory thickening obscuring >50% of large, deep tarsal vessels
- **TS = TRACHOMATOUS CICATRIZATION** (scarring): visible white lines or sheets of fibrosis (Arlt's line)
- **TT = TRACHOMATOUS TRICHIASIS:** at least one misdirected eyelash
- **CO = CORNEAL OPACITY:** obscuring at least part of pupil margin, causing vision worse than 20/60

Pathology: epithelial cells contain initial bodies (basophilic intracytoplasmic inclusions of Halberstaedter and Prowazek); Leber's cells (macrophages in conjunctival stroma with phagocytosed debris)

Treatment: 3 weeks of systemic and several months of topical antibiotics (tetracycline) during active disease; management of dry eyes; removal of misdirected lashes

Other Conjunctivitis

Ligneous

(See Ch. 5, Pediatrics/Strabismus)

Parinaud's Oculoglandular Syndrome

Monocular granulomatous conjunctivitis, with necrosis and ulceration of follicles; fever, malaise, lymphadenopathy; may have rash

Pathology: follicles and granulomas

DDx: cat-scratch disease (*Bartonella henselae*), tularemia, sporotrichosis, TB, syphilis, LGV, *Actinomyces*, mononucleosis, *Rickettsia*, coccidioidomycosis

Diagnosis: PCR assay

Reiter's Syndrome

Triad of urethritis, uveitis, and arthritis; mucopurulent discharge, conjunctivitis in 30%; may have keratoderma blenorrhagicum

Etiology: non-gonococcal urethritis, *Chlamydia*, *Shigella* and *Salmonella* bowel infection; 85% HLA-B27 positive

Staphylococcal Disease

Blepharitis, conjunctivitis, keratitis (SPK, marginal infiltrates), phlyctenule

Floppy Eyelid Syndrome

(See Ch. 6, Orbit/Lids/Adnexa)

Autoeversion of eyelids during sleep with mechanical irritation on bedsheets causes papillary reaction on tarsal conjunctiva

Associated with obesity, keratoconus, eyelid rubbing, and sleep apnea

Treatment: lubrication, tape/patch/shield lids during sleep; consider horizontal eyelid tightening

Tumors

Hamartoma: growth arising from tissue normally found at that site (e.g. nevus, neurofibroma, neurilemmoma, schwannomma, glioma, hemangioma, hemangiopericytoma, lymphangioma, trichoepithelioma)

Choristoma: growth arising from tissue not normally found at that site (e.g. dermoid cyst, dermatolipoma, ectopic lacrimal gland)

Congenital Tumors

(See Ch. 5, Pediatrics/Strabismus)

Cystic Tumors

Simple Cyst

Serous

Inclusion Cyst

Clear cyst lined by normal epithelium
Congenital or acquired (post surgery or trauma)

Dislodged epithelium undergoes cavitation within stroma

Lined by nonkeratinized stratified squamous epithelium; contains mucin (goblet cells)

Treatment: complete excision; recurs if not completely excised

Squamous Tumors

Squamous Papilloma

Benign proliferation of conjunctival epithelium, appears as sessile or pedunculated fleshy mass with prominent vascular tufts

Sessile: broad base, usually older patients, often located at limbus

Pedunculated: usually caused by HPV, occurs in children, often located near caruncle; frequently recurs after excision; can regress spontaneously

Pathology: vascular cores covered by acanthotic, nonkeratinized, stratified squamous epithelium (Figure 7-4)

Treatment:
  Adults: excisional biopsy with cryotherapy to rule out dysplastic or carcinomatous lesion; incomplete excision may result in multiple recurrences
Rare risk of malignant transformation

Conjunctival Intraepithelial Neoplasia (CIN)

Premalignant lesion

Replacement of conjunctival epithelium by atypical dysplastic squamous cells

Usually transluscent or gelatinous appearance; <10% exhibit leukoplakia (keratinization)

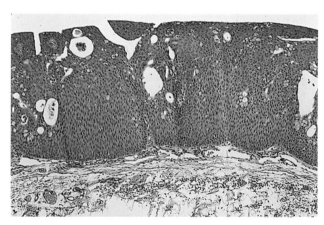

Figure 7-4. Squamous papilloma demonstrating acanthotic epithelium with blood vessels. (From Yanoff M, Fine BS: Ocular Pathology, 5th edn, St Louis, Mosby, 2002.)

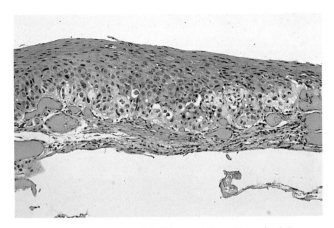

Figure 7-5. CIN demonstrating full-thickness atypia and loss of polarity. (From Yanoff M, Fine BS: Ocular Pathology, 5th edn, St Louis, Mosby, 2002.)

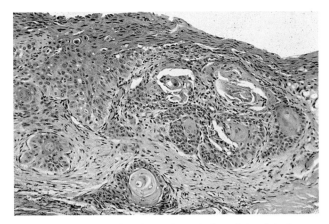

Figure 7-6. Squamous cell carcinoma demonstrating cells in substantia propria forming keratin pearls. (From Yanoff M, Fine BS: Ocular Pathology, 5th edn, St Louis, Mosby, 2002.)

Carcinoma in situ: total replacement of epithelium by malignant cells; BM intact; no invasion into substantia propria; characterized by leukoplakia, thickened epithelium, and abnormal vascularization

Usually begins at limbus and spreads onto cornea

Associated with HPV subtype 16 and 18 (check HIV in young patient), and actinic exposure

Men > women; occurs in older, fair-skinned individuals

Pathology: dysplastic epithelium spreads anterior to Bowman's membrane, fine vascularity with hairpin configuration (similar to papilloma), anaplastic cells, dyspolarity (Figure 7-5)

Treatment: wide local excision with cryotherapy; remove involved corneal epithelium (use fluorescein or rose bengal to delimit); excise until margins are clear. Consider topical or intralesional mitomycin C or interferon alpha-2b

Squamous Cell Carcinoma

Malignant cells have broken through epithelial basement membrane

Most common malignant epithelial tumor of conjunctiva; rarely metastasizes

Most common in Africa and Middle East

Appearance similar to carcinoma in situ

Pathology: invasive malignant squamous cells with penetration through basement membrane (Figure 7-6)

Treatment: wide excision (4 mm margin) with removal of surrounding conjunctiva and some scleral lamellae; cryotherapy (reduces recurrence rate from 40% to <10%); consider topical or intralesional mitomycin-C or interferon-alpha2b; enucleation for intraocular involvement; exenteration for intraorbital spread

Mucoepidermoid Carcinoma

Rare, aggresive variant of squamous cell carcinoma with malignant goblet cells

Typically occurs in individuals >60 years old

Very aggressive, can invade globe through sclera

Suspect in cases of recurrent squamous cell carcinoma

Pathology: epidermoid and mucinous components; stains with mucicarmine, Alcian blue, and colloidal iron

Treatment: wide local excision with cryotherapy; high recurrence rate

Melanocytic Tumors

Racial Melanosis

Light brown, flat, perilimbal pigmentation; increased melanin in basal epithelium

Most common in pigmented individuals

No malignant potential

Freckle

Congenital; increased melanin in basal epithelium; normal number of melanocytes

Nevus

Congenital nests of benign nevus cells along basal epithelial and/or substantia propria

20–30% amelanotic

Freely movable over globe

50% have epithelial inclusion cysts

Often enlarges or becomes more pigmented during puberty or pregnancy

Types (classified by location):
  Junctional: nevus cell confined to epithelial/subepithelial junction (anterior to basement membrane); often seen during 1st and 2nd decades of life; appearance similar to PAM with atypia
  Compound (most common): nevus cells in epithelial and subepithelial locations; cystic or solid epithelial rests are very common; epithelial inclusion cysts common
  Subepithelial: nevus cells confined to substantia propria; malignant transformation possible (Figure 7-7)

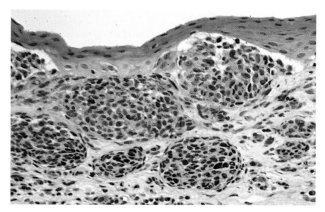

Figure 7-7. Nevus with subepithelial rests of nevus cells. (From Yanoff M, Fine BS: Ocular Pathology, 5th edn, St Louis, Mosby, 2002.)

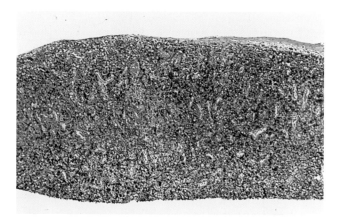

Figure 7-9. Malignant melanoma appears as pigmented tumor with loss of polarity. (From Yanoff M, Fine BS: Ocular Pathology, 5th edn, St Louis, Mosby, 2002.)

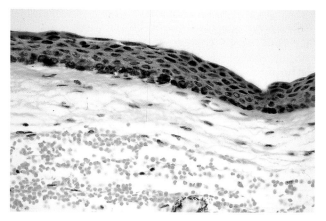

Figure 7-8. PAM with pigmentation throughout the epithelium. (From Yanoff M, Fine BS: Ocular Pathology, 5th edn, St Louis, Mosby, 2002.)

Primary Acquired Melanosis (PAM, Acquired Melanosis Oculi)

Unilateral, flat, diffuse, patchy, brown pigmentation; waxes and wanes

Proliferation of intraepithelial melanocytes; no cysts (Figure 7-8)

Most frequently on bulbar conjunctiva or in fornices, but can occur on palpebral (tarsal) conjunctiva

Analogous to lentigo maligna of skin
Occurs in middle-aged to elderly whites
20–30% risk of malignant transformation, nodular thickening is indication for excisional biopsy

PAM without atypia: very low risk for melanoma

PAM with atypia: high risk for melanoma (overall 46%)
   20% if atypical melanocytes confined to basal epithelium
   75% if epithelioid cells present
   90% if intraepithelioid pagetoid spread present

Treatment: observe with photographs; biopsy thickened areas (does not increase risk of metastasis); complete excision if malignant

Congenital Ocular Melanosis

(See Ch. 5, Pediatrics/Strabismus)

Secondary Acquired Conjunctival Melanosis

Addison's disease, radiation, pregnancy, topical epinephrine

Malignant Melanoma

Rare, variably pigmented, elevated mass most commonly on bulbar conjunctiva
May see feeder vessel
Arises from PAM (67%) or preexisting nevi (25%), or de novo

Pathology: intraepithelial pagetoid spread; need to bleach specimen to determine amount of atypia (Figure 7-9), stain with S-100 and HMB-45

Treatment: document with photos; complete excision (no touch technique) with clear margins, partial lamellar sclerectomy, and cryotherapy
Recurrence is usually amelanotic

Prognosis: 20% mortality; 25% risk of metastases (regional lymph nodes and brain); more likely to invade sclera than SCC

If more than 2 mm thick, increased risk of metastasis and mortality
Involvement of caruncle, fornices, palpebral conjunctiva has worst prognosis

Better prognosis than cutaneous melanoma

Exenteration does not improve survival

Vascular Tumors

Pyogenic Granuloma

Exuberant proliferation of granulation tissue

Vascular mass with smooth convex surface occurring at site of previous surgery (usually strabismus or chalazion excision)

Pathology: loose fibrous stroma containing multiple capillaries and inflammatory cells

Treatment: topical steroids; excision with conjunctival graft or cryotherapy

Kaposi's Sarcoma

Red mass, often multifocal

Stages 1 and 2: patchy and flat, <3 mm in height, <4 months in duration

Stage 3: more nodular, >3 mm in height, longer duration
Associated with AIDS (20%)

Pathology: proliferation of capillaries, endothelial cells, and fibroblast-like cells (Figure 7-10)

Treatment: excision, XRT, paclitaxel (Taxol) (inhibits mitosis)

Cavernous Hemangioma

Red patch; may bleed
Associated with other ocular hemangiomas or systemic disease

Pathology: endothelial lined canals with RBCs

Lymphangioma

Cluster of clear cysts; may have areas of hemorrhage

Pathology: dilated lymphatic vessels

Treatment: excision if small

Lymphoid Tumors

(See Ch. 6, Orbit/Lids/Adnexa)
Smooth, flat, fleshy, salmon-colored mass; single or multiple

Occurs in substantia propria; overlying epithelium is smooth; can be bilateral

Most commonly in fornix

20% associated with systemic disease (but systemic lymphoma rarely presents in conjunctiva)

Spectrum of disease from benign to malignant; cannot distinguish clinically; requires immunohistochemical studies (fresh, unfixed tissue specimen)

Requires systemic workup, including CT scan, bone scan, SPEP, medical consultation

DDx: leukemia, metastases

Treatment: low-dose XRT, surgery, local chemotherapy

Metastatic Tumors

Very rare to conjunctiva

Fleshy yellow-pink mass

Breast, lung, cutaneous melanoma (usually pigmented)

Other Tumors

Fibrous Histiocytoma

Yellow-white mass composed of fibroblasts and histiocytes
Extends from limbus to peripheral cornea

Pathology: storiform pattern

Treatment: local excision

Benign Hereditary Intraepithelial Dyskeratosis (BHID) (AD)

Mapped to chromosome 4q35

Originally seen in triracial families in Halifax County, North Carolina (Haliwa Indians)

Usually presents in 1st decade of life

Symptoms: itching, burning, photophobia

Findings: bilateral dyskeratotic lesions (plaques with gelatinous base and keratinized surface) involving bulbar conjunctiva near limbus; may have similar plaques on buccal mucosa or oropharynx

Pathology: acanthosis, dyskeratosis, prominent rete pegs; no malignant potential

DDx: Bitot's spot, pingueculum, squamous papilloma, squamous cell carcinoma

Treatment: observe; topical steroids (severe symptoms); excision (diagnostic; lesions recur)

Pseudoepitheliomatous Hyperplasia

Benign proliferation of conjunctiva onto corneal epithelium

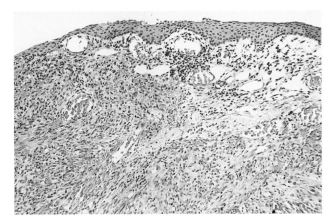

Figure 7-10. Kaposi's sarcoma demonstrating neoplastic cells and vascular spaces. (From Yanoff M, Fine BS: Ocular Pathology, 5th edn, St Louis, Mosby, 2002.)

Usually occurs away from limbus (in contrast to squamous hyperplasia or carcinoma)

Develops over weeks to months

Findings: raised, whitened hyperkeratotic surface (cannot differentiate clinically from dysplasia)

Pathology: thickened squamous epithelium; occasional mitotic figures; no atypia; no clear demarcation between normal and abnormal cells

Treatment: excision

Caruncle Tumors

Benign

Papilloma (30%), nevus (25%), inclusion cyst, sebaceous hyperplasia, sebaceous adenoma, pyogenic granuloma

Oncocytoma (oxyphilic adenoma): arises from metaplasia of ductal and acinar cells of accessory lacrimal glands; composed of polyhedral cells arranged in nests, cords, or sheets; eosinophilic cytoplasm correlates with abundance of mitochondria; more common in women

Malignant (5%)

Squamous cell carcinoma, malignant melanoma, sebaceous adenocarcinoma

CORNEAL DISORDERS

Congenital

(See Ch. 5, Pediatrics/Strabismus)

Trauma

Abrasion

Epithelial defect, most commonly traumatic (e.g. fingernail, plant branch)

Increased risk of infection, especially in contact lens wearer

Symptoms: foreign body sensation, pain, tearing, redness, photophobia

Findings: epithelial defect stains with fluorescein, conjunctival injection, ciliary flush; may have mild AC reaction

Treatment: topical antibiotic, consider topical NSAID, cycloplegic, bandage contact lens, or patching for pain control (never patch CL wearer because of increased risk of microbial keratitis)

Foreign Body (FB)

May be superficial or deep

Often metal (usually associated with adjacent rust ring), glass, or organic material

Treatment: removal of FB, topical antibiotic; old deep inert material may be observed

Laceration

Partial- or full-thickness cut in cornea

Requires surgical repair and topical antibiotic and steroid

Complications include scarring and irregular astigmatism, which if affect vision, may be treated with rigid contact lens or keratoplasty

Recurrent Erosion

Spontaneous epithelial defect

Associated with anterior basement membrane dystrophy (ABMD) in 50% or previous corneal abrasion; also occurs in other corneal dystrophies

Abnormal adhesion of epithelium to Bowman's membrane allows spontaneous sloughing

Symptoms usually occur in morning upon awakening (epithelium swells 4% overnight, and mechanical force of lids rubbing across corneal surface when open eyes or blink can dislodge epithelium)

Duration of symptoms depends on size of erosion

Findings: epithelial defect (may be partially healed), conjunctival injection; may have mild AC reaction and signs of corneal dystrophy (i.e. ABMD with irregular epithelium, areas of negative stain)

Treatment: lubrication, hypertonic saline (Muro 128 5% ointment qhs × 3-12 months); if recurs, consider bandage contact lens, epithelial débridement, anterior stromal puncture/reinforcement, diamond burr (débride and polish Bowman's membrane), laser (phototherapeutic keratectomy [PTK] with excimer laser, or micropuncture with Nd:YAG laser (1 mJ, aim just below epithelium)); also, consider treatment with matrix metalloproteinase-9 inhibitors (doxycycline 50 mg PO bid × 2 months and topical steroids tid × 2-3 weeks); débridement for subepithelial scarring

Burns

Acid: denatures and precipitates tissue proteins
   Sulfuric (batteries): most common
   Sulfurous (bleach): penetrates more easily than other acids
   Hydrofluoric (glass polishing/etching): increased penetration
   Hydrochloric: severe burn only with high concentration
   Acetic: mild burn if concentration <10%
   Pathology: superficial coagulative necrosis of conjunctiva and corneal epithelium

Alkali: denatures but does not precipitate proteins, also saponifies fat; therefore penetrates deeply
   Lime (plaster, cement): most common; toxicity increased by retained particulate matter; less penetration
   Ammonia (fertilizers), lye (drain cleaners): produce most serious injury

Also, MgOH (fireworks), KOH

Pathology: conjunctival and corneal epithelial loss with corneal clouding and edema; conjunctival and corneal necrosis; ischemia from thrombosis of conjunctival and episcleral vessels

Radiation: thermal burn (similar to acid burn)

UV light (snow blindness, arc-welding): punctate epithelial keratitis 8–12 hours after exposure; completely resolves

Ionizing radiation: superficial keratitis; then stromal disruption from keratocyte damage; corneal drying secondary to keratinization of conjunctiva

Grading systems:

Grade I: corneal epithelial damage, no ischemia; full recovery

Grade II: stromal haze but iris details seen, ischemia $<\frac{1}{3}$ of limbus; good prognosis, some scarring

Grade III: total corneal epithelial loss, stromal haze, obscuration of iris; ischemia from $\frac{1}{3}$ to $\frac{1}{2}$ of limbus; guarded prognosis

Grade IV: cornea opaque; ischemia $>\frac{1}{2}$ of limbus; poor prognosis, risk of perforation

McCulley Classification:

1. **IMMEDIATE PHASE:** extent of ocular surface involvement
2. **ACUTE PHASE:** 0–7 days
3. **EARLY REPARATIVE PHASE:** 7–21 days
4. **LATE REPARATIVE PHASE:** 3 weeks to several months

Treatment: Copious irrigation; débridement of necrotic conjunctiva and particulate matter; check pH level

Topical (10%) and oral sodium ascorbate (aids collagen synthesis and scavenges superoxide radicals)

Collagenase inhibitors (acetyl cysteine or EDTA)

Steroids for first 5–10 days only (reduce corneal and intraocular inflammation, help prevent symblepharon but can enhance collagenase-induced corneal melting, which often begins 1–2 weeks after injury)

Topical antibiotic

Ocular hypotensive medication for elevated IOP

Cycloplegic

Citrate (chelates calcium)

During first 1–3 weeks:

PROMOTE EPITHELIAL HEALING: artificial tears, tarsorrhaphy, bandage CL

LIMIT ULCERATION AND SUPPORT REPAIR: ascorbate × 21 days, steroids × 1 week; if epithelium does not heal, consider conjunctival flap, tissue glue, or keratoplasty to prevent perforation

TREAT SYMBLEPHARON: lyse with glass rod; consider vitamin A to improve goblet cell function

TREAT GLAUCOMA: topical medication; may eventually require surgery

SURGERY: limbal autograft or keratoepithelioplasty (if epithelium not healed after 3 weeks); penetrating keratoplasty (poor results; better if performed 1–2 years after injury; may need limbal stem cell transplant)

Complications: cataract, glaucoma, uveitis, symblepharon, entropion, xerosis, retrocorneal membrane, neurotrophic keratitis, corneal ulceration, anterior segment ischemia, and neovascularization

Ocular Surface Disease

Causes tear film disturbance and dry eye

Due to deficiency in tear film component(s)

Aqueous Deficiency

Lacrimal gland dysfunction (aplasia, surgical removal), infiltration (sarcoidosis, thyroid disease, lymphoma, amyloidosis, TB), inflammation (mumps, Sjögren's syndrome), denervation (Riley-Day [familial dysautonomia], Shy-Drager [adult dysautonomia, idiopathic autonomic dysfunction], Möbius' syndrome), drugs that decrease lacrimal secretion (antihistamines, diuretics, anticholinergics, psychotropics)

Keratoconjunctivitis Sicca

Adult women (95%), often associated with Sjögren's syndrome

Diagnostic criteria for Sjögren's syndrome: Keratoconjunctivitis sicca

Xerostomia (decreased parotid flow rate)

Lymphocytic infiltration on labial salivary gland biopsy

Laboratory evidence of systemic autoimmune disease (positive ANA titer, rheumatoid factor, or SS-A or SS-B antibody; associated with HLA-B8 [90%])

Symptoms: burning, dryness, foreign body sensation, tearing; worse later in day, with prolonged use of eye, and in dry or windy environments

Findings: decreased tear meniscus height (normal = 0.5 mm), decreased tear breakup time (<10 seconds), increased mucus, filaments in severe cases, interpalpebral corneal and conjunctival staining with rose bengal/lissamine green or fluorescein, Schirmer's test (<10 mm/5 min), increased tear osmolarity (>311 mOsm), Phenol red thread test (<9 mm/15 seconds)

Pathology: lymphocytic infiltration of lacrimal gland

Treatment: lubrication with artificial tears and ointments, punctal occlusion, humidifier, moisture chamber goggles; consider acetylcysteine (Mucomyst) or bandage contact lens for filaments; topical cyclosporine (Restasis)

Mikulicz's syndrome: lacrimal and parotid gland swelling and keratoconjunctivitis sicca due to sarcoidosis, TB, lymphoma, leukemia

Mucin Deficiency

Goblet cell dysfunction due to conjunctival scarring and keratinization (vitamin A deficiency, OCP, Stevens-Johnson syndrome, alkali burns, trachoma, GVH disease); impression cytology measures number of goblet cells

Xerophthalmia

Epithelial keratinization due to vitamin A deficiency

Vitamin A required for conjunctival goblet cell mucin production, corneal stromal metabolism, retinal photoreceptor metabolism, normal iron metabolism, normal growth, resistance to measles

Incidence 5 million new cases/year; affects 20-40 million children worldwide

Usually in developing countries (50% in India); in developed countries, due to lipid malabsorption (short bowel syndrome, chronic liver dysfunction, cystic fibrosis) and poor diet (chronic alcoholism)

Findings: night blindness (nyctalopia), conjunctival xerosis (leathery appearance) and Bitot's spots (gray foamy plaques), corneal xerosis with keratomalacia, ulceration, and scarring, xerophthalmic fundus (fine white mottling)

Treatment: 200,000 IU vitamin A (IM or PO)

Stevens-Johnson Syndrome

Young people; 25% recurrence, 10–33% mortality

Etiology: drugs (sulfa, antibiotics, barbituates, phenytoin [Dilantin]), infection (herpes, *Mycoplasma*), idiopathic

Findings: acute pseudomembranous conjunctivitis, symblepharon, persistent epithelial defects, dry eye, trichiasis, corneal scarring, vascularization, erosions, and ulcers

Other findings:
Erythema multiforme: cutaneous bullous eruptions (target lesions), crusting, rash involves face, mucosal ulceration and strictures, sore throat, fever, arthralgias
ERYTHEMA MULTIFORME MINOR: no mucous membrane involvement
ERYTHEMA MULTIFORME MAJOR: mucous membrane ulceration; 20% mortality from secondary infection

Pathology: occurs at mucocutaneous junction
Early: epithelial thinning with fibrinous exudate and stromal lymphocytic infiltration
Late: patchy epidermalization with keratinization and subepithelial fibrosis

Treatment: topical antibiotic, steroid, lubrication, symblepharon lysis

Ocular Cicatricial Pemphigoid

Bullous disease of mucous membranes resulting in scarring
Usually women age >60 years old

Etiology: probably autoimmune (immune complexes present in basement membrane zone)

Associated with HLA-B12 and with medications (pilocarpine, phospholine iodide, timolol, epinephrine, idoxuridine)

Findings: symblepharon, ankyloblepharon, trichiasis, entropion, subconjunctival fibrosis, severe dry eye, corneal ulcers, vascularization, and scarring

Other findings:
Skin: recurrent vesiculobullous lesions of inguinal region and extremities, scarring lesions on scalp and face
Mucous membranes (nose, pharynx, larynx, esophagus): strictures, dysphagia

Pathology: occurs at level of basement membrane (subepithelial bullae); epithelial thinning, loss of goblet cells, keratinization, subepithelial inflammation and fibrosis; IgA in conjunctival basement membrane zone; mostly polys; antigen-antibodies are deposited below epidermis
Pemphigus vulgaris: antigen-antibodies located within epithelium (intraepithelial acantholysis with epithelial bullae)

Conjunctival scraping: lymphocytes, plasma cells, eosinophils

Treatment: lubrication, immunosuppressive therapy, dapsone, cyclophosphamide, surgery
Penetrating keratoplasty: poor success rate
Keratoprosthesis: limited success for end-stage disease

Prognosis: remissions and excacerbations

Lipid Deficiency

Meibomian gland disease (blepharitis, meibomitis, acne rosacea) (see Ch. 6, Orbit/Lids/Adnexa)

Other Factors

Lid abnormalities: increased evaporative loss (lagophthalmos, Bell's palsy, ectropion, entropion, thyroid disease); treat with lid taping, tarsorrhaphy, surgical repair of underlying abnormality

Aging: reduced basal tear secretion

Environment: wind, low humidity

Medications: antihistamines, phenothiazines, anticholinergics, β-adrenergic blocking agents, diuretics, retinoids, estrogens, preservatives (benzalkonium chloride, thimerosal, polyquad)
Contact lens wear: can cause reduced tear production

Inflammation

Interstitial Keratitis

Etiology:

Bacteria: syphilis (congenital [90%; most common cause of bilateral IK] or acquired), relapsing fever (*Borrelia*), TB (unilateral, sectoral), leprosy, LGV

Virus: HSV, EBV, measles, mumps, rubella, influenza, smallpox, vaccinia

Protozoa: leishmaniasis, African sleeping sickness (*Taenia cruzi*), malaria, onchocerciasis, cysticercosis (*Taenia solium*)

Other causes: sarcoidosis, Hodgkin's disease, Kaposi's sarcoma, mycosis fungoides, incontinentia pigmenti, hidradenitis suppurativa, Cogan's syndrome (vertigo, tinnitus, hearing loss, IK)

Can be initiated by minor corneal trauma in patients with congenital syphilis

Findings: neovascularization appears as salmon patch, results in hazy corneal scarring, regression of vessels leaves ghost vessels (clear branching pattern within the scar); may develop secondary glaucoma from iris / angle damage

Pathology: diffuse lymphocytic infiltrate with thickened corneal stroma

Treatment: topical steroids

Cogan's Syndrome

Ocular inflammation (usually IK) with Meniere's-like vestibular dysfunction

Most likely autoimmune

Affects young adults, average age of onset is 29 years

Associated with antecedent upper respiratory illness (50%) and vascular inflammatory disease (10%; aortic insufficiency, aortitis, necrotizing large vessel [Takayasu's-like], and polyarteritis nodosa)

Symptoms: pain, redness, photophobia

Findings: SEIs, IK, conjunctivitis, iritis, scleritis, episcleritis

Other findings: sudden onset of Meniere's-like symptoms (nausea, emesis, tinnitus, decreased hearing, severe vertigo; may have nystagmus); 80% progress to deafness without systemic steroids

DDx of keratitis with vestibuloauditory symptoms: syphilis, polyarteritis nodosa, Wegener's granulomatosis, sarcoidosis, VKH, sympathetic ophthalmia, cerebellopontine angle tumor

Audiogram: most pronounced loss at extreme frequencies, relative sparing of midrange

Treatment: systemic steroids to prevent permanent hearing loss

Thygeson's Superficial Punctate Keratopathy

Associated with HLA-DR3; 90% bilateral; spontaneous remissions and exacerbations for years

Symptoms: photophobia, foreign body sensation, burning, tearing

Findings: coarse, punctate, gray-white snowflake opacities in corneal epithelium with faint subepithelial haze; raised center breaks through epithelial surface and stains with fluorescein during acute attack; during remissions, inactive lesions appear flat and do not stain; no associated conjunctivitis or iritis

Treatment: topical steroids (symptomatic relief and rapid resolution of lesions, but may prolong course of disease), therapeutic contact lens, trifluoridine (Viroptic; may help, but idoxuridine does not work and can cause subepithelial scarring), topical cyclosporine (may also be beneficial)

Without treatment symptoms last for 1–2 months, then remission; recurrences can begin 6–8 weeks later

Filamentary Keratitis

Strands composed of mucus and desquamated epithelial cells adherent to cornea at one end

Due to increased mucus production and abnormal epithelial turnover

Etiology: keratoconjunctivitis sicca, SLK, recurrent erosions, bullous keratopathy, prolonged patching, HSV keratitis, neurotrophic keratitis, neuroparalytic keratopathy, ectodermal dysplasia, trauma, atopic dermatitis, adenoviral keratoconjunctivitis, topical medication toxicity (medicamentosa), ptosis

No filaments in OCP because mucus production is diminished in this disorder

Treatment: acetylcysteine (Mucomyst), lubrication, remove filaments, bandage contact lens, treat underlying disorder

Degenerations

Pannus

Peripheral ingrowth of subepithelial fibrovascular tissue, usually superiorly

Inflammatory: destruction of Bowman's membrane (i.e. trachoma)

Degenerative: Bowman's membrane remains intact; may contain fatty plaque deposits (i.e. chronic edema)
Most commonly due to contact lens wear

White Limbal Girdle of Vogt

Small, white, fleck and needle-like deposits at temporal and nasal limbus

Pathology: subepithelial elastotic degeneration of collagen (sometimes with calcium particles)

Corneal Arcus

Arcus senilis: hazy white peripheral corneal ring with intervening clear zone between limbus

Arcus juvenilis: arcus in person <40 years old; associated with hyperlipoproteinemia types 2, 3, and 4

Pathology: lipid deposition in stroma

DDx: lecithin cholesterol acyltransferase (LCAT) deficiency, fish eye disease, Tangier's disease

Carotid ultrasound: for unilateral arcus senilis (may have stenosis on uninvolved side)

Furrow Degeneration

Thin area peripheral to arcus senilis, more apparent than real; nonprogressive; asymptomatic

Crocodile Shagreen

Mosaic, polygonal, hazy, gray opacities separated by clear zones; 'cracked-ice' appearance

Extends to periphery

Anterior crocodile shagreen: occurs at level of Bowman's membrane

Posterior crocodile shagreen: occurs at level of Descemet's membrane

Salzmann's Nodular Degeneration

Blue-white elevated nodules; more common in older females

Etiology: chronic inflammation (e.g. old phlyctenulosis, trachoma, IK, staph hypersensitivity)

Pathology: replacement of Bowman's membrane by hyaline and fibrillar material

Treatment: superficial keratectomy, PTK; may recur after

Polymorphic Amyloid Degeneration

Bilateral, symmetric, small stellate flecks or filaments in deep stroma

Slowly progressive; usually seen in patients >50 years old; asymptomatic

Not associated with systemic amyloid

Spheroidal Degeneration (Labrador Keratopathy, Actinic Keratopathy, Lipid Droplet Degeneration, Bietti's Hyaline Degeneration, Keratinoid Degeneration)

Bilateral; male > female

Etiology: combination of genetic predisposition, actinic exposure, and age

Types:
  Type 1 (most common): involves peripheral cornea in horizontal meridian; occurs after age 30
  Type 2: associated with other corneal pathology; may involve central cornea; occurs earlier in life
  Type 3: involves conjunctiva
Usually asymptomatic

Findings: translucent, golden brown, spherical, superficial, stromal and conjunctival proteinaceous deposits

Pathology: extracellular basophilic material

Cornea Farinata (AD)

Tiny, dot- and comma-shaped, deep stromal opacities; may contain lipofuscin (degenerative pigment)

Involutional change

Hassall-Henle Bodies

Small, peripheral, wart-like excrescences (gutatta) of Descemet's membrane (protrude toward AC)

Normal senescent change; rare before age 20 years

Depositions

Band Keratopathy

Interpalpebral band of subepithelial hazy white opacities with ground-glass, Swiss-cheese appearance; begins at limbus

Etiology: uveitis, interstitial keratitis (IK), superficial keratitis, phthisis, sarcoidosis, trauma, intraocular silicone oil, systemic disease (hypercalcemia, vitamin D intoxication, Fanconi's syndrome, hypophosphatemia, gout, 'milk-alkali' syndrome, myotonic dystrophy, chronic mercury exposure)

Pathology: calcification of epithelial basement membrane, Bowman's membrane, and anterior stroma, with destruction of Bowman's membrane; calcium salts are extracellular when process is due to local ocular disease, calcium salts are intracellular when process is due to alteration of systemic calcium metabolism

Treatment: chelation with topical disodium EDTA
Gout and hyperuricemia cause brown band from deposition of urate

Lipid Keratopathy

Diffuse or crystalline yellow stromal deposits

Due to lipid exudation from corneal vascularization

Coat's White Ring

Small, discrete, gray-white dots

Follows metallic foreign body

Mucopolysaccharidoses

(See Ch. 5, Pediatrics/Strabismus)

Sphingolipidoses

(See Ch. 5, Pediatrics/Strabismus)

Dyslipoproteinemias

Fish eye disease (AR): mapped to chromosome 16q22; diffuse corneal clouding, denser in periphery

Hyperlipoproteinemia types 2, 3, and 4: arcus

LCAT deficiency: mapped to chromosome 16; dense arcus and diffuse, fine, gray stromal dots

Tangier's disease (AR): HDL deficiency, relapsing polyneuropathy, small deep stromal opacities

Hypergammaglobulinemia

Crystals

Cystinosis

(See Ch. 5, Pediatrics/Strabismus)

Ochronosis (Alkaptonuria) (AR)

Mapped to chromosome 3q2

Melanin-like pigment (alkapton; peripheral epithelium and superficial stroma)

Tyrosinemia Type II (Richner-Hanhart Syndrome) (AR)

Mapped to chromosome 16q22

Deposits in epithelium and subepithelial space due to tyrosine aminotransferase deficiency

Refractile branching linear opacities, may have dendritic pattern

Triad of painful hyperkeratotic skin lesions (on palms and soles), keratitis, and mental retardation

Wilson's Disease (Hepatolenticular Degeneration) (AR)

Increased copper levels due to deficiency in ceruloplasmin

Copper deposition in
  Basal ganglia: spasticity, dysarthria, tremor, ataxia
  Liver: cirrhosis
  Eye: Kayser-Fleischer ring (copper deposition in peripheral Descemet's; starts superiorly, then inferiorly, medially, and temporally); sunflower cataract

DDx of Kayser-Fleischer ring: primary biliary cirrhosis, chronic active hepatitis, multiple myeloma, chronic cholestatic jaundice

Treatment: oral tetrathiomolybdate (penicillamine), followed by oral zinc maintenance; Kayser-Fleischer rings resolve with adequate treatment

Chalcosis

Copper (Descemet's), due to intraocular foreign body composed of <85% copper

Siderosis

Iron (stroma)

Iron Lines

Due to stagnation of tears (basal epithelium)

Fleischer ring: base of cone in keratoconus

Stocker's line: head of pterygium

Ferry's line: adjacent to filtering bleb

Hudson-Stähli line: horizontal at lower $\frac{1}{3}$ of cornea; normal aging, nocturnal exposure

Argyrosis

Silver (deep stroma/Descemet's)

Chrysiasis

Gold (peripheral deep stroma)

Krukenberg's Spindle

Melanin (on endothelium)

Plant Sap

From *Dieffenbachia*

Ulcers

Corneal Melt (Noninfectious Ulcer)

Nonimmune mediated: traumatic, eyelid abnormalities (entropion, ectropion, trichiasis, exposure, lagophthalmos), neurotrophic cornea, acne rosacea, keratomalacia, gold toxicity

Systemic immune mediated: primary keratoconjunctivitis sicca, Sjögren's syndrome, ocular cicatricial pemphigoid, Stevens-Johnson syndrome, rheumatoid arthritis, SLE, Wegener's granulomatosis, polyarteritis nodosa

Localized immune mediated: Mooren's ulcer, Staph marginal ulcer, vernal keratoconjunctivitis

Peripheral Corneal Ulcers

Mooren's Ulcer

Chronic, very painful, progressive ulceration
Typically begins nasally or temporally and spreads circumferentially (up to 360°)
Type II hypersensitivity reaction
Associated with hepatitis C, Crohn's disease, and hydradenitis

Symptoms: photophobia, decreased vision (irregular astigmatism)

Findings: undermined leading edge with overhanging margin, absent epithelium in active areas; may have conjunctival injection

Variants:
   USA: unilateral disease of elderly (males = females), usually less aggressive; perforation rare
   Africa: severe bilateral disease in young patients; rapidly progressive with risk of perforation
Diagnosis of exclusion (rule out rheumatologic and autoimmune diseases)

Pathology: adjacent conjunctiva contains increased plasma cells, immunoglobulin, and complement

Treatment: steroids, immunosuppressive agents (methotrexate, cyclosporine), NSAIDs, bandage contact lens, conjunctival recession or resection; may require corneal glue or penetrating or lamellar keratoplasty for perforation

Terrien's Marginal Degeneration

Painless, progressive, bilateral, trough-like stromal thinning; starts superiorly

Young to middle-aged men (75%), unknown etiology

Findings: leading edge of lipid, steep central edge, sloping peripheral edge, intact epithelium, superficial vascularization; can progress circumferentially or centrally; induces 'against-the-rule' astigmatism; may perforate with mild trauma, rarely spontaneously

Staph Marginal Ulcer

Hypersensitivity reaction

Findings: initial subepithelial infiltrate with peripheral clear zone, progresses to shallow ulcer; adjacent conjunctival injection; blepharitis

Treatment: resolves spontaneously, topical steroids may help; treat blepharitis

Marginal Keratolysis/Peripheral Ulcerative Keratitis (PUK)

Ulceration is typically peripheral and unilateral, can be central and bilateral

Due to elevated collagenase; melting stops when epithelium heals

Associated with dry eyes (Sjögren's) and sytemic disease:
   Rheumatoid arthritis: painless guttering or acute painful ulceration; also may have scleritis
   Wegener's granulomatosis: 60% have ocular involvement, most commonly PUK; also, may have scleritis, conjunctivitis, orbital involvement with proptosis, retinal vasculitis, and AION
   Polyarteritis nodosa: may be presenting feature; also may have pale yellow, waxy, raised, friable conjunctival vessels, scleritis, conjunctivitis, and retinal vasculitis
   SLE: rare manifestation
   Scleroderma: also may have keratoconjunctivitis sicca and trichiasis
   Others: relapsing polychondritis, inflammatory bowel disease, Behçet's disease

Diagnosis: blood tests as for scleritis (CBC, ESR, ANA, RF, ANCA)

Treatment: lubrication, punctal occlusion, tarsorrhaphy; consider immunosuppressive agents (topical cyclosporine), conjunctival recession or resection; treat underlying disease

Fuchs' Superficial Marginal Keratitis

Marginal infiltrates initially, then pseudopterygium with severe corneal thinning underneath

Risk of perforation with surgery or trauma

Microbial Keratitis (Infectious Ulcer)

Bacterial

Most common

Penetration of intact epithelium: *Neisseria, Corynebacterium diphtheriae, Shigella, Haemophilus aegyptus, Listeria monocytogenes*

Through epithelial defect: any organism; most commonly *Staphylococcus, Streptococcus,* and *Pseudomonas*

Risk factors: corneal trauma or surgery, contact lens wear, epithelial ulceration, dry eye, lid abnormalities

Signs of improvement: decrease in infiltrate (density/size), stromal edema, endothelial plaque, AC reaction, hypopyon; and reepithelialization

Treatment:
   Empiric: topical fortified antibiotics (vancomycin or cefazolin, plus tobramycin alternating q1h) or fluoroquinolone (Besivance, Zymaxid or Vigamox q15min for 2–3 hours, then q1h); consider subconjunctival antibiotic injection (if noncompliant)
   If no response to empiric therapy: antibiotic resistance (change regimen based on culture results); fungal, protozoal, or viral process; poor compliance (admit to hospital); anesthetic abuse
   Topical cycloplegic

Topical steroid (should be avoided until improvement is noted [usually after 48–72 hours], then dosed at lower frequency than topical antibiotic)

Complications:

Spread to adjacent structures: sclera (*Pseudomonas*), intraocular (rare in absence of corneal perforation; filamentous fungi may penetrate intact Descemet's membrane)

Corneal damage: scarring, neovascularization, endothelial dysfunction (corneal edema), descemetocele, perforation

Synechiae and secondary glaucoma

Cataract

Syphilis

(See Ch. 5, Pediatrics/Strabismus)

Crystalline Keratopathy

Often caused by *Streptoccus viridans*, also *Candida*

Associated with chronic topical steroid use (post corneal graft)

Branching, cracked-glass appearance without epithelial defect

Treat strep with vancomycin

Herpes Simplex (HSV)

Most common cause of infectious blindness and second most common cause of corneal blindness in United States (trauma is first); HSV-1 is more common for ocular infections than HSV-2 (genital)

Often asymptomatic primary infection before age 5 years, 3- to 5-day incubation period

Generally unilateral but can be bilateral (i.e. immunocompromised host)

Seropositivity to HSV is 25% by age 4 years and 100% by age 60 years

Congenital: (see Ch. 5, Pediatrics/Strabismus)

Vesicular blepharitis: primary or secondary HSV; lymphadenopathy does not occur in recurrences; perilimbal involvement is atypical, dendrite uncommon

Acute unilateral follicular conjunctivitis: primary or recurrent HSV; may mimic and often misdiagnosed as EKC; usually punctate epithelial keratitis near limbus, preauricular lymphadenopathy; may develop dendrite and pseudomembrane, may have vesicular skin eruption; bulbar conjuntival ulceration is rare but specific

Primary HSV epithelial keratitis: one or multiple small dendrites, stromal infiltrates; no conjunctivitis; heals in 1–2 weeks with corneal scarring; lid lesions occur (uncommon in recurrences except in children) but without scarring; may have lid margin ulceration (ulcerative blepharitis); associated with decreased corneal sensation and patchy iris atrophy near pupillary margin

Cultures: positive in 75%

Pathology: intranuclear viral inclusions and multinucleated giant cells with Giemsa stain

Prognosis: risk of recurrence is 30% within 2 years; can be induced by many stimuli (stress, sun exposure, hormonal changes, fever, corneal trauma or surgery)

Recurrent HSV: due to reactivation of latent virus in trigeminal (Gasserian) ganglion; 4 presentations:

Epithelial keratitis: infectious dendritic ulcer caused by live virus in basal epithelium

4 lesions:

VESICLES: clear cystic lesions that coalesce to form dendrite

DENDRITIC ULCER: branching linear lesion with central trough (stains with fluorescein), swollen heaped-up borders containing active virus (stain with rose bengal or lissamine green), and terminal bulbs (accumulations of vesicular cells); may have stromal edema or infiltrate, iritis (few KP).

GEOGRAPHIC ULCER: enlarged, nonlinear dendritic ulcer with scalloped borders containing live virus

MARGINAL ULCER: stromal infiltrate under a limbal dendrite with adjacent limbal injection (no clear zone as seen in staph marginal keratitis); may have conjunctival dendrite(s)

TREATMENT: topical antiviral (trifluridine [Viroptic] 9×/day, ganciclovir [Zirgan 5×.day, or vidarabine [Vira A] or idoxuridine 5×/day; use until ulcer heals (1–2 weeks), then taper for 1 week; beware of toxicity from overuse [>2–3 weeks]), cycloplegia, consider debridement and oral antivirals (acyclovir, famciclovir, or valacyclovir)

Dendrite usually resolves in 1 week; if still present after 10 days, possible resistance, so switch medication. As the lesion heals, a dendritic shape epitheliopathy persists for several weeks (which should not be treated with antiviral medication)

Antiviral toxicity (idoxuridine > vidarabine > trifluridine > acyclovir/ganciclovir): punctate epithelial keratopathy, follicular conjunctivitis, indolent corneal ulceration, preauricular lymphadenopathy with idoxuridine, punctal stenosis

Steroids reduce scarring; taper very slowly, critical dose variable (may need steroids for years); potentiate but do not activate live virus

Without treatment, 25% of epithelial keratitis resolves in 1 week and 50% resolves in 2 weeks but increased risk of stromal involvement with scarring, neovascularization, and decreased vision

Stromal keratitis (immune or interstitial keratitis): immunologic reaction due to recurrent infection in 20–30% of dendritic ulcer patients within 5 years. Hallmarks are stromal infiltrate, neovascularization, and scarring

NON-NECROTIZING (DISCIFORM) KERATITIS: inflammatory reaction within endothelium with secondary focal nummular stromal edema due to delayed hypersensitivity reaction

Localized fine keratic precipitates (KP), no necrosis; may have iritis, increased IOP (trabeculitis)

If severe: diffuse stromal edema, Descemet's folds; may have hypopyon, rarely corneal vascularization

Culture negative

PATHOLOGY: granulomatous reaction, sometimes with retrocorneal membrane

TREATMENT: topical steroid (cover with antiviral to prevent epithelial recurrence and antibiotic ointment to prevent secondary bacterial infection); consider topical cyclosporine

NECROTIZING KERATITIS: rare; antigen-antibody complement mediated reaction to rapid viral replication in stroma

Ulceration with infiltrate and thinning, stromal inflammation, epithelial defect, AC reaction; may perforate, may be difficult to distinguish from bacterial or fungal keratitis

TREATMENT: steroid and antiviral; consider cyclosporine or amniotic membrane transplant

Endotheliitis: inflammatory reaction to live virus in the endothelium with varying degrees of isolated stromal edema and stellate KP; can be disciform (round), linear, or diffuse (limbus to limbus); may develop hypopyon, rubeosis, spontaneous hyphema, elevated IOP

TREATMENT: topical steroid plus oral antiviral; consider oral steroid

Neurotrophic keratopathy (metaherpetic ulcer): chronic sterile macroulceration due to impaired corneal sensation and decreased tear production

Oval-shaped with smooth edges, no staining with rose bengal at edge; no stromal inflammation; may have thinning and scarring

TREATMENT: lubrication; may take months to heal owing to damaged basement membrane, impaired corneal innervation, and abnormal tear film; may require tarsorrhaphy, bandage contact lens

Diagnosis:

Papanicolaou smear: intranuclear inclusion bodies (Lipschütz bodies), Cowdry type A (eosinophilic) intranuclear inclusions

Tzanck's prep: multinucleated giant cells with Giemsa stain

Culture: only 60% positive if swab active dendrite

Immunofluorescence: detects HSV antigen

Treatment: depends on lesion (see earlier); preferred topical antiviral is now ganciclovir (Zirgan); corneal tranplant (PK) for visually significant scarring

Herpetic Eye Disease Study (HEDS):

STROMAL DISEASE: treatment with topical steroids and trifluridine (Viroptic) is better than Viroptic alone (prednisolone acetate 8×/day and viroptic qid for 1 week, then 10-week taper; supports immune mediated mechanism for stromal disease); no benefit to concomitant oral acyclovir

IRITIS: acyclovir (400 mg 5×/day), in addition to topical Viroptic and steroid, is better than topicals alone

PROPHYLAXIS: acyclovir (400 mg bid for 1 year) decreases by 50% risk of recurrent HSV keratitis

Complications: uveitis, glaucoma, episcleritis, scleritis, secondary bacterial keratitis, corneal scarring and neovascularization, corneal perforation, iris atrophy, punctal stenosis

MAJOR CLINICAL STUDY

Herpetic Eye Disease Study (HEDS)

Objective: Five trials to evaluate the role of steroids and antiviral medication in the treatment and prevention of ocular HSV disease:

1. Efficacy of oral acyclovir in treating stromal keratitis (non-necrotizing [disciform] and necrotizing): 10-week course of ACV 400 mg 5×/day or placebo, in addition to topical steroids and trifluridine
2. Efficacy of topical corticosteroids in treating stromal keratitis: 10-week tapering course of prednisolone phosphate or placebo in addition to topical trifluridine (prednisolone acetate 8×/day and trifluridine [Viroptic] qid × 1 week, then gradual taper over 10 weeks)
3. Efficacy of oral acyclovir (ACV) in treating iridocyclitis: 10-week course of ACV 400 mg 5 ×/day or placebo, in addition to topical steroids and trifluridine
4. Efficacy of oral acyclovir in preventing stromal keratitis or iritis in patients with epithelial keratitis: 3-week course of ACV 400mg 5 ×/day or placebo, in addition to topical trifluridine
5. Efficacy of oral acyclovir in preventing recurrent ocular HSV disease: 12-month course of ACV 400 mg bid or placebo and 6-month observation period for patients with a history of ocular HSV within the preceding year
6. Determinants of recurrent HSV keratitis: analyzed the placebo group from the acyclovir prevention trial

Results:

1. Oral acyclovir, in addition to topical steroids and trifluridine (Viroptic), for the treatment of stromal keratitis did not improve the number of treatment failures, time to resolution of keratitis, or 6-month best-corrected visual acuity
2. Topical corticosteroids reduced the risk of persistent or progressive stromal keratitis by 68% and shortened the duration of keratitis
3. Trial was stopped due to slow recruitment. Treatment failure occurred in 50% of the ACV group vs 68% of the placebo group
4. Oral acyclovir did not reduce the risk of stromal keratitis or iritis development in patients with epithelial keratitis. Stromal keratitis or iritis developed in 11% of patients in the ACV group vs 10% in the placebo group, and such an occurrence was more common in those with a previous history of stromal keratitis or iritis (23% vs 9% without previous history)

5. Oral acyclovir reduced the risk of recurrent ocular disease during the treatment period (19% vs 32%), especially in the stromal keratitis subset (14% vs 28%). Recurrence of nonocular HSV disease was also lower in the treated group (19% vs 36%). No rebound in the rate of disease was seen during the 6-month observation period after treatment

6. In the placebo group of the previous trial, 18% developed epithelial keratitis and 18% developed stromal keratitis. Previous epithelial keratitis did not significantly affect the subsequent risk of epithelial keratitis; previous stromal keratitis significantly increased the subsequent risk of stromal keratitis (10×)

Conclusions:

1. Oral ACV is not useful for the treatment of stromal keratitis

2. Topical corticosteroids are beneficial for the treatment of stromal keratitis

3. Results were not statistically significant but suggest a possible benefit of oral acyclovir for the treatment of iridocyclitis

4. In patients with epithelial keratitis, a 3-week course of oral acyclovir has no apparent benefit in preventing stromal disease or iritis

5. Oral acyclovir prophylaxis significantly reduces the risk of recurrent ocular and orofacial HSV disease, especially in patients with previous stromal keratitis

6. In patients with ocular HSV disease in the previous year, a history of epithelial keratitis is not a risk factor for recurrent epithelial keratitis, but a history of stromal keratitis increases the risk of subsequent stromal keratitis, and this risk is strongly associated with the number of previous episodes

Herpes Zoster Ophthalmicus (HZO)

Herpes zoster involvement of first branch of trigeminal nerve CN 5 (V_1)

Acute, painful, unilateral dermatomal vesicular eruption (obeys midline) with prodrome; new lesions occur for ~1 week with resolution in 2–6 weeks

May occur without rash (zoster sine herpete)

After chickenpox, 20–30% risk of developing herpes zoster (shingles); increased incidence and severity with age >60 years, up to 50% at age 85 years; 10–20% have HZO and 50% of these have ocular involvement if untreated

Most common single dermatome is CN 5: ophthalmic (V_1) > maxillary (V_2) > mandibular (V_3)

3 branches of ophthalmic division: frontal nerve > nasociliary nerve > lacrimal nerve

Hutchinson's sign: skin lesion on tip or side of nose (nasociliary nerve) is a strong indication of ocular involvement

Symptoms: 2- to 3-day prodrome (fever, malaise, headache, paresthesia)

Findings:

Lid: vesicles, cicatricial changes (ectropion, entropion, madarosis, ptosis), trichiasis, lagophthalmos, blepharitis

Conjunctiva: follicular conjunctivitis, vesicles, pseudomembranes, symblepharon

Cornea: keratitis (65%)

PUNCTATE EPITHELIAL: precursor to dendrite; viral replication with epithelial destruction

DENDRITIC: blunt ends, no terminal bulbs, no ulceration, minimal staining; self-limited (appears within a few days of rash, resolves in 4–6 days)

INFLAMMATORY ULCERATION: immune response; often peripheral; may lead to perforation

DENDRITIFORM EPITHELIAL PLAQUES (delayed mucous plaques): can occur at any time even weeks later; linear or branching, sharply demarcated gray-white lesion on epithelial surface; mild fluorescein staining, vivid rose bengal staining; interference with normal mucous–epithelial interaction, no active virus replication

STROMAL: occurs in 50% with epithelial disease within first 1–3 weeks; nummular subepithelial infiltrates and disciform keratitis beneath initial keratitis; immune response (may develop ring)

ENDOTHELIITIS: occurs in 10% with epithelial disease; bullous keratopathy (corneal edema out of proportion to stromal infiltrate), few KP, iritis

NEUROTROPHIC KERATOPATHY: occurs in 20%; due to decreased corneal sensation; leads to ulceration

Also, stromal scarring, pannus, exposure keratopathy (due to lid abnormalities)

Episcleritis/scleritis: limbal vasculitis, sclerokeratitis, scleral atrophy, posterior scleritis

Iris: segmental atrophy due to vasculitis with ischemia and necrosis; Argyll-Robertson pupil (ciliary ganglion involvement)

Uveitis: can occur months later; may have elevated IOP, 45% develop glaucoma; may develop cataract

Retina: central retinal artery occlusion, acute retinal necrosis (ARN); progressive outer retinal necrosis (PORN) in patients with AIDS

Optic nerve: ischemic optic neuropathy

CN palsies: CN 3, 4, or 6 palsy occurs in 25%; self-limited; may involve pupil; may have orbital apex syndrome (optic neuropathy, ophthalmoplegia, and anesthesia) from vasculitis

Syndromes:

RAMSAY HUNT SYNDROME: CN 5 and 7 involvement with facial paralysis

ZOSTER SINE HERPETAE: zoster-type dermatomal pain without rash

Diagnosis: characteristic skin lesions, Tzanck's prep, serology (IgG antibodies), culture, ELISA

Prevention: vaccination in patients age 60 years or older (safety and efficacy demonstrated in Shingles Prevention Study); reduces incidence (51%), severity and duration of zoster; reduces incidence of pain (61%) and postherpetic neuralgia (67%)

Treatment:

Oral antiviral within 72 hours of rash: acyclovir (800mg 5× /day), famciclovir (Famvir, 500 mg tid), or valacyclovir (Valtrex, 1000mg tid) × 7 days; IV acyclovir × 10-14 days if immunocompromised
Reduces time course (formation of new lesions, healing of lesions, period of viral shedding), and risk and severity of ocular involvement. Famvir and Valtrex reduce risk, duration, and severity of postherpetic neuralgia

Oral steroid: prednisone 60 mg qd × 1 week, then 30 mg qd × 1 week, then 15 mg qd × 1 week
Reduces time course, duration and severity of acute pain, and incidence of postherpetic neuralgia

For intraocular and ocular surface involvement: topical steroid, cycloplegic, and antibiotic; may require IOP control and treatment of ocular complications

For postherpetic neuralgia: capsaicin cream (Zostrix; depletes substance P), cimetidine, tricyclic antidepressants (amitriptyline, desipramine), carbamazepine (Tegretol), gabapentin (Neurontin), pregabalin (Lyrica), lidocaine (Lidoderm patch), opioids, benadryl; consider nerve block, botox map injections

Complications: occur in 50%; most common is postherpetic neuralgia

Postherpetic neuralgia (PHN): neuropathic pain syndrome that persists or occurs after resolution of rash; risk factors include age >60 years, severity of prodromal and acute pain, severity of rash, and HZO. Occurs in 10% of all zoster patients, 10–20% with HZO; 50% resolve within 1 month, 80% within 1 year

Meningoencephalitis and myelitis: rare; occurs 7–10 days after rash with fever, headache, cranial nerve palsies, hallucinations, altered sensorium; most common in patients with cranial zoster, dissemination, or immunocompromised (may be fatal in AIDS)

Granulomatous arteritis: contralateral hemiplegia weeks to months after acute disease; involves middle cerebral artery; 65% are >60 years old; 25% mortality

Table 7-1. Comparison of herpetic epithelial keratitis

Lesion	HSV Dendrite	HZV Pseudodendrite
Appearance	Delicate, fine, lacy ulcer	Coarse, ropy, elevated, 'painted-on' lesion Smaller, less branching than HSV dendrite
	Terminal bulbs	Blunt ends (no terminal bulbs)
	Epithelial cells slough	Epithelial cells are swollen and heaped-up
Staining	Base with fluorescein	Poor with fluorescein and rose bengal
	Edges with rose bengal	
Treatment	Do not use steroids	Good response to steroids

Note: Active viral replication in epithelial lesions occurs in both HSV and HZV

Other causes of pseudodendrite: Acanthamoeba, tyrosinemia II, epithelial healing ridge

Chickenpox

Findings: papillary conjunctivitis, 'pock' lesions on bulbar conjunctiva and at limbus, keratitis (dendritic, disciform, interstitial)

Fungi

Types:

Molds (filamentous): form hyphae
  SEPTATE: most common cause of fungal keratitis; most common in southern/southwestern United States – *Fusarium* (*F. solani* is most virulent), *Aspergillus, Cuvularia, Paecilomyces, Penicillium, Phialophora*
  NONSEPTATE: *Mucor* (rare cause of keratitis)

Yeast: Candida (most common cause of mycotic ocular infections in northern United States), *Cryptococcus* (associated with endogenous endophthalmitis; rarely keratitis)

Dimorphic fungi: grow as yeast or mold – *Histoplasma, Blastomyces, Coccidioides*

Risk factors:

Molds: corneal injury especially from tree branch or vegetable material, soft contact lens wear

Yeast: therapeutic soft contact lens wear, topical steroid use, nonhealing epithelial defect, decreased host resistance

Findings: satellite infiltrates, feathery edges, endothelial plaque; can penetrate Descemet's membrane

Treatment: topical antifungal (natamycin 5% [filamentous], clotrimazole [*Aspergillus*], amphotericin B 0.15% [yeast], flucytosine 1%, ketoconazole 2%, miconazole 1%, itraconazole 1%, fluconazole 0.5%); cycloplegic

Corneal epithelium is significant barrier to natamycin penetration

Acanthamoeba

22 species; exists as trophozoite or cyst

90% initially misdiagnosed as HSV

Risk factors: cleaning soft contact lenses with homemade saline solution; swimming or hot tubbing while wearing contact lenses

Prevention: heat disinfectant (75°C)

Findings: epithelial cysts (can look like EKC with subepithelial infiltrates and punctate keratopathy), perineural infiltrate (enlarged corneal nerves, decreased corneal sensation, pain [perineuritis]), ring-shaped infiltrate, corneal edema, pseudodendrite, iritis, hypopyon (30–40%), scleritis; may perforate

Diagnosis: calcofluor white, Giemsa stain, culture (non-nutrient agar with *E. coli* overlay; can grow on blood or chocolate agar but not as well), confocal microscopy

Pathology: oval amoebic double-walled cysts in stroma

Treatment: débridement if infection limited to epithelium (may be curative), topical agents
Antibacterial: neomycin, paromomycin (Humatin) 1% 6-8×/day
Antifungal: miconazole 1%, clotrimazole 1%; ketoconazole or itraconazole (oral)
Antiparasitic: propamidine isethionate (Brolene) 0.1% 6×/day, hexamidine (Desomedine) 0.1%, pentamidine (Biocide), polyhexamethylene biguanide (PHMB, Baquacil; swimming pool cleaner) 0.02%, chlorhexidine 0.02%
Steroid: controversial
30% recurrence after penetrating keratoplasty

Microsporidia

Obligate intracellular spore-forming parasite (*Encephalitozoon hellem, E. cuniculi*)

Keratitis in HIV-positive patients

Symptoms: blurred vision, photophobia, foreign body sensation

Findings: diffuse punctate epithelial erosions and intraepithelial opacities; may have sinusitis

Diagnosis: epithelial cells with cytoplasmic inclusions on Giemsa stain

Treatment: fumagillin (10 mg/mL), itraconazole, albendazole

Onchocerciasis

(See Ch. 8, Uveitis)

Leprosy

(See Ch. 8, Uveitis)

Epstein-Barr Virus (EBV)

Findings: multifocal stromal keratitis; may rarely have episcleritis, follicular conjunctivitis, uveitis, optic neuritis

Diagnosis:
Antibodies: viral capsid antigen IgM and IgG and early antigen-diffuse (EA-D) peak at 6–12 weeks; viral capsid antigen (VCA)-IgM and Epstein-Barr nuclear antigen (EBNA) are detectable for life; heterophile antibodies (IgM that reacts to horse and sheep blood cells) peak at 2–3 weeks and last 1 year (Monospot test)
Lymphocytosis: occurs in 70%; peaks at 2–3 weeks
Liver enzymes: elevated

Ectasias

Keratoconus

90% bilateral; onset typically around puberty

Associations:
Systemic conditions: atopy (eye rubbing), Down's syndrome, connective tissue disease (Ehlers-Danlos syndrome, Marfan's syndrome, osteogenesis imperfecta)
Ocular conditions: aniridia, retinitis pigmentosa, VKC, Leber's congenital amaurosis, ectopia lentis, floppy eyelid syndrome, CHED, posterior pPolymorphous dystrophy (PPMD)

Findings: inferior corneal protrusion, stromal thinning at cone apex (apical thinning), apical scarring, Fleischer ring (epithelial iron deposition at base of cone), Vogt's striae (fine deep striae anterior to Descemet's membrane; disappear with external pressure), prominent corneal nerves, scissors reflex on retinoscopy, Munson's sign (angulation of lower lid on downgaze due to corneal protrusion), Rizzutti's sign (conical reflection of light from temporal light source on nasal iris); may develop hydrops
Hydrops: acute corneal edema and clouding due to break in Descemet's membrane; painful or painless; decreased IOP; heals over 6–10 weeks; scarring can occur occasionally with stromal neovascularization

Pathology: breaks in Bowman's membrane, stromal folds, superficial scarring, stromal thinning; Descemet's is normal unless hydrops has occurred (breaks with curled edges covered by adjacent endothelial cells and new Descemet's)

DDx: contact lens-induced corneal warpage, pellucid marginal degeneration, keratoglobus

Diagnosis: corneal topography (irregular astigmatism, central or inferior steepening), keratometry (steep readings, irregular mires)

Treatment: contact lenses (rigid, piggyback) for visual improvement; rigid contact lenses do not stop progression of disease. Corneal collagen crosslinking, Intacs (to stop progression); penetrating keratoplasty for advanced cases; supportive for hydrops (topical steroids, cycloplegic, bandage contact lens)

Posterior Keratoconus

(See Ch. 5, Pediatrics/Strabismus)

Keratoglobus

Rare, sporadic, globular corneal deformity

Associated with connective tissue disorders, Leber's congenital amaurosis

Findings: bilateral corneal thinning, maximal in midperiphery at base of protrusion

Treatment: CL (rigid), penetrating keratoplasty

Pellucid Marginal Degeneration

Onset age 20–40 years old; no sex predilection; more common in Europeans and Japanese

Findings: bilateral, inferior corneal thinning with protrusion above thinnest area; no vascularization; acute hydrops rare

Pathology: resembles keratoconus

Diagnosis: corneal topography (irregular, against-the-rule astigmatism with inferior annular pattern of steepening)

Treatment: contact lenses for visual improvement; corneal collagen crosslinking to stop progression. If severe, a large penetrating keratoplasty may be required

Dystrophies

Inherited genetic disorders (usually defective enzyme or structural protein)

AD except macular, type 3 lattice, gelatinous, and nystagmus-associated form of CHED, which are AR

Genetics: many dystrophies have a mutation of the *BIGH3 (TGFBI)* gene on chromosome 5. These dystrophies tend to be AD and include granular, Avellino's, lattice types 1 and 3, Reis-Bucklers', and Thiel-Behnke's

Onset by age 20 years, except anterior basement membrane dystrophy (ages 30–40), pre-Descemet's (ages 30–40), and Fuchs' (ages 40–50)

Not associated with systemic diseases, except central crystalline dystrophy (associated with hypercholesterolemia with or without hyperlipidemia), and type 2 lattice (Meretoja's syndrome associated with systemic amyloidosis)

Affect central cornea, except Meesmann's, macular, fleck, CHED, and CHSD, which extend to limbus

Anterior

Anterior Basement Membrane (Cogan's Microcystic; Map-Dot-Fingerprint) (AD)

Most common anterior corneal dystrophy

Usually bilateral, can be asymmetric; primarily affects middle-aged women

Symptoms more common in those >30 years old

Symptoms: usually asymptomatic; may have pain, redness, tearing, irritation (recurrent erosions), or decreased vision (subepithelial scarring)

Findings: irregular and often loose epithelium with characteristic appearance (map, dot, fingerprint):
  Map lines: subepithelial connective tissue
  Microcysts: white, putty-like dots (degenerated epithelial cells trapped in abnormal epithelium)
  Fingerprints: parallel lines of basement membrane separating tongues of reduplicated epithelium

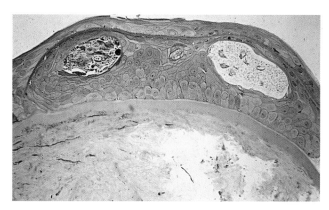

Figure 7-11. ABMD demonstrating cysts and aberrant production of basement membrane material in the epithelium. (From Yanoff M, Fine BS: Ocular Pathology, 5th edn, St Louis, Mosby, 2002.)

May develop recurrent erosions (10% with the dystrophy get erosions, 50% with erosions have the dystrophy) or decreased vision or monocular diplopia from subepithelial scarring (irregular astigmatism)

Pathology: epithelial reduplication with excess subepithelial and intraepithelial production of basement membrane material and collagen (due to poor epithelial adhesion to basement membrane) (Figure 7-11)

Treatment: none unless symptomatic. For erosions, treat with lubrication, hypertonic saline (Muro 128 5% ointment qhs × 3–12 months); if recurs, consider bandage contact lens, epithelial débridement, anterior stromal puncture/reinforcement, diamond burr (débride and polish Bowman's membrane), laser (PTK with excimer laser, or micropuncture with Nd:YAG laser (1 mJ, aim just below epithelium)); also, consider treatment with matrix metalloproteinase-9 inhibitors (doxycycline 50 mg PO bid × 2 months and topical steroids tid × 2–3weeks); débridement for subepithelial scarring

Meesmann's (AD)

Mapped to chromosomes 12q12 and 17

Appears early in life

Minimal symptoms, good vision

Findings: tiny epithelial vesicles, most numerous interpalpebrally, extend to limbus

Pathology: epithelial cells contain PAS-positive material (peculiar substance); thickened epithelial basement membrane (Figure 7-12)

No treatment

Gelatinous Drop–Like (AR)

Mapped to chromosome 1p32

Rare; occurs in 1st decade

Symptoms: decreased vision, photophobia, tearing

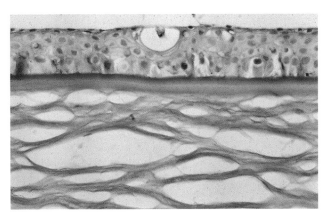

Figure 7-12. Meesmann's dystrophy with Periodic Acid-Schiff stain. (From Yanoff M, Fine BS: Ocular Pathology, 5th edn, St Louis, Mosby, 2002.)

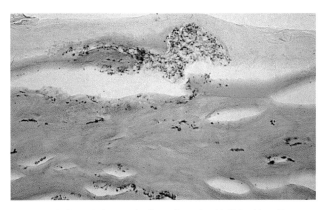

Figure 7-13. Deposits in macular dystrophy stain with Alcian blue. (From Yanoff M, Fine BS: Ocular Pathology, 5th edn, St Louis, Mosby, 2002.)

Findings: central, mulberry-like, subepithelial opacity

Pathology: absence of Bowman's layer; amyloid

Reis-Bucklers' (Corneal Dystrophy of Bowman's Membrane Type I) (AD)

Mapped to chromosome 5q31 (*BIGH3*)

Appears early in life

Findings: subepithelial, irregularly shaped rings with scalloped edges and geographic gray-white reticular opacification, greatest centrally; epithelial erosions, corneal scarring

Pathology: absence of Bowman's layer and replacement by connective tissue; irregular saw-toothed epithelium; curly filaments (electron microscopy); stain with Masson's trichrome

Treatment: penetrating keratoplasty (recurrence is common)

Thiel-Behnke's Dystrophy (Corneal Dystrophy of Bowman's Membrane Type II) (AD)

Mapped to chromosomes 5q31 and 10q24

Honeycomb pattern; *BIGH3* gene defect

Stromal

Mnemonic: Marilyn Monroe Always Gets Her Men in LA County

Refers to name of dystrophy, substance deposited in cornea, special stain (for the 3 classic dystrophies)
    Macular, Mucopolysaccharide, Alcian blue, Granular, Hyaline, Masson's trichrome
    Lattice, Amyloid, Congo red

Macular (AR)

Mapped to chromosome 16q22; error in synthesis of keratan sulfate

Most severe but least common of the 3 classic stromal dystrophies

Deposits present in 1st decade of life

Symptoms: decreased vision in 1st–2nd decade of life

Findings: gray-white stromal opacities at all levels extending to periphery with diffuse clouding (no intervening clear spaces), central thinning; may have guttata

Pathology: mucopolysaccharide deposits, stain with Alcian blue and colloidal iron (Figure 7-13)

Treatment: penetrating keratoplasty; PTK (less useful, lesions extend though entire stroma and erosions rare)

Granular (AD)

Most common stromal dystrophy
Mapped to chromosome 5q31 (*BIGH3*)
Deposits present in 1st decade of life, can remain asymptomatic for decades

Symptoms: mild irritation, decreased vision

Findings: discrete focal, white, granular deposits in central anterior stroma with intervening clear areas; recurrent erosions rare

Superficial variant: looks like Reis-Bucklers'

Pathology: hyaline deposits, stain with Masson's trichrome (Figure 7-14)

Treatment: penetrating keratoplasty, PTK

Lattice

Mapped to chromosome 5q31 (BIGH3)
Deposits present in 1st decade of life

Symptoms: pain, decreased vision in 2nd–3rd decade of life

Findings: branching refractile lines in anterior stroma (best seen in retroillumination), central subepithelial white

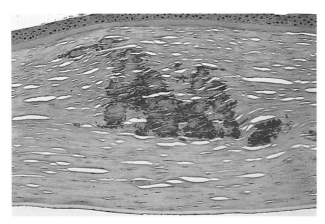

Figure 7-14. Deposits in granular dystrophy stain red with trichrome. (From Yanoff M, Fine BS: Ocular Pathology, 5th edn, St Louis, Mosby, 2002.)

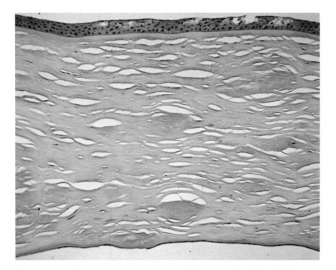

Figure 7-15. Deposits in lattice dystrophy. (From Yanoff M, Fine BS: Ocular Pathology, 5th edn, St Louis, Mosby, 2002.)

dots, stromal haze with ground-glass appearance, peripheral cornea typically clear (depends on type); eventually recurrent erosions with scarring

Types:
Type I (Biber-Haab-Dimmer) (AR): classic lattice dystrophy; starts centrally, spares periphery, no systemic amyloid; *BIGH3* gene defect
Type II (Meretoja's syndrome) (AR): Mapped to chromosome 9q32-34 (*GSN*); Finnish descent; systemic amyloidosis (facial mask; dry, lax skin; blepharochalasis, dermatochalasis; pendulous ears; cranial and peripheral nerve palsies); corneal involvement more peripheral and moves centrally
Type III (AR): Japanese descent, adult onset, thicker lattice lines, limbus to limbus, no recurrent erosions; *BIGH3* gene defect

Pathology: amyloid deposits, stain with Congo red, thioflavin T, metachromatic with crystal violet, apple-green birefringence and dichroism with polarization microscopy (Figure 7-15)

Treatment: penetrating keratoplasty (recurrence more likely than in macular or granular, but less likely than in Reis-Bucklers')

Avellino's

Mapped to chromosome 5q31 (*BIGH3*)
First identified in family from Avellino, Italy

Findings: appears like granular dystrophy with interspersed lattice lines; granular deposits occur early in anterior stroma, lattice findings occur later in deeper stroma; stromal haze; may get erosions

Pathology: hyaline and amyloid deposits; stain with Masson's trichrome and Congo red

Central Crystalline (Schnyder's) (AD)

Mapped to chromosome 1p36

Slowly progressive, rarely reduces vision enough to require corneal transplantation

Findings: minute yellow-white crystals just beneath Bowman's membrane in central doughnut-like pattern, diffuse stromal haze, dense arcus with age, limbal girdle of Vogt; no recurrent erosions; hyperlipidemia or hypercholesterolemia (33%); may have short forearms and genu valgum

Pathology: cholesterol and neutral fat deposits, stain with oil-red-O
Can recur in graft

Fleck (Francois-Neetans') (AD)

Congenital, nonprogressive, asymmetric or unilateral

Usually not present before age 15

Vision usually not affected

Findings: discrete, flat, gray-white, dandruff-like speck and ring-shaped opacities, extending to periphery; decreased corneal sensation
Associated with limbal dermoid, keratoconus, central cloudy corneal dystrophy (Francois'), punctate cortical lens changes, pseudoxanthoma elasticum, atopy

Pathology: glycosaminoglycan and lipid deposits, stain with Alcian blue and colloidal iron (GAGs), Sudan black and oil-red-O (lipid)

Central Cloudy (Francois') (AD)

Nonprogressive

Vision usually not affected

Findings: multiple, nebulous, polygonal gray areas separated by crack-like intervening clear zones (looks similar to crocodile shagreen); most dense centrally and posteriorly, fade anteriorly and peripherally

Posterior Amorphous Stromal (AD)

Early in life, minimally progressive or nonprogressive

Findings: diffuse gray-white stromal opacities concentrated in posterior stroma, mostly centrally but extends to periphery

Associated with hyperopia, central thinning, flat corneal topography, anterior iris abnormalities, fine iris processes extending to Schwalbe's line

Congenital Hereditary Stromal (CHSD)

(See Ch. 5, Pediatrics/Strabismus)

Endothelial

Cornea Guttata

Associated with aging and with corneal endothelial dystrophy

Beaten metal appearance

Most never develop corneal edema

Pathology: thickened Descemet's with localized excrescences of collagen; variable endothelial size and shape and reduced number on specular microscopy

Fuchs' (AD)

Early onset (mapped to chromosome 1p32-34) or late onset (mapped to chromosomes 13 and 18 (*TCF4*)

Variable penetrance, may be sporadic

Most common in postmenopausal women

Symptoms: blurred vision (initially, only in morning; later, all day); may have pain (ruptured bullae)

Findings: guttata, stromal edema, Descemet's folds, endothelial pigment dusting, epithelial bullae, subepithelial fibrosis; may develop degenerative pannus

Pathology: guttata, thickened BM, atrophic endothelium with areas of cell dropout, endothelial cell polymegathism and pleomorphism

Treatment: hypertonic ointment, contact lens or conjunctival flap (Gunderson) for comfort; may require Descemet's stripping endothelial keratoplasty (DSEK) or penetrating keratoplasty

Posterior Polymorphous (PPMD) (AD, Occasionally AR)

Mapped to chromosome 20p11

Minimally or nonprogressive; occurs early in life

Vision usually normal

Endothelium behaves like epithelium, forming multiple layers with occasional migration of cells into angle causing glaucoma (15%)

Findings: isolated grouped vesicles, geographically shaped discrete gray lesions, broad bands with scalloped edges; variable amounts of stromal edema, corectopia, and broad iridocorneal adhesions

Pathology: irregular blebs or vacuoles at level of Descemet's surrounded by gray opacification, thickened Descemet's, abnormal endothelial cells (resemble epithelial cells; contain keratin, microvilli, desmosomes)

DDx: Haab's striae in congenital glaucoma, ICE syndrome

Treatment: penetrating keratoplasty for endothelial decompensation, can recur in graft

Congenital Hereditary Endothelial (CHED)

(See Ch. 5, Pediatrics/Strabismus)

Miscellaneous

Delle(n)

Focal thinning(s) from dehydration due to adjacent area of elevation (i.e. pingueculum, pterygium, filtering bleb)

Treatment: lubrication; punctal occlusion to raise tear film; may require removal of inciting lesion

Descemetocele

Extreme focal thinning of cornea in which only Descemet's membrane remains

Due to corneal melt (see Corneal melt section)

High risk of perforation

Bullous Keratopathy

Corneal edema with epithelial bullae, thickened stroma, but no guttata

Due to loss or dysfunction of endothelial cells

May develop fibrovascular pannus

Etiology: aphakia, pseudophakia (rigid AC IOL), vitreocorneal touch, iridocorneal touch, sequela of severe or chronic keratitis

Pathology: blister-like elevations of corneal epithelium, damaged hemidesmosomes

DDx of corneal edema: aphakic bullous keratopathy (ABK), PBK, inflammation, infection, Fuchs' dystrophy, PPMD, CHED, hydrops, acute angle-closure glaucoma, congenital glaucoma, graft failure, contact lens overwear, hypotony, birth trauma, ICE syndrome, anterior segment ischemia, Brown-McLean syndrome

> *Brown-McLean Syndrome:* peripheral corneal decompensation in aphakic patients, central cornea clear
>> **ETIOLOGY:** uncertain, possibly mechanical irritation from floppy peripheral iris

Neurotrophic Keratitis

Corneal anesthesia due to CN 5 lesion

Disruption of reflex arc between CN V$_1$ and lacrimal gland in anesthetic eye causes epithelial abnormalities

Findings: conjunctival injection, corneal edema, nonhealing epithelial defects, risk of infection and perforation; may have AC reaction

DDx: familial dysautonomia, topical anesthetic abuse, 'crack' cornea (anesthesia from smoking crack cocaine), HSV, HZV

Diagnosis: decreased corneal sensation (test with cotton-tipped applicator or anesthesiometer)

Treatment: lubrication; consider prophylactic antibiotic, bandage CL, punctal plugs, tarsorrhaphy, Boston ocular surface keratoprosthesis

Familial Dysautonomia (Riley-Day Syndrome)

(See Ch. 5, Pediatrics/Strabismus)

Exposure Keratopathy

Desiccation of corneal epithelium due to CN 7 lesion (failure to close eyelids)

Findings: epithelial defects; may develop infection, melt, perforation

Treatment: lubrication, moisture chamber goggles, lid taping at bedtime; consider tarsorrhaphy, lid weights

Contact Lens-related Problems

SPK: mechanical or chemical (solutions)

3 and 9 o'clock staining: due to poor wetting of peripheral cornea; refit lens

Abrasion: increased risk of infection in CL wearers
  Treatment: topical antibiotics, never patch

Infiltrates: hypoxia, antigenic reaction to preservatives in CL solutions, infection
  Treatment: stop CL wear, topical antibiotics

Edema: epithelial microcystic edema due to altered metabolism; associated with extended wear CL
  Treatment: decrease wear time; switch to daily wear lenses

Giant papillary conjunctivitis (GPC): sensitivity to CL material, deposits on CL, or mechanical irritation
  Treatment: stop CL wear, topical allergy medication

Superior limbic keratoconjunctivitis (SLK): may be due to hypersensitivity or toxic reaction to thimerosal
  Treatment: resolves with discontinuation of lens wear

Neovascularization: superficial, deep, sectoral, or 360°; due to chronic hypoxia
  Treatment: refit lens with increased oxygen transmission; stop lens wear if significant vascularization

Corneal warpage: irregular astigmatism related to lens material (hard > rigid gas-permeable [RGP] > soft), fit, and length of time of wear; not associated with corneal edema. Usually asymptomatic; may have contact lens intolerance, blurred vision with glasses, loss of best spectacle-corrected visual acuity, or change in refraction (especially axis of astigmatism); corneal topography is abnormal (irregular astigmatism)
  Treatment: discontinue lens wear; repeat refraction and corneal topography until stable

Corneal Transplant Failure

Early (primary): poor tissue or surgery

Late: allograft rejection (delayed onset [at least 2 weeks]); homograft reaction

Risk factors: young age, stromal vascularization, previous graft failure, post chemical burns, inflammatory disease

Symptoms: decreased vision, redness, pain, irritation

Findings:
  Epithelial rejection line ('battle' line of host-versus-donor epithelium): occurs in 10%, often precedes more destructive rejection events
  Endothelial rejection: anterior chamber reaction, keratitic precipitates, graft edema, Khodadoust rejection line (moves across cornea destroying endothelium, resulting in stromal edema)
  Other findings: subepithelial infiltrates, new KP, increased IOP (trabeculitis from AC reaction)

Treatment:
  Endothelial rejection: IV steroids (methylprednisone 500 mg; reduces risk of subsequent rejection episodes [33% vs 67% for oral steroids]), topical steroids (40% reversal rate alone), oral steroids
  Epithelial rejection or stromal infiltrates with no graft swelling: treat with topical therapy alone

Prognosis: graft survival rate for treating endothelial rejections with a single pulse of IV steroids is 90% when presents within 1 week and 67% when presents later than 1 week (probably due to irreversible damage to endothelial cells despite reversal of rejection)

Epithelial Downgrowth

Can occur following almost any intraocular surgery; increased risk with complicated surgery associated with hemorrhage, inflammation, vitreous loss, or incarcerated tissue

Surface epithelium grows through wound into eye, covering anterior segment structures

Appears as advancing line on corneal endothelium

Epithelium can cover the endothelium (leading to edema) and the angle (resulting in glaucoma); contact inhibition by healthy endothelium may inhibit this

Pathology: multilayered nonkeratinized squamous epithelium; PAS stains conjunctival goblet cells (differentiates between corneal and conjunctival epithelium) (Figure 7-16)

DDx of retrocorneal membrane: mesodermal dysgenesis, ICE syndrome, trauma, posterior polymorphous dystrophy, disciform keratitis (HSV or HZV), alkali burn

Diagnosis: argon laser application to surface of iris produces white burn if iris involved; helps delineate extent of epithelial membrane

Treatment: excision of epithelial membrane and involved tissue with cryotherapy to remaining corneal membrane; high-power laser ablation of entire membrane may occasionally work; complete excision is difficult

Prognosis: poor, often develop secondary glaucoma

Fibrous Ingrowth

Fibrous proliferation through wound into AC

Less progressive and destructive than epithelial downgrowth

Fibroblasts originate from episclera or corneal stroma

Limbal Stem Cell Deficiency

Etiology: destruction of stem cells (chemical burn, Stevens-Johnson syndrome, corneal infections) or dysfunction of stem cells (aniridia, multiple endocrine deficiency, neurotrophic)

Symptoms: decreased vision, photophobia, pain, tearing, blepharospasm

Findings: conjunctivilization of cornea, corneal vascularization, poor epithelial integrity, chronic inflammation

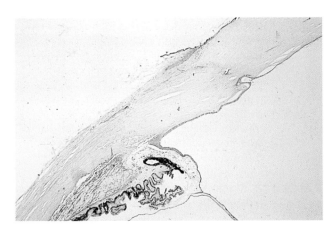

Figure 7-16. Epithelial downgrowth with epithelium present on corneal endothelium, angle, and iris, and into vitreous. (From Yanoff M, Fine BS: Ocular Pathology, 5th edn, St Louis, Mosby, 2002.)

Pathology: Bowman's membrane destruction, fibrous tissue ingrowth

Diagnosis: impression cytology (presence of goblet cells on cornea); corneal epithelium takes up fluorescein

Treatment: limbal stem cell transplant (autograft [from other eye if unilateral], allograft [amniotic membrane]); poor candidate for penetrating keratoplasty; risk of recurrent conjunctivilization

Graft-Versus-Host Disease (GVHD)

Ominous complication of bone marrow transplant (BMT)

3 requirements: Graft must contain immunologically competent cells
  Host must possess important transplantation isoantigens lacking in graft (so host appears foreign)
  Host must not be able to mount immunologic reaction against graft

Types of bone marrow transplants:
  Autologous: patient's own stored marrow
  Syngeneic: marrow from identical twin
  Allogeneic: marrow from HLA-matched donor

Complications:
  Acute: hemorrhage and infection (first 100 days following BMT [period of aplasia])
  Late: GVHD (T lymphocytes in transplanted marrow recognize antigens of host as foreign, become sensitized, and attack host's organs; minor histocompatability antigens are the inciting antigens, cytotoxic T cells are the effectors)

Occurs primarily in allogeneic grafts: 50% develop acute GVHD (50% mortality); 20–40% develop chronic GVHD

Acute GVHD is biggest risk factor for chronic GVHD

Findings: hemorrhagic cicatricial conjunctivitis, pseudomembranes, symblepharon, punctate keratitis, keratoconjunctivitis sicca, lagophthalmos, entropion, microvascular retinopathy (4–10%), optic neuropathy (2%; thought to be due to cyclosporine [ciclosporin], resolves with discontinuation)

Other findings:
  Acute GVHD: maculopapular rash on palms and soles, pruritus, GI involvement (diarrhea), elevated liver enzymes
  Chronic GVHD: sclerodermatoid or lichenoid skin changes, Sjögren's-like syndrome

Diagnosis: skin, liver, intestinal biopsy

Treatment: cyclosporine, high-dose systemic steroids; treat ocular complications

Prognosis: acute GVHD (stage 2 or higher) occurs in 12% and has a 90% mortality; chronic GVHD 10-year survival = 40%

Iridocorneal Endothelial Syndrome (ICE)

(See Ch. 10, Anterior Segment)

Multiple Endocrine Neoplasia (MEN)

MEN 1 (Werner's syndrome): Mapped to chromosome 11
Neoplasias of pituitary, parathyroid, and islet cells of pancreas
Findings: visual field defects from pituitary tumors

MEN 2a (Sipple's syndrome) (AD): Mapped to chromosome 10
Medullary thyroid carcinoma, pheochromocytoma, parathyroid adenomas
Findings: prominent corneal nerves
Pathology: thickened conjunctival nerves contain numerous Schwann cells and partially myelinated axons; thickened corneal nerves are due to an increased number of axons per nerve fiber bundle
Diagnosis: elevated calcitonin and vanillylmandelic acid

MEN 2b (Sipple-Gorlin syndrome) (AD): Mapped to chromosome 10
Medullary thyroid carcinoma, pheochromocytoma, mucosal and GI neuromas, marfanoid habitus
Eye findings: prominent corneal nerves, conjunctival neuroma (87%), eyelid neuroma (80%), dry eye (67%), prominent perilimbal blood vessels (40%)
DDx of prominent corneal nerves: leprosy, *Acanthamoeba*, Down's syndrome, neurofibromatosis, keratoconus, congenital glaucoma, Refsum's disease, Fuchs' corneal endothelial dystrophy, failed corneal graft, keratoconjunctivitis sicca, trauma, advanced age, ichthyosis, posterior polymorphous dystrophy

Tumors

Corneal Intraepithelial Neoplasia (CIN)

(See Conjunctiva section)

Squamous Cell Carcinoma (SCC)

(See Conjunctiva section)

SCLERAL DISORDERS

Episcleritis

Inflammation of episclera

Self-limited, usually young adults

33% bilateral; 67% recurrent

Associated with HZV, RA, gout

Signs: sectoral (70%) or diffuse (30%) injection with mild or no discomfort; may have nodule (20%), chemosis, AC reaction

Pathology: nongranulomatous vascular dilatation, perivascular lymphocytic infiltration; diffuse or nodular

(similar to rheumatoid scleritis but limited to episclera); palisade of epithelioid cells bordering central fibrinoid necrosis

Diagnosis: blanches with topical 2.5% phenylephrine; if lasts for >3 weeks, perform systemic workup

Treatment: topical vasoconstrictor (Naphcon A) or mild topical steroid (FML, loteprednol [Alrex, Lotemax])

Scleritis

Inflammation of sclera

More common in females; onset age 30–60 years

>50% bilateral

Etiology: 50% associated with systemic disease
Collagen vascular diseases (RA [20% of all cases of scleritis; only 3% of patients with RA develop scleritis; 75% of RA-related scleritis is bilateral], SLE, polyarteritis nodosa), vascular disease (Wegener's granulomatosis, giant cell arteritis, Takayasu's disease), relapsing polychondritis, sarcoidosis, ankylosing spondylitis, Reiter's syndrome, Crohn's disease, ulcerative colitis, infections (syphilis, TB, leprosy, HSV, HZV), gout, rosacea

Classification:
Anterior: 98%
  DIFFUSE (40%): most benign; widespread involvement
    PATHOLOGY: sclera thickened, diffuse granulomatous inflammation of scleral collagen
  NODULAR (44%): focal involvement; nodule is immobile
    PATHOLOGY: zonal necrotizing granuloma, fibrinoid necrosis, chronic inflammation, fusiform thickening, immune complex deposition with complement activation; once collagen has been destroyed, inflammation recedes, uvea herniates into defect
  NECROTIZING (14%): associated with life-threatening autoimmune disease (5-year mortality rate = 25%)
    WITH INFLAMMATION: focal or diffuse, progressive, pain and redness; vascular sludging and occlusion; underlying blue uveal tissue may be visible giving redness a 'violaceous' hue; 40% lose vision; 60% have ocular complications: anterior uveitis, sclerosing keratitis, cataract, glaucoma, peripheral corneal melt, scleral thinning
    WITHOUT INFLAMMATION (scleromalacia perforans): minimal symptoms, minimal injection; scleral thinning, marked ischemia; seldom perforate; females with severe rheumatoid arthritis; 8-year mortality rate = 21%
Posterior: 2%; usually unilateral; very painful
  Usually no associated systemic disorder
  80% have anterior scleritis
  FINDINGS: thickened and inflamed posterior sclera, chorioretinal folds, amelanotic fundus mass, ON edema; may have vitritis, macular edema, limitation of motility, ptosis, proptosis, exudative

RD, elevated IOP (forward shift of lens-iris diaphragm due to ciliochoroidal detachment)

B-SCAN ULTRASOUND: pocket of fluid in Tenon's space (sclerotenonitis), T sign, thickened sclera

FA: early patchy hypofluorescence, late staining, disc leakage

CT SCAN: thickening of posterior sclera with contiguous involvement of orbital fat (T sign)

DDX: choroidal tumor, orbital pseudotumor (IOI), uveal effusion syndrome, VKH, thyroid-related ophthalmopathy, orbital tumors

Symptoms: pain, redness, photophobia

Findings: diffuse or sectoral area of deep injection (violaceous hue), tender to touch, chemosis, scleral edema; may have scleral nodule, scleral thinning, AC reaction (33%), keratitis (acute stromal keratitis, sclerosing keratitis, marginal keratolysis); chorioretinal folds and serous RD in posterior scleritis

Diagnosis: does not blanch with topical phenylephrine

Lab tests: CBC, ESR, RF, ANA, ANCA (antineutrophil cytoplasmic antibody), VDRL, FTA-ABS, uric acid, blood urea nitrogen (BUN), PPD, CXR

ANCA (antineutrophil cytoplasmic antibodies): positive in Wegener's; also polyarteritis nodosa, Churg-Strauss, and crescentic glomerulonephritis

2 TYPES:

C-ANCA (cytoplasmic; positive in Wegener's)

P-ANCA (perinuclear; positive in polyarteritis nodosa [PAN])

Anterior segment fluorescein angiogram: may detect nonperfusion and vaso-obliteration

Treatment: oral NSAID, consider oral steroids or immunosuppressive agents; treat underlying disorder; topical steroids are not effective; sub-Tenon's steroid injection is contraindicated; may require patch graft for perforation

Complications: keratitis, cataract, uveitis, glaucoma

Wegener's Granulomatosis

Systemic disease of necrotizing vasculitis and granulomatous inflammation involving sinuses, respiratory system, kidneys, and orbit

Males > females

Findings (60%): nasolacrimal duct obstruction, proptosis, painful ophthalmoplegia, conjunctivitis, chemosis, KCS, episcleritis, necrotizing scleritis (most common type of ocular involvement), keratitis, cotton-wool spots, arterial narrowing, venous tortuosity, choroidal thickening, CME, CRAO, optic nerve involvement

Other findings: upper respiratory tract (hemoptysis), renal failure (major cause of death), hemorrhagic dermatitis, cerebral vasculitis, weight loss, peripheral neuropathy, fever, arthralgia, saddle nose (destruction of nasal bones)

Diagnosis: C-ANCA positive in 67%

Treatment: systemic steroids and immunosuppressives (cyclophosphamide)

Complications: fatal if untreated

Takayasu's Disease

Narrowing of large branches of aorta

Diminished pulsations in upper extremities

Decreased blood pressure in upper extremities, increased BP in lower extremities

Findings: scleritis, amaurosis fugax, ocular ischemia, AION

Polyarteritis Nodosa

Systemic vasculitis affecting medium-sized and small arteries

Males > females

Findings: necrotizing sclerokeratitis, vascular occlusions, ischemic optic neuropathy, rarely aneurysms of retinal vessels

Other findings: kidneys (nephritic or nephrotic syndrome, hypertension, renal failure), heart (MI, angina, pericarditis), intestines (pain, infarction), arthritis, peripheral neuropathy

Relapsing Polychondritis

Multisystem disorder characterized by recurrent episodes of inflammation in cartilaginous tissues throughout body

Findings (60%): episcleritis, scleritis, iritis, conjunctivitis, keratoconjunctivitis sicca (KCS), exudative RD, optic neuritis, proptosis, CN 6 palsies

Other findings: migratory polyarthritis, fever, diffuse inflammation of cartilage (nose, ear, trachea, larynx)

Treatment: topical or systemic steroids; dapsone

Discoloration

Blue sclera: sclera appears blue owing to thinning and visualization of underlying uvea

DDx: Ehlers-Danlos, Hurler's, Turner's, and Marfan's syndromes; osteogenesis imperfecta, scleromalacia perforans, congenital staphyloma

Scleral icterus: yellow sclera caused by hyperbilirubinemia

Ochronosis (alkaptonuria) (AR): homogentisic acid oxidase deficiency

Homogentisic acid accumulates, metabolized into melanin-like compound with brown pigmentation of cartilage (ear, nose, heart valves) and sclera; excreted in urine (dark)

Findings: triangular pigment deposits anterior to rectus muscle insertions, pinhead-sized peripheral corneal stromal deposits, pigmentation of tarsus and lids

Cogan's senile scleral plaque: blue-gray hyalinization of sclera anterior to horizontal rectus muscle insertions

SURGERY

Penetrating Keratoplasty (PK; PKP)

Full-thickness corneal graft/transplant

Most common indications: bullous keratopathy (pseudophakic, aphakic), keratoconus, graft failure, corneal scar; Peter's anomaly (children)

Success rate: 90% of grafts are clear at 1 year (>90% for keratoconus; 65% for HSV)

Complications: rejection (20%), failure, glaucoma, suprachoroidal or expulsive hemorrhage, endophthalmitis, recurrence of pathology

Collaborative Corneal Transplant Treatment Study (CCTS):
ABO blood type incompatability is a possible risk factor for rejection
HLA matching is not cost-effective or advantageous
High-risk status: vascularization of cornea in 2 quadrants, history of previous graft rejection, glaucoma, extensive PAS, traumatic or hereditary ocular surface disorders

Donor screening:
Contraindications for donor corneas: septicemia, lymphoma or leukemia, systemic malignancy with ocular metastasis, anterior segment tumors (choroidal melanoma is not a contraindication), Creutzfeldt-Jakob disease, rabies, subacute sclerosing panencephalitis, PML, HIV, hepatitis B and C (neither HIV nor hepatitis C has ever been transmitted)

Tissue preservation:
4°C moist chamber: use within 48 hours
M-K medium (McCarey-Kaufman): TC-199 medium with dextran (5% concentration) and gentamicin stored at 4°C; use within 48 hours
Chondroitin sulfate: acts as antioxidant and membrane growth factor
K-Sol (Kaufman): chondroitin sulfate in TC-199 at 4°C; discontinued
Corneal storage media (CSM): from Minnesota Lions Eye Bank researchers plus mercaptoethanol (antioxidant) and chondroitin sulfate; discontinued with introduction of dexsol and optisol
Dexsol: minimal essential medium with chondroitin sulfate and dextran 1% (osmotic agent to keep cornea thin)

Optisol: hybrid of K-Sol, Dexsol, and CSM, plus vitamins, amino acids, and antioxidants; as effective as dexsol but keeps cornea thinner
Many media contain pH indicators that change color with a change in pH (i.e. microbial contamination)

Lamellar Keratoplasty (ALK, DALK)

Partial or full-thickness stromal graft composed of epithelium, Bowman's membrane, and stroma. Anterior lamellar keratoplasty (ALK) involves a stromal dissection, while deep anterior lamellar keratoplasty (DALK) entails replacement of stromal tissue down to the level of Descemet's membrane. The dissection can be performed manually, with an air bubble or viscoelastic

Indications: stromal pathology (scar, dystrophy) and keratoconus (DALK)

Contraindications: corneal endothelial dysfunction

Complications: graft rejection, suture-related complications, and interface opacification can occur with both procedures; intraoperative Descemet's membrane tear or perforation can occur with DALK requiring conversion to penetrating keratoplasty.

Endothelial Keratoplasty (EK)

Descemet's Stripping and Automated Endothelial Keratoplasty (DSAEK): Endothelium is manually stripped and replaced by donor lenticule composed of endothelium, Descemet's membrane, and thin layer of stroma prepared with a microkeratome

Indications: corneal edema due to Fuchs' dystrophy and bullous keratopathy

Complications: endothelial rejection, lenticule separation or displacement

Alternatives: Descemet's Membrane Endothelial Keratoplasty (DMEK; requires peripheral iridotomy/iridectomy), Descemet's Membrane and Automated Endothelial Keratoplasty (DMAEK; lenticule has peripheral ring of stroma) require smaller incision and may have better vision

Keratophakia

Donor lenticule is placed between the cornea and a microkeratome created lamellar section to correct aphakia

Contraindications: thinned corneas, infants, glaucoma

Keratomileusis

Lamellar section is removed, frozen, shaped on a cryolathe, then replaced in stromal bed to correct myopia or hyperopia. Donor lenticule can be used instead (Figure 7-17)

Contraindications: glaucoma

Epikeratophakia (Epikeratoplasty)

Epithelium is removed and a lathed donor lenticule is placed to correct myopia or hyperopia (Figure 7-18)

Can be performed in children; reversible

Contraindications: blepharitis, dry eye, lagophthalmos

Pathology: 2 Bowman's membranes (donor lenticule and patient)

Astigmatic Keratotomy (AK)

99% depth arcuate or straight incisions typically placed at the 7 or 8 mm optical zone (OZ) to correct astigmatism

Various nomograms exist (i.e. Lindstrom ARC-T)

Do not make arcuate incisions >90° (decreased efficacy, increased instability)

When combined with RK, do not cross incisions (creates wound gape and instability)

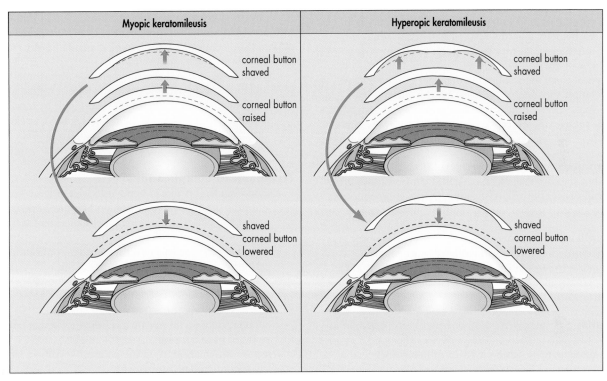

Figure 7-17. Keratomileusis. In a myopic keratomileusis, a corneal button is raised using a microkeratome, and it is reshaped using a cryolathe (*upper part*). When the button is replaced, the central cornea is flattened (*lower part*). (From Chang SW, Azar DT: Automated and manual lamellar surgical procedures and epikeratoplasty. In Yanoff M, Duker JS [eds]: Ophthalmology, London, Mosby, 1999.)

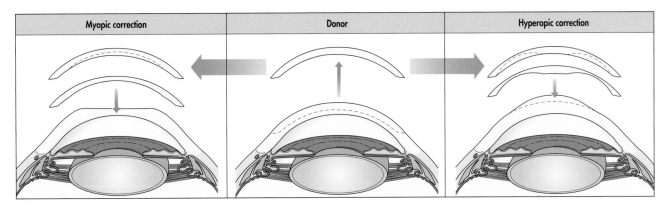

Figure 7-18. Epikeratoplasty. A preshaped donor lenticule is sutured to the recipient stromal bed to correct myopia and hyperopia. (From Chang SW, Azar DT: Automated and manual lamellar surgical procedures and epikeratoplasty. In Yanoff M, Duker JS [eds]: Ophthalmology, London, Mosby, 1999.)

Limbal/corneal relaxing incisions (LRI/CRI) are performed at 10–12 mm OZ, usually at time of cataract surgery with preset diamond knife (500–600 μm depth)

Radial Keratotomy (RK)

Deep radial corneal incisions to correct low to moderate myopia

Effect dependent on number of incisions, depth of incisions, size of optical zone, patient age

Number of incisions: the greater the number of incisions, the greater the effect; never use more than 8 incisions (additional incisions have limited effect and cause greater destabilization of the cornea)

Incision depth: the deeper the incision, the greater the effect; diamond knife is set at 100% of thinnest pachymetry measurement (usually paracentral inferotemporal region; temporal < inferior < nasal < superior)

Optical zone: the smaller the diameter of the OZ (the longer the incision), the greater the effect; do not make OZ <3 mm (visual aberrations [starburst])

Patient age: the older the patient, the greater the effect

Patient sex: greater effect in males than in females

Technique: American (downhill cut [toward limbus], safer but shallower) vs Russian (uphill cut [toward central cornea], deeper but risk of invading OZ); combined technique with special knife gives deep cut with safety

Complications: undercorrection or overcorrection, perforation, infection, scarring, irregular astigmatism, progressive hyperopia (in PERK study, 43% had ≥1.00 D of hyperopia after 10 years), glare/starburst, fluctuating vision

Results: 85% achieved 20/40 or better vision after initial procedure; 96% achieved 20/40 or better after enhancement, 85% achieved 20/25 or better after enhancement

Photorefractive Keratectomy (PRK)

Laser ablation of corneal surface to correct myopia, hyperopia, and astigmatism

Excimer (excited dimer) laser: argon-fluoride (wavelength = 193 nm; far ultraviolet), energy = 64 eV

Functions as a 'cold' laser (breaks molecular bonds to ablate tissue; no thermal damage)

Each pulse removes approximately 0.25 μm of corneal tissue

Depth of ablation is related to diameter of optical zone and amount of intended correction

Munnerlyn equation: depth = (refractive error/3) × OZ²
   Example: 12 μm for 6 mm OZ and 1 D of myopia

Advantages of PRK: precise removal of tissue, minimal adjacent tissue damage

Disadvantages of PRK: involves visual axis, risk of haze/scarring, regression, requires removal of epithelium

Contraindications: collagen vascular, autoimmune, or immunodeficiency disorders; pregnancy; corneal ectasia; keloid formation; isotretinoin (Accutane), amiodarone, sumatriptan (Imitrex)

Cautions: unstable refraction (change of >0.5 D/year), systemic diseases that affect wound healing (diabetes, atopy, connective tissue diseases, immunocompromised status), herpes keratitis (HSV or HZV), ocular inflammation (keratitis, acne rosacea, pannus that extends into visual axis)

Complications: undercorrection or overcorrection, haze/scarring, delayed reepithelialization, sterile infiltrates, infection, decentered ablation, central island, irregular astigmatism, keratectasia, regression, glare, halos, dry eye, glaucoma or cataract (from steroids)

Corneal haze: risk and severity increases with deeper ablations and postoperative ultraviolet (UV) radiation exposure; results in decreased vision with regression of effect. Oral vitamin C 1000 mg/day for 1 week before surgery and 2 weeks postoperatively, and avoidance of UV exposure may help prevent haze

Treatment of complications:

Enhancements: it is recommended to wait at least 3 months or until the refraction and corneal topography are stable before performing an enhancement for overcorrection or undercorrection

Haze: treat with topical steroids; consider application of mitomycin C 0.02% for 2 minutes along with scar débridement with either a diamond burr or a superficial excimer laser treatment (PTK). Once the haze is reduced, the refraction can change dramatically, so do not treat residual refractive error at time of haze removal

Irregular astigmatism: rigid gas-permeable contact lens, wavefront-guided retreatment

Laser in Situ Keratomileusis (LASIK)

Combination of keratomileusis and excimer laser ablation to correct myopia, hyperopia, and astigmatism

Corneal flap created with mechanical or laser microkeratome and laser ablation performed on underlying stromal bed

Advantages of LASIK: more rapid healing, less discomfort, less risk of haze, less postoperative medications

Disadvantages of LASIK: flap complications

Complications:

Intraoperative: flap complication (buttonhole, incomplete, or irregular flap, free cap) epithelial abrasion or sloughing, programming error, decentered ablation.

Immediate postoperative: diffuse lamellar keratitis (DLK, sands of Sahara), central toxic keratopathy, infection, flap dislocation, flap striae, epithelial ingrowth, central island, irregular astigmatism, dry eye, undercorrection or overcorrection, night vision problems (glare, halos)

Delayed postoperative: dry eye, late DLK, late flap slip, undercorrection or overcorrection, keratectasia, photophobia (from laser keratome, 1–3 weeks to 3 months postop, treat with topical steroids)

Treatment of complications:

Buttonhole (increased risk with steep corneas), incomplete or irregular flap: replace flap, do not perform ablation; when cornea stabilizes, either cut a new flap or perform surface ablation (PRK/PTK)

Free cap (increased risk in cases of flat corneas): place free cap in moisture chamber epithelial side down, perform ablation, then replace cap and let dry

Epithelial slough or corneal abrasion: increased risk with certain microkeratomes and in eyes with epithelial basement membrane dystrophy; increases risk of developing DLK and epithelial ingrowth
   Treat with bandage contact lens and close follow-up. If large defect occurs in first eye, consider postponing treatment of second eye

Flap striae or flap dislocation: replace flap and stretch; consider use of epithelial débridement, hypotonic saline or sterile water, ironing with a warm spatula, or suturing (interrupted radials or antitorque)

DLK: inflammation within flap interface; etiology often unknown; increased risk with epithelial defect. Late DLK may result from increased intraocular pressure, epithelial defect, and cornea ulcer
   Treat with frequent topical steroids for grades I and II, and flap lifting and interface irrigation for grades III and IV; consider a short pulse of oral steroids

Central toxic keratopathy: noninflammatory central corneal opacity and hyperopic shift; appears on postop day 3–5, usually preceded by DLK. No treatment. Spontaneously resolves in 2–18 months. May also occur after PRK

Epithelial ingrowth: nests of epithelium growing under the flap; more common in eyes with epithelial basement membrane dystrophy and after enhancements. Ingrowth that is progressive or affects the vision is treated with flap lifting and débridement of the stromal bed and flap undersurface. Consider radial sutures if ingrowth recurs, Consider Nd:YAG laser treatment

Irregular ablation (decentered, irregular astigmatism): requires custom or wavefront-guided retreatment

Corneal ectasia (keratectasia): treatment of eyes with a preexisting ectasia (keratoconus, forme fruste keratoconus, pellucid marginal degeneration) or excessive depth of ablation in normal corneas (residual stromal depth <250 μm) can result in progressive myopic astigmatism and corneal ectasia. Treat with corneal collagen crosslinking to halt progression. A rigid gas-permeable contact lens can help with visual improvement, but will not stop progression. Consider Intacs to improve the shape of the cornea, or penetrating keratoplasty for severe cases.

Dry eye: can worsen postoperatively if untreated prior to surgery; can also occur in patients without pre-existing dry eye. Superior hinged flap may cause greater dryness than is caused by nasal hinged flap. Treat with frequent lubrication; consider punctal occlusion and topical cyclosporine

Glare/halos: often due to residual refractive error. The role of scotopic pupil size as a contributing factor is controversial (may have been a risk with older laser ablations, but is not a risk factor with modern laser ablations). Treatment options include pharmacologic miosis (Alphagan-P or iilocarpine), or retreatment with larger optical zone or blend zone

Infectious keratitis: uncommon but serious complication; most common organisms are Gram-positive cocci and atypical *Mycobacteria*. Suspected infection requires lifting flap and culturing; treat with fortified topical antibiotics (vancomycin and amikacin); may require flap amputation

Laser-Assisted Epithelial Keratomileusis (LASEK)

Variation of PRK; epithelial flap is created with alcohol, excimer laser is applied, and epithelial flap is replaced

Advantages of LASEK: may have less risk of haze than PRK

Disadvantages of LASEK: slower visual recoevery than with PRK.

Complications: same as with PRK. undercorrection or overcorrection, haze/scarring, delayed reepithelialization, infection, decentered ablation, central island, irregular astigmatism, regression, glare/halos, dry eye, stromal incursion (with mechanical flap device)

Risk of haze can be reduced with oral vitamin C and avoidance of UV exposure

Phototherapeutic Keratectomy (PTK)

Use of excimer laser to ablate corneal pathology limited to anterior ⅓ of cornea

Indications: superficial scars, dystrophies, irregularities, residual band keratopathy, recurrent erosions

Can use confocal microscopy to determine depth of pathology

Complications: recurrence of pathology, reactivation of HSV, induced hyperopia or irregular astigmatism

Intracorneal Inlays

A thin, contact lens-like, implant placed in the central optical zone beneath a corneal flap to correct myopia, hyperopia, astigmatism, or presbyopia without removing corneal tissue

Potential technologies: implant thickness and shape alters the corneal curvature, implant has power, or implant acts as a pinhole.

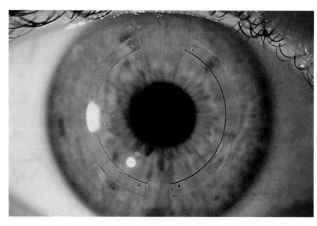

Figure 7-19. Slit-lamp photograph of the intrastromal corneal ring segments in position in patient's cornea. (Courtesy of Mr. Thomas Loarie. From Friedman NJ, Husain SE, Kohnen T et al: Investigational refractive procedures. In: Yanoff M, Duker JS [eds]: Ophthalmology, London, Mosby, 1999.)

Advantages: reversible, adjustable, no removal of tissue

Complications: undercorrection or overcorrection, irregular astigmatism, glare, halos, flap striae, epithelial ingrowth, DLK, infection, implant decentration or extrusion

Intrastromal Corneal Ring Segments (Intacs)

Ring segment implants placed into peripheral corneal channels outside the visual axis to correct low to moderate myopia. Implants flatten the cornea without cutting or removing tissue from the central optical zone. Also used to reshape corneas with keratoconus or post-LASIK ectasia (Figure 7-19)

Advantages: reversible, adjustable, spares visual axis, no removal of tissue

Complications: undercorrection or overcorrection, irregular astigmatism, glare, halos, infection, implant decentration or extrusion, stromal deposits

Conductive Keratoplasty (CK)

A contact probe directly delivers radiofrequency (thermal) energy to the peripheral cornea in a ring pattern to steepen the central corneal and correct low to moderate hyperopia

Advantages: spares visual axis, no removal of tissue

Complications: undercorrection or overcorrection, irregular astigmatism, regression

REVIEW QUESTIONS (Answers start on page 365)

1. Which is the least desirable method for corneal graft storage?
   a. moist chamber at 4°C
   b. glycerin
   c. Optisol
   d. cryopreservation

2. Presently in the United States, phlyctenule is most commonly associated with
   a. HSV
   b. tuberculosis
   c. *Staphylococcus*
   d. fungus

3. Which blood test is most helpful in the evaluation of a patient with Schnyder's crystalline corneal dystrophy?
   a. calcium
   b. uric acid
   c. immunoglobulins
   d. cholesterol

4. Which disease has never been transmitted by a corneal graft?
   a. CMV
   b. Creutzfeldt-Jakob
   c. rabies
   d. *Cryptococcus*

5. Which corneal dystrophy does not recur in a corneal graft?
   a. granular
   b. macular
   c. lattice
   d. PPMD

6. A conjunctival map biopsy is typically used for which malignancy?
   a. squamous cell carcinoma
   b. basal cell carcinoma
   c. sebaceous cell carcinoma
   d. malignant melanoma

7. Corneal clouding does not occur in which mucopolysaccharidosis?
   a. Hunter
   b. Hurler
   c. Scheie
   d. Sly

8. All of the following may cause follicular conjunctivitis except
   a. *Chlamydia*
   b. *Neisseria*
   c. Iopidine
   d. EKC

9. Which of the following tests is least helpful in determining the etiology of enlarged corneal nerves?
   a. EKG
   b. calcitonin
   c. urinary VMA
   d. acid-fast stain

10. Corneal filaments are least likely to be present in which condition?
    a. keratoconjunctivitis sicca
    b. Thygeson's SPK
    c. SLK
    d. medicamentosa

11. Which of the following is not an appropriate treatment for SLK?
    a. bandage contact lens
    b. conjunctival resection
    c. silver nitrate stick
    d. conjunctival cautery

12. In what level of the cornea does a Kayser-Fleischer ring occur?
    a. epithelium
    b. Bowman's membrane
    c. stroma
    d. Descemet's membrane
13. Cornea verticillata-like changes are associated with all of the following except
    a. indomethacin
    b. thorazine
    c. chloroquine
    d. amiodarone
14. The least common location for a nevus is
    a. bulbar conjunctiva
    b. palpebral conjunctiva
    c. caruncle
    d. lid skin
15. All of the following ions move across the corneal endothelium by both active transport and passive diffusion except
    a. Cl⁻
    b. K⁺
    c. Na⁺
    d. H⁺
16. Which organism is associated with crystalline keratopathy?
    a. S. aureus
    b. H. influenzae
    c. Enterococcus
    d. S. viridans
17. Which of the following conditions is associated with the best 5-year prognosis for a corneal graft?
    a. PBK
    b. Fuchs' dystrophy
    c. ABK
    d. HSV
18. The best strategy for loosening a tight contact lens is to
    a. increase the diameter
    b. increase the curvature
    c. decrease the diameter
    d. decrease the curvature
19. The type of contact lens that causes the least endothelial pleomorphism is
    a. soft daily wear
    b. soft extended wear
    c. rigid gas permeable
    d. hard/PMMA
20. Which of the following conditions is associated with the worst prognosis for a corneal graft?
    a. PBK
    b. Fuchs' dystrophy
    c. Reis-Bucklers' dystrophy
    d. keratoglobus
21. Which is not a treatment of acute hydrops?
    a. steroid
    b. homatropine
    c. bandage contact lens
    d. corneal transplant
22. Which organism cannot penetrate intact corneal epithelium?

    a. Corynebacterium diphtheriae
    b. N. gonorrhoeae
    c. Pseudomonas aeruginosa
    d. H. aegyptius
23. Which organism is most commonly associated with angular blepharitis?
    a. S. epidermidis
    b. Moraxella
    c. S. aureus
    d. Demodex folliculorum
24. Which of the following medications would be the best choice in the treatment of microsporidial keratoconjunctivitis?
    a. fumagillin
    b. chloramphenicol
    c. galardin
    d. paromomycin
25. All of the following agents are used in the treatment of Acanthamoeba keratitis except
    a. paromomycin
    b. natamycin
    c. chlorhexidine
    d. miconazole
26. Goblet cells are most abundant in which location?
    a. fornix
    b. plica
    c. bulbar conjunctiva
    d. limbus
27. Thygeson's superficial punctate keratopathy is best treated with topical
    a. cyclosporine (ciclosporin)
    b. idoxuridine
    c. loteprednol
    d. trifluridine
28. EKC is typically contagious for how many days?
    a. 5 days
    b. 7 days
    c. 10 days
    d. 14 days
29. A shield ulcer is associated with
    a. AKC
    b. SLK
    c. VKC
    d. GPC
30. Ulcerative blepharitis is most likely to be caused by
    a. Staphylococcus
    b. Herpes
    c. Moraxella
    d. Demodex
31. Which of the following is most likely to be associated with melanoma of the conjunctiva and uvea?
    a. dysplastic nevus syndrome
    b. melanosis oculi
    c. nevus of Ota
    d. secondary acquired melanosis
32. Which of the following is not associated with N. gonorrheae conjunctivitis?
    a. pseudomembrane
    b. preauricular lymphadenopathy
    c. purulent discharge
    d. corneal ulcer

33. Even spreading of the tear film depends most on which factor?
    a. lipid
    b. aqueous
    c. mucin
    d. epithelium
34. Neurotrophic ulcer should not be treated with
    a. tarsorrhaphy
    b. antiviral
    c. antibiotic
    d. bandage contact lens
35. Which layer of the cornea can regenerate?
    a. Bowman's membrane
    b. stroma
    c. Descemet's membrane
    d. endothelium
36. The most appropriate treatment for a patient with scleromalacia is
    a. topical steroid
    b. sub-Tenon's steroid injection
    c. oral NSAID
    d. oral immunosuppressive agent
37. The HEDS recommendation for treating stromal (disciform) keratitis is
    a. topical steroid alone
    b. topical steroid and topical antiviral
    c. topical steroid and oral antiviral
    d. topical steroid, topical antiviral, and oral antiviral
38. A satellite infiltrate with feathery edges is most characteristic of a corneal ulcer caused by
    a. *Pseudomonas*
    b. *Acanthamoeba*
    c. *Microsporidia*
    d. *Fusarium*
39. PTK would be most appropriate for treating which of the following corneal disorders?
    a. superficial granular dystrophy
    b. anterior stromal neovascularization
    c. mid-stromal herpes scar
    d. Fuchs' dystrophy
40. A 62-year-old woman with keratoconjunctivitis sicca is most likely to demonstrate corneal staining in which location?
    a. superior third
    b. middle third (interpalpebral)
    c. inferior third
    d. diffuse over entire cornea
41. Which of the following findings is most commonly associated with SLK?
    a. filaments
    b. giant papillae
    c. pseudomembrane
    d. follicles
42. Which lab test is most helpful to obtain in a 38-year-old man with herpes zoster ophthalmicus?
    a. ANCA
    b. Lyme titer
    c. chest x-ray
    d. HIV test
43. A patient with conjunctival intraepithelial neoplasia is most likely to have
    a. CMV
    b. EBV
    c. HSV
    d. HPV
44. Which of the following disorders is most likely to be found in a patient suffering from sleep apnea?
    a. iritis
    b. interstitial keratitis
    c. follicular conjunctivitis
    d. trichiasis
45. A patient with graft-vs-host disease is most likely to have which eye finding?
    a. scleritis
    b. symblepharon
    c. optic neuropathy
    d. iritis

SUGGESTED READINGS

American Academy of Ophthalmology: External Disease and Cornea, vol 8. San Francisco, AAO, 2012.

Arffa RC: Grayson's Diseases of the Cornea, 4th edn. St Louis, Mosby, 1998.

Brightbill FS, McDonnell PJ, McGhee CNJ, et al: Corneal Surgery Theory, Technique and Tissue, 4th edn. St Louis, Mosby, 2008.

Kaufman HE, Barron BA, McDonald MB: The Cornea, 2nd edn. Philadelphia, Butterworth-Heinemann, 1997.

Krachmer JH, Mannis MJ, Holland EJ: Cornea, 3rd edn. St Louis, Mosby, 2011.

Krachmer JH, Palay DA: Cornea Color Atlas, 2nd edn. St Louis, Mosby, 2006.

Leibowitz HM, Waring GO: Corneal Disorders: Clinical Diagnosis and Management, 2nd edn. Philadelphia, Saunders WB, 1998.

Foster CS, Azar DT, Dohlman CH: Smolin and Thoft's The Cornea: Scientific Foundations and Clinical Practice, 4th edn. , Lippincott Williams & Wilkins, 2005.

8

Uveitis

PATHOPHYSIOLOGY

Inflammatory reaction:

Acute: chemical mediators (histamine, serotonin, kinins, plasmin, complement, leukotrienes, prostaglandins)

Chronic: cellular infiltrates

  NONGRANULOMATOUS: lymphocytes, plasma cells

  GRANULOMATOUS: epithelioid and giant cells (Langhans', foreign body, Touton)

  3 PATTERNS: diffuse (e.g. VKH syndrome), discrete (e.g. sarcoidosis), zonal (e.g. lens-induced)

Retinal S-antigen:

Protein found in human retinal photoreceptors and pineal gland

Most potent uveitic antigen; thought to be an enzyme located in rod outer segments

In animal model: produces uveitis when injected into nonocular sites (experimental autoimmune uveitis [EAU]; type 4 hypersensitivity); removal of thymus prevents EAU (supports T cell-mediated basis of inflammatory response)

Human diseases that resemble EAU: VKH, sympathetic ophthalmia, birdshot retinochoroidopathy; lymphocytes from these patients develop an in vitro proliferative response to retinal S-antigen, suggesting an autoimmune basis for these diseases

CLASSIFICATION

Pathology: nongranulomatous, granulomatous

Etiology: infection, immune response, malignancy, trauma, chemical, idiopathic

Location: sclerouveitis, keratouveitis, anterior uveitis (iritis), iridocyclitis, lens-induced uveitis, intermediate uveitis, endophthalmitis (infection or inflammation of the vitreous, anterior chamber, ciliary body, and choroid), posterior uveitis (retinitis, choroiditis, vasculitis), panuveitis (endophthalmitis and involvement of the sclera)

ANTERIOR UVEITIS

Inflammation of iris (iritis) and ciliary body (cyclitis)

Most common cause of anterior uveitis in adults is idiopathic (followed by HLA-B27 associated)

Most common cause of acute, noninfectious, hypopyon iritis is HLA-B27-associated iritis

Etiology:

Children: JRA, ankylosing spondylitis, psoriatic arthritis, acute interstitial nephritis, Fuchs' heterochromic iridocyclitis, sarcoidosis, postviral, HSV, Lyme disease, trauma, Kawasaki's disease

50% have posterior component (toxoplasmosis in 50% with posterior component)

Young adults: HLA-B27 associated, sarcoidosis, syphilis, Fuchs', Behçet's disease, spillover from intermediate or posterior uveitis

Older adults: idiopathic, sarcoidosis, HZO, masquerade syndromes (peripheral RD, intraocular foreign body, JXG, multiple sclerosis, malignancies [retinoblastoma, leukemia, large cell lymphoma, malignant melanoma])

Classification:

Nongranulomatous:

  ACUTE: idiopathic, HLA-B27 associated (5% of general population; associated with acute, recurrent uveitis;

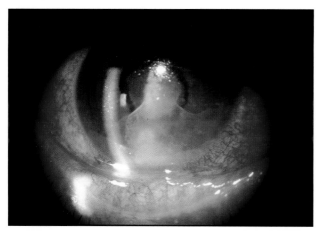

Figure 8-1. Severe idiopathic anterior uveitis with fibrinoid reaction. (From Hooper PL: Idiopathic and other anterior uveitis. In Yanoff M, Duker JS [eds]: Ophthalmology, London, Mosby, 1999.)

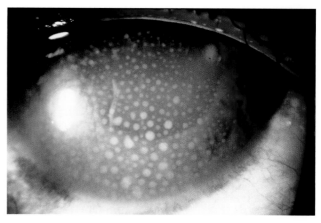

Figure 8-2. Keratic precipitates in anterior uveitis. (From Forster DJ: General approach to the uveitis patient and treatment strategies. In Yanoff M, Duker JS [eds]: Ophthalmology, London, Mosby, 1999.)

usually starts unilaterally; associated with the following 4 disorders: ankylosing spondylitis, Reiter's syndrome, psoriatic arthritis, inflammatory bowel disease), Behçet's disease, glaucomatocyclitic crisis (Posner-Schlossman syndrome), HSV, Kawasaki's disease, Lyme disease, traumatic, postoperative, other autoimmune diseases (lupus, relapsing polychondritis, Wegener's granulomatosis, interstitial nephritis)

CHRONIC (duration >6 weeks): JRA, Fuchs' heterochromic iridocyclitis

Granulomatous:

INFECTIOUS: syphilis, TB, leprosy, brucellosis, toxoplasmosis, *P. acnes*, fungal (*Cryptococcus, Aspergillus*), HIV

IMMUNE-MEDIATED: sarcoidosis, VKH syndrome, sympathetic ophthalmia, phacoanaphylactic

Symptoms: pain, photophobia, decreased vision, redness

Findings: conjunctival and episcleral injection, ciliary injection (circumcorneal flush from branches of anterior ciliary arteries), miosis (iris sphincter spasm), AC reaction; may have hypopyon, keratic precipitates, iris nodules, dilated iris vessels (occasionally, rubeosis), synechiae (posterior [iris adhesions to lens; seclusio pupillae is a complete adhesion that can result in iris bombe] or anterior [iris adhesions to cornea and angle]) (Figure 8-1)

Keratitic precipitates (KP): aggregates of white blood cells on corneal endothelium; typically located inferiorly and centrally (Figure 8-2)

May occur with any intraocular inflammation, most commonly with uveitis

May be white or pigmented, small or large, nongranulomatous (fine) or granulomatous (mutton fat), diffuse or focal

NONGRANULOMATOUS: composed of lymphocytes and PMNs

GRANULOMATOUS: composed of macrophages, lymphocytes, epithelioid cells, and multinucleated giant cells

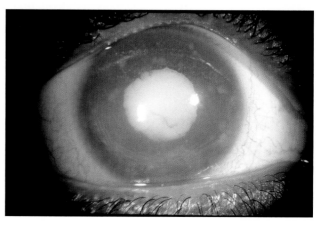

Figure 8-3. Chronic granulomatous uveitis demonstrating Busacca nodules. (From Forster DJ: General approach to the uveitis patient and treatment strategies. In Yanoff M, Duker JS [eds]: Ophthalmology, London, Mosby, 1999.)

DDX OF DIFFUSE KP: Fuchs' heterochromic iridocyclitis, sarcoidosis, syphilis, keratouveitis, toxoplasmosis (rarely)

Iris nodules:

KOEPPE: located at pupil margin; occur in granulomatous and nongranulomatous uveitis

BUSACCA: located on anterior iris surface; occur only in granulomatous uveitis (Figure 8-3)

BERLIN: located in anterior chamber angle; occur in granulomatous uveitis

DDx of hypopyon: HLA-B27 associated, infection (keratitis, endophthalmitis), foreign body, Behçet's disease, VKH syndrome, malignancy (leukemia, retinoblastoma), toxic (rifabutin)

DDx of uveitic glaucoma: HSV, HZV, Posner-Schlossman syndrome, Fuchs' heterochromic iridocyclitis, sarcoidosis; rarely toxoplasmosis, syphilis, sympathetic ophthalmia

Diagnosis:

Minimum: CBC with differential, urinalysis, VDRL and FTA-ABS

Expanded (for recurrent anterior [3 or more attacks], granulomatous, positive review of systems, or posterior involvement): ESR, ACE, ANA, ANCA, IL-10, PPD plus anergy panel, CXR or chest CT; consider Lyme test in endemic areas, HLA typing (25% with HLA-B27 develop sacroiliac disease, so obtain sacroiliac X-ray), HIV Ab test

Targeted approach:

RECURRENT UVEITIS, WITH BACK STIFFNESS UPON AWAKENING: rule out ankylosing spondylitis
   HLA-B27
   Lumbosacral spine imaging (CT)

GRANULOMATOUS UVEITIS: rule out TB and sarcoidosis
   CXR
   Upper body gallium scan
   Angiotensin-converting enzyme ([ACE]; elevated in 60% with sarcoidosis; also in Gaucher's disease, miliary tuberculosis, silicosis)
   Lysozyme
   Serum calcium
   Liver function tests and bilirubin
   PPD

CHILD WITH RECURRENT OR CHRONIC IRIDOCYCLITIS: rule out JRA (usually ANA-positive, RF-negative)
   ANA
   RF
   HLA-B8

RETINAL VASCULITIS, RECURRENT APHTHOUS ULCERS, PRETIBIAL SKIN LESIONS: rule out Behçet's disease
   Skin lesion biopsy
   HLA-B51 and -B27

PARS PLANITIS AND EPISODIC PARESTHESIAS: rule out multiple sclerosis (MS)
   Brain MRI
   Lumbar puncture

RETINOCHOROIDITIS ADJACENT TO PIGMENTED CR SCAR: rule out toxoplasmosis
   Toxoplasma IgM and IgG titers

RETINAL VASCULITIS AND SINUSITIS: rule out Wegener's granulomatosis
   ANCA
   CXR
   Sinus films
   Urinalysis

RECURRENT UVEITIS AND DIARRHEA: rule out inflammatory bowel disease (IBD)
   GI consult
   Endoscopy with biopsy

CHOROIDITIS, EXUDATIVE RD, EPISODIC TINNITUS: rule out Harada's disease/VKH syndrome
   FA
   Lumbar puncture
   Brain MRI
   Audiometry

ELDERLY FEMALE WITH VITRITIS: rule out intraocular lymphoma or infection
   Vitreal biopsy for culture or cytology

UNILATERAL IRIDOCYCLITIS, FINE WHITE KP, LIGHTER IRIS IN AFFECTED EYE: rule out Fuchs' heterochromic iridocyclitis
   IOP
   Gonioscopy (fine-angle vessels)

Treatment: topical steroids, cycloplegic; may require systemic steroids, immunosuppressive agents, antibiotics

Poor response to steroids: Fuchs', syphilis, toxoplasmosis, keratouveitis, Lyme disease, chronic postoperative endophthalmitis, ARN, CMV

Complications: iris atrophy, band keratopathy, cataract, glaucoma, cystoid macular edema

Ankylosing Spondylitis

90% HLA-B27-positive; typically young men

Symptoms: lower back pain and stiffness with inactivity (upon awakening in morning)

Findings: anterior uveitis (30%; recurrent in 40%), episcleritis, scleritis

Other findings: arthritis (sacroiliac and peripheral joints), heart (aortic insufficiency, heart block), colitis (10%), lungs (restricted chest expansion, apical fibrosis)

Sacroiliac X-ray: sclerosis and narrowing of joint space; ligamentous ossification can occur

Reiter's Syndrome

Triad of conjunctivitis, urethritis, and arthritis
75% HLA-B27; males > females
Associated with infections: *Chlamydia, Ureaplasma urealyticum, Yersinia, Shigella, Salmonella*

Findings: mucopurulent conjunctivitis, keratitis, acute anterior uveitis

Diagnosis: 3 major criteria, or 2 major and 2 minor criteria

Major:
   Urethritis
   Polyarthritis (knees, sacroiliac joints)
   Conjunctivitis
   Keratoderma blenorrhagicum (scaling skin lesion, often on feet and hands [20%]; similar to pustular psoriasis)

Minor:
   Plantar fasciitis and Achilles tendinitis
   Circinate balanitis
   Painless mouth ulcers
   Prostatitis
   Cystitis
   Spondylitis/sacroiliitis
   Tendinitis
   Recent history of diarrhea
   Iritis/keratitis

Psoriatic Arthritis

Associated with HLA-B17 and HLA-B27

Uveitis does not occur in psoriasis without arthritis

Findings: conjunctivitis, dry eyes, anterior uveitis

Other findings: arthritis (hands, feet, sacroiliac joints), psoriatic skin and nail changes

Inflammatory Bowel Disease (IBD)

Uveitis occurs in ulcerative colitis (10%) and Crohn's disease (3%)

Findings: conjunctivitis, keratoconjunctivitis sicca, episcleritis, scleritis, anterior uveitis, orbital cellulitis, optic neuritis

Other findings: arthritis, erythema nodosum, pyoderma gangrenosum, hepatitis, sclerosing cholangitis

Fuchs' Heterochromic Iridocyclitis

Occurs in young adults; unilateral

Associated with chorioretinal scars (toxo)

Symptoms: blurred vision

Findings: diffuse small white stellate KP, minimal AC reaction, no posterior synechiae, iris heterochromia (diffuse atrophy of stroma, loss of iris crypts; involved iris is paler; 15% bilateral), fine-angle vessels (may bleed during gonioscopy, cataract surgery, or paracentesis) (Figure 8-4)

DDx of iris heterochromia: trauma (intraocular metallic foreign body), inflammation, congenital Horner's syndrome, iris melanoma, Waardenburg's syndrome (iris heterochromia, telecanthus, white forelock, congenital deafness), Parry-Romberg syndrome (iris heterochromia, Horner's syndrome, ocular motor palsies, nystagmus, facial hemiatrophy), glaucomatocyclitic crisis, medication (topical prostaglandin analogues [Xalatan, Lumigan, Travatan]), nevus of Ota

Pathology: plasma cells in ciliary body

Treatment: poor response to steroids

Complications: glaucoma (60%), cataract (PSC; 50%)

Juvenile Rheumatoid Arthritis (JRA)

(See Ch. 5, Pediatrics/Strabismus)

Kawasaki's Disease

(See Ch. 5, Pediatrics/Strabismus)

Lyme Disease

Due to *Borrelia burgdorferi* (spirochete)

Ocular involvement is usually bilateral

Affected organ systems: skin, CNS, cardiovascular, musculoskeletal

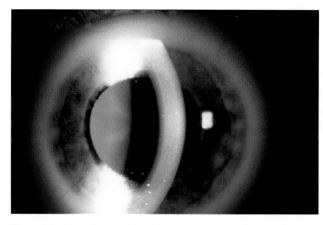

Figure 8-4. Fuchs' uveitis (From Hooper PL: Idiopathic and other anterior uveitis. In Yanoff M, Duker JS [eds]: Ophthalmology, London, Mosby, 1999.)

Findings (in stage 2 and 3 disease): cranial nerve palsies (CN 7 most common), orbital myositis, follicular conjunctivitis, symblepharon, episcleritis, keratitis (multiple nummular stromal infiltrates), chronic granulomatous iridocyclitis with posterior synechiae and vitreous cells, intermediate or posterior uveitis, pars planitis, chorioretinitis, exudative RD, CME, BRAO, retinal vasculitis, papilledema, pseudotumor cerebri, optic neuritis, optic atrophy

Posner-Schlossman Syndrome (Glaucomatocyclitic Crisis)

Recurrent anterior uveitis and increased IOP; episodes are typically self-limited

Symptoms: unilateral pain

Findings: mild AC reaction, few or no KP, elevated IOP

Treatment: may require topical glaucoma medications to control IOP, steroids to control inflammation

Phacoanaphylactic Endophthalmitis

Immune complex disease (type 3 hypersensitivity reaction) when normal tolerance to lens protein is lost

Previous rupture of lens capsule in same or fellow eye, followed by latent period; with re-exposure to lens protein during surgery, zonal granulomatous uveitis occurs

Associated with trauma (80%)

May develop severe uveitis with hypotony, secondary open-angle glaucoma

Pathology: zonal pattern (PMNs infiltrate central lens material; epithelioid histiocytes and mononuclear cells around nidus)

Treatment: remove lens

Interstitial Nephritis

Rare; can be idiopathic or triggered by allergic reaction to medicines (antibiotics, NSAIDs)

Associated with acute anterior uveitis

Pathology: interstitial edema with mononuclear inflammatory cells; eosinophils can be present

INTERMEDIATE UVEITIS

Etiology: pars planitis, multiple sclerosis (5–25% have periphlebitis and intermediate uveitis), Lyme disease, sarcoidosis, Fuchs' heterochromic iridocyclitis

Pars Planitis

Most common cause of intermediate uveitis (85–90%)
Usually young adults; females > males; 75% bilateral

Accounts for 25% of uveitis in children

Associated with HLA-DR15 and MS

Etiology: unknown; diagnosis of exclusion

Symptoms: floaters, decreased vision

Findings: light flare with a few KP, anterior vitritis, snowballs (white vitreous cellular aggregates near ora serrata; may coalesce to form peripheral fibrovascular accumulation [snowbank] over inferior pars plana and vitreous base), peripheral retinal periphlebitis, hyperemic disc, no chorioretinitis, no synechiae (Figure 8-5)

Pathology:
  Snowballs: epithelioid cells and multinucleated giant cells
  Snowbank: preretinal membrane of fibroglial and vascular elements
  Peripheral retinal veins: often have perivascular cuff of lymphocytes

DDx: sarcoidosis, toxoplasmosis, toxocariasis, syphilis, Lyme disease, MS
  Multiple sclerosis: bilateral pars planitis can occur (80% bilateral, 20% unilateral); may present with band keratopathy, mild AC reaction, vitreous cells in a young patient; can also have cataract (PSC), epiretinal membrane, CME, retinal phlebitis

Treatment: (main indication is CME with reduced vision): periocular and oral steroids; consider immunosuppressive agents, vitrectomy, cryotherapy to areas of peripheral NV (controversial; can decrease leakage and macular edema, but can lead to retinal tears)

Prognosis: 10% self-limited, 90% chronic (⅓ with exacerbations)

Complications: cataract, retrolenticular cyclitic membrane, VH (from peripheral retinal neovascularization), tractional RD, CME (primary cause of vision loss, followed by cataract), band keratopathy

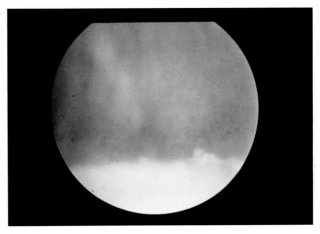

Figure 8-5. Inferior pars plana snowbank with attached snowballs. (From Zimmerman PL: Pars planitis and other intermediate uveitis. In Yanoff M, Duker JS [eds]: Ophthalmology, London, Mosby, 1999.)

POSTERIOR UVEITIS

Most common cause of posterior uveitis in adults is toxoplasmosis (followed by retinal vasculitis)

Signs: vitreous cells, membranes, opacities, inflammatory exudates ('snowballs'), vasculitis (opacification around vessels [sheathing {whole vessel}, cuffing {segment of vessel}]), exudates (candlewax drippings), retinitis, pigmentary changes (due to RPE inflammation), choroiditis (focal, multifocal, or diffuse), choroidal detachment

DDx of vitritis:
  Panuveitis: sarcoidosis, TB, syphilis, VKH, sympathetic ophthalmia, Behçet's disease
  Postsurgical/trauma: Irvine-Gass syndrome
  Endophthalmitis
  Choroiditis: acute posterior multifocal placoid pigment epitheliopathy (APMPPE), serpiginous, birdshot, multifocal choroiditis, *Toxocara*, POHS
  Retinitis: ARN, CMV, toxoplasmosis, candidiasis, cysticercosis, onchocerciasis
  Vasculitis: Eales disease
  Other infections: nematodes, Whipple's disease, EBV, Lyme disease
  Other: amyloidosis, ocular ischemia, masquerade syndromes, spillover from anterior uveitis
  Intermediate uveitis: pars planitis, MS

Complications: NV, CME, ON swelling and atrophy
  CME: common cause of vision loss in pars planitis, birdshot retinochoroidopathy, retinal vasculitis, and any iridocyclitis (especially chronic, recurrent cases); CME does not occur in VKH

Indications for cytotoxic therapy: Behçet's disease, sympathetic ophthalmia, VKH, pars planitis, Eales disease, retinal vasculitis, serpiginous choroidopathy, OCP, necrotizing scleritis, inflammations unresponsive to maximum steroid therapy

Infections

Toxoplasmosis

(See Ch. 5, Pediatrics/Strabismus)

Toxocariasis

(See Ch. 5, Pediatrics/Strabismus)

Presumed Ocular Histoplasmosis Syndrome (POHS)

(See Ch. 11, Posterior Segment)

Cytomegalovirus (CMV)

Progressive hemorrhagic necrotizing retinitis involving all retinal layers

Occurs in 15–46% of AIDS patients; usually when CD4 count <50 cells/mm^3

40% bilateral at presentation

Rare syndrome of neonatal cytomegalic inclusion disease

Symptoms: often asymptomatic; may have floaters, scotoma

Findings: well-circumscribed necrotizing retinitis (2 appearances), mild AC and vitreous reaction
  Brushfire: indolent, granular, yellow-white advancing edge with peripheral atrophic 'burned out' region
  Pizza-pie fundus: thick, yellow-white necrosis; hemorrhage, vascular sheathing (Figure 8-6)

Pathology: infected retinal cells are markedly enlarged, then necrotic, finally atrophic; large owl's eye intranuclear inclusions

Treatment: antiviral therapy (induction during first 2 weeks)
  Ganciclovir (Cytovene): virostatic
    TOXICITY: neutropenia and thrombocytopenia
    INDUCTION: 5–7.5 mg/kg IV bid × 2–4 weeks
    MAINTENANCE: 5–10 mg/kg IV qd
    INTRAVITREAL INJECTION: 200–2000 μg/0.1 mL 2–3 times a week × 2–3 weeks
  Foscarnet: virostatic
    TOXICITY: renal
    INDUCTION: 90 mg/kg IV bid or 60 mg/kg IV tid × 2 weeks
    MAINTENANCE: 90–120 mg/kg IV qd
    INTRAVITREAL INJECTION: 2.4 mg/0.1 mL 2–3 times a week × 2-3 weeks, then 1–2 times a week
  Cidofovir (Vistide): longer half-life
    TOXICITY: renal, uveitis (50%), hypotony
    INDUCTION: 3–5 mg/kg IV once a week × 2 weeks
    MAINTENANCE: 3–5 mg/kg IV once every 2 weeks
    Administered through peripheral line (central line required for ganciclovir and foscarnet)

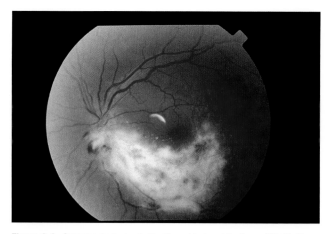

Figure 8-6. Cytomegalovirus retinitis. (From Hudson HL, Boyer DS, Martin DF, et al: Viral posterior uveitis. In Yanoff M, Duker JS [eds]: Ophthalmology, London, Mosby, 1999.)

    INTRAVITREAL INJECTION: 165–330 μg once a week × 3 weeks, then every 2 weeks
    Associated with lowering of IOP (about 2 mmHg), 20–50% develop iritis (about 5 days after last infusion)
    Probenecid and hydration with each dose to reduce renal toxicity and decrease iritis
    Median time to progression = 120 days
    B-scan ultrasound in patients with severe hypotony revealed CB atrophy
  Ganciclovir (Vitrasert):
    Median time to progression = 194 days (vs 72 days with IV ganciclovir and 15 days with no treatment)
    May be increased risk of RD with implantation
  Oral ganciclovir: poor bioavailability; only 6% absorbed with food, 9% absorption without food
  Surgery: vitrectomy with long-acting tamponade for RD repair

Complications: rhegmatogenous RD

Acute Retinal Necrosis (ARN)

Acute self-limited confluent peripheral necrotizing retinitis due to infection with VZV, HSV, or rarely CMV

Usually occurs in immunocompetent individuals; 33% bilateral (BARN), commonly in immunosuppressed

Association with HLA-DQw7 (50%)

Symptoms: rapid onset of ocular/periocular pain, pain on eye movement, redness, photophobia, floaters, decreased vision, constriction of visual field

Findings: diffuse episcleral injection, mild iritis with granulomatous KP, vitritis; 'thumbprint' nummular infiltrates posterior to equator with isolated peripheral patches of necrotizing retinitis that becomes confluent; sawtooth demarcation line between necrotic and healthy retina, generalized obliterative retinal arteritis (with

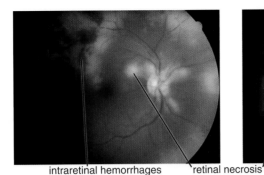
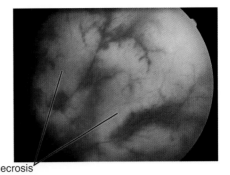

intraretinal hemorrhages   retinal necrosis

Figure 8-7. Acute retinal necrosis. (From Kaiser PK, Friedman NJ, Pineda II, R: Massachusetts Eye and Ear Infirmary Illustrated Manual of Ophthalmology, 2nd edn. Philadelphia, WB Saunders, 2004.)

peripheral vaso-occlusion), pale disc edema (Figure 8-7); within 2 months, retinitis gradually resolves and necrotic retina sloughs; coarse salt and pepper pigmentation

Pathology: necrosis occurs from virally induced cytolysis, arteriolar and choriocapillaris occlusion; necrotic cells slough into vitreous, leaving large areas devoid of retina

FA: focal areas of choroidal hypoperfusion early; late staining

Treatment: acyclovir (IV × 5–10 days, then oral × 6 weeks; decreases risk of development of ARN in fellow eye by approximately 50%; ganciclovir is an alternative); oral steroids; aspirin to inhibit vascular thrombosis

Prognosis: watch fellow eye closely (usually develops ARN within 4 weeks)

65–90% develop rhegmatogenous RD (usually within 3 months)

Progressive Outer Retinal Necrosis (PORN)

Variant of ARN in AIDS but painless with minimal intraocular inflammation

Often have history of cutaneous zoster

74% unilateral at presentation, 70% become bilateral

> *Findings*: multiple discrete peripheral or central areas of retinal opacification/infiltrates (deep with very rapid progression), 'cracked mud' appearance after resolution; vasculitis is not prominent (Figure 8-8)
> *Treatment*: combination of foscarnet and ganciclovir; poor response to antivirals
> *Prognosis*: 67% become NLP within 4 weeks; RD in 90%

Herpes Zoster

Uveitis typically develops during convalescence from acute *Varicella* infection

Reactivated uveitis (anterior and/or posterior), may have keratitis (epithelial or stromal)

May require chronic topical steroid treatment to prevent recurrence

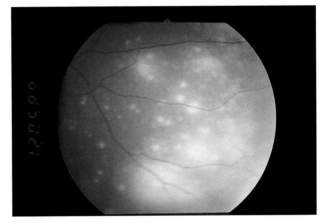

Figure 8-8. Progressive outer retinal necrosis, early stage. (From Hudson HL, Boyer DS, Martin DF, et al: Viral posterior uveitis. In Yanoff M, Duker JS [eds]: Ophthalmology, London, Mosby, 1999.)

Rubella

Sensorineural hearing loss, salt and pepper retinopathy; may develop cataract or glaucoma (rare to have both) (Figure 8-9)

Vision and electrophysiologic testing are usually normal

Live virus in an infant is found in the lens, as well as conjunctival swab, pharyngeal swab, and urine cultures

Measles

Pigmentary retinopathy due to infection acquired in utero

Acute blindness 6–12 days after measles rash appears

Findings: keratoconjunctivitis, retinal edema, vascular attenuation, macular star, no hemorrhages; Koplik's spots in mouth

Treatment: none; most infants recover, some develop pigmentary degeneration

Subacute sclerosing panencephalitis (SSPE): fatal measles slow virus infection of CNS
> *Findings:* macular or perimacular chorioretinitis, pigmentary changes with bone spicules, papilledema, optic atrophy, nystagmus, cortical blindness

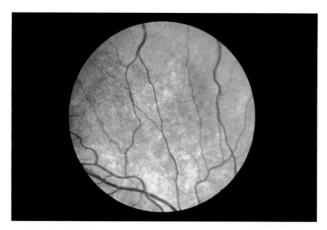

Figure 8-9. Rubella retinopathy. (Courtesy of George S. Novalis, MD. From Hudson HL, Boyer DS, Martin DF, et al: Viral posterior uveitis. In Yanoff M, Duker JS [eds]: Ophthalmology, London, Mosby, 1999.)

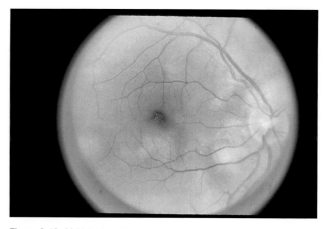

Figure 8-10. Multiple choroidal lesions in *Pneumocystis* choroiditis. (From Cowan CL: Sarcoidosis. In Yanoff M, Duker JS [eds]: Ophthalmology, London, Mosby, 1999.)

Other findings: personality or behavioral changes, dementia, seizures, myoclonus

Pathology: eosinophilic nuclear inclusions in neuronal and glial cells

Candidiasis

Yeast-like form (blastoconidia), or pseudohyphae or elongated branching structures (pseudomycelia)

Occurs in debilitated patients on hyperalimentation and in IV drug abusers

Most cases occur without positive blood cultures or ongoing fungemia

Approximately 10% with candidemia develop endophthalmitis

Findings: anterior uveitis, retinal hemorrhages, perivascular sheathing, chorioretinitis with fluffy white lesions (puff balls; may be joined by opaque vitreous stands ['string of pearls']), vitreous abscess; may have subretinal abscess

DDx of pale subretinal mass: metastasis, amelanotic melanoma, choroidal osteoma, old subretinal hemorrhage, granuloma

Culture: blood agar or Sabaraud's glucose (large, creamy white colonies)

Treatment: IV amphotericin B

Prognosis: 70% mortality within 1 year

Pneumocystis Choroiditis

Due to *Pneumocystis carinii*

Choroiditis with multifocal orange nummular lesions; lesions contain cysts of *Pneumocystis carinii* (Figure 8-10)

Associated with use of inhaled pentamidine (which is prophylaxis for pulmonary *Pneumocystis* only)

Cysticercosis

Due to infection with pork tapeworm *Taenia solium* or *T. saginata*; humans are definitive host, pigs are intermediate host

Adult worm lives in small intestine; larvae travel to eye, producing cystic subretinal or intravitreal lesion (cysticercus)

Findings: mass lesion or exudative RD (Figure 8-11)

Treatment: vitrectomy required for posterior segment disease

Leprosy

Due to *Mycobacterium leprae*

5–15 million infected; 250,000 blind

Findings:

Lids: lagophthalmos, madarosis, blepharochalasis, nodules, trichiasis, entropion, ectropion, reduced blinking

Lacrimal: acute and chronic dacryocystitis

Cornea: anesthesia, exposure keratopathy, band keratopathy, corneal leproma, interstitial keratitis, thickened nerves, superficial stromal keratitis

Sclera: episcleritis, scleritis, staphyloma, nodules

Iris: miosis, iritis, synechiae, seclusio pupillae, atrophy, iris pearls, leproma

Ciliary body: loss of accommodation, hypotony, phthisis

Fundus: peripheral choroidal lesions, retinal vasculitis

Complications: cataract, glaucoma

Diffuse Unilateral Subacute Neuroretinitis (DUSN)

Due to infection with small roundworm in subretinal space: dog hookworm (*Ancylostoma caninum*) or racoon nematode (*Baylisascaris procyonis*)

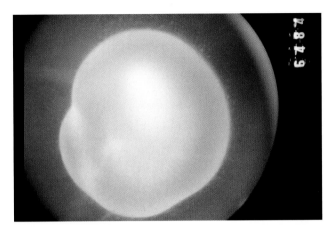

Figure 8-11. Cysticercus in the eye. (From Cowan CL: Sarcoidosis. In Yanoff M, Duker JS [eds]: Ophthalmology, London, Mosby, 1999.)

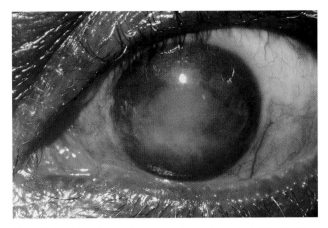

Figure 8-12. Sclerosing keratitis as a result of onchocerciasis. (Courtesy of Professor HR Taylor. From Cowan CL: Sarcoidosis. In Yanoff M, Duker JS [eds]: Ophthalmology, London, Mosby, 1999.)

Findings: deep, gray-white retinal lesions; optic nerve swelling; vitreous cells; late findings include retinal vascular narrowing, diffuse RPE pigmentary changes, optic atrophy; results in unilateral 'wipe-out' syndrome

ERG: decreased

Treatment: laser nematode

Cat-Scratch Disease

Due to *Bartonella henselae* (also causes oculoglandular syndrome)

Findings: retinal granuloma or neuroretinitis

Treatment: oral antibiotics (doxycycline 100 mg bid, and rifampin 300 mg bid × 4–6 weeks)

Onchocerciasis (River Blindness)

Due to *Onchocerca volvulus*; larvae mature in humans, forming adult worms that live in fibrous, subcutaneous nodules (usually in joints); female worms (100 cm long, live for up to 20 years) and male worms (5 cm long, live for much shorter time) reproduce sexually, females give birth to ~2000 microfilariae/day; microfilariae (300 μm long, live for 1–2 years) migrate all over body by direct invasion and hematogenous spread, prefer skin and eyes; live microfilariae induce little or no inflammation; death of organism causes severe granulomatous inflammation and scarring

Transmitted by black fly: breeds along fast-moving streams; bites infected host and acquires microfilariae, which mature into infectious larvae; transmits larvae to humans with bite; 17 million infected; 1–2 million blind (Africa and Latin America)

Second leading cause of corneal blindness in world (trachoma is first)

Findings: intraocular microfilariae (in AC), anterior uveitis, SPK, sclerosing keratitis, scleritis, chorioretinitis, optic neuritis and atrophy; may develop cataract, PAS, and glaucoma (Figure 8-12)

Other findings: pruritus, pigmentary changes (leopard-skin appearance), chronic inflammation, scarring, maculopapular rash, subcutaneous nodules

Diagnosis: skin snip (place piece of skin in tissue media, 20–100 microfilariae emerge)

Treatment: ivermectin, suramin, diethylcarbamazine (DEC)

Whipple's Disease

Due to *Tropheryma whipplei*; Gram-positive bacillus, Actinomycetes family; found intracellularly and extracellularly

Findings: uveitis, retinal vasculitis

Other findings: malabsorption (diarrhea, steatorrhea), migratory arthralgias

Pathology: PAS-positive macrophages within lamina propria of 'clubbed' (abnormal) microvilli of intestinal wall, or vitreous biopsy

Treatment: Bactrim may be helpful; may require a year of therapy as shorter courses lead to relapses

Propionibacterium Acnes

Gram-positive rod; anaerobic

May become sequestered in capsular bag following cataract surgery

Findings: delayed onset, chronic granulomatous uveitis, often with fibrin or hypopyon; white plaque on posterior capsule is characteristic

Treatment: intravitreal antibiotics (vancomycin, cephalosporins; resistant to aminoglycosides); usually also requires partial or total removal of capsular bag with/without IOL removal/exchange

Table 8-1. White Dot Syndrome

	APMPPE	MEWDS	Serpiginous	Birdshot	Multifocal choroiditis with panuveitis	PIC
Age	20–40	20–50	30–50	40–60	20–50	20–40
Sex	F = M	F > M	F = M	F > M	F > M	Female
Laterality	Bilateral	Unilateral	Bilateral	Bilateral		
HLA	B7, DR2	None	B7	A29	None	None
Vitritis	Mild	Mild	Mild	Chronic, moderate	Chronic, moderate	None
Lesions	Large, geographic, gray-white shallow pigmented scars within 1–2 weeks	Small, soft, gray-white dots; no scarring	Active, geographic, gray-white patches; deep scars with fibrosis	Deep, creamy spots; indistinct margins; yellow scars without pigmentation	50–350 μm gray-white yellow spots; mixture of old scars and new spots	100–300 μm yellow or gray spots; punched-out scars
Macula	Rare CNV	Granularity Rare CNV	Subretinal scars 25% CNV	CME Rare CNV	CME 35% CNV	Atrophic scars 40% CNV
Prognosis	Good	Good	Poor	Fair	Fair	Good
Treatment	None	None	Steroids Laser CNV	Steroids Cyclosporine	Steroids Laser CNV	None Laser CNV

Ophthalmomyiasis

Due to direct ocular invasion by fly larvae (maggots) that can invade AC, posterior segment, or subretinal space

Subretinal invasion: larvae travel through fundus, leaving criss-crossing tracks of atrophied RPE; death of organism causes ocular inflammation

Inflammations (Table 8-1)

Acute Posterior Multifocal Placoid Pigment Epitheliopathy (APMPPE)

Occurs in young, healthy adults; female = male; usually bilateral

Acute, self-limited; may be nonspecific choroidal hypersensitivity reaction

Possible HLA-B7 association

Associated with cerebral vasculitis

Flu-like prodrome (33%) followed by decreased vision

Findings: multiple creamy yellow-white plaque-like lesions (usually <1 DD) at level of RPE or choriocapillaris (possibly due to choroidal hypoperfusion); lesions fade over 2–6 weeks, leaving geographically shaped RPE changes (hypopigmentation and hyperpigmentation); may have vitreous cells, mild AC reaction; rarely vascular sheathing, disc edema, CNV (Figures 8-13)

Other findings: thyroiditis, erythema nodosum, cerebral vasculitis, regional enteritis

FA: initial blockage with late hyperfluorescence; window defects in old cases (Figures 8-14, 8-15)

Treatment: none

Prognosis: vision recovers in most patients to >20/40; rarely recurs

APMPPE lesions

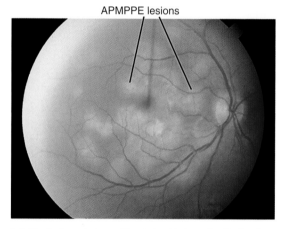

Figure 8-13. Acute posterior multifocal placoid pigment epitheliopathy demonstrating multiple posterior pole lesions. (From Kaiser PK, Friedman NJ, Pineda II R: Massachusetts Eye and Ear Infirmary Illustrated Manual of Ophthalmology, 2nd edn. Philadelphia, WB Saunders, 2004.)

Multiple Evanescent White Dot Syndrome (MEWDS)

Onset between age 14 and 50; female > male; unilateral > bilateral

Symptoms: decreased vision, dark spots in the periphery (peripheral scotomas), shimmering photopsias

Findings: granular retinal appearance with small (100–200 μm) white spots in posterior pole at level of RPE; may have vitreous cells, positive RAPD, mild optic disc swelling (Figure 8-16)

VF: enlarged blind spot

FA: early hyperfluorescence in wreath-like configuration; late staining of lesions and optic nerve (Figure 8-17)

ERG: reduced a wave (involvement of RPE and outer retina)

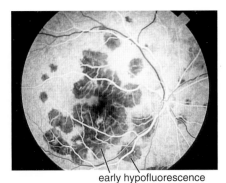

early hypofluorescence

Figure 8-14. Fluorescein angiogram of same patient as shown in Figure 8-13 demonstrating early hypofluorescence of the lesions. (From Kaiser PK, Friedman NJ, Pineda II, R: Massachusetts Eye and Ear Infirmary Illustrated Manual of Ophthalmology, 2nd edn. Philadelphia, WB Saunders, 2004.)

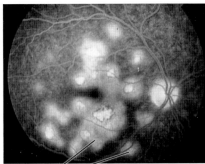

late staining

Figure 8-15. Fluorescein angiogram of same patient as shown in Figure 8-14 demonstrating late staining of the lesions. (From Kaiser PK, Friedman NJ, Pineda II, R: Massachusetts Eye and Ear Infirmary Illustrated Manual of Ophthalmology, 2nd edn. Philadelphia, WB Saunders, 2004.)

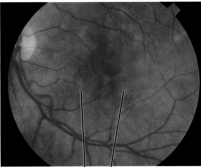

multiple evanescent white dot syndrome

Figure 8-16. Multiple evanescent white dot syndrome demonstrating faint white spots. (From Kaiser PK, Friedman NJ, Pineda II, R: Massachusetts Eye and Ear Infirmary Illustrated Manual of Ophthalmology, 2nd edn. Philadelphia, WB Saunders, 2004.)

Prognosis: vision recovers over weeks but may be permanently decreased due to pigmentary changes in fovea; 10% have recurrent episodes in same or fellow eye

Serpiginous Choroidopathy

Chronic, recurrent, indolent disease of unknown etiology

Onset between age 40–60; female = male; usually bilateral

Affects inner chorioretinal pigment epithelium

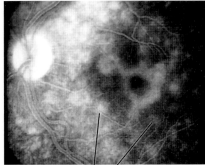

dot syndrome   early hyperfluorescence

Figure 8-17. Same patient as shown in Figure 8–16 demonstrating early fluorescein angiogram appearance. (From Kaiser PK, Friedman NJ, Pineda II, R: Massachusetts Eye and Ear Infirmary Illustrated Manual of Ophthalmology, 2nd edn. Philadelphia, WB Saunders, 2004.)

Symptoms: painless loss of vision

Findings: geographic (map-like) pattern of scars with active edges (yellow-gray, edematous), usually beginning in posterior pole (often extending from disc); active areas become atrophic over weeks to months; new lesions occur contiguously or elsewhere (often in snake-like pattern); may have mild AC reaction, vitritis, vascular sheathing, RPE detachment, NVD, CNV (rare) (Figure 8-18)

VF: absolute scotomas corresponding to atrophic scars

FA: acute lesions stain

Treatment: may respond to oral steroids, immunosuppressive drugs

Prognosis: fair to poor; commonly recurs months to years later

Birdshot Choroidopathy (Vitiliginous Chorioretinitis)

Occurs after 4th decade of life; female > male; usually bilateral
Associated with HLA-A29 (90%)

Symptoms: decreased vision, nyctalopia, decreased color vision, peripheral visual field loss

Findings: cream-colored depigmented spots scattered throughout fundus; may have mild AC reaction, vitritis, retinal vasculitis, disc edema, optic atrophy, CME, epiretinal membrane, CNV (Figure 8-19)

FA: pronounced perifoveal capillary leakage with CME

ERG: diminished scotopic response (rod dysfunction)

Multifocal Choroiditis with Panuveitis

Onset between age 20–50; female > male

Findings: multiple gray-white to yellow lesions (50–350 µm) at level of choroid or RPE; vitreous and AC cells;

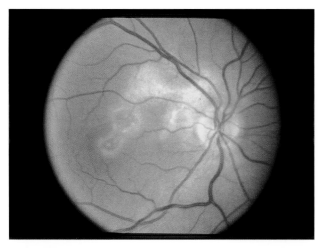

Figure 8-18. Fundus view of the right eye of a 57-year-old woman with early serpiginous choroiditis. (From Moorthy RS, Jampol LM: Posterior uveitis of unknown cause. In Yanoff M, Duker JS [eds]: Ophthalmology, London, Mosby, 1999.)

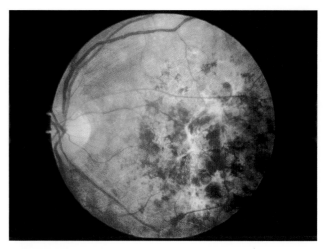

Figure 8-20. Fundus view of the left eye of a 50-year-old woman who has progressive subretinal fibrosis and uveitis syndrome. (From Moorthy RS, Jampol LM: Posterior uveitis of unknown cause. In Yanoff M, Duker JS [eds]: Ophthalmology, London, Mosby, 1999.)

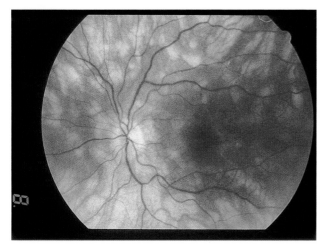

Figure 8-19. Birdshot retinochoroidopathy. (From Moorthy RS, Jampol LM: Posterior uveitis of unknown cause. In Yanoff M, Duker JS [eds]: Ophthalmology, London, Mosby, 1999.)

chronic lesions become atrophic with punched-out margins, variable amounts of pigmentation, and occasionally fibrosis (Figure 8-20)

FA: acute lesions block or fill early and stain late; older lesions behave like window defects with early hyperfluorescence and late fading

Treatment: steroids

Complications: CNV (most common cause of vision loss), CME

Punctate Inner Choroidopathy (PIC)

Onset between age 20 and 40; healthy, moderately myopic women

Symptoms: acute scotomas and photopsias

Findings: small (100–300 μm) yellow or gray inner choroidal lesions; resolve over weeks to form atrophic scars that may enlarge and become pigmented; new lesions do not appear; may have serous RDs; 40% risk of CNV; no AC or vitreous cells (Figure 8-21)

Treatment: none

Acute Retinal Pigment Epitheliitis (Krill's Disease)

Rare, occurs in young adults; usually unilateral

Symptoms: sudden decrease in vision

Findings: clusters of hyperpigmented spots (300–400 μm) in macula surrounded by yellow-white halos; with resolution, the spots lighten or darken, but halos remain; no vitritis (Figure 8-22)

DDx: central serous retinopathy, acute macular neuroretinopathy (wedge-shaped or cloverleaf dark red perifoveal dots; paracentral scotoma; normal ERG)

FA: blockage of spots with halos of hyperfluorescence

Treatment: none

Prognosis: resolves completely in 6–12 weeks

Frosted Branch Angiitis

White spots along retinal arterioles (Figure 8-23)

DDx: CMV retinitis, toxoplasmosis (Kyrieleis' plaques)

Acute Zonal Occult Outer Retinopathy (AZOOR)

Usually bilateral; females > males

Symptoms: rapid loss of function in 1 or more regions of visual field, photopsias

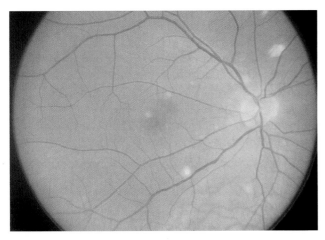

Figure 8-21. Punctate inner choroidopathy. (From Moorthy RS, Jampol LM: Posterior uveitis of unknown cause. In Yanoff M, Duker JS [eds]: Ophthalmology, London, Mosby, 1999.)

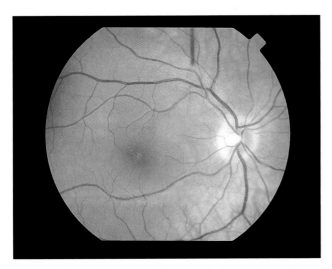

Figure 8-22. Retinal pigment epitheliitis. (From Moorthy RS, Jampol LM: Posterior uveitis of unknown cause. In Yanoff M, Duker JS [eds]: Ophthalmology, London, Mosby, 1999.)

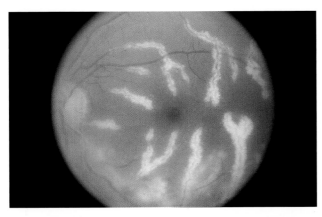

Figure 8-23. 'Frosted branch angiitis' secondary to cytomegalovirus retinitis. (From Hudson HL, Boyer DS, Martin DF, et al: Viral posterior uveitis. In Yanoff M, Duker JS [eds]: Ophthalmology, London, Mosby, 1999.)

Findings: minimal changes initially; retinal degeneration/ pigmentary changes late

DDx: MEWDS, acute macular neuroretinopathy, multifocal choroiditis

VF: scotomas (may enlarge)

ERG: decrease rod and cone

Idiopathic Uveal Effusion Syndrome

Occurs in healthy, middle-aged males
Chronic, recurrent disorder

Symptoms: decreased vision, metamorphopsia, scotomas

Findings: serous retinal, choroidal, and ciliary body detachments; mild vitritis, RPE changes (leopard spots), conjunctival injection; key finding is shifting subretinal fluid

B-scan ultrasound: thickened sclera, serous RD, choroidal detachments

FA: no discrete leakage

Treatment: steroids and immunosuppressive agents are not effective; consider scleral resection in nanophthalmic eyes, or quandrantic partial-thickness scleral windows

ENDOPHTHALMITIS

Inflammation involving 1 or more coats of the eye and adjacent ocular cavities

Etiology: infectious or sterile; must rule out infection

Symptoms: pain, decreased vision

Findings: lid edema, chemosis, AC reaction, hypopyon (pink hypopyon = *Serratia*), vitritis

Classification:

Acute postoperative (<6 weeks after surgery; 90% in 1st week):
  RISK FACTORS: blepharitis, wound leak, iris prolapse, vitreous loss, contaminated IOL, diabetes, chronic alcoholism
  ORGANISMS: *S. epidermidis, S. aureus, Streptococci, Pseudomonas*
  INCIDENCE:
  Extracapsular extraction (ECCE) or intracapsular cataract extraction (ICCE) (with or without IOL): 0.072%
  Secondary IOL: 0.3%
  PPV: 0.51%
  PK: 0.11%
  Glaucoma filter: 0.061% (*Streptococcus [Enterococcus] faecalis*, Streptococci [57%], *H. influenzae* [23%])

PREVENTION:

TREAT BLEPHARITIS: 85% of responsible organisms (*S. epidermidis* and *S. aureus*) are found on lids; hot compresses, lid hygiene, Polysporin ointment × 1 week preop; add doxycycline 100 mg bid × 1 week for acne rosacea or seborrheic dermatitis

STERILIZE OPERATIVE FIELD: 5% povidine iodine (Betadine); preoperative topical antibiotics (fluoroquinolone)

AVOID INOCULATION: drape eyelashes

ANTIBIOTICS: intracameral (injection or in irrigating solution); topical preop for 1–3 days and postop for 7–10 days; consider subconjunctival antibiotics with broken posterior capsule or vitreous loss

Delayed postoperative:

Propionibacterium acnes (anaerobic gram + rod) or fungal

Trauma:

Incidence of 2%–7% after penetrating trauma

RISK FACTORS: retained intraocular FB, delayed surgery (>24 hours), rural setting (soil contamination), and disruption of the crystalline lens

25% CULTURE POSITIVE: *Bacillus* (30%), *S. epidermidis* (25%), *Streptococci* (13%), *S. aureus* (8%), Gram-negative and mixed flora

Poor visual outcome

Endogenous:

RISK FACTORS: immunosuppression, indwelling venous catheters, IVDA, following intra-abdominal surgery

30% of patients with *Candida* septicemia develop endophthalmitis

Sterile: culture negative

Treatment: rule out infection (AC and vitreous taps)

Intravitreal antibiotics: vancomycin 1 mg/0.1 mL, ceftazidime 2.25 mg/0.1 mL (consider intravitreal dexamethasone 400 μg/0.1 mL)

Systemic antibiotics: in severe cases, most traumatic cases, and endogenous bacterial cases; vancomycin 1 g IV q12 hours or cefazolin 1 g IV q8 hours; ceftazidime 1 g IV q12 hours

Topical fortified antibiotics: vancomycin 25–50 mg/mL, ceftazidime 50 mg/mL q1 hour

Topical steroids and cycloplegics

MAJOR CLINICAL STUDY

Endophthalmitis Vitrectomy Study (EVS)

Objective: to evaluate the treatment of acute (<6 weeks) postoperative (cataract or secondary IOL surgery) endophthalmitis with immediate vitrectomy vs 'tap and inject,' and whether intravenous antibiotics (ceftazidime and amikacin) are necessary

Methods: patients with clinical evidence of acute (<6 weeks) postoperative (cataract or secondary IOL surgery) endophthalmitis and visual acuity of LP or better, and sufficient clarity to see at least some part of the iris were randomly assigned to emergent AC and vitreous taps alone or with vitrectomy and with injection of intravitreal antibiotics (0.4 mg amikacin and 1.0 mg vancomycin). Patients were also given subconjunctival injections of antibiotics (25 mg vancomycin, 100 mg ceftazidime, and steroid [6 mg dexamethasone phosphate]), topical fortified antibiotics (50 mg/mL vancomycin and 20 mg/mL amikacin) and steroid (prednisolone acetate), and oral steroid (prednisone 30 mg bid × 5–10 days). Patients were also randomly assigned to receive systemic IV antibiotics (2 g ceftazidime IV q8h and 7.5 mg/kg amikacin IV followed by 6 mg/kg q12h) or no systemic antibiotics. Intravitreal steroids were not used

Results:

420 patients enrolled

On average, signs and symptoms occurred 6 days after surgery (75% presented within 2 weeks of surgery)

69% had positive cultures; 94% were Gram-positive bacteria (70% coagulase-negative *Staphylococcus*, 10% *S. aureus*, 9% *Streptococci* species)

IV antibiotics were of no benefit

Immediate vitrectomy had significant benefits only when patients presented with light perception vision or worse

Conclusions:

For endopthalmitis after cataract or secondary IOL surgery, perform emergent treatment with AC tap and injection of intravitreal antibiotics when vision is better than LP

Vitrectomy should be reserved for patients presenting with light perception vision or worse

IV antibiotics do not improve the outcome

PANUVEITIS

Sarcoidosis

Multisystem granulomatous disease characterized by noncaseating granulomas; unknown etiology
Females > males; more common among African Americans (10 : 1)
25–50% have systemic sarcoidosis
Ocular disease: 30% unilateral, 70% bilateral; 40% acute, 60% chronic

Findings (25–30%): uveitis in 60% of patients with ocular involvement; 66% of uveitis is anterior (2 forms: acute granulomatous [responds well to corticosteroids] and

1. Lung (most commonly involved organ): hilar adenopathy (most common), diffuse fibrosis

2. Skin: erythema nodosum, skin granulomas (subcutaneous nodules)

3. Bones: arthralgias

4. Hepatosplenomegaly

5. Peripheral neuropathy

6. Diabetes insipidus

7. Hypercalcemia (vitamin D metabolism abnormality)

8. Elevated serum gamma globulin (abnormality in immunoregulation)

9. Parotid gland infiltration (may cause facial nerve palsy from compression)

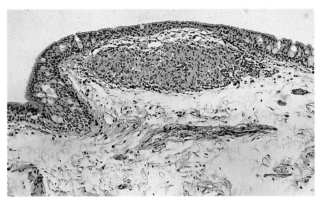

Figure 8-24. Sarcoidosis demonstrating conjunctival granuloma with giant cells surrounded by lymphocytes and plasma cells. (From Yanoff M, Fine BS: Ocular Pathology, 5th edn, St Louis, Mosby, 2002.)

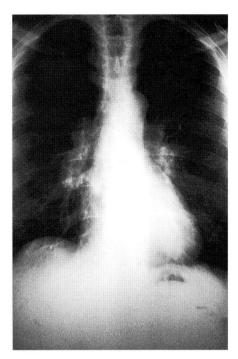

Figure 8-25. Bilateral hilar adenopathy in a patient without pulmonary symptoms. (From Cowan CL: Sarcoidosis. In Yanoff M, Duker JS [eds]: Ophthalmology, London, Mosby, 1999.)

chronic recurrent [difficult to control with corticosteroids]), KP, iris nodules, lacrimal gland infiltration (25%; painless bilateral enlargement), conjunctival follicles, keratoconjunctivitis sicca, episcleritis and scleritis with nodules, choroiditis with yellow or white nodules, retinal periphlebitis with candlewax drippings (granulomas along retinal venules), pars planitis, vitritis, retinal neovascularization, optic nerve granuloma; secondary cataracts, glaucoma, and band keratopathy

Other findings: pulmonary (50%), constitutional (40%; malaise, fever, weight loss), skin (15%), lymphadenopathy (20%) (Box 8-1)

Pathology: noncaseating granulomas (caseating granulomas occur in TB) with Langhans' multinucleated giant cells (Figure 8-24)

Diagnosis:

Lab tests: angiotensin-converting enzyme (ACE; elevated in any diffuse granulomatous disease affecting the lung), serum lysozyme (more sensitive than ACE, but less specific)

Chest X-ray or chest CT: hilar adenopathy (Figure 8-25)

Gallium scan: look for parotid, lacrimal, or pulmonary involvement

Biopsy: skin lesion, conjunctival nodule, lymph node, salivary or lacrimal gland, lung; if elevated ACE and positive CXR, 60–70% of blind conjunctival biopsies will be positive

Treatment: topical, periocular, and systemic steroids, immunosuppressive therapy

Lofgren's Syndrome

Hilar lymphadenopathy, erythema nodosum, anterior uveitis, arthralgia

Mikulicz's Syndrome

Lacrimal and parotid gland swelling, sicca syndrome

Etiology: sarcoidosis, TB, lymphoma/leukemia

Heerfordt's Syndrome

Fever, parotid gland enlargement, anterior uveitis, facial nerve palsy

Behçet's Disease

Chronic recurrent multisystem condition characterized by relapsing inflammation and occlusive vasculitis

Triad of oral ulcers, genital ulcers, and inflammatory eye disease

Associated with HLA-B51; males > females, usually young adults; more common in Japan and Mediterranean countries

Findings (75%): recurrent, explosive inflammatory episodes with active episodes lasting 2–4 weeks

Uveitis (posterior more common than anterior); can present with nongranulomatous anterior uveitis (usually bilateral; may have transient hypopyon); occasionally, conjunctivitis, episcleritis, or keratitis can occur; posterior involvement with recurrent vascular occlusions, retinal hemorrhages, exudates, CME, vitritis, traction RD, ischemic optic neuropathy; may develop glaucoma and cataract (Figure 8-26)

Other findings: oral (aphthous) ulcers, genital ulcers, skin lesions (erythema nodosum, acne-like lesions, folliculitis), arthritis (50%; especially wrists and ankles), thrombophlebitis, large vessel occlusion; GI pain, diarrhea, constipation; CNS involvement (25%; meningoencephalitis, strokes, palsies, confusional states)

Pathology: obliterative vasculitis with activation of both cellular and humoral limbs of immune system; circulating immune complexes in >50%

Diagnosis:
Clinical: (see Box 8-2)
Behcetine skin test (cutaneous hypersensitivity): intradermal puncture; positive test = pustule formation within minutes
HLA-B51

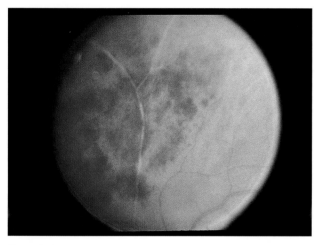

Figure 8-26. Fundus view of a patient who has Behçet's disease. (From Yanoff M, Fine BS: Ocular Pathology, 5th edn, St Louis, Mosby, 2002.)

Box 8-2. Criteria for Behçet's Disease

Major criteria

1. Oral aphthous ulcers (round, discrete borders; heal without scarring)
2. Genital ulcers
3. Skin lesions (erythema nodosum)
4. Ocular disease (75%): nongranulomatous iridocyclitis with sterile hypopyon, necrotizing retinal vasculitis (may cause vascular occlusion), posterior synechiae, glaucoma (pupillary block, uveitic), cataract, TRD

Minor criteria

1. Arthritis (50%)
2. GI lesions
3. Occlusive vascular lesions of major vessels (vena cava)
4. Migratory thrombophlebitis (33%)
5. CNS involvement (25%; neuro-Behçet's; meningoencephalitis, involvement of brain stem, spinal cord, peripheral nerves)
6. Pulmonary artery aneurysm (pathognomonic CXR finding)
7. Interstitial lung changes

Treatment: systemic steroids, cytotoxic agents (chlorambucil most effective for retinal vasculitis, meningoencephalitis), colchicine (prevents recurrences), cyclosporine (ciclosporin); plasmapheresis

Vogt-Koyanagi-Harada Syndrome (VKH)

Uveoencephalitis: bilateral diffuse granulomatous panuveitis, serous RDs, disc edema, meningeal irritation, skin pigmentary changes, and auditory disturbance

Harada's disease: if only eye findings
Presumed autoimmune process against melanocytes

Typically occurs in Asians, American Indians, and Hispanics between ages 30 and 50 years; female > male

Associated with HLA-DR4

Symptoms: decreased vision, pain, redness, photophobia, stiff neck, headache, deafness, tinnitus, vertigo

Findings: bilateral diffuse granulomatous panuveitis, serous RDs, vitritis, exudative choroiditis, CB detachment, CME, ON hyperemia and edema, poliosis; later develop perilimbal vitiligo (Sugiura's sign), Dalen-Fuchs nodules (yellow-white retinal spots), sunset fundus (RPE disturbance with focal areas of atrophy and hyperpigmentation [healing phase])

Other findings: temporary deafness, tinnitus, vertigo, meningeal irritation, skin changes (30%; alopecia, vitiligo, poliosis)

Clinical course:
Prodrome: headache, meningismus, seizures, bilateral decreased vision with pain, redness, photophobia
Syndrome: uveitis with serous RDs
Chronic stage: sunset fundus, Dalen-Fuchs nodules, perilimbal vitiligo
Recurrent stage: AC reaction, pigment changes; 60% retain vision >20/30

Pathology: inflammation of choriocapillaris and retina; Dalen-Fuchs nodules (epithelioid cells between Bruch's membrane and RPE) (Figure 8-27)

DDx: sympathetic ophthalmia, posterior scleritis, syphilis, lupus choroiditis, hypotony, uveal effusion syndrome

Diagnosis:
LP: CSF pleocytosis
FA: multiple focal areas of subretinal leakage ('1000 points of light')

Treatment: steroids (6 months), cycloplegic, immunosuppressive agents

Prognosis: 60% retain vision >20/30

Complications: cataracts (25%), glaucoma (33%), CNV (10%)

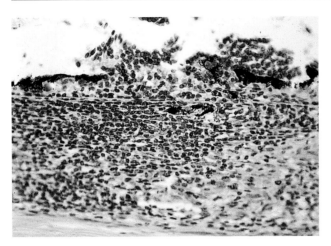

Figure 8-27. VKH demonstrating granulomatous inflammation in choroid extending into choriocapillaris and through RPE. (From Yanoff M, Fine BS: Ocular Pathology, 5th edn, St Louis, Mosby, 2002.)

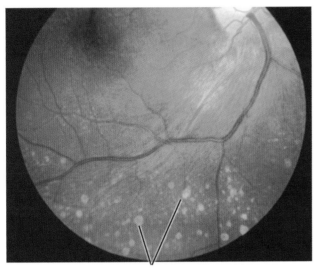

Dalen-Fuchs nodules

Figure 8-28. Dalen-Fuchs nodules in a patient with sympathetic ophthalmia. (From Kaiser PK, Friedman NJ, Pineda II, R: Massachusetts Eye and Ear Infirmary Illustrated Manual of Ophthalmology, 2nd edn, Philadelphia, WB Saunders, 2004.)

Sympathetic Ophthalmia

Bilateral granulomatous panuveitis following penetrating eye trauma

Due to immune sensitization to melanin or melanin-associated proteins in uveal tissues; T-cell mediated (delayed hypersensitivity reaction); latency of 10 days to 50 years after injury

Incidence: 0.1–0.3% of penetrating injuries; 0.015% of intraocular surgery

Findings: Koeppe nodules, mutton fat KP, retinal edema, Dalen-Fuchs nodules; may have disc edema (Figure 8-28)

Pathology: diffuse lymphocytic infiltration of choroid with ill-defined patchy accumulations of epithelioid (giant) cells that contain phagocytosed uveal pigment;

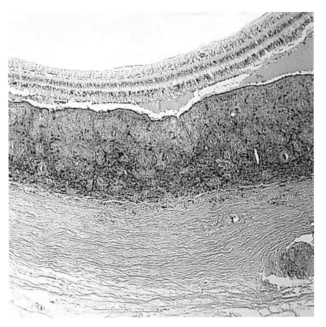

Figure 8-29. SO demonstrating thickened choroid with epithelioid cells and lymphocytes; the choriocapillaris is spared. (From Yanoff M, Fine BS: Ocular Pathology, 5th edn, St Louis, Mosby, 2002.)

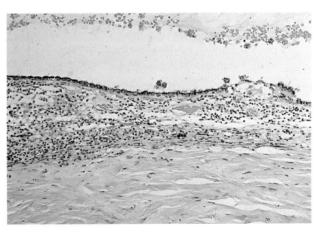

Figure 8-30. Higher magnification of Figure 8-29 shows a Dalen-Fuchs nodule between RPE and Bruch's membrane. (From Yanoff M, Fine BS: Ocular Pathology, 5th edn, St Louis, Mosby, 2002.)

inflammation can extend into optic nerve, causing granulomatous optic neuritis; Dalen-Fuchs nodules (epithelioid giant cells between Bruch's membrane and RPE that appear as small, round, yellow depigmented spots in peripheral retina [also seen in VKH, sarcoidosis, TB]); no involvement of choriocapillaris (Figure 8-29, 8-30)

FA: multiple hyperfluorescent sites of leakage

Treatment: steroids, immunosuppressive agents; consider enucleation of injured eye within 10–14 days if NLP vision, but once inflammation has started in fellow eye, removal of inciting eye is controversial

Prognosis: Many patients retain very good vision

Syphilis

Panuveitis ('great mimic') due to infection with spirochete *Treponema pallidum*

Acquired:

Findings (secondary and tertiary): panuveitis, iris papules and gummata (yellow-red nodules), chorioretinitis (salt and pepper changes), optic neuritis, optic atrophy, Argyll-Robertson pupil, ectopia lentis, interstitial keratitis (Figure 8-31)

Other findings:

    SECONDARY: chancre, rash, lymphadenopathy, condyloma lata

    TERTIARY: CNS, aortic aneurysm, gummas

Diagnosis: serology (VDRL or RPR, and FTA-ABS); must rule out neurosyphilis with LP

    FALSE-POSITIVE VDRL: rheumatoid arthritis, anticardiolipin antibody, SLE

Treatment: as for neurosyphilis

    Penicillin G 12–24 million units/day IV × 2 weeks, followed by penicillin G 2.4 million units/week IM × 3 weeks

    In penicillin-allergic patients: doxycycline, erythromycin

Congenital:

Findings: interstitial keratitis (new vessels meet in center of cornea [salmon patch]); then atrophy (ghost vessels), anterior uveitis, ectopia lentis, Argyll-Robertson pupil, optic atrophy, chorioretinitis (salt and pepper fundus)

Other findings: death (in utero or perinatal), inflammation of internal organs, dental abnormalities (Hutchinson's teeth), facial deformities (saddle nose), saber shins

Tuberculosis

Due to infection with *Mycobacterium tuberculosis*

Findings: lupus vulgaris on eyelids, phlyctenule, primary conjunctival TB, interstitial keratitis, scleritis, lacrimal gland

involvement, orbital periostitis, granulomatous panuveitis, secondary glaucoma and cataract, chorioretinal plaque or nodule (tuberculoma), exudative RD, cranial nerve palsies (often due to basal meningitis)

Treatment: isoniazid, rifampin, ethambutol, pyrazinamide; systemic steroids may cause a flare-up; ethambutol and isoniazid can cause a toxic optic neuropathy

MASQUERADE SYNDROMES

Conditions that present as uveitis: peripheral RD, intraocular foreign body, JXG, multiple sclerosis, malignancies (retinoblastoma, acute lymphoblastic eukemia [ALL], large cell lymphoma, malignant melanoma), RP

Intraocular Foreign Body

Findings: AC reaction; may have signs of ocular trauma, visible FB, iris heterochromia

Diagnois: X-ray, B-scan ultrasound

Juvenile Xanthogranuloma

Findings: small fleshy iris tumors, AC reaction, spontaneous hyphema

Diagnosis: skin lesions, iris biopsy

Multiple Sclerosis

Findings: periphlebitis, pars planitis, optic neuritis

Diagnosis: neurologic examination, head MRI

Retinoblastoma

Findings: pseudohypopyon, vitreous cells

Diagnosis:

    AC tap: lactate dehydrogenase (LDH) levels, cytology

    B-scan ultrasound: calcifications

Leukemia

Retina is most common ocular tissue affected clinically
Choroid is most common ocular tissue affected histopathologically

Findings: AC reaction, iris heterochromia, Roth spots, retinal hemorrhages, cotton wool spots, peripheral NV, serous RDs, vascular dilation and tortuosity, optic nerve infiltration

Diagnosis: bone marrow, peripheral blood smear, aqueous cytology

    FA with serous retinal detachment: multiple areas of hyperfluorescence (similar to VKH)

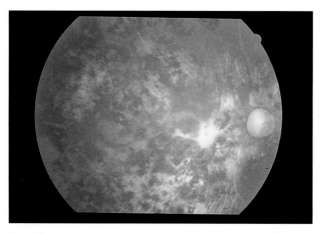

Figure 8-31. Extensive chorioretinal damage with hyperplasia of retinal pigment epithelium due to syphilis. (From Dugel PU: Syphilitic uveitis. In Yanoff M, Duker JS [eds]: Ophthalmology. London, Mosby, 1999.)

Primary Intraocular Lymphoma (Reticulum Cell Sarcoma)

Findings: bilateral vitreous cells, retinal hemorrhage and exudates, retinal and choroidal infiltrates

Diagnosis: cytology (aqueous and vitreous)

Treatment: radiation therapy (ocular and CNS), intrathecal chemotherapy

Malignant Melanoma

Necrotic tumor may seed tumor cells into the vitreous and anterior segment, causing an inflammatory response

Findings: AC reaction, iris heterochromia, vitreous hemorrhage; may have brown pseudohypopyon (melanin-laden macrophages) and melanomalytic glaucoma

Diagnosis: FA, B-scan ultrasound

Retinitis Pigmentosa

Findings: vitreous cells, pigmentary retinopathy with vascular attenuation and optic nerve pallor

Diagnosis: ERG, electro-oculography (EOG), visual fields

DIFFERENTIAL DIAGNOSIS OF UVEITIS AND ASSOCIATED SIGNS

Band keratopathy: JRA, sarcoidosis, multiple sclerosis

Hyphema: Fuchs' heterochromic iridocyclitis, trauma, JXG, HZV

Vitreous hemorrhage: VKH, POHS

Iris nodules: TB, syphilis, sarcoidosis, leprosy

Bell's palsy (bilateral): Lyme disease, sarcoidosis

Genitourinary involvement: Reiter's syndrome, gonococcal disease, Behçet's disease

Jaundice: leptospirosis, inflammatory bowel disease (IBD), CMV, schistosomiasis

Liver enlargement: toxocariasis, toxoplasmosis, CMV

CNS involvement: TB, VKH, congenital toxoplasmosis, congenital CMV, Behçet's disease, large cell lymphoma

Skin rash: secondary syphilis, sarcoidosis, Behçet's disease, psoriasis, Reiter's syndrome, VKH, POHS

Erythema nodosum: sarcoidosis, TB, IBD, POHS, Behçet's disease, APMPPE

Oral ulcers: Behçet's disease, Reiter's syndrome, HSV, IBD, OCP, Stevens-Johnson syndrome (SJS), SLE

Genital ulcers: syphilis, Reiter's syndrome, Behçet's disease, OCP

Pulmonary involvement: TB, sarcoidosis, Churg-Strauss syndrome, *Toxocara*, aspergillosis, coccidioidomycosis, POHS, Wegener's granulomatosis

SURGERY AND UVEITIS

Usually wait at least 3 months for cataract surgery, 6 months for corneal transplant

JRA: no IOL; can develop cyclitic membranes and CB detachments; consider lensectomy with partial vitrectomy

Pars planitis: increased risk of complications, higher risk for CME; vitreous opacities may limit vision, therefore, consider lensectomy with pars plana vitrectomy

Fuchs' heterochromic iridocyclitis: cataract surgery is safe; increased risk of transient postoperative hyphema

REVIEW QUESTIONS (Answers start on page 366)

1. The most effective antibiotic for the treatment of *P. acnes* endophthalmitis is
   a. amikacin
   b. gentamicin
   c. vancomycin
   d. ceftazidime
2. For the diagnosis of granulomatous inflammation, which cell type must be present?
   a. Langhans' cell
   b. lymphocyte
   c. Touton giant cell
   d. epithelioid histiocyte
3. All of the following are true concerning sarcoidosis except
   a. Touton giant cells are common
   b. lymphocytes surround the granuloma
   c. histiocytes are abundant
   d. necrosis is rare
4. Which of the following is not characteristic of Fuchs' heterochromic iridocyclitis?
   a. iris neovascularization
   b. cataract
   c. posterior synechiae
   d. vitreous opacities
5. The most common organism causing endopthalmitis following cataract surgery is
   a. *S. pneumoniae*
   b. *H. influenzae*
   c. *S. aureus*
   d. *S. epidermidis*

6. MEWDS can be differentiated from APMPPE by
   a. age of onset
   b. female predilection
   c. paracentral scotomas
   d. viral prodrome
7. All of the following disorders are correctly paired with their HLA associations except
   a. POHS, B9
   b. Behçet's disease, B51
   c. Birdshot retinochoroidopathy, A29
   d. Reiter's syndrome, B27
8. Decreased vision in a patient with intermediate uveitis is most likely due to
   a. cataract
   b. macular edema
   c. papillitis
   d. glaucoma
9. A 71-year-old woman with a 6-month history of fatigue, anorexia, and 10-pound (4 kg) weight loss is found to have left-sided weakness, visual acuity of 20/80 OD and 20/60 OS, and vitreous cells. The most helpful workup is
   a. LP and vitrectomy
   b. ESR and temporal artery biopsy
   c. CBC and lymph node biopsy
   d. PPD and chest X-ray
10. The most common organisms causing endophthalmitis following trauma are
    a. *Enterococcus* species and *S. aureus*
    b. *Bacillus* species and *S. epidermidis*
    c. *Pseudomonas* species and *S. aureus*
    d. *S. aureus* and *S. epidermidis*
11. All of the following are features common to both sympathetic ophthalmia and Vogt-Koyanagi-Harada syndrome except
    a. serous retinal detachments
    b. Dalen-Fuchs nodules
    c. pathology localized to choroid
    d. vitritis
12. Which disorder is more common in males?
    a. MEWDS
    b. uveal effusion syndrome
    c. APMPPE
    d. Birdshot choroidopathy
13. EVS findings include all of the following except
    a. vitrectomy was beneficial only in patients with LP vision
    b. intravitreal corticosteroids were helpful
    c. IV antibiotics were not helpful
    d. the most common organism was *S. epidermidis*
14. Which of the following is not characteristic of MEWDS?
    a. enlargement of the blind spot
    b. bilaterality
    c. flu-like illness
    d. female preponderance
15. The most common cause of posterior uveitis is
    a. sarcoidosis
    b. syphilis
    c. CMV
    d. toxoplasmosis
16. All of the following are causes of HLA-B27-associated uveitis except
    a. ankylosing spondylitis
    b. ulcerative colitis
    c. Crohn's disease
    d. psoriasis
17. Which of the following is not part of the classic triad of findings in Reiter's syndrome?
    a. iritis
    b. arthritis
    c. conjunctivitis
    d. urethritis
18. Which of the following laboratory tests is most commonly found in JRA-related iritis?
    a. RF–, ANA–
    b. RF+, ANA–
    c. RF–, ANA+
    d. RF+, ANA+
19. Phacoantigenic endophthalmitis is characterized by which pattern of granulomatous inflammation?
    a. zonal
    b. diffuse
    c. discrete
    d. necrotizing
20. Which combination of findings is least likely to occur in rubella?
    a. retinopathy and cataract
    b. glaucoma and cataract
    c. glaucoma and retinopathy
    d. cataract and deafness
21. A 35-year-old man with decreased vision OD is found to have optic nerve edema and a macular star. The causative organism most likely is
    a. *Onchocerca volvulus*
    b. *Bartonella henselae*
    c. *Treponema pallidum*
    d. *Borrelia burgdorferi*
22. Which is least helpful for the diagnosis of toxocariasis?
    a. ELISA test
    b. AC tap
    c. vitrectomy
    d. stool examination
23. A person living in which area of the US would be most likely to develop POHS?
    a. southwest
    b. northwest
    c. midwest
    d. southeast
24. All of the following are true of birdshot choroidopathy except
    a. more common in males
    b. usually bilateral
    c. CME is common
    d. associated with HLA-A29
25. Which of the following is least commonly associated with *Treponema pallidum* infection?
    a. interstitial keratitis
    b. chorioretinitis
    c. ectopia lentis
    d. glaucoma

26. The HLA association for pars planitis with multiple sclerosis is
    a. B8
    b. B51
    c. DR4
    d. DR15

27. Retinal S antigen is found in
    a. ganglion cells
    b. retinal pigment epithelium
    c. photoreceptors
    d. Mueller cells

28. Features of Harada's disease include all of the following except
    a. vitritis
    b. deafness
    c. serous retinal detachments
    d. Dalen-Fuchs nodules

29. Larva cause all of the following infections except
    a. cysticercosis
    b. diffuse unilateral subacute neuroretinitis
    c. onchocerciasis
    d. cat-scratch disease

30. Which of the following signs of pars planitis is most associated with multiple sclerosis?
    a. subretinal neovascularization
    b. snowbank
    c. periphlebitis
    d. CME

31. CSF abnormalities are associated with all of the following disorders except
    a. VKH syndrome
    b. ocular sarcoidosis
    c. APMPPE
    d. pars planitis

32. All of the following can present as uveitis except
    a. retinoblastoma
    b. choroidal hemangioma
    c. leukemia
    d. juvenile xanthogranuloma

33. Which of the following is not associated with inflammatory bowel disease?
    a. conjunctivitis
    b. episcleritis
    c. interstitial keratitis
    d. iritis

34. Anterior vitreous cells are least likely to be found in
    a. retinitis pigmentosa
    b. CMV
    c. serpiginous choroidopathy
    d. chronic cyclitis

35. Gastrointestinal disorders associated with uveitis include all of the following except
    a. ulcerative colitis
    b. Whipple's disease
    c. diverticulitis
    d. Crohn's disease

36. All of the following may occur in ocular sarcoidosis except
    a. optic disc nodules
    b. pars planitis
    c. CN palsies
    d. low serum gamma globulin

37. The choroid is the primary location of the pathologic process in
    a. toxoplasmosis
    b. CMV
    c. Coat's disease
    d. VKH syndrome

38. Which of the following is least likely to be found in a patient with sympathetic ophthalmia?
    a. onset after a latent period of 40 years
    b. granulomatous nodules in the retina
    c. history of evisceration of the traumatized eye
    d. iris nodules in the sympathizing eye

39. Band keratopathy is least likely to occur in a patient with
    a. sarcoidosis
    b. JRA
    c. Behçet's disease
    d. multiple sclerosis

40. A patient with APMPPE is most likely to have
    a. unilateral involvement
    b. enlarged blind spot
    c. viral prodrome
    d. CNV

SUGGESTED READINGS

American Academy of Ophthalmology: Intraocular Inflammation and Uveitis, vol 9. San Francisco, AAO, 2012.

Foster CS, Vitale AT: Diagnosis and Treatment of Uveitis. Philadelphia, WB Saunders, 2002.

Jones NP: Uveitis: An Illustrated Manual. Philadelphia, Butterworth-Heinemann, 1998.

Michelson JB: Color Atlas of Uveitis, 2nd edn. St Louis, Mosby, 1992.

Nussenblatt RB, Whitcup SM: Uveitis: Fundamentals and Clinical Practice, 4th edn. Philadelphia, Mosby, 2010.

Tabbara KF, Nussenblatt RB: Posterior Uveitis Diagnosis and Management. Philadelphia, Butterworth-Heinemann, 1994.

9

Glaucoma

ANATOMY/PHYSIOLOGY
TESTING
PATHOLOGY
DISORDERS
TREATMENT

Ciliary body (CB)

6-mm-wide structure located between the scleral spur anteriorly and the ora serrata posteriorly; composed of the pars plicata (anterior 2 mm with ciliary processes) and the pars plana (posterior 4 mm, flat)

Pars plicata consists of

Ciliary muscle: longitudinal fibers (insert into scleral spur and affect outflow facility), circular fibers (anterior inner fibers oriented parallel to limbus and affect accommodation), and radial fibers (connect longitudinal and circular fibers)

Ciliary vessels: major arterial circle of the iris (in CB near iris root) formed by anastomosis of branches of anterior and long posterior ciliary arteries

Ciliary processes: 70 finger-like projections composed of pigmented and nonpigmented epithelial cell bilayer, capillaries, and stroma

Functions

Suspends and alters shape of lens: zonular fibers that originate between the ciliary processes of the pars plicata, attach to the crystalline lens, and suspend it. Helmholtz's theory of accommodation explains the changes in lens shape and thus refractive power with contraction and relaxation of the ciliary muscle. Contraction of the longitudinal fibers pulls the lens forward, shallowing the anterior chamber. Contraction of the circular fibers relaxes the zonules making the lens more spherical with greater focusing power. Relaxation of circular fibers (or cycloplegia) tightens the zonules, stretching the lens and making it thinner with less focusing power.

Produces aqueous humor: production of aqueous is primarily by active secretion (also diffusion and ultrafiltration); both an Na^+/K^+ pump and carbonic anhydrase are involved. β-blockers act through adenylcyclase to inhibit the Na^+/K^+ pump; glucose enters by passive diffusion.

Rate = 2–3 μL/min, AC volume = 250 μL, posterior chamber volume = 60 μL (AC volume turnover is approximately 1%/min). Rate measured by fluorophotometry (direct optical measurement of decreasing fluorescein concentration) or tonography (indirect calculation from outflow measurement). Diurnal production of aqueous (may be related to cortisol levels) decreases with sleep (45%), age (2%/decade; counterbalanced by the decreased outflow with age), inflammation, surgery, trauma, and drugs

AQUEOUS COMPOSITION: slightly hypertonic and acidic (pH 7.2) compared with plasma; 15× more ascorbate than plasma; lower protein (0.02% vs 7% in plasma); lower calcium and phosphorus (50% of the level in plasma); chloride and bicarbonate vary (from 25% above or below plasma levels); sodium, potassium, magnesium, iron, zinc, and copper levels similar to those in plasma

FUNCTIONS OF AQUEOUS: maintains intraocular pressure, provides metabolic substrates (glucose, oxygen, electrolytes) to the cornea and lens, and removes metabolic waste (lactate, pyruvate, carbon dioxide)

Affects aqueous outflow: contraction of ciliary muscle causes traction on the trabecular meshwork, increasing outflow

Synthesizes acid mucopolysaccharide component of vitreous: occurs in nonpigmented epithelial cells of pars plana and enters vitreous body at its base

Maintains blood–aqueous barrier: within the ciliary processes, plasma enters from thin fenestrated endothelium of capillary core → passes through stroma → 2 layers of epithelium with apposing apical surfaces (which forms the ciliary epithelial bilayer):

OUTER PIGMENTED LAYER: continuous with the RPE (basal lamina continuous with Bruch's membrane), contains zonula occludens

---

INNER NONPIGMENTED LAYER: equivalent to the sensory retina (basal lamina continuous with ILM), site of active secretion

Both layers have basal basement membranes with their apices facing each other. During passage from the bloodstream to the posterior chamber, a molecule must pass through capillary basement membrane, pigmented epithelium basement membrane, pigmented epithelium, nonpigmented epithelium, nonpigmented epithelium basement membrane

Cryodestruction and inflammation cause loss of barrier function (tight junctions open), resulting in flare (proteins in aqueous); atropine reduces flare by closing tight junctions

Outflow Pathways

Trabecular meshwork (traditional pathway): represents major aqueous drainage system; uveoscleral meshwork → corneoscleral meshwork → juxtacanalicular connective tissue → Schlemm's canal → collector channels → aqueous veins → episcleral and conjunctival veins → anterior ciliary and superior ophthalmic veins → cavernous sinus

The pore size of the meshwork decreases towards Schlemm's canal:

Uveal meshwork: collagenous core surrounded by endothelial cells; pore size up to 70 μm; linked to ciliary muscle

Corneoscleral meshwork: sheet-like beams insert into scleral spur; pore size up to 30 μm

Juxtacanalicular tissue: links corneoscleral trabeculae with Schlemm's endothelium; pore size = 4–7 μm; site of greatest aqueous outflow resistance

Canal of Schlemm is lined by a single layer of endothelial cells (mesothelial cells) and connects to the venous system by 30 collector channels

Uveoscleral outflow (15–20% of total outflow): aqueous passes through face of ciliary body in the angle, enters the ciliary muscle and suprachoroidal space, and is drained by veins in the ciliary body, choroid, and sclera

Cyclodialysis cleft increases aqueous outflow through the uveoscleral pathway (without reducing aqueous production); cycloplegics and prostaglandin analogues increase uveoscleral outflow; miotics decrease uveoscleral outflow and increase trabecular meshwork outflow

Angle Structures

Visible only by gonioscopy because of total internal reflection at the air/cornea interface (Figure 9-1)

Schwalbe's line: peripheral/posterior termination of Descemet's membrane, which corresponds to apex of corneal light wedge (optical cross section of the cornea with narrow slit beam reveals 2 linear reflections, 1 from external and 1 from internal corneal surfaces, which meet at Schwalbe's line)

Trabecular meshwork (TM): anterior nonpigmented portion appears as a clear white band; posterior pigmented portion has variable pigmentation (usually darkest inferiorly). Increased pigmentation of trabecular meshwork occurs with pseudoexfoliation syndrome (Sampaolesi's line), pigment dispersion syndrome, uveitis, melanoma,

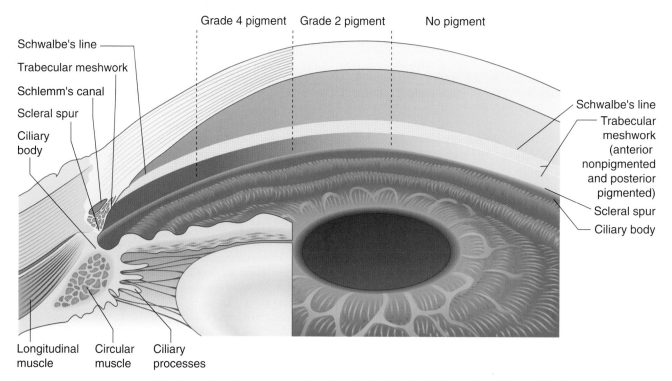

Figure 9-1. Composite drawing of the microscopic and gonioscopic anatomy. (From Becker B, Shaffer RN: Diagnosis and Therapy of the Glaucomas, St Louis, Mosby, 1965.)

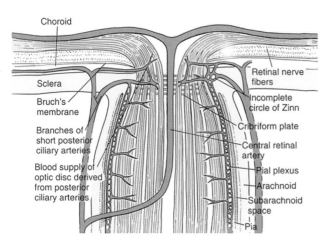

Figure 9-2. Vascular supply and anatomy of the anterior optic nerve. (From Hart WM Jr: In Podos SM, Yanoff M [eds]: Textbook of Ophthalmology, vol 6, London, Mosby, 1994.)

trauma, surgery, hyphema, darkly pigmented individuals, and increasing age

Schlemm's canal: usually not visible or only faintly visible as a light gray band at the level of posterior TM; elevated venous pressure or pressure from the edge of the gonioscopy lens may cause blood to reflux, making Schlemm's canal visible as a faint red band

DDx of blood in Schlemm's canal: elevated episcleral venous pressure, oculodermal melanocytosis (nevus of Ota), neurofibromatosis, congenital ectropion uveae, hypotony, secondary to gonioscopy

Scleral spur (SS): narrow white band that corresponds to the site of insertion of longitudinal fibers of ciliary muscle to sclera

Ciliary body (CB): pigmented band that represents the anterior face of the ciliary body; iris processes may be seen as lacy projections crossing this band but not the scleral spur (occur in 33% of population)

Angle Abnormalities

Peripheral anterior synechia (PAS): any pigmented structure that crosses scleral spur

> *Etiology:* angle-closure, uveitis, neovascularization, flat anterior chamber, ICE syndrome, ciliary body tumors, mesodermal dysgenesis

Normal vessels: radial iris vessels, portions of arterial circle of CB, and rarely, vertical vessels deep in CB; do not branch or cross the scleral spur; present in 7% of patients with blue irides and 10% with brown

Abnormal vessels: fine, often branch, no orientation, cross-scleral spur

> *DDx:* neovascularization (rubeosis iridis), iris neoplasm, Fuchs' heterochromic iridocyclitis (sparse, faint, and delicate; bleed easily on decompression of AC)

Angle recession: tear between longitudinal and circular fibers of the ciliary muscle. Because longitudinal fibers are still attached to the scleral spur, miotics still work, but because they decrease uveoscleral outflow, IOP may actually increase. Breaks in posterior TM result in scarring and a nonfunctional TM; aqueous drains primarily through uveoscleral outflow; 60–90% of patients with traumatic hyphemas have angle recession; 5% of eyes with angle recession will develop glaucoma

> *Gonioscopic findings:* widened ciliary body band, increased visibility of scleral spur, torn iris processes, sclera visible through disrupted ciliary body tissue, marked variation in CB width in different quadrants of same eye

Cyclodialysis cleft: separation of ciliary body from scleral spur; often from trauma. Results in direct communication between AC and suprachoroidal space causing hypotony; spontaneous closure may occur (unlikely after 6 weeks) with marked IOP rise; shortly thereafter, the TM should begin to function normally again

> *Gonioscopic findings:* cleft at junction of scleral spur and CB band
>
> *Treatment:* cycloplegic to relax ciliary body in an attempt to close cleft (avoid pilocarpine, which may open the cleft through ciliary muscle traction); laser (argon induces inflammation to close the cleft; spot size = 50–100 μm, duration = 0.1–0.2 s; power = 0.5–1.0 watts to uvea and 1–3 watts to sclera); cryotherapy; suture CB to sclera (direct cyclopexy); intravitreal air bubble for a superior cleft; YAG laser can be used to open a closed cleft

Iridodialysis: tear/disinsertion of iris root. If large or symptomatic, consider surgical repair with mattress sutures

Optic Nerve (Figure 9-2)

Approximately 1.2 million axons; cell bodies of ganglion cells are located in the ganglion cell layer

4 layers of optic nerve head based on blood supply:

> *Nerve fiber:* supplied by branches of central retinal artery
>
> *Prelaminar:* supplied by capillaries of the short posterior ciliary arteries
>
> *Laminar* (lamina cribrosa): supplied by dense plexus from short posterior ciliary arteries
>
> *Retrolaminar:* supplied by both ciliary (via recurrent pial vessels) and retinal (via centripetal branches from pial region) circulations

Optic nerve blood flow is influenced by mean blood pressure, IOP, blood viscosity, blood vessel caliber, and blood vessel length

TESTING

Intraocular Pressure

Goldmann equation: $IOP = F/C + EVP$ relates 3 factors important in determination of IOP

> F = rate of aqueous formation = 2–3 μL/min

C = facility of outflow = 0.28 μL/min/mmHg; <0.20 is abnormal; decreases with age, increases with medication; measured by tonography

EVP = episcleral venous pressure = 8–12 mmHg; increases with venous obstruction or A-V shunt; measured by manometry

IOP = 8–21 mmHg is considered normal; average = 16 +/−2.5 mmHg; distribution is not Gaussian and is skewed to higher IOPs

IOP is influenced by age (may increase with age), genetics, race (higher in African Americans), season (higher in winter, lower in summer), blood pressure, obesity, exercise (lower after exercise), Valsalva, time of day (diurnal variation [2–6 mm/day]; peak in morning), posture (higher when lying down vs sitting up), various hormones, and drugs. Also ocular factors: refractive error (higher in myopes) and eyelid closure

Tonometry

IOP measurement can be performed with a variety of devices (tonometers)

Indentation

Schiøtz tonometer: known weight indents cornea and displaces a volume of fluid within the eye; amount of indentation estimates pressure; falsely low readings occur with a very elastic eye (low scleral rigidity as with high myopia, buphthalmos, retinal detachment, treatment with cholinesterase inhibitors, thyroid disease, and previous ocular surgery) or a compressible intraocular gas (e.g. SF_6 and C_3F_8); falsely high readings occur with scleral rigidity and hyperopia

Applanation: based on the Imbert-Fick principle: $P = F/A$ (for an ideal thin-walled sphere, pressure inside sphere equals force necessary to flatten its surface divided by the area of flattening). The eye is not an ideal sphere: the cornea resists flattening, and capillary action of the tear meniscus pulls the tonometer to the eye. However, these 2 forces cancel each other when the applanated diameter is 3.06 mm

Goldmann tonometer: biprism attached to a spring; fluorescein semicircles align when area applanated has a diameter = 3.06 mm; unaffected by ocular rigidity; error can occur with squeezing, Valsalva, irregular or edematous cornea, corneal thickness (thick corneas overestimate IOP [~5 mmHg per 70 μm], and thin corneas underestimate IOP [~5 mmHg per 70 μm]), amount of fluorescein, external pressure on or restriction of globe, and astigmatism >1.5 D (must align red mark on tip with axis of MINUS cylinder)

Perkins tonometer: portable form of Goldmann device

Mackay-Marg tonometer: applanates small area; good for corneal scars and edema. Examples of this style tonometer include the tonopen and the pneumotonometer

TONOPEN: probe indents cornea, and microprocessor calculates IOP and reliability

PNEUMOTONOMETER: central sensing device is controlled by air pressure

Noncontact

Air puff tonometer: noncontact device; time required for air jet to flatten cornea is proportional to IOP; varies with cardiac cycle

Gonioscopy

Classification systems

Scheie:

Grade I = wide open (CB visible)

Grade II = SS visible; CB not visible

Grade III = only anterior TM visible

Grade IV = closed angle (TM not visible)

Schaffer: opposite of Scheie (Grade 0 is closed; Grade IV is wide open) (Figure 9-3)

Grade I = 10% open

Grade II = 20% open

Grade III = 30% open

Grade IV = 40% open

Spaeth: most descriptive; 4 elements

FIRST ELEMENT: level of iris insertion (capital letter A-E)

A = Anterior to TM

B = Behind Schwalbe's line or at TM

C = At scleral spur

D = Deep angle, CB visible

E = Extremely deep, large CB band

Perform indention gonioscopy: if true insertion is more posterior, place original impression in parentheses followed by true insertion location

SECOND ELEMENT: number that denotes the iridocorneal angle width in degrees from 5 to 45

THIRD ELEMENT: peripheral iris configuration (lower case letter r, s, or q)

r = regular (flat)

s = steep (convex)

q = queer (concave)

FOURTH ELEMENT: pigmentation of posterior TM (graded from 0 [none] to 4 [maximal])

Example: (A)B15 r, 1+ (appositionally closed 15° angle that opens to TM with indentation, regular iris configuration, and mildly pigmented posterior TM)

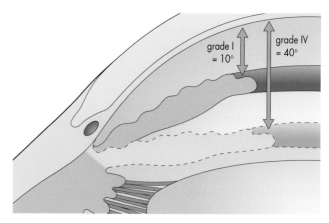

Figure 9-3. Shaffer's angle-grading system. (From Fran M, Smith J, Doyle W: Clinical examination of glaucoma. In Yanoff M, Duker JS [eds]: Ophthalmology, 2nd edn. St Louis, Mosby, 2004.)

Types of lenses

Koeppe lens: direct view
Goldmann 3-mirror lens: requires coupling solution (Goniosol)
Zeiss, Posner, and Sussman 4-mirror lenses: can perform indentation gonioscopy to determine whether angle closure is appositional or synechial

Grading system of shallow/flat anterior chamber

Grade I: Contact between cornea and peripheral iris
Grade II: Contact between cornea and iris up to pupil (consider reforming AC with BSS or viscoelastic)
Grade III: Contact between cornea and crystalline lens (surgical emergency)

Visual Fields

Perimetry measures the 'island of vision' or topographic representation of differential light sensitivity. Peak = fovea; depression = blind spot; extent = 60° nasally, 60° superiorly, 70–75° inferiorly, and 100–110° temporally

Central field tests points only within a 30° radius of fixation

Types:
(Figure 9-4)
Kinetic: uses a moving stimulus of constant intensity to produce an isopter or points of equal sensitivity (horizontal cross section of the hill of vision)
Static: uses a fixed stimulus with constant or variable intensity to produce a profile (vertical cross section of the hill of vision)

Goldmann (kinetic and static):

Test distance: 0.33 m
Test object size: I–V (each increment doubles the diameter [quadruples the area] of test object; III4e test object will have 2× the diameter and 4× the area of II4e)
Light filters: 1–4 (increments of 5db), a–e (increments of 1db)

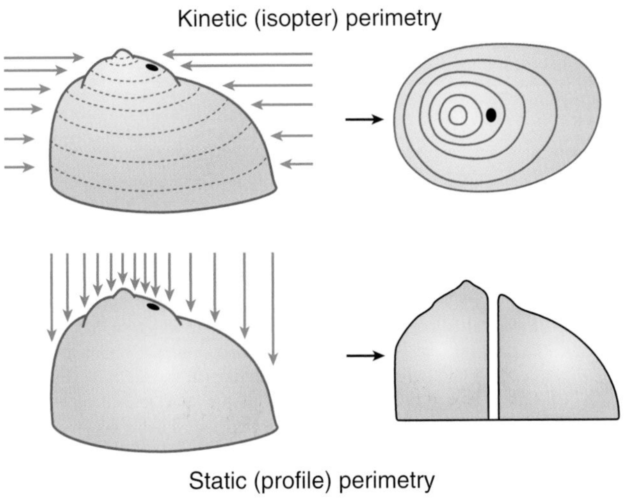

Kinetic (isopter) perimetry

Static (profile) perimetry

Figure 9-4. Kinetic and static perimetry. (From Bajandas FJ, Kline LB: Neuro-Ophthalmology Review Manual, 3rd edn, Thorofare, NJ, Slack, 2004.)

Humphrey (static):

Test distance = 0.33 m; background illumination = 31.5 apostilbs (asb); stimulus size = III; stimulus duration = 0.2 s; various programs (i.e. central 30°, 24°, 10°, neuro fields, ptosis fields, etc.)
Reliability indices:
FIXATION LOSS: patient responds when a target is displayed in blind spot. There is also a gaze tracking printout at the bottom of the page that shows the deviation of fixation during each stimulus presentation
FALSE-POSITIVE: patient responds when there is no stimulus (nervous or trigger-happy; causes white areas)
FALSE-NEGATIVE: patient fails to respond to a superthreshold stimulus at a location that was previously responded to (indicates loss of attention or fatigue; causes cloverleaf pattern)
Global indices:
MEAN DEVIATION (MD): average departure of each test point from the age-adjusted normal value. This represents the overall deviation (mean elevation or depression) of the visual field from the normal reference field
PATTERN STANDARD DEVIATION (PSD): standard deviation of the differences between the threshold and expected values for each test point. This represents the change in shape of the field from the expected shape for a normal field
SHORT-TERM FLUCTUATION (SF): variability in responses when the same 10 points are retested; measure of consistency
CORRECTED PATTERN STANDARD DEVIATION (CPSD): PSD adjusted for patient reliability (correcting for SF)
Patient vision ≤20/80 will cause a scotoma to appear larger and deeper
Pupil <3 mm will cause reduction in total deviation

Tangent screen (usually kinetic): test distance is 1m, test object may vary in size and color; tests only central field. Magnifies scotoma and is of low cost; however, poor reproducibility and lack of standardization

VF defect: a scotoma is an area of partial or complete blindness
Corresponds to a defect that is 3° wide and 6 decibels (dB) deep; also 1 point on Humphrey testing that is depressed >10 dB or at least 2 points that are depressed at least 5 Db
Typical localized glaucomatous scotomas: (Figure 9.5)
PARACENTRAL: within central 10°
ARCUATE (Bjerrum): isolated, nasal step of Rönne and Seidel (connected to blind spot)
TEMPORAL WEDGE
Glaucomatous scotomas do not respect the vertical meridian (vs neurologic VF defects, which do)
VF should correlate with optic nerve appearance; otherwise, consider refractive error, level of vision, media opacities, pupil size, and other causes of VF

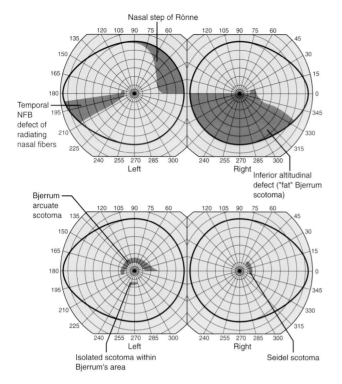

Figure 9-5. Composite diagram depicting different types of field defects. (From Bajandas FJ, Kline LB: Neuro-Ophthalmology Review Manual, 3rd edn, Thorofare, NJ, Slack, 2004.)

defects (tilted ON head, ON head drusen, retinal lesions, etc.)

Optic Nerve Head (ONH) Analyzers

Various digital and video cameras that capture ONH image; computer then calculates cup area in an attempt to objectively quantify ONH appearance (Table 9-1)

Confocal scanning laser ophthalmoscopy (CSLO; Heidelberg retinal tomograph [HRT]; TopSS): low-power laser produces digital 3D picture of ON head by integrating coronal scans of increasing tissue depth; indirectly measures nerve fiber layer (NFL) thickness (Figures 9-6, 9-7)

Optical coherence tomography (OCT): measures optical backscattering of light to produce high-resolution, cross-sectional image of the NFL (Figure 9-8)

Scanning laser polarimetry (SLP; Nerve Fiber Analyzer, GDx): uses a confocal scanning laser ophthalmoscope with an integrated polarimeter to detect changes in light polarization from axons to measure the NFL thickness; quantitative analysis of NFL thickness to detect early glaucomatous damage (Figure 9-9)

Optic nerve blood flow measurement: color Doppler imaging and laser Doppler flowmetry (Figure 9-10)

TABLE 9-1	Summary of Techniques for Retinal Nerve Fiber Layer Analysis			
Technique	**Equipment Needed**	**Governing Principles**	**Advantages**	**Disadvantages**
Ophthalmoscopy	Direct ophthalmoscope or slit lamp and 78D or 90D lens Red-free light	Nerve fiber layer visibility is enhanced with shortwavelength light	Easy to perform using readily available equipment	May be difficult without clear media Nerve fiber layer not easily seen in lightly pigmented fundi
Red-free, highcontrast fundus photography	Fundus camera with red-free filter High contrast black-and-white film and paper	Nerve fiber layer visibility is enhanced with shortwavelength light	Nerve fiber layer defects may be easy to detect	Requires skilled photographer Requires dilated pupil Limitations of ophthalmoscopy apply
Retinal contour analysis	Scanning laser ophthalmoscope that can perform tomographic topography	Three-dimensional construction of retinal surface can measure retinal height above a reference plane – height is related to nerve fiber layer thickness	Easy to perform through undilated pupil No discomfort to patient Can image through most media opacities unless very dense	Equipment is expensive Height measurements depend upon location of reference plane Retinal thickness may not be true indirect measure of nerve fiber layer thickness
Optical coherence tomography	Optical coherence tomography unit	Uses reflected and backscattered light to create images of various retinal layers (analogous to the use of sound waves in ultrasonography)	Can differentiate layers within the retina, including the nerve fiber layer, with a 10 µm resolution Correlates with known histology	Equipment is expensive Requires dilated pupil Resolution may not be high enough to detect small changes
Scanning laser polarimetry	Scanning laser polarimeter	Birefringent properties of the nerve fiber layer cause a measurable phase shift of an incident polarized light proportional to the tissue thickness	Easy to perform through undilated pupil No discomfort to patient Can image through most media opacities, unless very dense Resolution limited to size of a pixel (possibly as small as 1 µm) Reproducibility 5–8 µm	Equipment is expensive Measurements not correlated histologically in humans Requires compensation for other polarizing media, e.g. cornea

From Chopin NT: Retinal nerve fiber layer analysis. In Yanoff M, Duker JS [eds]: Ophthalmology, London, Mosby, 1999.

PATHOLOGY

Glaucoma

Dropout of ganglion cells, replacement of NFL with dense gliotic tissue and some glial cell nuclei; partial preservation of inner nuclear layer with loss of Müller's and amacrine cells (normal 8–9 cells high; in glaucoma, 4–5 cells high); earliest histologic changes occur at level of lamina cribrosa; advanced cases may show backward bowing of lamina or 'beanpot' appearance (Figures 9-11, 9-12)

Schnabel's Cavernous Optic Atrophy

Histologic finding in eyes with increased IOP or atherosclerosis and normal IOP; hyaluronic acid infiltration of nerve from vitreous due to imbalance between perfusion pressure in the posterior ciliary arteries and IOP; also occurs in eyes with ischemic optic neuropathy

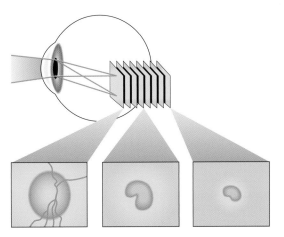

Figure 9-6. Confocal scanning laser ophthalmoscopy. (Adapted from Schuman JS, Noeker RJ: Imaging of the optic nerve head and nerve fiber layer in glaucoma. Ophthalmol Clin North Am 8:259–279, 1995.)

Pathology: atrophy of neural elements with cystic spaces containing hyaluronic acid (mucopolysaccharides derived from vitreous), which stains with colloidal iron (Figure 9-13)

Gliosis of the Optic Nerve

With optic atrophy, glial cells replace nerve cells and assume a random distribution throughout the optic nerve

DISORDERS

Childhood Glaucoma

(See Ch. 5, Pediatrics/Strabismus)

Primary Open-Angle Glaucoma (POAG)

Progressive, bilateral, optic neuropathy with open angles, typical pattern of nerve fiber bundle visual field loss, and increased intraocular pressure (IOP >21 mmHg) not caused by another systemic or local disease

Epidemiology: second leading cause of blindness in US; most common form of glaucoma (60–70%); 7% of population has ocular hypertension; 3% of population in Baltimore Eye Study had glaucomatous VF defects. If damage in one eye, untreated fellow eye has 29% risk over 5 years. Steroid responders have 31% risk of developing glaucoma within 5 years

Genetics: juvenile-onset POAG has been mapped to chromosome 1q21-q31 (*GLC1A*, *MYOC/TIGR*). Adult POAG has been mapped to chromosomes 2qcen-q13 (*GLC1B*), 2p15-p16 (*GLC1H*), 3q21-q24 (*GLC1C*), 8q23 (*GLC1D*), 10p14 (GLC1E, OPTN [optineurin]). A mutation in the *OPTN* gene accounts for ~17% of POAG

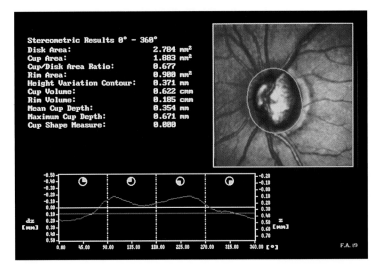

Figure 9-7. Confocal scanning laser ophthalmoscopy printed report. (From Zangwill L, de Souza K, Weinrob RN: Confocal scanning laser ophthalmoscopy to detect glaucomatous optic neuropathy. In Shuman JS [ed]: Imaging in Glaucoma. Thorofare, NJ, Slack, 1997.)

Stereometric Results 0° - 360°
Disk Area: 2.784 mm²
Cup Area: 1.883 mm²
Cup/Disk Area Ratio: 0.677
Rim Area: 0.900 mm²
Height Variation Contour: 0.371 mm
Cup Volume: 0.622 cmm
Rim Volume: 0.185 cmm
Mean Cup Depth: 0.354 mm
Maximum Cup Depth: 0.671 mm
Cup Shape Measure: 0.000

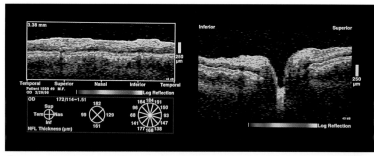

A

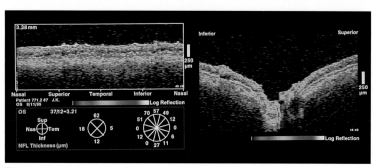

B

Figure 9-8. Optical coherence tomography. (From Pedut-Kloizman TP, Schuman JS: Disc analysis. In Yanoff M, Duker JS [eds]: Ophthalmology, London, Mosby, 1999.)

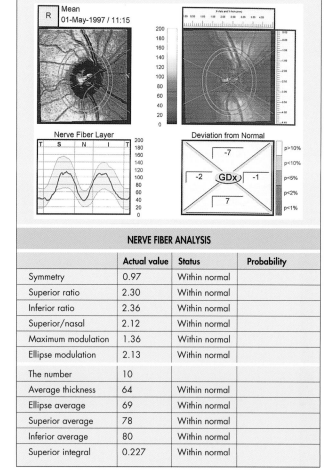

NERVE FIBER ANALYSIS

	Actual value	Status	Probability
Symmetry	0.97	Within normal	
Superior ratio	2.30	Within normal	
Inferior ratio	2.36	Within normal	
Superior/nasal	2.12	Within normal	
Maximum modulation	1.36	Within normal	
Ellipse modulation	2.13	Within normal	
The number	10		
Average thickness	64	Within normal	
Ellipse average	69	Within normal	
Superior average	78	Within normal	
Inferior average	80	Within normal	
Superior integral	0.227	Within normal	

Figure 9-9. Printout from the GDx software of the Nerve Fiber Analyzer; normal eye. (From Chopin NT: Retinal nerve fiber layer analysis. In Yanoff M, Duker JS [eds]: Ophthalmology, London, Mosby, 1999.)

Risk factors: increased IOP, increased cup-to-disc ratio, thinner central corneal thickness (less than ~550 μm), positive family history (6× increase in first-degree relatives), age (increased in patients >60 years old; 15% of those >80 years old have glaucoma), race (6× increase in African Americans vs Caucasians); other possible risk factors include DM, myopia, hypertension, migraines

Pathogenesis: unknown
Theories of optic nerve damage:
  Mechanical: resistance to outflow, trabecular meshwork dysfunction
  Vascular: poor optic nerve perfusion; ischemia occurs with systemic hypotension; possible contribution of vasospasm; increased IOP reduces blood flow to optic nerve
  Ganglion cell necrosis or apoptosis: excitotoxicity (glutamate), neurotrophin starvation, autoimmunity, abnormal glial-neuronal interactions (tumor necrosis factor [TNF]), defects in endogenous protective mechanisms (heat shock proteins)

Findings: increased IOP, large cup-to-disc ratio (especially vertical elongation of optic cup; notching of rim; asymmetry of C/D ratio), nerve fiber layer loss (evaluate with red-free light), disc splinter hemorrhage (often followed by notching in region of hemorrhage), characteristic visual field defects. Peripapillary atrophy is not a sign of glaucoma damage
  With optic nerve damage, loss of yellow-blue color axis occurs first
  Combined sensitivity of tonometry and disc exam = 67%

Visual fields: sensitivity (% of diseased properly identified) = 85%; specificity (% of normals properly

Figure 9-10. Color Doppler imaging of the ophthalmic artery. (From O'Brien C, Harris A: Optic nerve blood flow measurement. In Yanoff M, Duker JS [eds]: Ophthalmology, London, Mosby, 1999.)

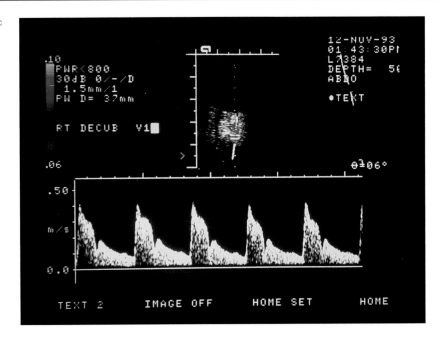

Figure 9-11. POAG demonstrating cupping of the optic nerve head. (From Yanoff M, Fine BS: Ocular Pathology, 5th edn. St Louis, Mosby, 2002.)

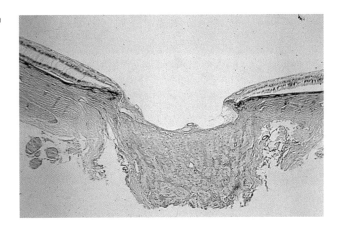

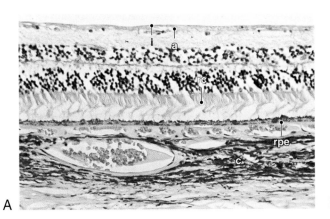

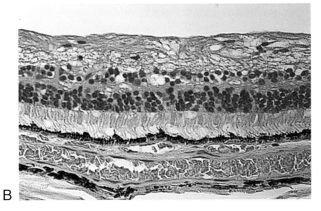

Figure 9-12. POAG demonstrating atrophy of the inner retinal layers. **A,** low power, **B,** higher magnification. (From Yanoff M, Fine BS: Ocular Pathology, 5th edn, St Louis, Mosby, 2002.)

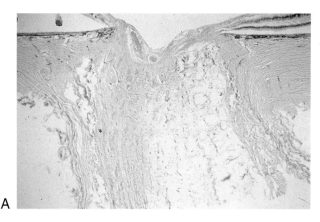
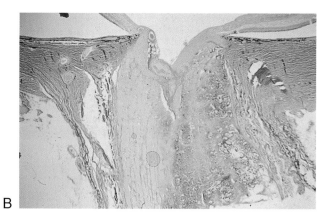

A | B

Figure 9-13. Schnabel's cavernous optic atrophy demonstrating cystic spaces in optic nerve parenchyma. **A,** H&E stain, **B,** colloidal iron stain. (From Yanoff M, Fine BS: Ocular Pathology, 5th edn. St Louis, Mosby, 2002.)

identified) = 85%. Risk of initial field loss is 1–2%/year for ocular hypertensive patients, risk of field loss increases with increasing IOP

Secondary Open-Angle Glaucoma

Mechanism/Etiology:
   Clogging of TM: RBCs (hyphema, sickle cell, ghost cells), macrophages (hemolytic, phacolytic, melanocytic, melanomalytic), neoplastic cells (malignant tumors, neurofibromatosis, juvenile xanthogranuloma), pigment (pigmentary glaucoma, pseudoexfoliation, chronic uveitis, malignant melanoma), lens protein (lens-particle glaucoma), photoreceptor segments (Schwartz's syndrome), zonular fragments (α-chymotrypsin induced), viscoelastic
   Toxic/medication: steroid-induced, siderosis, chalcosis
   Inflammation: uveitis, IK
   Increased episcleral venous pressure
   Trauma: angle recession, chemical injury, hemorrhage, postoperative

Hyphema

27% risk of glaucoma if hyphema >50% of AC volume; 52% risk with total hyphema
   Surgical intervention for uncontrolled IOP, corneal blood staining, prolonged presence of clot (>15 days), rebleed, 8-ball hyphema (see Ch. 10, Anterior Segment)

Sickle cell

Sickled cells are rigid; therefore, even small hyphemas can obstruct TM and raise IOP; acetazolamide (Diamox) contraindicated (increases ascorbic acid in AC causing greater sickling, also causes hemoconcentration and systemic acidosis, both of which favor sickling)

Ghost cells

Weeks to months after vitreous hemorrhage, degenerated RBCs pass through hyaloid face. These khaki-colored, spherical cells are less pliable than RBCs and do not pass through trabecular meshwork; layer of cells forms a pseudohypopyon

Lytic glaucomas

Macrophages laden with various materials

Hemolytic: hemosiderin-laden macrophages deposit in TM

Phacolytic: denatured lens proteins escape from hypermature or morgagnian cataract; proteins and macrophages that have ingested lens material clog the outflow tract; appears as milky substance in AC; requires surgical removal of lens. Reduce the inflammation preoperatively with topical steroid, cycloplegic, and ocular hypotensive medications

Melanomalytic: melanin from malignant melanoma is engulfed by macrophages, which clog TM

Melanocytomalytic: melanin from necrotic melanocytoma

Tumor cells

Deposition of tumor cells, inflammatory cells, and cellular debris; also macrophages laden with melanin from melanomas, direct infiltration of trabecular meshwork, or neovascularization with subsequent intraocular hemorrhage or neovascular glaucoma (NVG). 45% of anterior uveal melanomas and 15% of choroidal melanomas are associated with glaucoma. Retinoblastoma causes glaucoma in 25–50% from NVG, pupillary block, or tumor material; also lymphoma

Pigmentary glaucoma (PG) (AD)

Mapped to chromosome 7q35-q36 (*GLC1F*)

Typically young myopic males; up to 50% of patients with pigment dispersion syndrome (PDS) develop glaucoma

Mechanism: reverse pupillary block bows iris against zonules, and iris movement results in pigment liberation; pigment obstructs TM

Findings: halos and blurry vision with IOP spikes (pigment may be released with exercise); Krukenberg spindle (melanin phagocytized by corneal endothelium); heavy TM pigmentation; iridodonesis; iris transillumination defects (radial midperipheral spoke-like appearance); associated with lattice degeneration (20%) and retinal detachment (5%) (Figure 9-14)

Treatment: miotics minimize iris-zonule touch; very good response to laser trabeculoplasty; laser peripheral iridotomy may help reduce posterior bowing of iris

Pseudoexfoliation glaucoma (PXG)

Mapped to chromosome 15q24 (*LOXL1*).

High incidence (up to 50%) of secondary open-angle glaucoma in patients with pseudoexfoliation syndrome

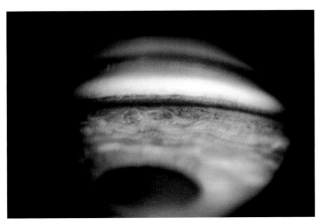

Figure 9-14. Gonioscopic view of pigmentary glaucoma. (From Ball SF: Pigmentary glaucoma. In Yanoff M, Duker JS [eds]: Ophthalmology, London, Mosby, 1999.)

(PXS); more common among Scandinavians. Amyloid-like substance deposits in eye and clogs TM, also found in other organs (Figure 9-15)

Findings: iridopathy (blood-aqueous barrier defect, pseudouveitis, iris rigidity, posterior synechiae, poor pupillary dilation), keratopathy (reduced endothelial cell count, endothelial decompensation, corneal endothelial proliferation over trabecular meshwork), Sampaolesi's line (scalloped band of pigmentation anterior to Schwalbe's line), weak zonules (phacodonesis, risk of lens dislocation during cataract surgery, and angle closure from anterior movement of lens), lens capsule (white fibrillar material)

Treatment: very good response to laser trabeculoplasty. PXS usually presents with higher initial IOP and is more difficult to control with medical treatment alone vs POAG

Lens-particle glaucoma

Lens material blocks TM following trauma or cataract surgery. Greater inflammation than with phacolytic; PAS, posterior synechiae, and inflammatory membranes are common; IOP can be very high

Treatment: cycloplegics, steroids (careful because steroids slow absorption of lens material), and ocular hypotensive medications

Schwartz's syndrome

High IOP associated with rhegmatogenous RD. Photoreceptor outer segments migrate transvitreally into aqueous and block trabecular meshwork; outflow obstruction is also due to pigment released from RPE and glycosaminoglycans released from photoreceptors. Usually resolves after repair of RD

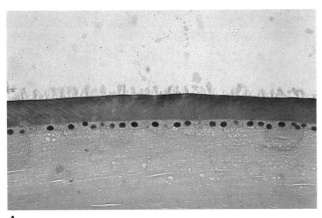 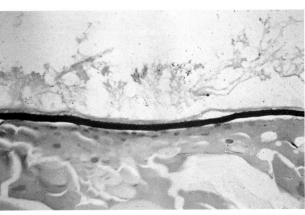

A   B

Figure 9-15. Pseudoexfoliative syndrome demonstrating exfoliative material on lens capsule. (From Samuelson TW, Shah G: Pseudoexfoliative glaucoma. In: Yanoff M, Duker JS [eds]: Ophthalmology, London, Mosby, 1999.)

Alpha-chymotrypsin induced

Zonular fragments accumulate in trabecular meshwork after intracapsular cataract extraction (ICCE) with enzymatic zonulysis. Alpha-chymotrypsin itself does not cause damage

Corticosteroid-induced

Risk factors include open-angle glaucoma, family history of glaucoma, increasing age, diabetes, and high myopia. Topical steroids have greater pressure-raising effects than do systemic steroids:

> In response to topical dexamethasone 0.1% qid for 6 weeks, 65% had IOP rise of <5 mmHg, 30% had a rise of 5–14 mmHg, and 5% had a rise of at least 15 mmHg
>
> Fluoromethalone, rimexolone (Vexol), and loteprednol (Lotemax, Alrex) are less likely to increase IOP

Siderosis (iron) or chalcosis (copper)

TM toxicity and scarring from intraocular foreign body

Uveitic

Normally, a decrease in aqueous production by the ciliary body occurs due to inflammation (trabeculitis); however, aqueous outflow is acutely impaired by the disruption of the blood-aqueous barrier and inflammatory cells. Chronic inflammation may cause TM scarring

JRA-associated uveitis: glaucoma occurs in about 20% of cases

Glaucomatocyclitic crisis (Posner-Schlossman syndrome): episodic trabeculitis (mononuclear cells in TM) with high IOP for hours to weeks; minimal inflammatory signs

Fuchs' heterochromic iridocyclitis: up to 60% develop high IOP (glaucoma occurs more commonly in patients with bilateral disease and spontaneous hyphema); may persist after resolution of uveitis

Uveitis-glaucoma-hyphema syndrome: nongranulomatous inflammation. IOL physically irritates iris and ciliary body

Traumatic

Angle recession: glaucoma develops in 10% of cases with >180° of involvement due to scarring of the angle and TM

Chemical burn: can damage trabecular meshwork or uveal circulation, or cause shrinkage of scleral collagen

After vitrectomy: most common complication is glaucoma; caused by intraocular gas, hyphema, ghost cells, uveitis, silicone oil

Elevated episcleral venous pressure

Causes resistance to aqueous outflow

Etiology: carotid-cavernous sinus fistula, cavernous sinus thrombosis, Sturge-Weber syndrome, neurofibromatosis, orbital mass (tumor, varices), thyroid-related ophthalmopathy (false elevation of IOP can be caused by IR fibrosis with increased resistance in upgaze), superior vena cava obstruction, mediastinal tumors and syndromes, idiopathic. May see blood in Schlemm's canal

Primary Angle-Closure Glaucoma

Glaucoma caused by peripheral iris obstructing the trabecular meshwork, most commonly due to pupillary block; classified as acute, intermittent, or chronic. Plateau iris syndrome is a form of primary angle-closure without pupillary block

Mechanism of pupillary block: in susceptible patients, iridolenticular touch causes resistance of aqueous flow from posterior to anterior chamber, causing increased posterior pressure. When the pupil is mid-dilated (i.e. stress, low ambient light levels, sympathomimetic or anticholinergic medications), the elevated posterior chamber pressure causes peripheral iris tissue to bow forward and occlude the TM

Epidemiology: acute form is most common in Eskimos and Asians, followed by Caucasians, then African Americans; highest risk is between age 55 and 65 years old; more common in women only among Caucasians. Chronic form is more common in African Americans than Asians, who have a higher risk than Caucasians. 5% of population older than 60 years of age have angles that can be occluded; 0.5% of these individuals develop angle closure. Usually bilateral (75% risk in untreated fellow eye within 5 years)

Anatomic features predisposing to angle closure: small anterior segment (hyperopia, nanophthalmos, microcornea, microphthalmos); hereditary narrow angle; anterior iris insertion (Eskimos, Asians, and African Americans); shallow AC (large lens, plateau iris configuration, loose or dislocated lens)

Acute angle closure

Symptoms: blurred vision, colored halos around lights, pain, redness, nausea and vomiting, headache

Findings: high IOP, corneal epithelial edema, conjunctival injection, mid-dilated pupil, shallow anterior chamber, mild AC cell and flare, closed angle (perform indentation gonioscopy to differentiate between appositional and synechial angle closure; glycerin can be used to clear corneal edema; evaluate angle in other eye), ON swelling and hyperemia; with rapid rise in IOP, may see arterial pulsations (retinal ischemia can occur)

Sequelae of ischemia: segmental iris atrophy (focal iris stroma necrosis), dilated irregular pupil (sphincter and dilator necrosis), glaukomflecken (focal anterior lens opacities due to epithelial necrosis)

Late findings: decreased vision, PAS, chronic corneal edema

Provocative tests: prone test, darkroom test, prone darkroom test, pharmacologic pupillary dilation; positive if IOP rises >8 mmHg

Thymoxamine test: α-adrenergic antagonist used to distinguish angle closure from glaucoma with narrow angles; thymoxamine blocks iris dilator muscle producing miosis; however, it does not affect trabecular meshwork and normally does not decrease IOP; therefore, decrease in IOP suggests miosis has removed iris from the outflow channel reversing angle closure

Treatment of acute angle-closure glaucoma: peripheral iridotomy or iridectomy (PI, definitive treatment); compression gonioscopy (may force aqueous through block and open angle); pilocarpine (may not be effective at IOP >40 mmHg due to sphincter ischemia; may also cause lens–iris diaphragm to move forward, worsening pupillary block); reduce IOP with β-blocker, α_2-agonist, topical or oral CAI, or hyperosmotic agent (isosorbide, glycerin [contraindicated in diabetics], or IV mannitol [risk of cardiovascular adverse effects]); topical steroids for inflammation; laser PI in fellow eye (75% chance of attack in untreated fellow eye; pilocarpine lowers risk to 40% but may lead to chronic angle closure)

If attack of angle closure is broken medically, consider waiting a few days before performing laser PI because corneal edema, iridocorneal touch, and iris congestion make the procedure more difficult

Persistently increased IOP following laser PI may be due to PAS, incomplete iridotomy, underlying open-angle glaucoma, or secondary angle closure

Intermittent angle closure

2 : 1 ratio of nonacute-to-acute presentations; may be asymptomatic or have similar presentation as acute angle closure but less severe, and occurs over days to weeks; often complain of headaches, episodes resolve spontaneously, especially by entering a well-lit area (induces miosis); IOP may be normal, glaukomflecken and PAS are evidence of previous attack. Treat with laser PI

Chronic angle closure

Gradual closure of angle by apposition or development of PAS leads to slow rise in IOP; variable IOP, but less than with acute angle closure. Often asymptomatic; cornea usually clear due to gradual rise in IOP, but can have extensive visual field loss

Plateau iris

Configuration: angle anatomy resulting in deep central AC and shallow peripheral AC

Syndrome: angle closure in an eye with plateau iris configuration; usually occurs in 4th to 5th decade of life, and in individuals with less hyperopia than typical angle-closure patient

Findings: may present with acute or chronic angle closure; anteriorly positioned ciliary processes force the peripheral iris more anteriorly than normal; deep chamber centrally; flat iris contour with sharp dropoff peripherally; with dilation, peripheral iris folds into the angle and occludes TM; with compression gonioscopy, angle is more difficult to open and does not open as widely as in primary angle closure

Treatment: laser peripheral iridotomy, laser iridoplasty, and miotics; plateau iris appearance remains

Secondary Angle-Closure Glaucoma

Mechanism/Etiology

With pupillary block: phacomorphic (lens enlargement in elderly; urgent surgery needed to remove lens); dislocated lens; seclusio pupillae; nanophthalmos; aphakic and pseudophakic pupillary block; silicone oil (prevent by performing an inferior PI because oil is lighter than water)

Without pupillary block:

POSTERIOR 'PUSHING' MECHANISM (mechanical/anterior displacement of lens–iris diaphragm)

ANTERIOR ROTATION OF CILIARY BODY: inflammation (scleritis, uveitis, after scleral buckle or panretinal photocoagulation [PRP]), congestion (postscleral buckling, nanophthalmos), choroidal effusion (hypotony; uveal effusion), suprachoroidal hemorrhage

AQUEOUS MISDIRECTION (MALIGNANT GLAUCOMA)

PRESSURE FROM POSTERIOR SEGMENT: tumor, expanding gas, exudative retinal detachment (RD)

CONTRACTION OF RETROLENTAL TISSUE: persistent hyperplastic primary vitreous (PHPV), retinopathy of prematurity (ROP)

ANTERIOR 'PULLING' MECHANISM (adherence of iris to trabecular meshwork/membranes over TM)

EPITHELIAL: epithelial downgrowth, fibrous ingrowth

ENDOTHELIAL: iridocorneal endothelial (ICE) syndrome, posterior polymorphous dystrophy (PPMD)

NEOVASCULAR: neovascular glaucoma (NVG)

PERIPHERAL ANTERIOR SYNECHIAE (PAS) ADHESION FROM TRAUMA

Associated with RD surgery

Anterior rotation of CB around the scleral spur secondary to swelling from excessive PRP or tight scleral buckle

Treatment: cycloplegics, PI, consider cutting encircling band

Nanophthalmos

>10 D hyperopia; small eye (<20 mm) with small cornea (mean diameter = 10.5 mm), shallow AC, narrow angle, and high lens/eye volume. Pupillary block or uveal effusion produces angle-closure glaucoma. Thick sclera (about 2× thicker than normal) may impede vortex venous drainage, as well as decrease uveoscleral outflow, and can also result in spontaneous uveal effusion with anterior rotation of CB leading to angle closure

Treatment: weak miotics, cycloplegics (if no angle crowding), laser PI, laser iridoplasty, trabeculectomy after prophylactic sclerotomy. Because there is a high complication rate with surgery (uveal effusion), first use medical therapy, then laser

Increased risk of complications with cataract surgery (RD, choroidal effusion, angle-closure glaucoma, flat AC, CME, corneal decompensation, malignant glaucoma, IOL miscalculations). If shallow AC and thickened choroid preoperatively, perform prophylactic anterior sclerotomies with surgery

Malignant glaucoma (aqueous misdirection syndrome, ciliolenticular or ciliovitreal block)

Mechanism: tips of ciliary processes rotate forward against lens (ciliolenticular block); can also have a trapdoor tear in the anterior hyaloid; causes anterior displacement of lens-iris diaphragm

Risk factors: uveitis, angle closure, nanophthalmos, hyperopia; occurs postoperatively (usually 5 days) following a variety of laser or incisional surgeries; usually in patients with PAS or chronic angle closure following intraocular surgery if the hyaloid face has not been broken (follows 2% of surgical cases for angle closure); can also occur in unoperated eye when mydriatics are stopped or miotics are added

Findings: entire AC shallow (versus angle closure in which the AC is deeper centrally than peripherally), IOP higher than expected, presence of patent iridectomy, absence of suprachoroidal fluid or blood

DDx: pupillary block (no patent iridectomy; moderate depth of central AC), suprachoroidal hemorrhage (acute severe pain and choroidal elevation), choroidal effusion (usually low IOP and choroidal elevation), annular peripheral choroidal detachment

Treatment

Medical: cycloplegic (relaxes ciliary muscle and pulls lens-iris diaphragm posteriorly; continued indefinitely to prevent recurrence), aqueous suppressants, peripheral iridotomy in both eyes (eliminate any component of pupillary block); miotics are contraindicated

50% resolve within 5 days with medical therapy alone

Surgical: argon laser photocoagulation of ciliary processes (requires shrinkage of at least 2–4 ciliary processes), Nd:YAG laser rupture of hyaloid face (for pseudophakic and aphakic patients; 4–6 mJ; best to perform peripherally [through PI]), vitrectomy (for phakic patients; debulk vitreous and overdeepen AC with air)

Intraocular tumors

Can push angle closed from posteriorly

Malignant melanoma of the anterior uveal tract can cause glaucoma by direct extension of tumor into trabecular meshwork, inducing neovascularization of the angle, obstructing TM with melanin-laden macrophages (melanomalytic), or seeding of tumor cells in outflow channels; other mechanisms include pigment dispersion, inflammation, and hemorrhage

PHPV

Contraction of retrolenticular membrane and swelling of cataract can cause angle closure

Treatment: remove lens and membrane via limbal approach (pars plana approach may be dangerous in that retina can extend up to the pars plicata)

ROP

Due to contraction of retrolental tissue

Epithelial downgrowth

Due to epithelium growing over angle

Fibrous ingrowth

Due to fibrous proliferation through wound into AC

ICE syndrome

Due to descemetization of TM and angle closure from contraction of endothelial membrane; PAS are prominent but less responsible for glaucoma

PPMD

Due to abnormal corneal endothelial cells that migrate into angle causing glaucoma (15%)

NVG

Due to widespread retinal or ocular ischemia; clinically transparent fibrovascular membrane flattens anterior iris surface; myofibroblasts provide motive force for angle closure and ectropion uveae

Etiology: proliferative retinopathy (diabetes [33% of all forms of NVG], ischemic CRVO [33%], carotid occlusive disease [13%], ciliary artery occlusion, sickle cell, Norrie's disease, ROP); intraocular inflammation (uveitis, postoperative); neoplasms (retinoblastoma [50% develop NVG], malignant melanoma, large cell lymphoma [reticulum cell sarcoma], metastatic); chronic retinal detachment

Treatment: aqueous suppressants and hyperosmotics; increase uveoscleral outflow (atropine; avoid miotics); panretinal photocoagulation; peripheral retinal cryotherapy (if poor visualization of retina; 50% develop phthisis with cyclocryotherapy); glaucoma drainage implant (70% success rate)

Normal Tension Glaucoma (NTG)

Glaucoma with open angles and IOP <22 mmHg

Proposed mechanisms

Nocturnal systemic hypotension: diurnal curve of BP similar to IOP. 66% of patients will have a BP drop of greater than 10% during early morning hours ('dippers'); patients with HTN have an even greater swing in BP (26% average drop); patients with HTN treated with β-blockers can have diastolic BP <50 mmHg, which may compromise blood supply to optic nerve

Autoimmune: increased incidence of proteinemia and autoantibodies in patients with NTG

Vasospasm

Previous hemodynamic crisis: excessive blood loss or shock

Findings: VF defects in NTG have steeper slopes, greater depths, and closer proximity to fixation than in POAG; splinter hemorrhages are more common

DDx: POAG with large diurnal variation, 'burned-out' secondary open-angle glaucoma, chronic angle closure. Must rule out intracranial processes and other causes of optic neuropathy

Cupping can occur with neurologic disease: AION (arteritic 50%; nonarteritic 10%), chiasmal compressive lesions (5%), optic neuritis (<5%), methanol toxicity. These entities are more likely to have early loss of central vision and color vision; pallor may be worse than cupping

Diagnosis: diurnal curve, neurologic workup (CBC, ESR, ANA, VDRL and FTA-ABS, carotid evaluation, brain neuroimaging)

Prognosis: more difficult to treat than POAG

TREATMENT

Generally, medications are tried first, followed by laser treatment, and then surgery; however, the choice and timing of various treatment modalities are dependent on the type of glaucoma, severity of optic nerve damage, level of control, and many other factors. Therapy must also be directed to any preexisting or underlying process

Medication

Ocular hypotensive agents (see Ch. 2, Pharmacology)

Laser

Argon Laser Trabeculoplasty (ALT) (Figure 9-16)

Power 400–1200 mW; spot size 50 μm; duration 0.1 s; titrate power to generate small bubble at junction of nonpigmented and pigmented TM; 50 applications/180°; average of 30% reduction in IOP; can be repeated Iopidine immediately postoperatively to avoid pressure spike, and treat with steroids for 1 week. Assess efficacy of treatment at 6 weeks postoperatively
Anterior burns have poor effect; posterior burns more likely to develop PAS

Results: 25% fail to control IOP at 1 year; 10% per year failure rate thereafter. Repeating ALT may provide IOP control in 33–50%, but sustained elevation in 10%
Best predictor of success is type of glaucoma: PXG (best) > PG > POAG > NTG > aphakic (worst)

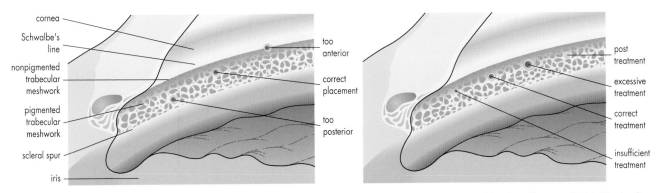

Figure 9-16. ALT. (From Schwartz AL: Argon Laser Trabeculoplasty in Glaucoma: What's Happening (Survey Results of American Glaucoma Society Members), J Glaucoma 2:329-336, 1993.)

The greater the amount of pigment in the angle, the better the result; poorer response in patients <50 years of age. ALT is ineffective (and may worsen IOP) in inflammatory glaucoma, angle recession, angle-closure glaucoma (membranes in angles), congenital glaucoma, and steroid-induced glaucoma. Contraindicated in patients with large amounts of PAS

Complications: IOP spike (increases with energy and number of laser burns), iritis, PAS

Selective Laser Trabeculoplasty (SLT)

Time and spot size (400 μm) are fixed, power 0.6–0.9 mJ; 50 confluent applications/180°, straddling TM
  Produces less tissue destruction than ALT, and is repeatable. Beware IOP spikes in patients with pigment dispersion syndrome and pigmentary glaucoma

Laser Iridotomy

Perform in eyes with narrow angles (prophylactically), iris bombe, synechial angle closure, pigmentary glaucoma (due to configuration of iris), plateau iris, and malignant glaucoma

YAG: power 1–12 mJ; bleed more, but close less than with argon

Argon: reaction is pigment-related and requires more energy and total applications than with YAG; less bleeding because of thermal effect; extensive tissue destruction at margins of treatment; iritis more pronounced

Iridoplasty

For narrow angles; aim at peripheral iris; stretch iris away from angle; power 200–400 mW; spot size 500 μm; duration 0.5–1.0 s

Surgery

Trabeculectomy

Consider use of antimetabolite in patients at risk for bleb failure

Risk factors for bleb failure: previous surgical failure, darker skin pigmentation, history of keloid formation, neovascular changes, younger age, intraocular inflammation, scarred conjunctiva, high hyperopia, inability to use corticosteroids, shallow AC

Antimetabolites
  Mitomycin-C (MMC): antineoplastic antibiotic (isolated from *Streptomyces caespitosus*)
    MECHANISM: intercalates with DNA and prevents replication; suppresses fibrosis and vascular ingrowth after exposure to the filtration site. Toxic to fibroblasts in all stages of cell cycle; 100∞ more potent than 5-FU

TOXICITY: intraocular causes corneal decompensation (damages endothelium), AC inflammation, and necrosis of ciliary body and iris; can develop scleral necrosis; retinal toxicity with intravitreal injection
  5-FU: specifically affects the S-phase of the cell cycle; requires postoperative injections (30–35 mg in 5 mg doses over 1–3 weeks); corneal epithelial toxicity may occur

Complications: block ostium during surgery in hyperopia, nanophthalmos, or chronic angle closure, the ciliary processes can roll anteriorly

Treatment: suture wound and reinflate eye allowing ciliary processes to revert to normal position; if still present, use cautery to remove the processes
  High IOP immediately postoperatively: attempt digital massage or laser suture lysis
  Shallow or flat AC: (Table 9-2)
  Blebitis: photophobia, discharge, marked conjunctival injection around an opalescent filtering bleb; often Seidel-positive, moderate AC cells and flare, but no involvement of the vitreous. Organism usually *Staphylococcus*
    TREATMENT: intensive topical antibiotics, repair wound leak, observe daily for endophthalmitis
  Bleb-associated endophthalmitis: pain, decreased vision, AC cells and flare, hypopyon, and vitreous cells; often Seidel-positive. Organism usually *Streptococcus* species or *H. influenzae*
    TREATMENT: emergent, as for endophthalmitis
  Suprachoroidal hemorrhage: usually occurs several days after trabeculectomy surgery with acute pain, often

Table 9-2. Treatment of shallow or flat anterior chamber following trabeculectomy

Bleb Height	IOP	DDx	Treatment
Elevated	Low	Excessive filtration	Bleb revision
Flat	Low	Choroidal detachment	Cycloplegic, steroid, drainage
		Bleb leak	Antibiotic, aqueous suppressants, stop steroid, AC reformation, pressure patch, Simmons' scleral compression shell, large diameter soft contact lens, trichloroacetic acid, glue, laser, or autologous blood injection. Consider surgical intervention (drainage of choroidals and repair of wound) for impending failure of bleb, flat anterior chamber with corneal decompensation, kissing choroidals, progressive cataract
Flat	Elevated	Suprachoroidal hemorrhage	Drainage
		Pupillary block	Cycloplegic, steroid, PI
		Malignant glaucoma	Cycloplegic, aqueous suppressants, PI, YAG anterior vitreolysis or vitrectomy
Elevated	Elevated	Encapsulated bleb	Needling, aqueous suppressants, bleb revision

while straining; also, nausea, vomiting, and decreased vision

MECHANISM: progressive serous choroidal detachment, stretching the long posterior ciliary artery until it ruptures

RISK FACTORS: aphakia, hypertension, cardiovascular disease, and increased age

Hypotony: generally seen in young myopic patients, especially with antimetabolites

DDx: wound leak, overfiltration, iridocyclitis, cyclodialysis, ciliochoroidal effusion, RD

TREATMENT: wound revision

COMPLICATIONS: corneal edema, cataract, choroidal effusion, optic disc edema, chorioretinal folds, maculopathy

Exuberant bleb: bleb can enlarge, spread onto cornea, and interfere with vision due to astigmatism, dellen, or encroachment into visual axis

TREATMENT: recess or amputate bleb; usually a cleavage plane is present

Drainage Implants (Setons/Tubes)

Seton is from Latin 'seta' or bristle (original surgery used horse hair)

Types

Nonvalve: Molteno (single or double plate), Schocket, Baerveldt; must temporarily occlude tube lumen with suture or biodegradable collagen plug

Valve: Ahmed (1-way valve maintains IOP at 8 mmHg or higher), Krupin, and Baerveldt (pressure-sensitive valve)

Anterior chamber glaucoma drainage implant: for patients with scleral buckles who do not have adequate scleral surface for placement of a seton; a silicone implant shunts fluid from AC or PC to the fibrous capsule surrounding the episcleral encircling element

Non-penetrating Filtration Surgery

Less invasive alternatives

Ab externo: Ex-Press minishunt, canaloplasty, viscocanalostomy

Ab interno: iStent, CyPass, DeepLight Gold micro-shunt, trabectome

Goniosynechialysis

Direct lysis of PAS with cyclodialysis spatula or other microinstrument; consider for angle-closure glaucoma of less than 12 months' duration

Cyclophotocoagulation

Laser treatment of ciliary body with argon (transpupillary or endoprobe), Nd:YAG (contact or noncontact), or diode (contact); useful in many types of refractory glaucomas, including aphakic, neovascular, and inflammatory, and in eyes with failed filtering blebs

Mechanism: reduced aqueous production by destruction of ciliary epithelium

Procedure is painful; therefore, requires peribulbar or retrobulbar block

Cyclocryotherapy

First treatment: 2.5 mm cryo tip, with anterior edge 1 mm from inferior limbus and 1.5 mm from superior limbus. Provide 6 freezes on the clock hours of the inferior 180°. Maintain each freeze for 60 seconds at −80°C. The iceball will encroach upon cornea for about 0.5 mm. Wait 1 month for the IOP to reach new baseline

Second treatment: if first treatment does not lower IOP sufficiently, treat superior temporal quadrant with 2–4 freezes. Always leave at least 1 quadrant (usually superonasal) free to prevent hypotony. Give subconjunctival steroid postoperatively

Procedure is painful; therefore, requires peribulbar or retrobulbar block

Surgical Iridectomy

Perform through 3 mm clear corneal wound for angle-closure glaucoma

Indications: if severe corneal edema precludes adequate iris visualization, AC is extremely shallow, or patient is unable to cooperate for laser iridotomy

MAJOR GLAUCOMA CLINICAL STUDIES

Advanced Glaucoma Intervention Study (AGIS)

Objective: to evaluate argon laser trabeculoplasty (ALT) vs trabeculectomy as the initial surgery in patients with advanced open-angle glaucoma not controlled by medical treatment

Main outcome variable was visual function (field and acuity)

Results

7-year data

In African Americans, the best results were obtained when ALT was performed 1st, followed by trabeculectomy (ATT sequence)

In Caucasians, the best results occurred when trabeculectomy was performed 1st, followed by ALT, and finally by a 2nd trabeculectomy (TAT sequence)

Visual field defects were more severe in African American patients

Eyes with IOP <18 mmHg at all visits had almost no progression of VF loss

Trabeculectomy increased the risk of cataract by 78% (47% if no complications occurred vs 104% if complications occurred, especially severe inflammation and flat anterior chamber)

Conclusions

In patients with advanced POAG, ALT should be considered as the first surgical treatment in African American patients; trabeculectomy should be considered first in Caucasians

Risk factors for ALT failure are younger age and higher IOP

Risk factors for trabeculectomy failure are younger age, higher IOP, diabetes, and postoperative complications (particularly elevated IOP and marked inflammation)

Risk factors for bleb encapsulation include male sex and previous ALT (but this was not statistically significant)

Low IOP reduces VF deterioration

Trabeculectomy is associated with an increased risk of cataract formation

Ocular Hypertension Treatment Study (OHTS)

Objective: to evaluate the effect of topical medication in delaying or preventing POAG in patients with ocular hypertension (IOP between 24 and 32 mmHg in one eye and between 21 and 32 mmHg in the fellow eye; normal visual fields and optic nerves)

The goal in the treatment group was to reduce the IOP by at least 20% from baseline and obtain a target pressure of ≤24 mmHg

The primary outcome variable was visual field loss or optic nerve damage

Results

Mean IOP reduction in the medicine group was 22.5% vs 4.0% in the observation group

At 5 years, the cumulative risk of developing POAG was 4.4% in the medicine group vs 9.5% in the observation group

Conclusions

Topical ocular hypotensive medication is effective in delaying or preventing POAG in eyes with ocular hypertension

Predictive factors for developing POAG include baseline IOP, age, cup-to-disc ratio, and central corneal thickness (CCT ≤555 μm)

Collaborative Initial Glaucoma Treatment Study (CIGTS)

Objective: to evaluate medicine (stepped regimen) vs trabeculectomy (with or without 5-fluorouracil) for the treatment of newly diagnosed open-angle glaucoma (primary, pigmentary, or pseudoexfoliative)

The primary outcome variable was progression of visual field loss

Secondary outcomes were quality of life, visual acuity, and intraocular pressure

Results

5-year data

VF loss was not significantly different with either treatment

Surgery had an initially increased risk of significant visual loss, but by 4 years, the average VA was equal in the 2 groups

IOP averaged 17–18 mmHg in the medicine group vs 14–15 mmHg in the surgery group

The rate of visually significant cataract was greater in the surgery group

Conclusions

Initial treatment of open-angle glaucoma with medicine or surgery results in similar VF outcome

Although VA loss was initially greater in the surgery group, the differences converged with time

Early Manifest Glaucoma Trial (EMGT)

Objective: to evaluate the effectiveness of reducing IOP (vs no treatment) on the progression of newly diagnosed open-angle glaucoma

The treatment group received argon laser trabeculoplasty plus topical betaxolol

The primary outcome measures were progression of visual field loss and optic disc changes

A secondary aim was to assess risk factors for progression

Results

6-year data

53% of patients progressed

Treatment reduced the IOP on average 5.1 mmHg (25%)

Progression was less common in the treatment group (45% vs 62%) and occurred later

Each 1 mmHg of IOP lowering from baseline to the first follow-up visit (3 months) reduced the risk of progression by approximately 10%

Increased nuclear lens opacity occurred with treatment

Conclusions

Treatment of early glaucoma halves the risk of progression

Risk factors for progression included higher baseline IOP, exfoliation, bilateral disease, older age, and frequent disc hemorrhages

Glaucoma Laser Trial (GLT)

Objective: to evaluate the efficacy and safety of starting treatment for POAG with ALT vs topical medication (Timoptic 0.5% bid)

Results

Eyes treated initially with ALT had lower IOP and better VF and optic nerve status than fellow eyes treated initially with topical medication

Conclusions

Initial treatment of POAG with ALT is at least as efficacious as initial treatment with Timoptic

Collaborative Normal Tension Glaucoma Study (CNTGS)

Objective: to evaluate whether IOP is a causative factor in NTG

The goal in the treatment group was to reduce the IOP by 30% with medication, laser, and/or surgery

Results

Lowering IOP by 30% or more reduced the rate of visual field loss in NTG. However, the rate of progression without treatment is variable and usually slow since half of untreated patients showed no progression in 5 years

Factors that increase the rate of progression include: female gender, migraine headaches, and presence of disc hemorrhage

Conclusions

IOP is a factor in the pathogenesis of NTG and lowering the IOP by 30% is beneficial

REVIEW QUESTIONS *(Answers start on page 368)*

1. Which form of glaucoma is associated with Down syndrome?
   a. congenital
   b. pigmentary
   c. Axenfeld-Rieger
   d. POAG

2. What is the most appropriate initial treatment of pupillary block in a patient with microspherophakia?
   a. acetazolamide
   b. laser iridotomy
   c. pilocarpine
   d. cyclopentolate

3. Which of the following statements is true? Uveoscleral outflow is
   a. inversely proportional to intraocular pressure
   b. measured clinically by fluorophotometry
   c. increased by atropine
   d. responsible for about 10% of total outflow

4. Risk factors for angle-closure glaucoma include all of the following except
   a. pseudoexfoliation
   b. myopia
   c. Eskimo ancestry
   d. nanophthalmos

5. Which of the following would cause the greatest elevation in IOP?
   a. blinking
   b. decreased blood cortisol levels
   c. change from supine to sitting position
   d. darkening the room

6. The most likely cause of a large filtering bleb and a shallow chamber is
   a. aqueous misdirection
   b. bleb leak
   c. pupillary block
   d. overfiltration

7. A change in Goldmann visual field stimulus from I4e to II4e is equivalent to
   a. 1 log
   b. 2 log
   c. 3 log
   d. 4 log

8. An Amsler grid held at 33 cm measures approximately how many degrees of central vision?
   a. 5
   b. 10
   c. 20
   d. 30

9. The most decreased sensitivity in an arcuate scotoma occurs in which quadrant?
   a. inferotemporal
   b. superonasal
   c. superotemporal
   d. inferonasal

10. The best gonioscopy lens for distinguishing appositional from synechial angle closure is
    a. Goldmann 3-mirror
    b. Zeiss
    c. Koeppe
    d. Goldmann 1-mirror

11. Which is not a risk factor for POAG?
    a. myopia
    b. CVO
    c. diabetes
    d. CRAO

12. ALT would be most effective in a patient with which type of glaucoma?
    a. congenital
    b. inflammatory
    c. pigmentary
    d. aphakic

13. In which direction should a patient look to aid the examiner's view of the angle during Zeiss gonioscopy?
    a. up
    b. toward the mirror
    c. away from the mirror
    d. down

14. The best parameter for determining the unreliability of a Humphrey visual field is
    a. fixation losses
    b. false-positives
    c. false-negatives
    d. fluctuation

15. Which of the following does not cause angle-closure glaucoma?
    a. ICE syndrome
    b. PHPV
    c. RD
    d. choroidal effusion

16. Factors producing increased IOP 2 days postoperatively include all of the following except
    a. retained viscoelastic
    b. red blood cells
    c. macrophages
    d. steroid drops

17. Treatment of malignant glaucoma may include all of the following except
    a. laser iridotomy
    b. pilocarpine
    c. atropine
    d. vitrectomy

18. The most common organism associated with bleb-related endophthalmitis is
    a. *Streptococcus* species
    b. *S. epidermidis*
    c. *H. influenzae*
    d. Gram-negative organisms

19. Which visual field defect is least characteristic of glaucoma?
    a. paracentral scotoma
    b. nasal defect
    c. central scotoma
    d. enlarged blind spot

20. The type of tonometer most greatly affected by scleral rigidity is
    a. Goldmann
    b. tonopen
    c. Schiøtz
    d. pneumotonometer

21. As compared with plasma, aqueous has a higher concentration of
    a. calcium
    b. protein
    c. ascorbate
    d. sodium

22. The rate of aqueous production per minute is approximately
    a. 0.2 μL
    b. 2 μL
    c. 20 μL
    d. 200 μL

23. The location of the greatest resistance to aqueous outflow is
    a. corneoscleral meshwork
    b. uveal meshwork
    c. juxtacanalicular connective tissue
    d. Schlemm's canal

24. Facility of aqueous outflow is best measured by
    a. tonography
    b. manometry
    c. tonometry
    d. fluorophotometry

25. A patient recently had an acute angle closure attack in the right eye. What is the most appropriate treatment for her left eye?
    a. synechiolysis
    b. laser peripheral iridotomy
    c. laser iridoplasty
    d. pilocarpine

26. The most likely gonioscopic finding in a patient with glaucoma and radial midperipheral spoke-like iris transillumination defects is
    a. concave peripheral iris
    b. anterior iris insertion
    c. peripheral anterior synechiae
    d. plateau iris configuration

27. A 60-year-old myope with early cataracts and enlarged cup-to-disc ratios of 0.6 OU is found to have an abnormal Humphrey visual field test OS. He has no other risk factors for glaucoma. What is the most appropriate next step for this patient?
    a. repeat visual fields
    b. diurnal curve (serial tonometry)
    c. monocular trial of latanoprost
    d. laser trabeculoplasty

28. Bilateral scattered PAS in an elderly hyperope with no past ocular history is most likely due to
    a. ICE syndrome
    b. uveitis
    c. chronic angle-closure glaucoma
    d. Axenfeld's anomaly

29. According to the CIGTS 5-year results, initial treatment of POAG with which two methods had similar visual field outcomes?
    a. medicine or laser trabeculoplasty
    b. medicine or trabeculectomy
    c. laser trabeculoplasty or trabeculectomy
    d. trabeculectomy or drainage implant

30. Which of the following medications should not be used to treat a patient with HSV keratouveitis and elevated IOP?
    a. pilocarpine
    b. timolol
    c. brimonidine
    d. dorzolamide

31. A patient undergoes multiple subconjunctival injections of 5-FU after glaucoma filtration surgery. The most common reason for discontinuing these injections is if the patient develops toxicity of which tissue?
    a. lens
    b. sclera
    c. cornea
    d. conjunctiva

32. A patient with retinoblastoma develops glaucoma. The most likely mechanism is
    a. secondary angle closure
    b. uveitic
    c. neovascular
    d. tumor cell

33. Glaucoma due to elevated episcleral venous pressure occurs in all of the following except
    a. carotid-cavernous fistula
    b. hyphema
    c. Sturge-Weber syndrome
    d. thyroid-related ophthalmopathy

34. The earliest color deficit in glaucoma is loss of
    a. yellow-green axis
    b. red-green axis
    c. red-blue axis
    d. blue-yellow axis

35. Blood in Schlemm's canal is not associated with
    a. Fuchs' heterochromic iridocyclitis
    b. thyroid-related ophthalmopathy
    c. hypotony
    d. Sturge-Weber syndrome

SUGGESTED READINGS

American Academy of Ophthalmology: Glaucoma, vol 10. San Francisco, AAO, 2012.

Anderson DR, Patella VM: Automated Static Perimetry, 2nd edn. St Louis, Mosby, 1999.

Campbell DG, Netland PA: Stereo Atlas of Glaucoma. St Louis, Mosby, 1998.

Higginbotham EJ, Lee DA: Clinical Guide to Glaucoma Management. Amsterdam, Butterworth-Heinemann, 2003.

Netland PA, Mandal AK: Pediatric Glaucoma. Philadelphia, Elsevier Butterworth-Heinemann, 2006.

Ritch R, Shields MB, Krupin T: The Glaucomas, 2nd edn. St Louis, Mosby, 1996.

Allingham RR, Moroi SE: Shields Textbook of Glaucoma, 6th edn. Philadelphia, Lippincott Williams and Wilkins, 2010.

Weber J, Caprioli J: Atlas of Computerized Perimetry. Philadelphia, WB Saunders, 2000.

Zimmerman TJ, Kooner KS: Clinical Pathways in Glaucoma. New York, Thieme Medical, 2001.

10

Anterior Segment

IRIS, CILIARY BODY, AND ANTERIOR CHAMBER (AC) ANGLE
LENS

Anatomy

Limbus

Transition zone between cornea and sclera; 1–2 mm wide

Conjunctiva and Tenon's capsule are fused over this area; contains corneal epithelial stem cells, goblet cells, lymphoid cells, Langerhans' cells, mast cells

Definitions:
Anatomist's: termination of Descemet's and Bowman's membranes
Pathologist's: anterior limbus corresponds to termination of Bowman's and Descemet's membranes, and posterior limbus corresponds to line between iris root and Schlemm's canal
Surgeon's: anterior blue zone (1 mm) and posterior white zone (1 mm); a perpendicular incision through the conjunctival insertion enters the AC through Descemet's membrane; a perpendicular incision through the posterior aspect of the limbus will enter the AC through the trabecular meshwork (Figure 10-1)

Ciliary Body and Angle Structures

(See Ch. 9, Glaucoma)

Disorders

Trauma

Hyphema

Blood in anterior chamber

Etiology: trauma, surgery (incisional or laser), spontaneous (neovascularization, Fuchs' heterochromic iridocyclitis, intraocular tumors, juvenile xanthogranuloma), clotting abnormalities (leukemia, hemophilia, anemia, coumadin, aspirin, ethanol)

Findings: layer of blood and/or clot with suspended RBCs in AC; called microhyphema if only suspended cells; damage to other structures may be seen

Diagnosis: sickle prep, consider hemoglobin electrophoresis, rule out ruptured globe, gonioscopy (wait 4–6 weeks in traumatic cases)

Treatment: cycloplegic, topical steroid, control IOP (avoid miotics); consider Amicar (aminocaproic acid), protective shield; elevate head, bed rest, no aspirin-containing products, control systemic BP, antiemetics (if needed); may require surgery (AC washout)
Indications for surgical intervention: large hyphema that persists for longer than 10 days, total hyphema that persists for longer than 5 days, corneal blood staining, uncontrolled IOP, 8-ball hyphema; best to perform washout 4–7 days after injury (clot has time to solidify, reducing rate of rebleed)

Complications:
8-Ball hyphema: hyphema that has clotted and taken on a black or purple color because of impaired aqueous circulation and deoxygenated blood, which prevents resorption; total hyphema is differentiated from 8-ball hyphema by retention of bright red color, which indicates aqueous circulation
Corneal blood staining: passage of erythrocyte breakdown products into stroma, creates yellow-brown discoloration; occurs in about 5%, especially with recurrent hemorrhage, compromised endothelial cell function, large hyphemas that remain for extended periods, elevated IOP
Recurrent hemorrhage: usually larger than initial hyphema; incidence 5–35% with greatest risk at 2–5 days
Secondary glaucoma:
   EARLY: due to TM obstruction, pupillary block by clot, hemolytic, steroid-induced
   LATE: due to angle recession, ghost cell, PAS formation, posterior synechiae with iris bombe
Central retinal artery occlusion

Sickle cell and hyphema: higher elevation in IOP (sickled RBCs cannot pass through TM), and higher risk of

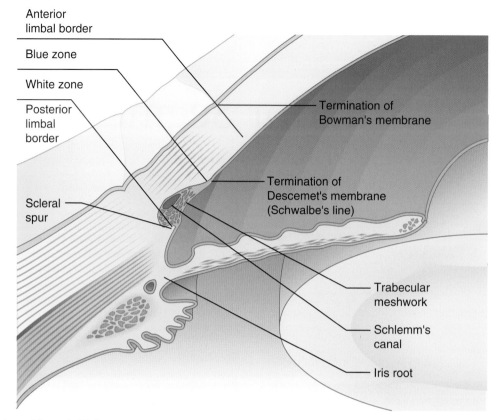

Figure 10-1. Anatomy of the surgical limbus.

central retinal artery occlusion and optic nerve infarction due to vascular sludging

Factors that increase sickling: acidosis, hypoxia, hemoconcentration

Ocular hypotensive medications in sickle cell: β-blockers are safe; avoid CAIs (increases concentration of ascorbic acid in aqueous, decreasing pH and leading to sickling), epinephrine and α-agonists (cause vasoconstriction with subsequent deoxygenation and sickling); hyperosmotics (lead to hemoconcentration with vascular sludging and sickling)

Iris and Angle Trauma (Figure 10-2)

Iris sphincter tear: small tear at pupillary margin; asymptomatic

Traumatic mydriasis: dilated, poorly reactive pupil; may cause glare or photophobia; consider cosmetic contact lens or surgical repair

Iridodialysis: tear in iris root; consider cosmetic contact lens or surgical repair if large or symptomatic

Angle recession: tear in anterior face of ciliary body between the longitudinal and circular ciliary muscles; most common source of hemorrhage in blunt trauma, occurs in more than 60% of hyphemas; 10% of patients with greater than 180° of angle recession will develop chronic glaucoma

Cyclodialysis: separation of ciliary body from scleral spur; allows free passage of aqueous into suprachoroidal space; can result in hypotony; treat with atropine, laser, and/or surgical repair

Open Globe/Intraocular Foreign Body

Full-thickness defect in cornea or sclera

Usually due to trauma (penetrating or blunt), may also occur from melt (chemical injury, autoimmune disorder, infection)

Penetration: entrance wound only

Perforation: entrance and exit wounds (double penetrating injury)

Risk of infectious endophthalmitis (3–7%) increases if retained foreign body, delayed surgery (>24 hours), rural setting (soil contamination), and lens disruption

S. aureus is the most common organism to cause post-traumatic endophthalmitis; *Bacillus cereus* is also common and causes severe damage

Findings: wound with positive Seidel test, hemorrhage (conjunctiva, hyphema, vitreous, retina), decreased IOP, shallow or flat AC, peaked pupil (toward wound), cataract, retinal tear//detachment, prolapsed intraocular contents (uvea, vitreous), foreign body (small high-velocity FB may cause self-sealing wound or intermittently positive Seidel; iris transillumination defect, capsule/lens disruption)

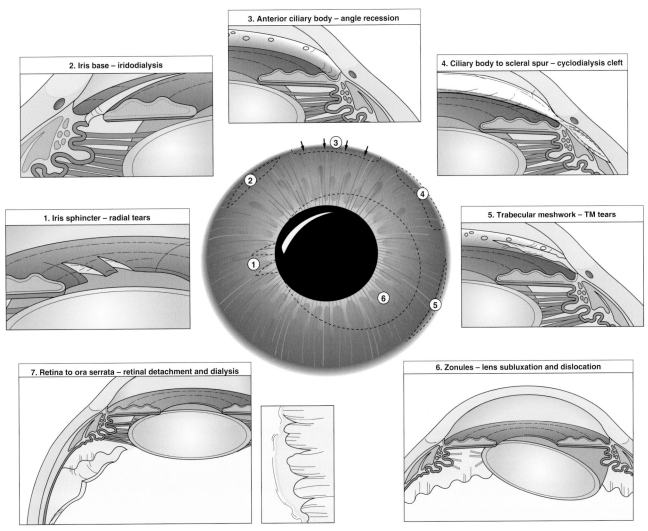

Figure 10-2. Seven areas of traumatic ocular tears (shown in yellow) with the resultant findings. (Adapted with permission from Campbell DG: Traumatic glaucoma. In Shingleton BJ, Hersh PS, Kenyon KR [eds]: Eye Trauma. St Louis, Mosby, 1991.)

Types of foreign bodies:

Inert: glass, plastic, sand, stone, ceramic, gold, platinum, silver, aluminum

Reactive:

COPPER: severity of inflammation is directly proportionate to amount of copper in foreign body (≥85% copper causes severe endophthalmitis; <85% causes chalcosis; <70% is relatively inert)

CHALCOSIS: mild intraocular inflammation, deposition of copper in anterior lens capsule (sunflower cataract) and Descemet's membrane (Kayser-Fleisher ring), retinal degeneration, iris may become green and sluggishly reactive to light

ERG: decreased amplitude (suppressed by copper ions)

IRON (siderosis): iris heterochromia (hyperchromatic on involved side), mid-dilated minimally reactive pupil, lens discoloration (brown-orange dots from iron deposition in lens epithelium, generalized yellowing from involvement of cortex), vitritis, pigmentary RPE degeneration with sclerosis of vessels, retinal thinning, and atrophy

ERG: initial a wave increased, may eventually become flat

WOOD: significant inflammation; plant matter has higher risk of endophthalmitis

Treatment: rule out FB with CT or MRI (contraindicated for metallic FB); surgical exploration and repair, remove reactive material as soon as possible

Prophylactic antibiotics: IV (aminoglycoside plus cephalosporin or vancomycin; consider clindamycin) and intravitreal (vancomycin [1 mg/0.1 mL], amikacin [0.4 mg/0.1 mL], or ceftazidime [2.25 mg/0.1 mL]) reduces risk of endophthalmitis; consider intravitreal dexamethasone 0.4 mg/0.1 mL

Prognosis: variable; poor if endophthalmitis or PVR develops (7–21 days later)

Congenital Abnormalities

(See Ch. 5, Pediatrics/Strabismus)

Mesodermal Dysgenesis Syndromes

(See Ch. 5, Pediatrics/Strabismus)

Other Disorders

Corectopia

Displacement of pupil

Isolated or associated with Axenfeld-Rieger syndrome, ICE syndrome, uveitis, trauma, or ectopia lentis et pupillae

Iris Heterochromia

Iris of different colors

May be congenital or acquired, unilateral (heterochromia iridis) or bilateral (heterochromia iridum)

DDx:
> *Congenital:*
> > **INVOLVED IRIS HYPOCHROMIC:** Horner's syndrome, Waardenburg's syndrome, Hirschsprung's disease, Parry-Romberg hemifacial atrophy
> > **INVOLVED IRIS HYPERCHROMIC:** ocular or oculodermal melanocytosis, iris pigment epithelium hamartoma
> *Acquired:*
> > **INVOLVED IRIS HYPOCHROMIC:** Horner's syndrome, Fuchs' heterochromic iridocyclitis, iris atrophy, metastatic carcinoma, juvenile xanthogranuloma
> > **INVOLVED IRIS HYPERCHROMIC:** iris nevus or melanoma, ICE syndrome, rubeosis, siderosis, hemosiderosis, medication (prostaglandin analogues)

Treatment: rule out tumor or intraocular foreign body

Rubeosis Iridis

Neovascularization of the iris

Etiology: ischemia (usually proliferative diabetic retinopathy [PDR], CRVO, carotid occlusive disease; also CRAO, sickle cell retinopathy, anterior segment ischemia), tumor, uveitis, chronic RD.

Findings: abnormal iris vessels; perform gonioscopy to assess presence of angle neovascularization; may have elevated IOP (neovascular glaucoma [NVG])
Treatment: often requires panretinal photocoagulation (PRP) for ischemia; NVG often needs glaucoma drainage implant for IOP control

Pigment Dispersion Syndrome

Pigment liberation from posterior iris surface (due to contact with zonules)

More common in young Caucasian males
Associated with myopia and lattice degeneration (20%)

Findings: pigment deposits on lens capsule, anterior iris, angle structures, and corneal endothelium (Krukenberg spindle); midperipheral, radial, iris transillumination defects; pigmentary glaucoma may develop

Iridocorneal Endothelial (ICE) Syndrome

Nonhereditary, progressive abnormality of corneal endothelium

Abnormal corneal endothelium grows across angle and iris, producing membrane that obstructs trabecular meshwork, distorts iris, and may contract around iris stroma to form nodules

Unilateral, mostly women, occurs during middle age

Findings: fine, beaten metal appearance of endothelium; secondary angle-closure glaucoma may develop due to angle endothelialization and PAS

Syndromes: common features of iris distortion, corneal edema, secondary angle-closure glaucoma
> *Iris nevus (Cogan-Reese) syndrome:* flattening and effacement of iris stroma, pigmented iris nodules (pseudonevi) composed of normal iris cells that are bunched up from the overlying membrane, corectopia, ectropion uveae
> *Chandler's syndrome:* corneal edema often with normal IOP, mild or no iris changes (minimal corectopia, iris atrophy, peripheral anterior synechiae)
> *Essential iris atrophy:* proliferating endothelium produces broad PAS, corectopia, ectropion uveae, and iris holes (stretch holes [area away from maximal pull of endothelial membrane is stretched so thin that holes develop] and melting holes [holes in areas without iris thinning due to iris ischemia])

Pathology: growth of endothelium and Descemet's membrane over trabecular meshwork and onto iris

DDx: posterior polymorphous dystrophy, mesodermal dysgenesis syndromes

Iridoschisis

Separation of iris stroma due to senile changes
Bilateral; onset in 6th-7th decade of life
Glaucoma in 50%

Iris Nodules

Brushfield's Spots

(See Ch. 5, Pediatrics/Strabismus)

Juvenile Xanthogranuloma (JXG)

(See Ch. 5, Pediatrics/Strabismus)

Epithelial Invasion, Serous Cyst, Implantation Membrane, Solid or Pearl Cyst

Serous or solid cysts after surgery or injury

Koeppe Nodules

Along pupillary border in granulomatous uveitis

Pathology: inflammatory cells and debris

Busacca Nodules

On anterior surface of the iris in granulomatous uveitis

Pathology: inflammatory cells and debris

Berlin Nodules

In anterior chamber angle in granulomatous uveitis

Pathology: inflammatory cells and debris

Iris Nevus Syndrome (Cogan-Reese)

(See above)

Iris Tumors

Perform transillumination to differentiate cyst from solid tumor

Freckle

No distortion of iris architecture

Nevus

Localized or diffuse variably pigmented lesion of stroma; obscures crypts

Pathology: usually low-grade spindle cells
Small risk of transformation into melanoma (~5% of suspicious iris lesions grow during first 5 years after detection)

Melanocytosis

Congenital ocular: usually unilateral with diffuse iris nevus causing iris heterochromia

Oculodermal (nevus of Ota): ocular plus periorbital skin involvement

Melanocytoma

Form of nevus; darkly pigmented, very discohesive (like black, wet sand)

May have necrotic center

5% risk of melanoma

Malignant Melanoma

Elevated, vascular, darkly pigmented or amelanotic lesion; usually located inferiorly

Can be diffuse (appearing as iris heterochromia) and associated with glaucoma, localized, annular, or tapioca (dark tapioca appearance)

Common in Caucasians with light irides

Findings suggestive of melanoma: growth (only 6.5% of iris melanomas enlarge over 5-year period), spontaneous hyphema, large size, vascularity, ectropion uveae, iris heterochromia, elevated IOP, angle involvement, glaucoma, sector cataract

Pathology: low-grade spindle B cells; epithelioid cells are rare

Treatment: resection (sector iridectomy), may require enucleation if extensive

Prognosis: 4–10% mortality; 14% overall risk of metastasis (associated with tumor extension into TM, glaucoma, older age, poorly defined margins)

Tumors of Iris Pigment Epithelium

Adenoma (benign) or adenocarcinoma (malignant) Rare compared with melanomas

Deeply pigmented, circumscribed or multinodular mass; can cause secondary glaucoma by involvement of angle

Treatment: chemotherapy, radiation, or excision

Lisch Nodules

Benign, tan, iris hamartomas; associated with neurofibromatosis type 1

Metastasis

Most commonly, breast, lung, lymphoma

Findings: fluffy, friable iris mass; may have pseudohypopyon, anterior uveitis, hyphema, rubeosis, and glaucoma

Leiomyoma

Well localized or pedunculated, often diffuse and flat

Pathology: very similar to amelanotic spindle cell melanoma

Leukemia

Rare nodular or diffuse milky lesions with intense hyperemia

Findings: iris thickening with loss of normal architecture; iris heterochromia and pseudohypopyon

Cystic Lesions

IPE: can be AD; flocculi around pupillary margin; associated in certain families with aortic dissection; midperipheral cysts, peripheral cysts (usually clear; can push iris forward)

Stroma: congenital or acquired (after trauma or surgery)

Ciliary Body Tumors

Melanoma

Pigmented mass
May be very large before detection, producing lenticular astigmatism, cataract, or shallow AC; may have classic sentinel vessel or nodule of extrascleral extension

Pathology: spindle, epithelioid, or mixed cells

Treatment: local resection, XRT, enucleation

Ciliary Body Leiomyoma

Similar to fibroid; myogenic origin

Schwannoma

Looks like amelanotic melanoma

Ciliary Body Adenoma or Adenocarcinoma

Arises from neuroepithelial cells

Occurs during adulthood

May metastasize

Fuchs' Adenoma (Fuchs' Reactive Hyperplasia, Benign Ciliary Epithelioma)

Proliferation of basement membrane material (type IV collagen and laminin) and nonpigmented ciliary body epithelial cells located at ciliary crest

Occurs in 25% of older patients

Rarely causes localized occlusion of anterior chamber angle

Medulloepithelioma

(See Ch. 5, Pediatrics/Strabismus)

LENS

Anatomy/Physiology (Figures 10-3 and 10-4)

Lens capsule: basement membrane secreted by epithelium; thickest peripherally near the equator, thinnest posteriorly. Thickening of lens capsule can occur with anterior chamber inflammation or pathologic proliferation of lens epithelium

Epithelium: present anteriorly, ending just posterior to the lens equator. Derived from cells of original lens vesicle. In the germinative zone, just anterior to equator, lens epithelial cells divide, elongate, and differentiate into lens fibers. During this transformation, epithelial cells lose their nuclei and most organelles. Lens fibers do not contain nuclei except in rubella, Lowe's syndrome, and trisomy 13. The embryonal nucleus develops by proliferation and

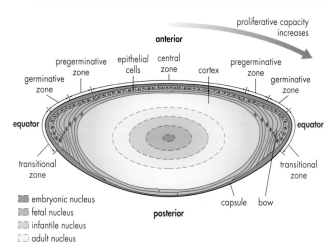

Figure 10-3. Typical photographic procedure. (From Mandava N, Reichel E, Guyer D, et al: Fluorescein and IGC angiography. In Yanoff M, Duker JS [eds]: Ophthalmology, London, Mosby, 1999.)

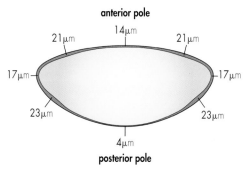

Figure 10-4. Thickness of the lens capsule. (From Saxby LA: Anatomy. In Yanoff M, Duker JS [eds]: Ophthalmology, London, Mosby, London, 1999.)

migration of epithelial cells from the equator. Acute IOP elevation may cause patches of epithelium degeneration and necrosis beneath the capsule, which appear as white flecks (glaukomflecken). Chronic iritis may cause liquefaction of the nucleus, peripheral cortical changes, and degeneration and necrosis, as well as proliferation of anterior lens epithelium

Sutures: upright Y suture anteriorly and inverted Y suture posteriorly represent the ends of lens fibers; sutures appear during the 2nd month of gestation because of unequal growth of new lens fibers

Zonules: attach from pars plicata to anterior and posterior lens capsule in midperiphery (inserting more centrally on anterior capsule). During the 5th month of gestation, nonpigmented ciliary epithelium of ciliary body secretes collagen fibers that become zonules. Equatorial zonules are lost with aging

Tunica vasculosa lentis: vascular network that surrounds lens during embryogenesis; derived from hyaloid and long ciliary arteries. Remnants of tunica vasculosa lentis include Mittendorf's dot, epicapsular star, persistent pupillary membrane, and capsular whorls

Properties of the crystalline lens

Composed of proteins: highest protein content in body (up to 60% wet weight and most of dry weight)

WATER SOLUBLE:

ALPHA CRYSTALLINS: largest of all water-soluble proteins, composed of 4 subunits; approximately 35% of lens protein by weight; involved in transforming epithelial cells into lens fibers

BETA CRYSTALLINS: most abundant lens protein by weight; composed of 3 subunits; approximately 55% of lens protein by weight; first appears in cortex

GAMMA CRYSTALLINS: smallest lens protein

WATER INSOLUBLE:

MAIN INTRINSIC POLYPEPTIDE: correlates with nuclear brunescence

Potassium-rich tissue: due to Na^+/K^+ pumps found on lens epithelial cells, which pump Na^+ out and K^+ in; concentrations of Na^+ and K^+ in aqueous are inverse to those in lens ($10\times$ as much Na^+ in aqueous as in lens)

Grows throughout life: weight at maturity is $3\times$ that at birth, anterior-posterior diameter increases from 3.5 mm at birth to 5 mm at maturity, equatorial length increases from 6.4 mm at birth to 9.0 mm at maturity; also increase in curvature with greater refractive power

Refractive index: increase in lens curvature and thickness with age is offset by change in gradient of refractive index due to increased concentration of main intrinsic polypeptide; associated with increased brunescence, resulting in greater absorption of blue and violet wavelengths, as well as UV light (aiding in retinal protection)

Metabolism: anaerobic; 80% of glucose metabolized by glycolysis, 10% metabolized by pentose phosphate pathway, 5% reduced to sorbitol, and 5% converted to glucuronic acid; highest metabolic rate is in cortex; energy is required for ion transport and glutathione production

Lens fiber structure: fibers contain few intracellular organelles and no nuclei; appear hexagonal in cross section

Average lens power: at birth = 37 diopters (D), at age 2 years = 23 D, at adulthood = 20 D

Protective mechanisms against free radical damage and oxidation: glutathione peroxidase, superoxide dismutase, catalase, and vitamins C and E

Accommodation: parasympathetic fibers of CN 3

Generally accepted theory is that of von Helmholtz: ciliary muscle contraction causes zonules to relax, allowing the lens to become more spherical and increasing its focusing power; presbyopia is therefore due to loss of lens elasticity with age

Disorders

Congenital Anomalies

(See Ch. 5, Pediatrics/Strabismus)

Cataracts

Congenital Cataracts

(See Ch. 5, Pediatrics/Strabismus)

Acquired Cataracts

Classified by location or etiology

Cortical: lens fiber fragments, degenerated protein, liquefaction

Spokes and vacuoles: radial lines and dots (Figure 10-5)

Mature: completely white

Hypermature: leakage of degenerated cortical material, wrinkled capsule; may have calcium deposits

Morgagnian: total liquefaction of lens cortex; nucleus floats freely within capsule; lens material can leak through intact capsule (Figure 10-6)

Pathology: hydropic swelling of lens fibers; morgagnian globules (eosinophilic, globular material between lens fibers)

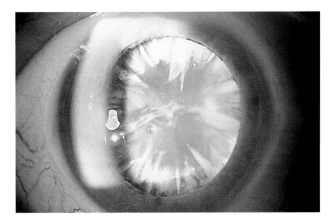

Figure 10-5. Cortical cataract. (From Collin J: The morphology and visual effects of lens opacities. In Yanoff M, Duker JS [eds]: Ophthalmology, London, Mosby, 1999.)

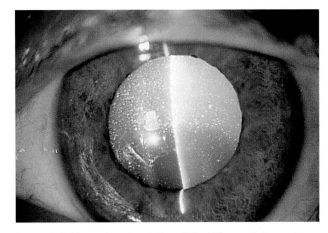

Figure 10-6. Morgagnian cataract. (From Collin J: The morphology and visual effects of lens opacities. In Yanoff M, Duker JS [eds]: Ophthalmology, London, Mosby, 1999.)

Nuclear sclerosis: increased nuclear density, then opacification occurs with aging; lenticular myopia results from increased index of refraction; 'second sight' (presbyopes can often read again without spectacles)

> Cataract brunescens (poor blue discrimination), cataract nigrans, calcium oxalate crystals in nucleus
>
> *Pathology:* inwardly sequestered lens fibers degenerate (analogous to desquamating skin); homogenous loss of cellular laminations

Posterior subcapsular (PSC): posterior migration of lens epithelium, and bladder (Wedl) cell formation (eosinophilic globular cells with nuclei; swell to 5–6× normal size)

> *Etiology:* age, trauma, steroids, inflammation, ionizing radiation, retinitis pigmentosa, atopic dermatitis, Werner's syndrome, Rothmund's syndrome, diabetes
>
> *Symptoms:* glare and poor vision from bright lights; affects near vision more than distance vision
>
> *Pathology:* posterior migration of lens epithelial cells, which swell along posterior capsule (swollen cells are called Wedl cells)

Anterior subcapsular (ASC): fibrous plaque beneath folded anterior capsule, secreted by irritated metaplastic anterior epithelial cells (due to trauma or uveitis), can also occur in atopic dermatitis

> *Pathology:* cells surrounded by basement membrane

Glaukomflecken: necrosis of lens epithelial cells due to ischemia from elevated IOP (angle closure); appears as central subcapsular small white dots and flecks

Traumatic and toxic cataracts

> *Contusion:* petalliform or rosette pattern due to separation of lens fibers around lens sutures
>
> *Vossius' ring:* with blunt injury, pigment from pupillary ruff is imprinted onto anterior lens capsule
>
> *Soemmering's ring:* doughnut of residual equatorial cortex; after cataract surgery or trauma; can be associated with an adherent leukoma
>
> *Siderosis lentis:* iron deposits in lens epithelium; anterior subcapsular orange deposits; photoreceptor and RPE degeneration resulting in pigmentary retinopathy with peripheral visual field loss; iris heterochromia (involved iris darker)
>
> *Chalcosis lentis:* copper deposits in lens capsule; green discoloration of anterior lens capsule and cortex in petaloid configuration occurs in Wilson's disease, forming a sunflower cataract; also Kayser-Fleischer ring (copper deposition in peripheral Descemet's membrane); can also occur in multiple myeloma and lung carcinoma
>
> *Other intraocular foreign bodies:* gold, silver, platinum, aluminum are inert; lead and zinc may cause mild nongranulomatous reaction
>
> > **COPPER:** if concentration ≥85%, an acute inflammatory reaction occurs; if concentration between 70 and 85%, chalcosis develops; lesser concentrations are relatively inert

Mercurial lentis: mercury deposits in lens capsule (occupational)

Electrical: lens vacuoles in anterior midperiphery; linear opacities (stellate pattern) in anterior subcapsular cortex; burns >200 volts cause conjunctival hyperemia, iritis, hyphema, iris atrophy, sphincter changes

Argon laser: blue light absorbed by yellow sclerotic nucleus

Nonionizing radiation: infrared causes true exfoliation (glassblower's cataract) with splitting and scrolling of anterior lens capsule; ultraviolet (UV-B) causes cortical cataracts

Ionizing radiation: a threshold level of radiation is required to induce cataract development (PSC)

Medications:

> **CORTICOSTEROIDS:** PSC from long-term use of any form of steroids, most commonly topical; develop in 33% of patients on long-term daily dose of 10 mg; also associated with inhaled steroids
>
> **MIOTICS:** echothiophate iodide and demecarium bromide cause anterior subcapsular vacuoles in adults (not children)
>
> **PHENOTHIAZINES AND AMIODARONE:** pigmented deposits in anterior lens capsule; axial, spoke-like configuration; dose and duration dependent
>
> **BUSULFAN:** PSC

Cataracts associated with systemic disease

> *Atopic dermititis:* PSC and ASC shield-like plaque Also associated with chronic keratoconjunctivitis, keratoconus, vernal keratoconjunctivitis
>
> *Diabetes:* osmotic cataract due to high glucose levels and aldose reductase, which results in high sorbitol levels
>
> > Snowflake cataract (punctate white subcapsular opacities) can occur rapidly with high blood sugar
>
> *Myotonic dystrophy* (AD): mapped to chromosome 19
>
> > **FINDINGS:** characteristic presenile 'Christmas tree' cataract consisting of polychromatic cortical crystals; ptosis, lid lag, light-near dissociation, mild pigmentary retinopathy; ERG – low voltage
> >
> > **OTHER FINDINGS:** myotonia (bilateral facial weakness, difficulty relaxing grip, muscle wasting), testicular atrophy, frontal baldness, cardiac abnormalities, mental retardation; excessive contractility of muscles
>
> *Neurofibromatosis type 2:* presenile PSC opacities
>
> *Werner's syndrome:* syndrome of premature aging, scleroderma-like matting of skin, and bilateral PSC cataracts in 3rd to 4th decade of life
>
> *Wilson's disease* (hepatolenticular degeneration): deficiency of ceruloplasmin (alpha-2 globulin)
>
> > **FINDINGS:** green sunflower cataract due to deposition of copper in anterior lens capsule and cortex in petaloid configuration; Kayser-Fleischer ring (copper in peripheral Descemet's membrane)
> >
> > **OTHER FINDINGS:** cirrhosis, renal impairment, degeneration of basal ganglia

TREATMENT: penicillamine to lower serum copper

Lens Capsule Abnormalities

True Exfoliation

Delamination/schisis of anterior lens capsule, forming scrolls; often due to infrared radiation (glassblowers), can be an aging change; not associated with glaucoma

Pseudoexfoliation Syndrome (PXS)

Material produced by lens epithelial cells and extruded through lens capsule
Appears to be an ocular sign of systemic elastosis; also found in conjunctiva, skin, lung, and liver
Usually elderly, Caucasian females; increased incidence in Scandinavians and with increasing age

Findings: white fibrillar material on anterior lens capsule, iris, ciliary body, zonules, anterior vitreous with characteristic pattern of deposition on lens surface (central disc, clear zone, then peripheral annulus, often with bridging strands to central disc); may see flakes on pupillary margin; Sampaolesi's line (pigment band anterior to Schwalbe's line) on gonioscopy; up to 50% develop glaucoma (PXG); poor dilation due to iris muscle degeneration or lack of iris stromal elasticity; peripupillary transillumination defects; weak zonules (phacodonesis, increased incidence of angle closure, lens subluxation, and complications during and after cataract surgery [vitreous loss, IOL and capsular dislocation])

Posterior Capsular Opacification (PCO; Secondary Cataract)

Proliferation of residual lens epithelial cells (Elschnig's pearls) and fibrosis

Incidence: up to 50% of patients within 2 years of extracapsular cataract surgery; influenced by optic material (acrylic < silicone < PMMA) and edge design (square edge < round edge); with newer IOLs, the incidence has decreased to ~10%. Incidence approaches 100% in children and patients with uveitis

Treatment: Nd:YAG laser posterior capsulotomy when visually significant

In young children, primary posterior capsulotomy and anterior vitrectomy are performed at the time of cataract surgery

Ectopia Lentis

Displacement of lens

Subluxation: partial displacement, remains in pupillary axis

Dislocation (luxation): complete displacement from pupil

Findings: decreased vision, astigmatism, monocular diplopia, iridodonesis, phacodenesis, malpositioned lens

DDx: trauma (most common acquired cause), Marfan's syndrome, homocystinuria, aniridia, congenital glaucoma, megalocornea, Ehlers-Danlos syndrome, hyperlysinemia, sulfite oxidase deficiency, hereditary ectopia lentis (AD >> AR; bilateral; may not present until 3rd–5th decade), ectopia lentis et pupillae (AR; lens and pupil are displaced in opposite directions; bilateral, asymmetric), tertiary syphilis, Weill-Marchesani syndrome, medulloepithelioma, Stickler's syndrome, pseudoexfoliation (rare)

Marfan's Syndrome (AD)

Mapped to chromosome 15q; defect in fibrillin (elastic microfibrillar glycoprotein, major constituent of zonules); 15% have no family history

Findings: ectopia lentis (65%; usually superotemporal); glaucoma, keratoconus, cornea plana, axial myopia, retinal degeneration (salt and pepper fundus), high risk of retinal detachment

Other findings: tall stature, spidery digits, arm span is larger than height, cardiac disease, dissecting aneurysm of the aorta

Homocystinuria (AR)

Deficiency of cystathionine β-synthase, which converts homocysteine to cystathionine; methionine and homocysteine accumulate; zonules are deficient in cysteine and weakened because of reduced sulfhydryl cross-linkage; degeneration of entire zonule occurs

Findings: bilateral ectopia lentis (90%; usually inferonasal; 30% in infancy, 80% by age 15), enlarged globe, myopia, peripheral RPE degeneration, increased risk of retinal detachment after cataract surgery, early loss of accommodation due to disintegration of zonules

Other findings: blonde, tall (marfinoid habitus with arachnodactyly), osteoporosis, fractures, seizures, mental retardation (50%), cardiomegaly, platelet abnormality with hypercoagulability (risk of thromboembolic problems, especially with general anesthesia); infants appear normal at birth; 75% mortality by age 30 years

Hyperhomocystinemia occurs in patients heterozygous for homocystinemia: high serum homocysteine increases risk of arterial and venous thrombosis (CRAO and CVO) and cardiovascular disease, especially in type 2 diabetic patients. In nondiabetic patients younger than 55 years of age who have had a stroke or MI, 25% have elevated homocysteine levels (5% in normal population)

Diagnosis: increased urinary excretion of homocysteine (nitroprusside urine test), amino acid assays; check renal function (homocysteine levels rise with elevated creatinine levels); subnormal or low levels of folate are associated with elevated levels of homocysteine

Treatment: vitamin B$_6$ (folate), methionine-restricted diet, supplementary cysteine (this diet can reduce lens dislocation); certain medications (methotrexate, phenytoin, carbamazepine) can elevate homocysteine levels by interfering with folate metabolism

Weill-Marchesani Syndrome (AR)

Findings: ectopia lentis (usually inferiorly or anteriorly), microspherophakia, high lenticular myopia, cataract, microcornea, glaucoma (pupillary block)

Other findings: short stature; short, stubby fingers with broad hands; hearing defects; inflexible joints; mental retardation

Ehlers-Danlos Syndrome (AD, AR, or X-Linked)

Defect in type III collagen; at least 9 types

Findings: ectopia lentis, easy lid eversion (Metenier's sign), epicanthal folds, myopia, microcornea, blue sclera, keratoconus, angioid streaks, retinal detachment

Other findings: hyperextensible joints and skin, poor wound healing, easy bruising

Sulfite Oxidase Deficiency (AR)

Enzymatic defect causing molybdenum deficiency and increased urinary sulfite

Findings: ectopia lentis (50%), enophthalmos, Brushfield's spots

Other findings: seizures, mental retardation, frontal bossing

Hyperlysinemia (AR)

Deficiency of lysine dehydrogenase

Findings: ectopia lentis, microspherophakia

Other findings: growth, motor and mental retardation

Surgery

Nd:YAG Laser

Posterior Capsulotomy

Open visually significant posterior capsule opacity
　　Power: 1.0–2.0 mJ; make an opening equal to the size of the pupil in ambient light
　　Treatment: pretreat with Iopidine (apraclonidine), then topical steroid qid × 1 week

Complications: increased IOP (glaucoma patients – 17% have rise after 2 hours; 14% with high IOP at 1 week; nonglaucoma patients – 6% have rise after 2 hours, 3% with high IOP at 1 week), retinal detachment (RD), cystoid macular edema (CME), rupture of the anterior hyaloid face, IOL dislocation, iritis, pitting of IOL, corneal or retinal burn

Vitreolysis

Disrupt anterior vitreous face in aphakic and pseudophakic eyes with malignant glaucoma
　　Power: 3–11 mJ, focused on anterior hyaloid; deepening of anterior chamber signifies success
　　Treatment: topical steroid qid × 1 week and cycloplegic; vitrectomy if regimen described here fails and in phakic eyes
Relieve CME due to vitreous wick
　　Power: 5-10 mJ bursts, often best to aim near wound or pigmented area of incarcerated vitreous; success occurs with a change in the pupil shape back to round
　　Treatment: pretreat with pilocarpine to induce miosis and stretch the strand, then topical steroid × 1 week

Cataract Surgery

Indications: altered vision (based on patient's functional impairment; when patient is having visual difficulty performing tasks and does not achieve adequate improvement from corrective lenses), also medical indications (phacolytic glaucoma, phacomorphic glaucoma, phacoantigenic uveitis, dense cataract that obscures view of fundus in patients who require regular retinal evaluation [i.e. diabetes, glaucoma])

IOL Calculations (see Ch. 1, Optics):
Formulas: rough estimation, use IOL power (D) = A constant of IOL – 2.5 (axial length) – 0.9 (average keratometry)
　　ACD (anterior chamber depth) approximately 3.5 mm
　　First generation: ACD is constant
　　Second generation: ACD is based on axial length (AL)
　　Third generation (Holladay 1, Hoffer Q, SRK/T): ACD is based on AL and keratometry (K)
　　Fourth generation (Holladay 2): variables include AL, K, corneal diameter, ACD, lens thickness, refraction, and patient age. (Haigis): ELP (effective lens position) derived from a function rather than a single number; used in the IOLMaster instrument
Most accurate formulas according to axial length
　　Long eyes ($AL > 26.0$ mm): SRK/T, Holladay 2, Haigis (customized)
　　Medium-long eyes (AL 24.6–26.0 mm): Holladay 1 or 2
　　Medium eyes (AL 22.0–24.5 mm): Hoffer Q, Holladay 1 or 2, SRK/T, Haigis
　　Short eyes ($AL < 22.0$ mm): Hoffer Q, Holladay 2

A scan: error of 0.1 mm = 0.3 D error in lens power; however, the shorter the axial length, the greater the effect of a measurement error
　　Myopia: 1.75 D error per mm of AL error
　　Emmetropia: 2.35 D error per mm of AL error
　　Hyperopia: 3.75 D error per mm of AL error

Ultrasound waves travel faster through lens (1640 m/s) than either aqueous or vitreous (1532 m/s)

To correct any AL, use the formula: $AL_{corrected} = AL_{measured} \times (V_{correct}/V_{measured})$

Average measurements

Axial length: 23.5 mm (22.0–24.5 mm)

Keratometry: 43.0–44.0 D

Anterior chamber depth (ACD): 3.25 mm

Lens thickness: 4.6 mm

Ultrasound speeds:

PHAKIC EYE = 1550 m/s (avg)

APHAKIC EYE = 1532 m/s

PSEUDOPHAKIC EYE (depends on IOL material and thickness) = 1556 m/s for PMMA lens, 1487 m/s for silicone lens, and 1549 m/s for acrylic lens

More accurate method for calculating pseudophakic AL is to measure at 1532 m/s and to use correction factors:

PMMA: $AL_{corrected} = AL_{1532} + 44\%$ IOL thickness + 0.04

SILICONE: $AL_{corrected} = AL_{1532} - 56\%$ IOL thickness + 0.04

ACRYLIC: $AL_{corrected} = AL_{1532} + 75\%$ IOL thickness + 0.04

SILICONE OIL = 980–1040 m/s (this is only for the portion of the eye containing silicone); thus to find the correct AL, the previous formula can be used, or the eye can be measured using an average velocity: phakic eye with silicone oil = 1140 m/s. Alternatively, use optical biometry (IOLMaster or Lenstar)

If silicone oil is to be left in the eye, the index of refraction of the oil will cause a hyperopic refraction; therefore, adjust the IOL power by adding 3.0–3.5 D

Immersion technique is more accurate than contact because of corneal compression (0.1–0.2 mm) for the later method. Optical biometry is most accurate.

Contact A scan:
5 spikes corresponding to beam reflection from interfaces: cornea, anterior lens surface, posterior lens surface, retina, sclera (Figure 10-7)

Causes of falsely long axial length:

Posterior staphyloma in high myopia; fovea may be located more anteriorly than the staphyloma

Measurement of the sclera rather than the retina

Wrong ultrasonic velocity (too fast)

Fluid meniscus between probe and cornea

Wrong gate position

Causes of falsely short axial length:

Excessive indentation of cornea with contact probe

Nonperpendicular measurement

Choroidal thickening or effusion

Vitreous opacity

Wrong ultrasonic velocity (too slow)

Wrong gate position

Keratometry in patient following refractive surgery:
need to determine accurate central corneal curvature; keratometer measures at 3 mm from center of cornea

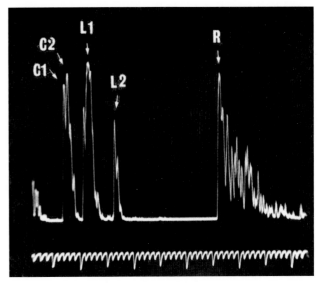

Figure 10-7. A-scan pattern of a phakic eye with the initial spike removed from the screen display. Identified are the 2 corneal peaks (Cl and C2), the anterior lens spike (L1), the posterior lens spike (L2), and the retinal spike (R). (From Shammas HJ: Intraocular lens power calculations. In Azar DT [ed]: Intraocular Lenses in Cataract and Refractive Surgery, Philadelphia, WB Saunders, 2001.)

Methods:

CLINICAL HISTORY: K = preopK + (refraction preop – refraction postop)

Convert for vertex distance: refraction (corneal surface) = refraction (spectacle plane)/(1 – 0.012 refraction [spectacle plane])

CONTACT LENS: use plano rigid gas-permeable contact lens with known base curve

K = base curve of CL + power + refraction (with CL) – refraction (without CL)

Convert for vertex distance

CORNEAL TOPOGRAPHY: use central 1 mm effective power reading from the Holladay diagnostic summary map (not sim K readings)

FORMULAS: numerous methods; online calculators available

Presence of cataract may induce myopia, causing error in first method, and may cause poor vision with inability to perform adequate CL overrefraction; therefore, a variety of methods should be used, then take flattest K to use in IOL calculation and consider using a final IOL 1–2 D stronger to avoid a hyperopic result

Piggyback IOL

Hyperopia (1.5 D per 1.0 D of hyperopia): if patient is +6.00, place a +9.00 D piggyback IOL.

Myopia (1.0 D per 1.0 D of myopia): if patient is –6.00, place a –6.00 D piggyback IOL

Interface membranes have been reported between piggyback lenses

Viscoelastic Device (Ophthalmic Viscosurgical Device [OVD])

Variety of clear gel-like materials composed of sodium hyaluronate and chondroitin sulfate

Used intraocularly to maintain and preserve space, displace and stabilize tissue, and coat and protect corneal endothelium

Vary in molecular weight, viscosity, clarity, ease of removal, and potential for IOP spike if retained in eye (peak usually 4–6 hours postoperatively)

Classification

Cohesive agent (ability to adhere to itself): long-chain, high-molecular-weight, high surface tension (low coating capability), high degree of pseudoplasticity (ability to transform from high viscosity at rest [zero shear rate] to lower viscosity at high shear rate)

   ADVANTAGES: capsulorhexis, insert IOL, ease of viscoelastic removal

   Examples: Healon, Healon GV, Amvisc, Amvisc Plus, Provisc

Dispersive agent: short-chain, low-molecular-weight, low surface tension (high coating ability), low to moderate pseudoplasticity

   ADVANTAGES: corneal coating, less IOP rise if retained, maintain space, move tissue

   Examples: Viscoat, Vitrax, Ocucoat

Viscoadaptive agent: ultrahigh-molecular-weight, superviscous and cohesive at low shear rates, more dispersive at increasing shear rates; thus combines the advantages of cohesive and dispersive agents

   Example: Healon 5

Phacodynamics

Irrigation: rate of fluid delivery; determined by bottle height above eye (34–110 cm); not adjusted by machine; depends on aspiration rate and wound leakage; maintains anterior chamber depth

Flow (aspiration rate [AFR]): rate of fluid removal (0–60 mL/min); determines how quickly vacuum is created; attracts material to tip

Vacuum (aspiration level): negative pressure created at tip by pump (0–500 mmHg); holds material onto occluded tip

Pump systems

Flow-based: independent, direct control of AFR and vacuum; vacuum rise requires tip occlusion; physically contacts and regulates aspiration line fluid

   PERISTALTIC: rollers compress tubing; AFR not smooth because of peristaltic wave; less accurate, especially at higher vacuum levels

   SCROLL: scroll element orbits against housing; more accurate; can act clinically like Venturi pump

Vacuum-based: direct control of vacuum only; AFR indirectly controlled by vacuum level; vacuum not affected by changes in tip occlusion; indirectly contacts aspiration line fluid by the induced vacuum in rigid drainage cassette between line and pump

   VENTURI: compressed air flows through tube; rapid, precise aspiration and vacuum response; requires external air supply

   DIAPHRAGM: flexible membrane moves like a piston; outmoded, large noisy system

   ROTARY VANE: wheel with vanes rotates; does not require external air supply

Hybrid: programmable like peristaltic or Venturi

Vacuum rise time: time for vacuum to reach preset limit; affected by aspiration rate; requires tip occlusion with peristaltic pump

Postocclusion surge (vacuum rush): collapse of AC due to increase in aspiration rate to level of pump speed; during occlusion, vacuum builds to preset level, no flow occurs, and tubing collapses; when occlusion breaks, pump pulls fluid at preset rate and rebound of tubing pulls additional fluid through tip. Prevented by venting, rigid tubing, microprocessor in pump

Followability: ability to bring material to tip; function of flow and vacuum

Holdability: ability to keep material at tip; function of vacuum and power

Phaco power (0–100%): depends on frequency and stroke length; surgeon (linear) or panel control; pushes material away from tip; generates heat.

   Power factors: amplitude (fixed vs linear) and duration (continuous vs intermittent)

   Power modulation: pulse, burst, bimodal, dual linear

Ultrasound effect

   Fragmentation: mechanical (jackhammer effect)

   Cavitation: sound waves expand and compress liquid, creating shock wave and microbubbles, which implode, forming cavity and dissolving nucleus in front of needle tip

Ultrasound instrument

   Handpiece: produces vibration of needle

     MAGNETORESTRICTIVE: converts magnetic energy into motion

     PIEZOELECTRIC CRYSTAL: converts electricity into motion

   Needle: oscillation produces phaco power

     FREQUENCY: rate of oscillation (25–62 kHz)

     STROKE LENGTH: distance of travel (0.002–0.004 inch [0.05–0.1 mm])

     BEVEL: occlusion vs cutting (0–45°)

     TIP SIZE/BORE: 0.9, 1.1, flared

     SHAPE: straight, angled

INNOVATIONS: microflow, microseal, aspiration bypass (ABS), torsional, elliptical

Footpedal: usual settings; can be programmed differently

KICK LEFT: reflux

POSITION 0: resting

POSITION 1: irrigation

POSITION 2: aspiration

POSITION 3: ultrasound

Audible clues:

METALLIC CLICK: irrigation (plunger opens)

HUMMING: aspiration

BUZZING: ultrasound (harmonic overtones)

BELLS: occlusion (no flow)

Customized tones

Alternative systems: Sonic, Fluid, Laser

Complications of Cataract Surgery

Preoperative (retrobulbar/peribulbar injection):

Globe perforation

Retrobulbar hemorrhage

Strabismus (inferior rectus fibrosis or myotoxicity)

Central anesthesia

Intraoperative:

Wound burn

Iris prolapse

Iris damage

Intraoperative floppy iris syndrome (IFIS)

Descemet's membrane detachment

Capsule damage (radial tear, posterior rupture, zonulolysis)

Retained material (nucleus, cortex)

Vitreous loss

Choroidal effusion

Suprachoroidal hemorrhage

Phototoxicity

Postoperative:

Wound leak

Inadvertent filtering bleb

Epithelial downgrowth

Corneal edema

Corneal melt

Secondary glaucoma

Uveitis, glaucoma, hyphema (uveitis-glaucoma-hyphema [UGH]) syndrome

Sputtering hyphema (vascularization of posterior wound lip; malpositioned IOL)

Pupillary capture of IOL

IOL decentration

Capsular block syndrome

Anterior capsular contraction syndrome

Posterior capsular opacification (PCO)

Cystoid macular edema (CME)

Retinal detachment (RD)

Endophthalmitis

Mydriasis

Ptosis

Retrobulbar Hemorrhage

May occur following retrobulbar injection or trauma; risk of CRAO as orbital pressure rises

Findings: marked proptosis, rapid orbital swelling and congestion, limited extraocular motility, hemorrhagic chemosis, lid ecchymosis and edema

Treatment: consider emergent surgical decompression with lateral canthotomy and cantholysis, hyperosmotic agents to lower IOP

Strabismus

Due to inferior rectus damage

Paralysis or fibrosis result from anesthetic injection

Central Anesthesia Following Retrobulbar Block

Agent spreads along meningeal cuff of optic nerve to enter CSF

Increased risk with 4% lidocaine

Findings: mental confusion, dysphagia, dyspnea, apnea, amaurosis of fellow eye

Wound Burn

Thermal injury from phaco needle due to lack of irrigation

Etiology: excessively tight incision, low or empty infusion bottle, low-flow settings, occluded phaco tip (with dispersive viscoelastic agent or impaled nucleus), phaco needle without thermal protective design

Findings: wound whitening, distortion, and astigmatism

Treatment: scleral relaxing incision, horizontal suture, bandage contact lens; if severe, may require astigmatic surgery after stabilization or patch graft

Iris Prolapse During Phaco

Wound too large or too posterior, bottle too high, posterior pressure, suprachoroidal hemorrhage

Intraoperative Floppy Iris Syndrome (IFIS)

Altered iris dilator tone due to systemic α-1 blocker medications (most commonly tamsulosin [Flomax]) with varying degrees of poor iris dilation and atonic floppy iris tissue (billows and prolapses), which may increase the risk of intraoperative complications during cataract surgery

Treatment: one or a combination of approaches depending on the severity of IFIS including preoperative topical atropine, intraoperative use of preservative free epinephrine, Healon 5, pupil expansion devices (i.e. Malyugin ring, Graether expander, Morcher dilator), iris hooks. Stopping the medication does not prevent IFIS and may lead to urinary retention

Descemet's Membrane Detachment

Due to inadvertent stripping of Descemet's from instrument insertion during surgery or viscoelastic injection; causes corneal edema or decompensation

Treatment: air or gas bubble, may require suture repair

Expulsive Suprachoroidal Hemorrhage

May occur during intraocular surgery or days later; incidence of 0.5%

Risk factors: elderly patient, hypertension, atherosclerosis, diabetes, sudden drop in IOP during surgery, high myopia, vitreous loss or previous vitrectomy, previous expulsive hemorrhage in fellow eye, glaucoma, aphakia, postoperative Valsalva maneuver

Findings: forward movement of intraocular contents during surgery and loss of red reflex (ominous sign), subretinal hemorrhage, choroidal detachment, and extrusion of intraocular contents; delayed hemorrhage presents with severe eye pain, nausea, vomiting, and rapid loss of vision

Treatment: close wound rapidly; may require surgical drainage

Prevention: decompress eye preoperatively, small wound, control BP during surgery, prevent bucking in patients under general anesthesia

Phototoxicity

Occurs in up to 39% for surgical time >100 minutes

Prevention: dim light, oblique light, pupil shield

Corneal Edema

Etiology: trauma to endothelium, elevated IOP, endothelial chemical toxicity, Descemet's detachment, decompensation in patient with Fuchs' corneal endothelial dystrophy

Corneal Ulceration and Melting

Occurs most commonly after cataract surgery in patients with keratoconjunctivitis sicca and rheumatoid arthritis; melting several weeks after uncomplicated cataract surgery due to collagenase release from surrounding inflammatory cells

Uveitis-Glaucoma-Hyphema (UGH) Syndrome

Due to repeated trauma to angle structures and iris by IOL; scarring and degeneration occur

Treatment: atropine, topical steroids, ocular hypotensive medications; consider argon laser of bleeding site; usually requires IOL explantation

Hyphema

Result of fine neovascularization of scleral incision (Swan syndrome) or mechanical trauma from IOL haptics

Occurs with more posteriorly located incisions

IOP can become dangerously elevated

Pupillary Capture

Portion of IOL optic anterior to iris

Risk factors: large or incomplete capsulorhexis, sulcus haptic placement, nonangulated IOL, upside-down IOL placement, vitreous pressure

Treatment: observe if long-standing and stable without symptoms; dilate and place patient supine if occurs early postoperatively; may require lens repositioning with microhook

IOL Decentration

Causes diplopia or polyopia because of prismatic effect

Sunset syndrome: inferior displacement of IOL within capsular bag; occurs with unrecognized zonular dialysis, capsular tears, or asymmetric IOL haptic implantation (1 in bag and other in sulcus)

Sunrise syndrome: asymmetric IOL haptic placement

Treatment: consider pilocarpine; IOL repositioning or exchange may be required

Capsular Block Syndrome

Due to retained viscoelastic behind IOL

Causes myopic shift

Treatment: Nd:YAG laser anterior capsulotomy

Anterior Capsular Contraction Syndrome (Capsular Phimosis)

Due to small capsulorhexis with retention of lens epithelial cells

Treatment: Nd:YAG laser radial anterior capsulotomies

CME (Irvine-Gass Syndrome)

More common with intracapsular (ICCE) than extracapsular cataract extraction (ECCE)
50% angiographically for ICCE vs 15% for ECCE

Clinically significant (visual loss) in <1% of patients with ECCE

Risk factors: capsular rupture, dislocated IOL, iris-supported IOL, iris tuck, vitreous adhesion to pupil or wound; also patients with diabetes, epiretinal membrane, and retinal vein occlusion

FA: petalloid hyperfluorescence, late leakage; late staining of optic nerve helps to differentiate postoperative CME from other forms of CME

OCT: increased foveal thickness; intraretinal cystoid spaces

Treatment: topical steroid and NSAID, consider posterior sub-Tenon's steroid injection with kenalog

Endophthalmitis

(See Ch. 8, Uveitis)

Rhegmatogenous Retinal Detachment

Incidence: 1–2%

Risk factors: high myopia, lattice degeneration, history of RD in fellow eye, vitreous loss

Mydriasis

Due to sphincter damage (mechanical from iris stretching or ischemic from elevated IOP (Urrets-Zavalia syndrome))

Ptosis

Due to trauma from lid speculum

REVIEW QUESTIONS *(Answers start on page 369)*

1. The most helpful test for evaluating macular function in a patient with advanced cataract is
   a. blue field entoptic phenomenon
   b. 2-light separation
   c. red-light discrimination
   d. directional light projection

2. Ectopia lentis is least likely to be associated with
   a. cleft palate
   b. pectus excavatum
   c. short stature
   d. mental retardation

3. Anterior segment signs of ciliary body melanoma include all of the following except
   a. corneal edema
   b. increased IOP
   c. astigmatism
   d. cataract

4. Which of the following is least characteristic of ICE syndrome?
   a. corneal edema
   b. increased IOP
   c. ectropion uveae
   d. PAS

5. The crystalline lens is formed from which embryologic tissue?
   a. neural crest
   b. ectoderm
   c. mesoderm
   d. endoderm

6. A stellate anterior subcapsular cataract is most likely to be found in a patient with
   a. Fabry's disease
   b. atopic dermatitis
   c. myotonic dystrophy
   d. electrical injury

7. The most useful diagnostic test in an infant with an oil-droplet cataract is
   a. urine amino acids
   b. calcium
   c. TORCH titers
   d. urine reducing substances

8. Which of the following does not occur in siderosis bulbi?
   a. glaucoma
   b. retinal atrophy
   c. sunflower cataract
   d. fixed pupil

9. A patient has a history of increased IOP with exercise; which finding is associated with this condition?
   a. Krukenberg spindle
   b. PAS
   c. phacodenesis
   d. pars plana snowbank

10. Separation between the longitudinal and circumferential fibers of the ciliary muscle is called
    a. iridoschisis
    b. angle recession
    c. iridodialysis
    d. cyclodialysis

11. Characteristics of pigment dispersion syndrome include all of the following except
    a. increased IOP with exercise
    b. Krukenberg's spindle
    c. phacodenesis
    d. radial iris transillumination defects

12. Genetics of aniridia are best summarized as
    a. ⅓ AR, ⅔ AD
    b. ⅓ sporadic, ⅔ AR
    c. ⅓ AD, ⅔ sporadic
    d. ⅓ sporadic, ⅔ AD

13. A sickle cell patient with a hyphema develops increased IOP; which of the following treatment choices is best?
    a. pilocarpine
    b. Diamox
    c. hyperosmotic
    d. Timoptic

14. A pigmentary retinopathy occurs in which mesodermal dysgenesis syndrome?
    a. Axenfeld's anomaly
    b. Alagille's syndrome
    c. Rieger's syndrome
    d. Peter's anomaly

15. Of the following causes of iris heterochromia, the involved iris is hyperchromic in
    a. ICE syndrome
    b. Horner's syndrome
    c. Waardenburg's syndrome
    d. Fuchs' heterochromic iridocyclitis

16. Which of the following iris lesions is a true tumor?
    a. Kunkmann-Wolffian body
    b. Koeppe nodule
    c. Lisch nodule
    d. juvenile xanthogranuloma
17. At which location is the lens capsule thinnest?
    a. anterior capsule
    b. posterior capsule
    c. equatorial capsule
    d. anterior paracentral capsule
18. The iris sphincter is derived from what embryologic tissue?
    a. neural crest cells
    b. surface ectoderm
    c. neural ectoderm
    d. mesoderm
19. Which of the following is not associated with sunset syndrome?
    a. asymmetric IOL haptic placement
    b. polyopia
    c. pseudoexfoliation
    d. hyphema
20. Lens epithelial cells differentiate into lens fibers
    a. anterior to the equator
    b. at the equator
    c. posterior to the equator
    d. in the fetal nucleus
21. Light of which wavelength is absorbed greatest by a dense nuclear sclerotic cataract?
    a. red
    b. green
    c. yellow
    d. blue
22. A patient with background diabetic retinopathy and clinically significant macular edema desires cataract surgery. The most appropriate management is
    a. cataract surgery
    b. focal laser treatment then cataract surgery
    c. cataract surgery then panretinal photocoagulation
    d. cataract surgery with intraoperative laser treatment
23. After finishing phacoemulsification on a dense cataract, the surgeon notes whitening of the clear corneal incision. The most likely cause is
    a. tight incision
    b. high aspiration flow rate
    c. high phaco power
    d. 45° bevel phaco needle
24. Nuclear brunescence increases with higher concentrations of which lens protein?
    a. alpha crystallin
    b. beta crystallin
    c. gamma crystallin
    d. main intrinsic polypeptide
25. Lens fibers contain nuclei in all of the following conditions except
    a. trisomy 13
    b. syphilis
    c. rubella
    d. Lowe's syndrome
26. The most likely cause of an intraoperative complication during cataract surgery in a patient with pseudoexfoliation syndrome is
    a. small pupil
    b. thin posterior capsule
    c. weak zonules
    d. shallow anterior chamber
27. The majority of glucose metabolism in the lens is by
    a. glycolysis
    b. pentose phosphate pathway
    c. reduction to sorbitol
    d. conversion to glucuronic acid
28. The most appropriate systemic treatment for a patient with a sunflower cataract is
    a. insulin
    b. penicillamine
    c. steroids
    d. methotrexate
29. Which of the following is the least likely cause of decreased vision 2 years after cataract surgery?
    a. subluxed IOL
    b. retinal detachment
    c. posterior capsular opacity
    d. cystoid macular edema
30. Which type of cataract is most closely associated with UV-B exposure?
    a. anterior subcapsular
    b. cortical
    c. nuclear sclerotic
    d. posterior subcapsular

SUGGESTED READINGS

Abelson MB: Allergic Diseases of the Eye. Philadelphia, WB Saunders, 2001.

American Academy of Ophthalmology: Lens and Cataract, vol 11. San Francisco, AAO, 2012.

Boruchoff SA: Anterior Segment Disorder: A Diagnostic Color Atlas. Boston, Butterworth-Heinemann, 2001.

Elander RE, Rich LF, Robin JB: Principles and Practice of Refractive Surgery. Philadelphia, WB Saunders, 1997.

Jaffe NS, Jaffe MS, Jaffe GF: Cataract Surgery and Its Complications, 6th edn. St Louis, Mosby, 1997.

Mackie IA: External Eye Disease. Boston, Butterworth-Heinemann, 2003.

Watson P, Hazleman B, Pavesio C: Sclera and Systemic Disorders. Philadelphia, Butterworth-Heinemann, 2003.

11
Posterior segment

ANATOMY
PHYSIOLOGY
ELECTROPHYSIOLOGY
RETINAL IMAGING
DISORDERS
LASER TREATMENT

ANATOMY

Vitreous

Composed of 99% water and a few type II (mainly) and type IX collagen fibers; viscous, gel-like quality from mucopolysaccharide and hyaluronic acid that is folded into coiled chains and holds water like a sponge; volume ~4 cm^3; syneresis (liquefaction) occurs with aging (Figures 11-1, 11-2).

Vitreous base: portion of vitreous that attaches to peripheral retina and pars plana; 6 mm width – 2 mm anterior and 4 mm posterior to the ora serrata; straddles ora serrata; avulsion is pathognomonic for trauma

Vitreoretinal junctions: arise from footplates of Müller's cells at internal limiting membrane; provide firm vitreoretinal attachment, especially at vitreous base, macula, optic nerve, and retinal vessels; also at edge of lattice degeneration, chorioretinal scars, degenerative remodeling, enclosed oral bays; weak attachments at fovea and disc, and over areas of lattice

Retina (Figure 11-3)

Neurosensory Retina (9 Layers): Inner refers to proximal or vitreous side of retina

1. **Internal limiting membrane** (ILM): foot processes of Müller's cells (PAS-positive basement membrane); true basement membrane; clinically visible as small yellow-white spots (Gunn's dots) at ora serrata; continuous with inner bordering membrane of ciliary body
2. **Nerve fiber layer** (NFL): unmyelinated ganglion cell axons; also contains glial cells (astrocytes); myelination by oligodendrites occurs at lamina cribrosa; axons synapse with nuclei of cells in LGB

3. **Ganglion cell layer**: usually a single cell layer with cells packed tightly near the optic disc and more scattered in the periphery; nuclei are multilayered in macula
4. **Inner plexiform layer**: synaptic processes between bipolar and ganglion cells, as well as amacrine with bipolar cells; outermost layer completely nourished by retinal arteries
5. **Inner nuclear layer**: outermost retinal layer; inner $\frac{2}{3}$ of retina receives its nourishment from retinal vasculature (outer $\frac{1}{3}$ from choroid); contains cell bodies of bipolar, amacrine (confined to inner surface), horizontal (confined to outer surface), and Müller's (span from ILM [foot processes] to ELM [microvilli, which point toward RPE]) cells
6. **Outer plexiform layer**: synaptic processes between photoreceptors and dendritic processes of bipolar cells; cone axons = Henle fibers
   Middle limiting membrane (MLM): synapses; forms approximate border of vascular inner portion and avascular outer portion of the retina
   Central retinal artery supplies retina internally (MLM to ILM)
   Choriocapillaris supplies retina externally (MLM to RPE)
   Interior to MLM: dendrites of bipolar cells along with horizontally coursing processes of horizontal cells
   External to MLM: basal aspect of photoreceptors
   In macula, outer plexiform layer is called Henle's fiber layer; radial orientation of fibers (responsible for macular star configuration and cystic spaces in cystoid macular edema)
7. **Outer nuclear layer**: photoreceptor cell bodies and nuclei; most cone nuclei lie in single layer immediately internal to ELM
8. **External limiting membrane** (ELM): fenestrated intercellular bridges, situated external to

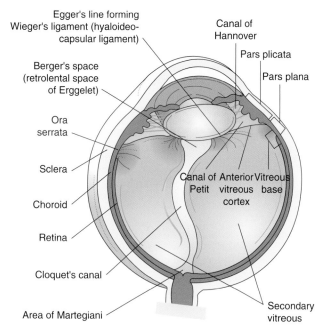

Figure 11-1. Vitreous anatomy according to classic anatomic and histologic studies. (From Schepens CL, Neetens A: The Vitreous and Vitreoretinal Interface. New York, Springer-Verlag, 1987.)

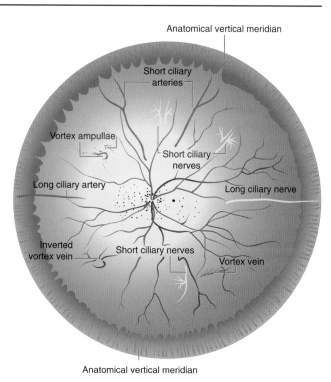

Anatomical vertical meridian

Figure 11-3. Normal fundus as seen through indirect ophthalmoscope. (From A Manual for the Beginning Ophthalmology Resident. 3rd edn, edited by James M. Richard. 1980, p. 122 Figure 60.)

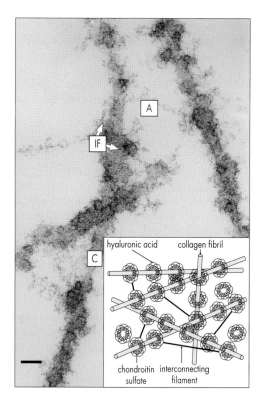

Figure 11-2. Ultrastructure of hyaluronan–collagen interaction in the vitreous. C, collagen; IF, interconnecting filament. (Courtsey of Dr Akiko Asakura. From Askura A: Histochemistry of hyaluronic acid of the bovine vitreous body as studied by electron micoscopy. Acta Soc Ophthalmol Jpn 89:179–191, 1985.)

photoreceptor nuclei; interconnects photoreceptor cells to Müller's cells; not a true basement membrane but an illusion caused by tight junctions between Müller's cells and photoreceptors

9. **Photoreceptor layer**: rods and cones; number equal in macula; 11-*cis* retinal converted to all-*trans* retinol in PR outer segments (not in RPE where it is converted back) (Figure 11-4)

100 million rods: rods account for 95% of photoreceptors; rhodopsin; density maximal in a ring 20–40° around fovea; when dark adapted, rods are 1000 times more sensitive than cones; rod disks are not attached to cell membrane, discrete structures; provide dark adapted vision

5 million cones (50% in macula): 3 types of visual pigment (blue [make up only 10%], green, red); density maximal in fovea; cone disks are attached to cell membrane and undergo membranous replacement; provide high acuity and color vision

Peripheral Retina: Extends from macula to ora serrata, nonpigmented epithelium is contiguous with pars plana; defined as any area of the retina with a single layer of ganglion cells (Figure 11-5)

Macula: Area of retina in which ganglion cell layer is more than 1 cell thick (5–6 mm in diameter)

Centered 4 mm temporal and 0.8 mm inferior to optic nerve

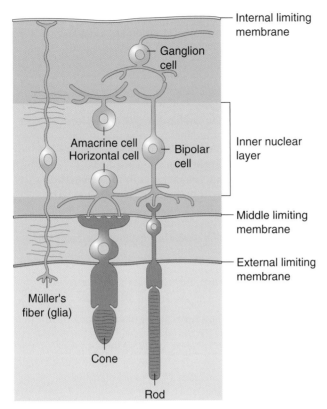

Figure 11-4. Neuronal connections in the retina and participating cells. (From Schubert HD: Structure and function of the neural retina. In: Yanoff M, Duker JS (eds) Ophthalmology. London, Mosby, 1999.)

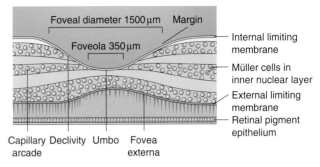

Figure 11-6. Foveal margin, foveal declivity, foveola, and umbo. (From Schubert HD: Structure and function of the neural retina. In: Yanoff M, Duker JS (eds) Ophthalmology. London, Mosby, 1999.)

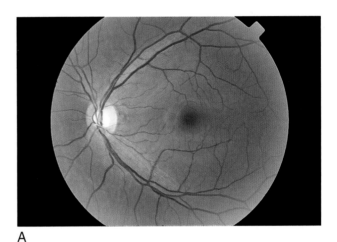

A

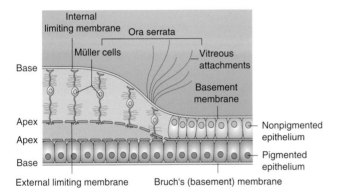

Figure 11-5. Transition of neural retina to nonpigmented epithelium at the ora serrata. (From Schubert HD: Structure and function of the neural retina. In: Yanoff M, Duker JS (eds) Ophthalmology. London, Mosby, 1999.)

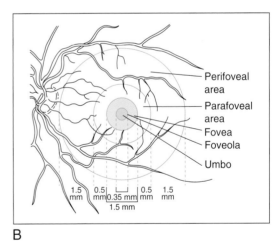

B

Figure 11-7. Normal fundus with macula encompassed by major vascular arcades. (From Schubert HD: Structure and function of the neural retina. In: Yanoff M, Duker JS (eds) Ophthalmology. London, Mosby, 1999.)

Differentiation of the macula does not occur until age 4–6 months old

Predominantly red and green cones in macula

High levels of carotenoids (100-1000× more than anywhere else): lutein (antioxidant) and zeaxanthin (light screening)

Fovea (Figures 11-6, 11.7): Central depression of inner retinal surface (1.5 mm in diameter) within macula

Corresponds to the foveal avascular zone (FAZ)

Contains taller RPE cells and xanthophyll pigment (blocks choroidal fluorescence during fluorescein angiography)

Initially, ganglion cell nuclei are present in fovea but are gradually displaced peripherally, leaving fovea devoid of accessory neural elements

Foveola: Central area of fovea (350 μm in diameter)

Absence of ganglion cells and other nucleated cells; avascular

Mechanisms to prevent foveal detachment:
  Microvilli of RPE, which surround tips of photoreceptors
  Viscous mucopolysaccharides, which bathe photoreceptors and RPE
  Intraocular pressure

Intercellular Junctions

Blood–retinal barrier:
  INNER BARRIER: tight junctions (zonula occludens) between retinal vascular endothelial cells
  OUTER BARRIER: tight junctions between RPE cells
Other intercellular junctions:
  ZONULA ADHERENS (external limiting membrane): no barrier to passage of fluids
  MACULA ADHERENS (desmosomes): no barrier to passage of fluids

Clinical Correlation

Collateral vessels: occur at site of obstruction, across horizontal raphe, and at disc

Hemorrhages

Flame or splinter: superficial; blood tracks along NFL
Blot or dot: deep; blood confined by axons oriented perpendicular to Bruch's membrane
Boat-shaped (scaphoid):
  SUB-ILM: hemorrhagic detachment of ILM
  SUB-HYALOID: blood between ILM and posterior hyaloid
Dark hemorrhage: sub-RPE; can be confused with choroidal melanoma

RPE: Monolayer of hexagonal cells with apical microvilli and basement membrane at base

RPE and outer segments of photoreceptors have apex-to-apex arrangement, resulting in a potential subretinal space

Merges anteriorly with pigmented epithelium of ciliary body

  Functions:
  Helps with development of photoreceptors during embryogenesis
  Involved in vitamin A cycle (uptake, transport, storage, metabolism, and isomerization)
  Provides nourishment for outer half of retinal cells
  Receives waste products: phagocytoses photoreceptor outer segments; photoreceptors renew outer segments every 10 days
  Forms outer blood–retinal barrier (tight junctions between RPE cells)
  Secretes basement membrane material (deposits on inner basal lamina of Bruch's membrane)
  Produces melanin granules in 6th week of gestation (first cells of body to melanize); melanization may induce further differentiation of retinal layers (may explain why macula fails to develop properly in albinism); melanin helps absorb excess light; macular RPE cells contain larger and a greater number of melanosomes than those in periphery

Contributes to adhesion of sensory retina
ATP-dependent Na+/K+ pump on apical surface maintains environment of subretinal space
Heat exchange
Light absorption
RPE cells may undergo hypertrophy, hyperplasia, migration, atrophy, and metaplasia
  HYPERTROPHY: flat, jet-black subretinal lesion
  HYPERPLASIA: intraretinal pigment deposition
    Migrate into retina to form bone spicules around blood vessels in retinitis pigmentosa
    Migrate through retinal holes to form preretinal membranes in proliferative vitreoretinopathy
  METAPLASIA: nonspecific reaction, observed most often in phthisis; fibrous (component of disciform scars in AMD) or osseous (intraocular ossification)

Bruch's Membrane: Permeable to small molecules

  Layers:
  1. Basement membrane (inner basal lamina of RPE)
  2. Collagen
  3. Elastic tissue
  4. Collagen
  5. Basement membrane (outer basal lamina of choriocapillaris)

RPE and Bruch's membrane are continuous with the pigmented ciliary epithelium

Neuroglial Cells

Astrocytes: branching neural cells in retina and CNS; proliferation leads to gliosis; cell of origin for optic nerve glioma; provide structural support to optic nerve and retina; contribute to nourishment of neuronal elements; foot processes ensheath blood vessels within nerve, contributing to blood–brain barrier

Müller's cells: modified astrocytes; footplates form ILM, nuclei in inner nuclear layer; provide skeletal support; contribute to gliosis; extend from ILM to ELM

Microglia: phagocytic cells of the CNS

Arachnoidal cells: cell of origin for meningioma

Oligodendrocytes: produce myelin in the CNS; cell of origin for oligodendroglioma

Schwann cells: produce myelin in peripheral nervous system

Choroid

Posterior part of uveal tract that extends from ora serrata (outer layers end before inner) to optic nerve. Attached to sclera by strands of connective tissue at optic nerve, scleral spur, vortex veins, and long and short posterior ciliary vessels; derived from mesoderm and neuroectoderm; 0.22 mm thick posteriorly and 0.1–0.15 mm thick anteriorly

Layers:

1. **Bruch's membrane** (innermost layer): PAS stain positive, 2 μm thick centrally and increases in thickness with age
2. **Choriocapillaris**: capillary layer of choroid with fenestrations (leak fluorescein dye); lobular pattern in posterior pole, more parallel in periphery (Figure 11-8)
3. **Stroma**: mainly blood vessels; outer, unfenestrated large vessel layer (Haller's layer) and unfenestrated, medium vessel layer (Sattler's layer)
4. **Suprachoroidal space** (outermost layer): 30 μm thick, darkly pigmented

Blood supply from 1–2 long and 15–20 short posterior ciliary arteries (from internal carotid to ophthalmic artery)

Endothelium is permeable to large molecules

Choriocapillaris arranged in segmental pattern; major source of nutrition for RPE and outer retinal layers

Drains via vortex veins to superior and inferior ophthalmic veins

Contain both parasympathetic and sympathetic nerves (autoregulatory function to keep blood flow constant) via short (mainly) and long posterior ciliary nerves

PHYSIOLOGY

Visual pigments: 4 types, each composed of 11-*cis*-retinal (vitamin A aldehyde) + a protein (opsin); 3 cone pigments and 1 rod pigment (Table 11-1)

Rod photoreceptor membranes: lipid bilayer in which rhodopsin is an integral component

Chromophore 11-*cis*-retinaldehyde is oriented parallel to the lipid bilayer (perpendicular to the path of photons)

Bleaching releases all-*trans*-retinaldehyde from the visual pigment (opsin) with conversion to all-*trans*-retinol; this initiates an electrical impulse that travels to visual cortex; rhodopsin is then resynthesized, and vitamin A is stored in liver and transported to RPE by serum retinol–binding protein and prealbumin

Rods shed outer segments during the day

Cones shed outer segments during the night

Luminosity curves:

Light-adapted: cone peak sensitivity is to light of 555 nm; yellow, yellow-green, and orange appear brighter than blue, green, and red

Dark-adapted: rod peak sensitivity is to light of 505 nm (blue)

Purkinje shift: shift in peak sensitivity that occurs from light- to dark-adapted states (Figure 11-9)

ELECTROPHYSIOLOGY

Electroretinogram (ERG)

Measures mass retinal response; useful for processes affecting large areas of retina

Photoreceptors, bipolar and Müller's cells contribute to flash ERG; ganglion cells do not

Light is delivered uniformly to entire retina, and electrical discharges are measured with a corneal contact lens electrode

Components (Figure 11-10):

a-wave: photoreceptor cell bodies (negative waveform)

b-wave: Müller's and bipolar cells (positive waveform)

Amplitude: bottom of a-wave to top of b-wave; measured in microvolts

Measures response of entire retina; proportionate to area of functioning retina

Decreased in anoxic conditions (diabetes, CRAO, ischemic CVO)

Table 11-1. Visual pigments

Photoreceptor	Pigment	Peak sensitivity
Rod	Rhodopsin	505 nm
Red cones	Erythrolabe	575 nm
Green cones	Chlorolabe	545 nm
Blue cones	Cyanolabe	445 nm

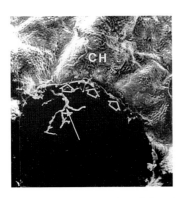
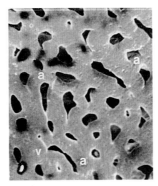
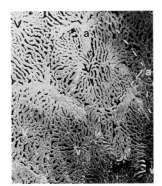
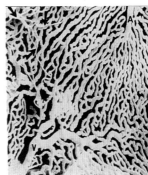

Figure 11-8. Human choriocapillaris, retinal view. (From Fryczkowski AW: Anatomical and functional choroidal lobuli. Int Ophthalmol 18:131–141, 1994.)

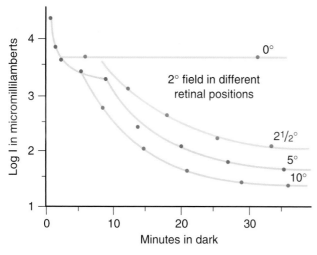

Figure 11-9. Normal dark-adaptation curves measuring retinal sensitivity to a small spot of light whose intensity is varied until the threshold value is found; a 2° test spot was placed at different distances from the foveal center. Note the cone–rod break at 9 minutes, middle graph. (From Hecht S, Haig C, Wald G: The dark adaptation of retinal fields of different size and location. J Gen Physiol 19:321–337, 1935.)

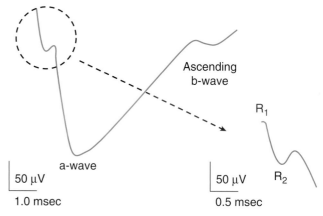

Figure 11-11. Normal human early receptor potential (ERP). This rapid response is complete within 1.5 ms and is believed to be generated by the outer segments. An intense, bright stimulus in the dark-adapted state is needed for an ERP to be obtained. (Redrawn from Berson EL, Goldstein EG: Early receptor potential in dominantly inherited retinitis pigmentosa. Arch Ophthalmol 83:412–420, 1970. From Slamovits TL: Basic and Clinical Science Course: Section 12: Orbit, Eyelids, and Lacrimal System. San Francisco, American Academy of Ophthalmology, 1993.)

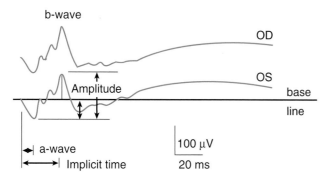

Figure 11-10. The photopic (cone-mediated) ERG is a light-adapted, bright flash-evoked response from the cones of the retina; the rods do not respond in the light-adapted state. (From Slamovits TL: Basic and Clinical Science Course: Section 12: Orbit, Eyelids, and Lacrimal System. San Francisco, American Academy of Ophthalmology, 1993.)

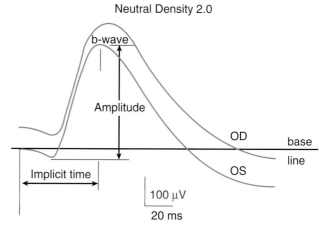

Figure 11-12. The scotopic (rod-mediated) ERG is a dark-adapted, dim flash (below cone threshold)-evoked response that records the signal from the rods. The test should be performed after at least 30 minutes of dark adaptation. (From Slamovits TL: Basic and Clinical Science Course: Section 12: Orbit, Eyelids, and Lacrimal System. San Francisco, American Academy of Ophthalmology, 1993. In: Yanoff M, Duker JS (eds) Ophthalmology. London, Mosby, 1999.)

Implicit time: time from light flash to peak of b-wave; measured in milliseconds
  Increased in various hereditary conditions
Oscillatory potential: wavelets on ascending b-wave of scotopic and photopic bright flash ERG
  Generated in middle retinal layers (inner plexiform layer): may be inhibitory potentials from amacrine cells
  Reduced in conditions of retinal hypoxia or microvascular disease
c-wave: RPE; late (2–4 seconds) positive deflection; occurs in dark-adapted state
Early receptor potential (ERP) (Figure 11-11): outer segments of photoreceptors; completed within 1.5 ms
  Represents bleaching of visual pigment; requires intense stimulus in dark-adapted state
  Ganglion cells are not measured; therefore, flash ERG is not useful in glaucoma

Photopic (light adapted): measures cone function; light adapted to bleach out rods
  Flicker ERG: flashing light at 30 flashes/second isolates cone response
    Small wave follows each flash
    Cone response because rods cannot recycle rhodopsin this quickly
    Poor response at 30 cycles/second indicates abnormal cone function; rods can respond up to 20 Hz
    Cones also respond to repetitive light

Scotopic (dark adapted): measures rod function; dark adapted for 30 min (Figure 11-12)
  Dim white or blue flash below cone threshold

At low intensity: small a- and b-waves

At increasing intensity: implicit time shortens, b-wave amplitude increases

Bright-flash ERG (in scotopic state; measures combined maximal rod and cone response): deep a-wave and large b-wave; oscillatory potentials are present (Figure 11-13)

Indications:

Diagnose generalized retinal degeneration

Assess family members for heritable retinal degeneration

Assess decreased vision and nystagmus present at birth

Assess retinal function in presence of opaque ocular media or vascular occlusion

Evaluate functional visual loss

Disease states (Figure 11-14, Table 11-2):

CRAO: normal a-wave (perfused by choroid), absent b-wave

Ischemic CVO: reduced b-wave amplitude, reduced b : a-wave ratio, prolonged b-wave implicit time

Retinitis pigmentosa: early, reduced amplitude (usually b-wave) and prolonged implicit time; later, extinguished with no rod or cone response to bright flash

Female carriers of X-linked RP: prolonged photopic b-wave implicit time, reduced scotopic b-wave amplitude

Sector RP: normal b-wave implicit time

Cone dystrophy: abnormal photopic and flicker, normal scotopic

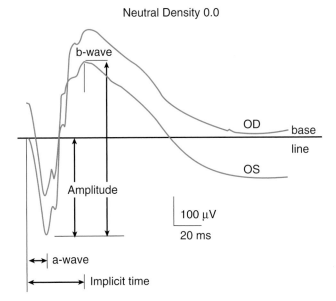

Figure 11-13. The bright flash, dark-adapted ERG stimulates both the cone and rod systems and gives large a and b-waves, with oscillatory potentials in the ascending b-wave. Some testing centers call this a 'scotopic ERG,' but the rods are not isolated by this method. (From Slamovits TL: Basic and Clinical Science Course: Section 12: Orbit, Eyelids, and Lacrimal System. San Francisco, American Academy of Ophthalmology, 1993. In: Yanoff M, Duker JS (eds) Ophthalmology. London, Mosby, 1999.)

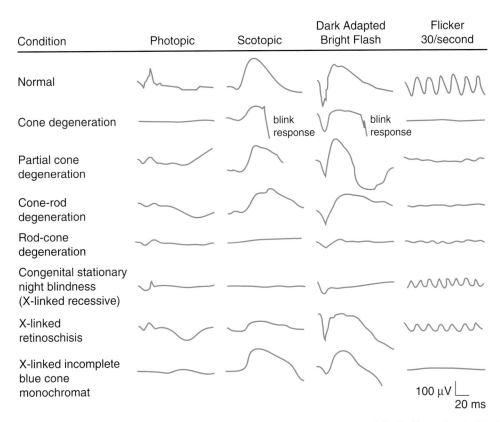

Figure 11-14. Electroretinogram patterns. (From Slamovits TL: Basic and Clinical Science Course: Section 12: Orbit, Eyelids, and Lacrimal System. San Francisco, American Academy of Ophthalmology, 1993.)

X-linked foveal retinoschisis: normal a-wave until late, reduced b-wave (especially scotopic)

Retinal detachment: reduction in amplitude corresponds to extent of neurosensory loss (50% decrease in amplitude = 50% of neurosensory retina is functionally detached)

Diffuse progressive retinal disease: increased b-wave implicit time

Nonprogressive retinal disease: decreased b-wave amplitude

MEWDS: reduced a-wave

Chalcosis: reduced amplitude (suppressed by intraocular copper ions)

Retinal microvascular disease (diabetes, hypertension, CVO): loss of oscillatory potentials

Achromotopsia: absent cone function; normal rod function

Leber's congenital amaurosis: flat ERG

CSNB: normal a-wave, poor b-wave

Congenital rubella: normal ERG

Glaucoma: normal ERG

Optic neuropathy/atrophy: normal ERG

Pattern ERG (PERG): waveform similar to flash ERG, but different test to measure ganglion cell activity; stimulus is an alternating checkerboard pattern that gives a constant illumination to the retina (Figure 11-15)

Normal response is composed of 3 waves:

N_{35}: cornea-negative wave at 35 ms

P_{50}: cornea-positive wave peak at 50 ms

N_{95}: negative trough at 95 ms

Electro-oculogram (EOG)

Indirect measure of standing potential of eye (voltage difference between inner and outer retina) (Figure 11-16)

Table 11-2. ERG patterns for various ocular diseases

Extinguished ERG abnormal photopic, normal ERG	Normal a-wave, reduced b-wave	Abnormal photopic, normal scotopic ERG
RP	CSNB; Oguchi's disease	Achromotopsia
Ophthalmic artery occlusion	X-linked juvenile retinoschisis	Cone dystrophy
DUSN	CVO	
Metallosis	CRAO	
RD	Myotonic dystrophy	
Drug toxicity (phenothiazine; chloroquine)	Quinine toxicity	
Cancer-associated retinopathy		

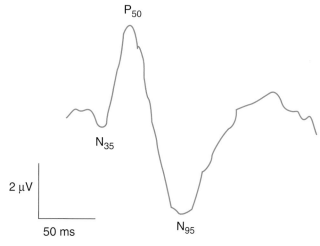

Figure 11-15. Pattern ERG with components labeled. This waveform measures retinal ganglion cell function and is not related to the flash ERG test. (After Treat GL: The pattern electroretinogram in glaucoma and ocular hypertension. In: Heckenlively JR, Arden GB (eds) Principles and Practice of Clinical Electrophysiology of Vision. St Louis, Mosby-Yearbook, 1991.)

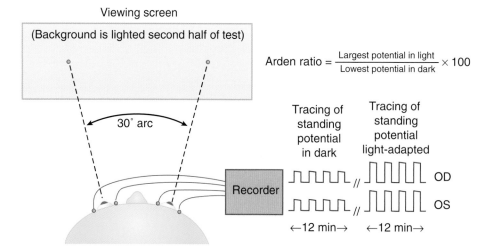

$$\text{Arden ratio} = \frac{\text{Largest potential in light}}{\text{Lowest potential in dark}} \times 100$$

Figure 11-16. Diagram illustrating technique used in recording the electro-oculogram test; the patient is positioned so that the eyes will traverse a 30° arc between 2 blinking red lights. The skin electrodes are positioned at the lateral and inner canthi. The standing potential is measured as the patient moves his eyes between the lights, first in the dark and then in the light. The maximum amplitude from the light condition is compared with minimum value from the dark to give a light peak-to-dark trough ratio. (From Heckenlively JR: Retinitis Pigmentosa. Philadelphia, JB Lippincott, 1988.)

Depolarization of basal portion of RPE produces light peak; normal result requires that both RPE and sensory retina be normal

Arden ratio: ratio of light-to-dark peak (2:1 is normal; <1.65 is abnormal); decreased ratio is due to photoreceptor or RPE disorder

Procedure: light adapt, dark adapt × 20 min, light adapt × 10 min

- Dark adaptation causes progressive decrease in response reaching a trough at 8–12 minutes
- Light adaptation causes progressive rise in amplitude over 6–9 minutes
- Measure lowest voltage with dark adaptation and highest voltage with light adaptation
- Amplitude is higher with light adaptation than dark adaptation

ERG is abnormal in all cases in which EOG is abnormal except:

- *Best's disease and carriers:* normal ERG but abnormal EOG
- *Pattern dystrophies*
- *Chloroquine toxicity*

Abnormal ERG, normal EOG: conditions with abnormal bipolar region but normal rods

- *CSNB*
- *X-linked retinoschisis*

RETINAL IMAGING

Optical Coherence Tomography (OCT)

Creates cross-sectional image of tissue using light
Provides retinal thickness measurements and cross-sectional retinal imaging to ~5–10 μm depending on light source; anterior segment spectral domain OCT is useful to image anterior segment, in particular the cornea and angle

Superluminescent diode fires beam of infrared light through fiberoptic Michelson interferometer at both the eye and a reference mirror; the reflected light from the retina is compared with the light from the reference mirror and analyzed so that the tissue reflectivity (similar to ultrasound) and density can be determined. With time-domain OCT (TDOCT), the reference mirror moves; with spectral-domain OCT (SDOCT) the mirror does not move and a Fourier transform is used to obtain imaging information (this makes SDOCT much faster than TDOCT)

Useful for optic nerve (glaucoma) and macular pathology (edema, hole, pucker); can compare thickness in cases of macular edema from one visit to next; can diagnose and differentiate vitreomacular pathology e.g. stage 1 macular hole vs full-thickness hole (≥stage 2) vs pseudohole or lamellar holes (Figures 11-17, 11-18)

Heidelberg Retinal Tomograph (HRT)

Laser tomography

Confocal scanning laser produces 3-dimensional sections of optic nerve and retina through undilated pupil

670 nm diode laser that is periodically deflected by oscillating mirrors; laser scans retina, and instrument measures reflectance and constructs series of 2-dimensional images at different depths, which are combined to create a multilayer 3D topographic image

Measures surface height to within 20 μm

Retinal Thickness Analyzer (RTA)

Creates thickness contour map

HeNe laser scans central 2 × 2 mm area; receives 2 reflections, 1 from ILM and 1 from RPE, then maps distance between these layers

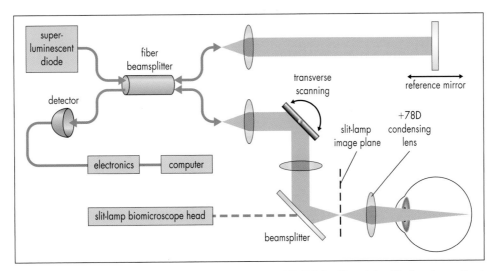

Figure 11-17. Optical coherence tomography principle. (Adapted from Shuman JS, Hee MR, Puliafito CA et al: Quantification of nerve fiber layer thickness in normal and glaucomatous eyes using optical coherence tomography. Arch Ophthalmol 113:586-596, 1995. From: Yanoff M, Duker JS (eds) Ophthalmology. London, Mosby, 1999.)

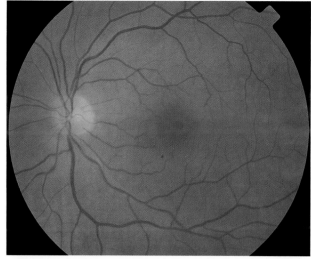

A

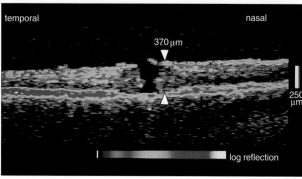

B

Figure 11-18. Stage 2 macular hole. **A,** fundus photograph, **B,** OCT. (From: Yanoff M, Duker JS (eds) Ophthalmology. London, Mosby, 1999.)

Scanning Laser Ophthalmoscope (SLO)

Modulated red light laser (633 nm)

Performs funduscopy and automated perimetry simultaneously

Ultrasound

Acoustic imaging of globe and orbit

A-scan: 1-dimensional display (amplitude of echoes plotted as vertical height against distance) (Figures 11-19 to 11-21)

B-scan: 2-dimensional display (amplitude of echoes represented by brightness on a grey scale image) (Figure 11-22)

Reflectivity: height of spike on A-scan and signal brightness on B-scan
  Internal reflectivity refers to amplitude of echoes within a lesion or tissue

Internal structure: degree of variation in histologic architecture within a mass lesion

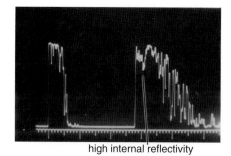

high internal reflectivity

Figure 11-19. A-scan ultrasound demonstrating high internal reflectivity. (From Friedman NJ, Kaiser PK, Pineda R II: The Massachusetts Eye and Ear Infirmary Illustrated Manual of Ophthalmology. 3rd ed. Philadelphia, Elsevier, 2009.)

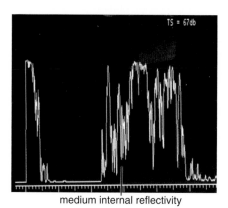

medium internal reflectivity

Figure 11-20. A-scan ultrasound demonstrating medium internal reflectivity. (From Friedman NJ, Kaiser PK, Pineda R II: The Massachusetts Eye and Ear Infirmary Illustrated Manual of Ophthalmology. 3rd ed. Philadelphia, Elsevier, 2009.)

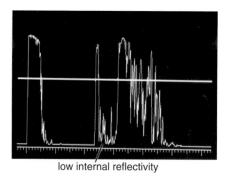

low internal reflectivity

Figure 11-21. A-scan ultrasound demonstrating low internal reflectivity. (From Friedman NJ, Kaiser PK, Pineda R II: The Massachusetts Eye and Ear Infirmary Illustrated Manual of Ophthalmology. 3rd ed. Philadelphia, Elsevier, 2009.)

Regular internal structure indicates homogenous architecture (minimal or no variation in the heights of spikes in A-scan and uniform appearance of echoes on B-scan)

Sound attenuation: occurs when acoustic wave is scattered, reflected, or absorbed by tissue
  Decrease in strength of echoes within or posterior to lesion; may produce a void posterior to lesion called

'shadowing' (caused by dense substances [bone, calcium, foreign body])

After movement: dynamic features of lesion echoes
Observe B-scan echoes for motion after cessation of eye movements (i.e. rapid movement of vitreous hemorrhage distinguished from slower, undulating movement of rhegmatogenous retinal detachment)

Vascularity: spontaneous motion of echoes within lesion corresponds to blood flow; may be visualized with Color doppler

Specific lesions: (Tables 11-3 and 11-4) (Figures 11-22 to 11-27)

Asteroid hyalosis:
A-SCAN: medium to high internal reflectivity
B-SCAN: bright echoes in vitreous due to calcium soaps; area of clear vitreous usually present between opacities and posterior hyaloid face

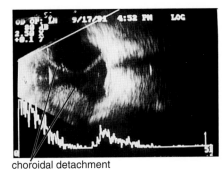

choroidal detachment

Figure 11-22. B-scan ultrasound demonstrating choroidal detachment. (From Kaiser PK, Friedman NJ, Pineda R II: Massachusetts Eye and Ear Infirmary Illustrated Manual of Ophthalmology, 2nd edn. Philadelphia, Saunders, 2004.)

Intraocular foreign body:
B-SCAN: high reflectivity when ultrasound probe is perpendicular to reflective surface of foreign body; bright echo persists when gain turned down; shadowing often present

Intraocular calcification:
A-SCAN: high amplitude peak due to strong acoustic interface
B-SCAN: white echoes; partial or complete shadowing
DDx: tumors (retinoblastoma, choroidal osteoma, optic nerve meningioma, choroidal hemangioma, choroidal melanoma), *Toxocara* granuloma, chronic retinal detachment, optic nerve head drusen, vascular occlusive disease of optic nerve, phthisis bulbi, intumescent cataractous lens

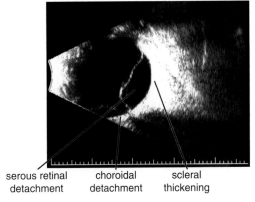

serous retinal detachment   choroidal detachment   scleral thickening

Figure 11-23. B-scan ultrasound demonstrating serous retinal detachment with shifting fluid, shallow peripheral choroidal detachment, and diffuse scleral thickening. (From Kaiser PK, Friedman NJ, Pineda R II: Massachusetts Eye and Ear Infirmary Illustrated Manual of Ophthalmology, 2nd edn. Philadelphia, Saunders, 2004.)

Table 11-3. Ultrasound characteristics of various lesions

Pathology	Location	Shape	Internal reflectivity	Internal structure	Vascularity
Melanoma	Choroid and/or CB	Dome or collar button	Low to medium	Regular	Yes
Choroidal hemangioma	Choroid; posterior pole	Dome	High	Regular	Yes
Metastasis	Choroid; posterior pole	Diffuse, irregular	Medium to high	Irregular	No
Choroidal nevus	Choroid	Dome or flat	High	Regular	No
Choroidal hemorrhage	Choroid	Dome	Variable	Variable	No
Disciform lesion	Macula	Dome, irregular	High	Variable	No

Table 11-4. Ultrasound characteristics of different types of detachments

Pathology	Topographic (B-scan)	Quantitative (A-scan)	After movement
Retinal detachment	Smooth or folded surface Open or closed funnel Inserts at ON and ora serrata May see intraretinal cysts	Steep spike (100% high)	Moderate to none
Posterior vitreous detachment	Smooth surface Open funnel With or without ON or fundus insertion Inserts at ora serrata or ciliary body	Variable spike height (<100%)	Marked to moderate
Choroidal detachment	Smooth, dome, or flat surface No ON insertion Inserts at ciliary body and vortex veins	Steeply rising, thick, double peaked spike (100% high)	Mild to none

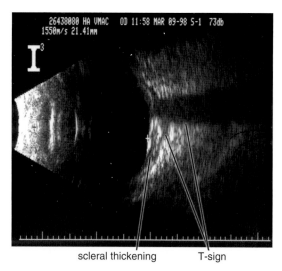

Figure 11-24. B-scan ultrasound demonstrating scleral thickening and the characteristic peripapillary T sign. (From Kaiser PK, Friedman NJ, Pineda R II: Massachusetts Eye and Ear Infirmary Illustrated Manual of Ophthalmology, 2nd edn. Philadelphia, Saunders, 2004.)

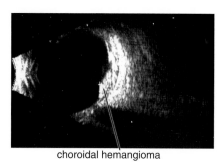

Figure 11-25. B-scan ultrasound demonstrating elevated mass with underlying thickened choroid. (From Kaiser PK, Friedman NJ, Pineda R II: Massachusetts Eye and Ear Infirmary Illustrated Manual of Ophthalmology, 2nd edn. Philadelphia, Saunders, 2004.)

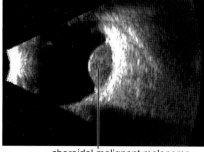

Figure 11-26. B-scan ultrasound demonstrating dome-shaped choroidal mass. (From Kaiser PK, Friedman NJ, Pineda R II: Massachusetts Eye and Ear Infirmary Illustrated Manual of Ophthalmology, 2nd edn. Philadelphia, Saunders, 2004.)

Fluorescein Angiogram (FA)

Phases: choroidal filling, arterial, venous, recirculation
Sodium fluorescein in a hydrocarbon based yellow-red dye with a molecular weight of 376 daltons (Da). Dye enters choroidal circulation via short posterior ciliary

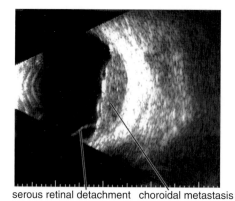

Figure 11-27. B-scan ultrasound of a patient with choroidal metastasis demonstrating elevated choroidal mass with irregular surface and overlying serous retinal detachment. (From Kaiser PK, Friedman NJ, Pineda R II: Massachusetts Eye and Ear Infirmary Illustrated Manual of Ophthalmology, 2nd edn. Philadelphia, Saunders, 2004.)

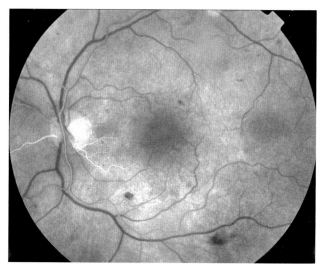

Figure 11-28. FA demonstrating choroidal and early arterial filling.

arteries 10-15 seconds after injection; choroidal flow is very rapid; choriocapillaris filling is usually completed in the AV or early venous phase; cilioretinal artery is filled at time of choroidal filling; central retinal artery takes more circuitous route, resulting in dye arriving 1–2 seconds after choroidal filling; AV phase occurs 1–2 seconds after arterial phase; veins fill in 10–12 seconds (Figures 11-28 to 11-32)
Exciter filter emits blue light that stimulates fluorescein to emit yellow-green light (barrier filter transmits only green light) so two filters are required to image: fluorescein absorbs light at 465–490 nm (blue), emits at 520–530 nm (green)
80% bound to albumin and other serum proteins
90% excreted from kidney (also liver) within 24–36 hours
Transient yellowing of skin and conjunctiva that lasts 8–12 hours; most common adverse events: nausea (3–15%), vomiting (5%), pruritus (5%); anaphylactic reaction in 1:100,000; death occurs in 1:220,000;

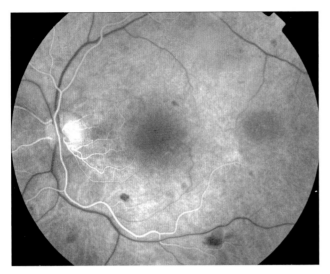

Figure 11-29. FA demonstrating arterial phase.

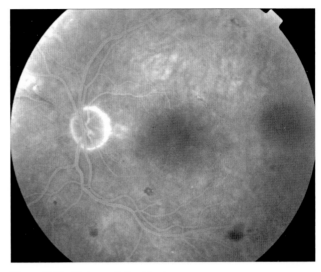

Figure 11-32. FA demonstrating late phase.

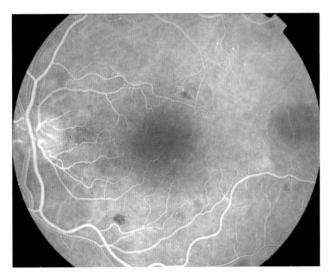

Figure 11-30. FA demonstrating early venous phase with laminar filling.

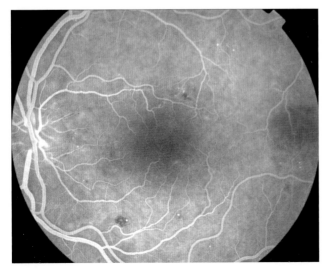

Figure 11-31. FA demonstrating peak AV transit.

pregnancy in first trimester is a relative contraindication

Characteristics:

Hyperfluorescence: leakage (fenestrated choriocapillaris, iris vessels), staining (structures such as collagen), pooling (pockets of fluid), window defects (RPE defects)

Hypofluorescence: blockage (opacity that reduces fluorescence; e.g. RPE, blood, xanthophyll) or filling defect (ischemia)

Macular dark spot is due to blockage by xanthophyll in outer plexiform layer and tall RPE cells with increased melanin and lipofuscin

Fluorescein passes through Bruch's membrane, cannot pass through RPE or retinal capillaries

Autofluorescence: fluorescence prior to fluorescein dye injection; seen in optic nerve drusen, astrocytic hamartomas, and large deposits of lipofuscin

Choroidal filling: choroidal lesions (malignant melanoma, cavernous hemangioma) and cilioretinal artery

Arterial phase filling: retinal lesions (capillary hemangioma, NVD)

Indocyanine Green (ICG)

Sterile, water-soluble, tricarbocyanine dye with a molecular weight of 775 Da. Absorbs light at 805 nm, emits at 835 nm (near infrared), which penetrates RPE, blood, and other ocular pigments to greater extent than visible light and fluorescein

98% bound to serum proteins (80% to globulins); therefore, leaks very slowly from choroidal circulation allowing enhanced imaging of the choroidal circulation; CNV often appears as hot spot (bright area; occurs within 3–5 min, lasts 20 min) (Figure 11-33)

Excreted via liver into bile

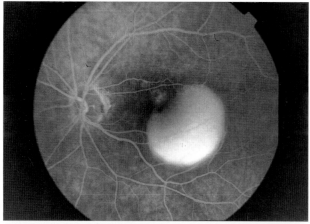

A

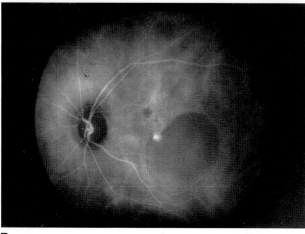

B

Figure 11-33. Serous retinal pigment epithelial detachment seen on FA: **A,** with associated hot spot seen on ICG **(B).** (From Reichel E: Indocyanine green angiography. In: Yanoff M, Duker JS (eds) Ophthalmology. London, Mosby, 1999.)

Safer than fluorescein angiography; nausea and vomiting uncommon; should not be done in patients allergic to iodide, uremic, or with liver disease

DISORDERS

Vitreous Abnormalities

Asteroid Hyalosis

Refractile particles (calcium soaps) suspended in vitreous

More common in older patients and those with diabetes; 25% bilateral

Rarely affects vision, but may prevent visualization of posterior pole, use FA to look for abnormalities in these patients

Pathology: gray spheres with 'Maltese cross' birefringence on polarization

Synchisis Scintillans (Cholesterol Bulbi)

Cholesterol crystals derived from old vitreous hemorrhage; with PVD crystals settle inferiorly

Rare, unilateral

Occurs after blunt or penetrating trauma in blind eyes

Crystals sink to bottom of globe because no fixed vitreous framework

Primary Amyloidosis

Vitreous involvement in familial amyloidotic polyneuropathies (FAP I and II get systemic manifestations)

Amyloid enters via retinal vessels

Patients have cardiac disease and amyloid neuropathy

Posterior Vitreous Detachment (PVD)

Separation of posterior hyaloid face from retina

Mechanism: vitreous syneresis (liquefaction) and contraction with age

Symptoms: floaters; may see flashes (due to traction on retina)

Findings: acute symptomatic PVD may have retinal tear (10–15% of acute symptomatic PVDs), vitreous hemorrhage (hemorrhagic PVD; 7.5% of PVDs) if vessel is torn during vitreous separation (70% risk of retinal tear), retinal detachment (RD) especially when pigmented vitreous cell is present

Vitreous Hemorrhage (VH)

Etiology: diabetes (most common), other proliferative retinopathies, trauma, PVD, Terson's syndrome (blood from subarachnoid hemorrhage travels along optic nerve and into eye), ruptured retinal arterial macroaneurysm, retinal angioma; in children, consider child abuse, pars planitis, X-linked retinoschisis

Ochre membrane: results from chronic hemorrhage accumulating on posterior surface of detached vitreous

Persistent Hyperplastic Primary Vitreous (PHPV)

(See Ch. 5, Pediatrics/Strabismus.)

Retinal Abnormalities

Congenital

(See Ch. 5, Pediatrics/Strabismus.)

Trauma

Commotio Retinae (Berlin's Edema)

Transient retinal whitening at level of deep sensory retina due to disruption (probably photoreceptor outer segments) with photoreceptor loss and thinning of outer nuclear and plexiform layers; not true edema

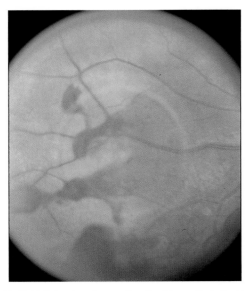

Figure 11-34. Berlin's edema (commotio retinae) in a patient after blunt ocular trauma. (From Rubsamen PE: Posterior segment ocular trauma. In: Yanoff M, Duker JS (eds) Ophthalmology. London, Mosby, 1999.)

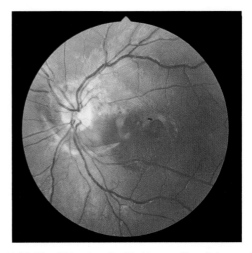

Figure 11-35. Choroidal rupture after blunt trauma. (From Rubsamen PE: Posterior segment ocular trauma. In: Yanoff M, Duker JS (eds) Ophthalmology. London, Mosby, 1999.)

Pigmentary changes can occur (RPE hyperplasia); traumatic macular hole may develop; usually resolves without sequelae (Figure 11-34)

Contusion of RPE

Blunt trauma can cause RPE edema with overlying serous RD

Choroidal Rupture

Tear in choroid, Bruch's membrane, and RPE due to blunt or penetrating trauma

Mechanism: mechanical deformation results in rupture of choroid; sclera is resistant due to high tensile strength, retina is resistant due to elasticity; Bruch's membrane is less elastic and breaks with choroid and RPE

Direct: occurs anteriorly at site of impact; oriented parallel to ora serrata

Indirect: occurs posteriorly away from site of impact; usually crescent-shaped, concentric with and temporal to optic disc; often associated with VH

Findings: choroidal neovascular membrane (CNV) can develop during healing process (months to years after trauma; can regress spontaneously), scar forms by 3–4 weeks, hyperplasia of RPE at margin of lesion (Figure 11-35)

Retina Sclopetaria

Trauma to retina and choroid caused by transmitted shock waves and necrosis from high-velocity projectile

Findings: rupture of choroid and retina with hemorrhage and commotio; vitreous hemorrhage can occur; lesion heals with white fibrous scar and RPE changes (Figure 11-36)

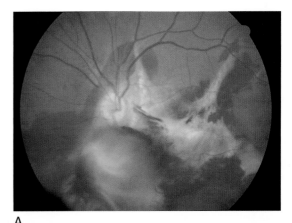

A

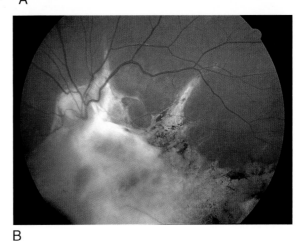

B

Figure 11-36. Gunshot wound to the periocular region demonstrating appearance of retina sclopetaria: **A,** acute; **B,** chronic. (From Rubsamen PE: Posterior segment ocular trauma. In: Yanoff M, Duker JS (eds) Ophthalmology. London, Mosby, 1999.)

Low risk of RD in young patients with formed vitreous; posterior vitreous face usually intact; choroid and retina tightly adherent

Traumatic Retinal Tear

Most patients are young with formed vitreous that tamponades the tear
As vitreous liquefies over time, fluid passes through breaks, causing retina to detach
Trauma is associated with 10–20% of all phakic RDs

4 types of traumatic retinal breaks: horseshoe tear, operculated tear, retinal dialysis, macular hole (rare)

Dialysis: most common type of retinal tear associated with traumatic RD; usually inferotemporal (31%) or superonasal (22%); 50% have demarcation line; 10% of dialysis-related RDs are present on initial examination, 30% occur within 1 month, 50% within 8 months, 80% within 2 years

Avulsion of vitreous base: separation of vitreous base from ora serrata; pathognomonic for trauma

Oral tear: at ora serrata; due to split of vitreous; fish-mouth appearance

Preoral tear: anterior border of vitreous base; most often superotemporal

Treatment: laser therapy or cryotherapy for horseshoe tear, operculated tear, and retinal dialysis without RD; vitrectomy with gas for macular hole; scleral buckle for RD due to retinal tear; proliferative vitreoretinopathy (PVR) is uncommon

Purtscher's Retinopathy

Due to head trauma or compressive injury to trunk
Unilateral or bilateral

Findings: retinal whitening, hemorrhages, cotton wool spots, papillitis; may have positive RAPD (Figure 11-37)

DDx: pancreatitis, fat emboli, lupus, leukemia, amniotic fluid emboli, dermatomyositis

FA: leakage from retinal vasculature, late venous staining
May take up to 3 months to resolve

Terson's Syndrome

Vitreous hemorrhage following subarachnoid or subdural hemorrhage due to intracranial hypertension blocking venous return from eye; patients have acute neck stiffness
20% of patients with spontaneous or traumatic subarachnoid hemorrhage will present with vitreous hemorrhage; bleeding can also occur between ILM and retina (Figure 11-38)

Valsalva Retinopathy

Rise in intrathoracic or intra-abdominal pressure against a closed glottis (Valsalva maneuver) causes superficial veins to rupture with hemorrhage under ILM
Preretinal hemorrhage in macula causes sudden decreased vision

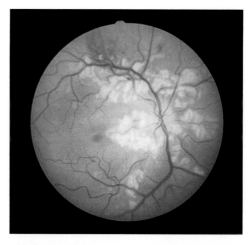

Figure 11-37. Purtscher's retinopathy. (From Regillo CD: Distant trauma with posterior segment effects. In: Yanoff M, Duker JS (eds) Ophthalmology. London, Mosby, 1999.)

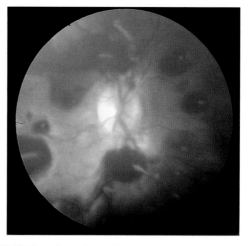

Figure 11-38. Terson's syndrome. (From Regillo CD: Distant trauma with posterior segment effects. In: Yanoff M, Duker JS (eds) Ophthalmology. London, Mosby, 1999.)

Fat Emboli Syndrome

Follows fracture of medullated bones; occurs in 5% of patients with long-bone fractures
Affects multiple organ systems

Findings (in 50%): cotton wool spots, small blot hemorrhages; rarely intravenous fat or CRAO
20% mortality

Whiplash Retinopathy

Associated with severe flexion/extension of head and neck without direct eye injury

Findings: mild reduction in vision (to 20/30); gray swelling of fovea, foveal pit (50–100 μm)

FA: may have tiny focal area of early hyperfluorescence

Macular Diseases

Epiretinal Membrane (Cellophane Maculopathy, Macular Pucker)

Proliferations at vitreoretinal junction, may contract and cause retinal folds and macular edema
12% prevalence in individuals 43–86 years old; 20% bilateral; 2% associated with retinal folds (decreased vision)
Associated with diabetes, retinal vascular occlusions, PVD, high myopia, retinal hole/tear, previous ocular or laser surgery, and increasing age

OCT: epiretinal membrane visible on surface of retina, distortion of retinal surface may be evident

Treatment: consider surgery for decreased vision (<20/50), marked retinal distortion, or metamorphopsia

Macular Hole

Due to tangential traction on foveal region by posterior cortical vitreous
Most commonly idiopathic (senile); may develop after trauma, surgery, CME, or inflammation
Female > male; bilateral in 25–30%; prevalence = 0.33%; average age of onset is 67 years; risk of developing in fellow eye <1% (no risk if PVD present)
Macular cyst may be precursor

Gass classification (Figure 11-39):
1. Premacular or impending hole with foveal detachment and macular cyst (yellow spot [1a] or ring [1b])
2. Full-thickness eccentric hole; usually <400 μm in width
3. Full-thickness hole with operculum, cuff of subretinal fluid, yellow deposits at base, positive Watzke-Allen sign
4. Full-thickness hole with PVD

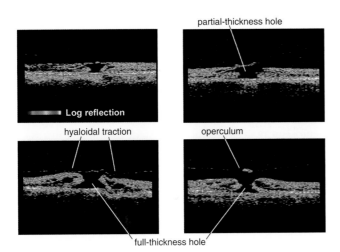

Figure 11-39. Optical coherence tomography scans demonstrating cross-sectional image of all stages of macular hole formation and the full-thickness retinal defect characteristic of stage 3 and 4 holes. (From Kaiser PK, Friedman NJ, Pineda R II: Massachusetts Eye and Ear Infirmary Illustrated Manual of Ophthalmology, 2nd edn. Philadelphia, Saunders, 2004.)

Watzke-Allen sign: shine narrow-slit beam over macular hole, positive if patient perceives 'break' in slit beam

DDx: epiretinal membrane with pseudohole, lamellar hole, vitreomacular traction/detachment; for stage 1: drusen, CME, CSR

FA: window defect corresponding to the hole (hyperfluorescence during choroidal filling)

OCT: differentiates between various stages and other disease, hole always evident on scan; often have rim of SRF and cysts within edges of hole, occasionally operculum can be seen over the hole

Treatment: stage 1 may close spontaneously so observation; consider vitrectomy with peeling of posterior hyaloid and gas tamponade for stage 2 through stage 4; microplasmin enzyme recently found to close smaller MH in up to 40% of cases with intravitreal ocriplasmin (Thrombogenics) injection (experimental)
    Complications of surgery: increased size of hole, RPE mottling, light toxicity, cataract, retinal tear, retinal detachment

Prognosis: good if recent onset and hole width < 400 μm, poor if >1 year duration

Traumatic macular hole

Rare (5%); due to disruption and necrosis of retinal photoreceptors with subsequent loss of retinal tissue; results from pre-existing commotio retinae in macula

Solar Retinopathy (Figure 11-40)

Photochemical retinal damage can occur after ~90 seconds or longer of sungazing, thought to be caused by blue (441 nm) and near UV light (325–250 nm)
With foveal fixation, retinal image of sun is 160 μm and is usually within the foveola and FAZ
Associated with solar eclipse, psychiatric disorders, religious rituals, or ingestion of hallucinogens

Symptoms: vision can range from normal to 20/100; usually returns to 20/20 to 20/40 within 6 months

Findings: yellow-white spot in fovea; later, red foveolar depression or lamellar hole

FA: intense staining of damaged RPE, particularly in acute phase of injury, but no leakage; as RPE heals, window defects develop (Figure 11-41)

Central Serous Retinopathy/Chorioretinopathy (CSR)/Idiopathic Central Serous Choroidopathy (ICSC)

Serous retinal detachment ± retinal pigment epithelium detachment (PED) (Figure 11-42)
Males (80%), typically in 4th–5th decade

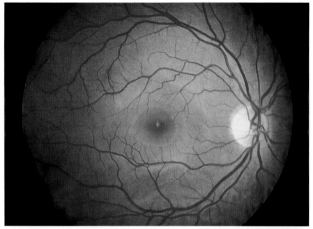

A

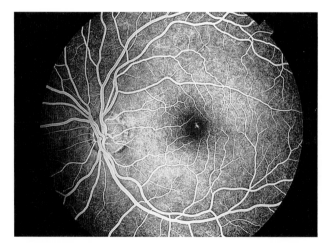

B

Figure 11-40. Solar retinopathy of both eyes. (Courtesy of William E. Benson. From Baumal CR: Light toxicity and laser burns. In: Yanoff M, Duker JS (eds) Ophthalmology. London, Mosby, 1999.)

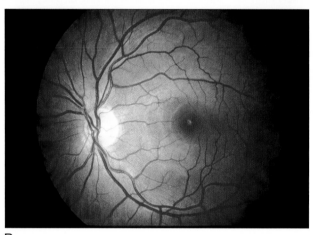

Figure 11-41. Fluorescein angiography of solar retinopathy in the left eye. (Courtesy of William E. Benson. From Baumal CR: Light toxicity and laser burns. In: Yanoff M, Duker JS (eds) Ophthalmology. London, Mosby, 1999.)

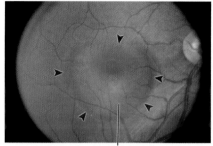

pigment epithelial detachment

Figure 11-42. Idiopathic central serous retinopathy with large serous retinal detachment. (From Kaiser PK, Friedman NJ, Pineda R II: Massachusetts Eye and Ear Infirmary Illustrated Manual of Ophthalmology, 2nd edn. Philadelphia, Saunders, 2004.)

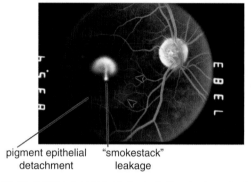

pigment epithelial   "smokestack"
detachment   leakage

Figure 11-43. Fluorescein angiogram demonstrating classic smokestack appearance. (From Kaiser PK, Friedman NJ, Pineda R II: Massachusetts Eye and Ear Infirmary Illustrated Manual of Ophthalmology, 2nd edn. Philadelphia, Saunders, 2004.)

Associated with hypertension, steroid use, psychiatric medication use, and type A personality

Findings: blurred vision, micropsia, paracentral scotoma; poor color vision; induced hyperopia, absent foveal reflex; after resolution, may have yellow subretinal deposits, RPE changes

DDx: AMD, VKH syndrome, uveal effusion syndrome, toxemia of pregnancy, optic nerve pit, pigment epithelial detachment from other causes (CNV)

FA: small focal hyperfluorescent dot (leakage of dye from choroid through RPE); later, dye accumulates beneath neurosensory detachment; 'smokestack' appearance in 10%; expanding dot of hyperfluorescence in 80%, diffuse leakage in the rest (Figure 11-43)

OCT: sensory retinal elevation, may have PED (usually within or near subretinal fluid accumulation)

ICG: can be useful in helping to distinguish atypical diffuse CSR in older patients from occult CNV in exudative AMD and idiopathic polypoidal choroidal vasculopathy

Treatment: observation in most cases, consider laser to focal hot spots outside fovea or verteporfin (Visudyne)

photodynamic therapy (PDT) for subfoveal spots or diffuse leakage (off label); rifampin and RU-486 have been used experimentally with limited success

Treatment indications:

1. Persistent serous detachment (>3 months)
2. Previous episode of CSR, with permanent vision reduction
3. Episode in fellow eye with vision loss
4. Demand for rapid recovery of binocular function for occupational reasons

Laser and PDT accelerate resolution of fluid, but does not result in better final vision or reduce rate of recurrence; laser may rarely cause CNV

Prognosis: 90% spontaneous resorption in 1–6 months; 50% recur; 66% achieve 20/20; 14% with bilateral vision loss over 10 years

Retinal Pigment Epithelial Detachment (PED)

Appears as discrete, blister-like elevation; sometimes outlined by orange-pink rim of subretinal fluid

DDx:

In patient <50 years old: probably due to central serous retinopathy

In patient >50 years old: PED associated with drusen may indicate occult CNV, especially if PED has a notch

FA: discrete early hyperfluorescence of entire serous PED with late pooling into PED

Complications: 33% develop CNV (FA shows slower, more homogenous filling with sharp border)

Age-Related Macular Degeneration (ARMD, AMD)

Leading cause of central visual loss in patients >60 years old in the United States and Western world

Risk factors: age, heredity, sex (female), race (white), smoking, nutrition, photic exposure, hypertension, light iris color, hyperopia

Symptoms: decreased vision, central scotoma, metamorphopsia

Forms:

1. **Nonexudative or dry** (80–90%): drusen, pigment changes, RPE atrophy (Figures 11-44 to 11-47)
2. **Exudative, neovascular, or wet** (10-20%): characterized by CNV (Figures 11-48 to 11-50)

Drusen: clinical marker for sick RPE; PAS-positive, mildly eosinophilic hyaline excrescences of abnormal basement membrane material between RPE basement membrane and inner Bruch's membrane

Types of drusen:

Hard (nodular/cuticular/hyaline): small yellow-white spots 50 μm in diameter

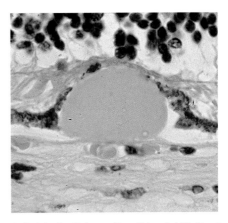

Figure 11-44. Nodular 'hard' drusen. (From Edwards MG, Bressler NM, Raja SC: Age-related macular degeneration. In: Yanoff M, Duker JS (eds) Ophthalmology. London, Mosby, 1999.)

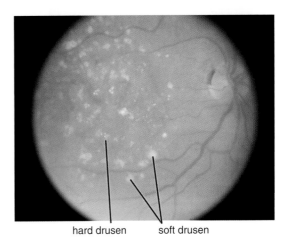

hard drusen   soft drusen

Figure 11-45. Dry, age-related macular degeneration demonstrating drusen and pigmentary changes (category 3). (From Kaiser PK, Friedman NJ, Pineda R II: Massachusetts Eye and Ear Infirmary Illustrated Manual of Ophthalmology, 2nd edn. Philadelphia, Saunders, 2004.)

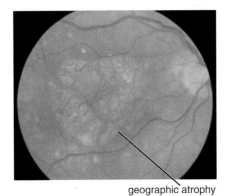

geographic atrophy

Figure 11-46. Advanced, atrophic, nonexudative, age-related macular degeneration demonstrating subfoveal geographic atrophy (category 4). (From Kaiser PK, Friedman NJ, Pineda R II: Massachusetts Eye and Ear Infirmary Illustrated Manual of Ophthalmology, 2nd edn. Philadelphia, Saunders, 2004.)

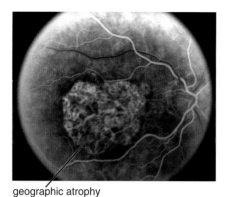

geographic atrophy

Figure 11-47. Fluorescein angiogram of same patient as in Figure 11-46, demonstrating well-defined window defect corresponding to the area of geographic atrophy. (From Kaiser PK, Friedman NJ, Pineda R II: Massachusetts Eye and Ear Infirmary Illustrated Manual of Ophthalmology, 2nd edn. Philadelphia, Saunders, 2004.)

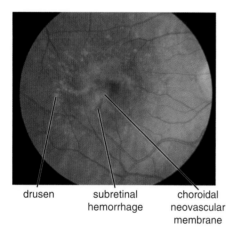

drusen   subretinal   choroidal
    hemorrhage   neovascular
            membrane

Figure 11-48. Exudative age-related macular degeneration, demonstrating subretinal hemorrhage from classic choroidal neovascular membrane. (From Kaiser PK, Friedman NJ, Pineda R II: Massachusetts Eye and Ear Infirmary Illustrated Manual of Ophthalmology, 2nd edn. Philadelphia, Saunders, 2004.)

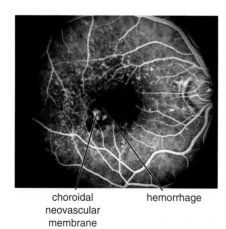

choroidal   hemorrhage
neovascular
membrane

Figure 11-49. Fluorescein angiogram of same patient as in Figure 11-48, demonstrating leakage from the CNV and blockage from the surrounding subretinal blood. (From Kaiser PK, Friedman NJ, Pineda R II: Massachusetts Eye and Ear Infirmary Illustrated Manual of Ophthalmology, 2nd edn. Philadelphia, Saunders, 2004.)

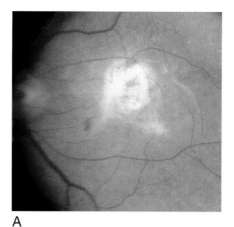

A

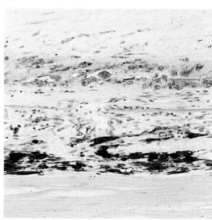

B

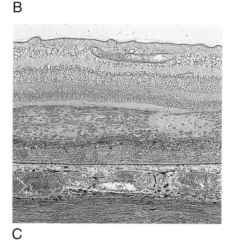

C

Figure 11-50. A-C, Neovascular, age-related macular degeneration. (From Edwards MG, Bressler NM, Raja SC: Age-related macular degeneration. In: Yanoff M, Duker JS (eds) Ophthalmology. London, Mosby, 1999.)

Soft: larger, less dense, more fluffy, with tapered edges; may resemble PED; associated with thickened inner Bruch's membrane and wet AMD

Basal laminar: diffuse, confluent (blocks early, stains late on FA)

Calcific: sharply demarcated, glistening; associated with RPE atrophy

Drusen size classification:

Small: <64 μm in diameter

Intermediate: 64–124 μm in diameter

Large: ≥125 μm in diameter (approximately equal to vein width at disk margin)

Also classified based on drusen extent:

Small drusen considered extensive if the cumulative area within 2 disc diameters of the center of the macula equal to at least that of the AREDS standard circle C-1 (with diameter $\frac{1}{12}$ that of the average disc) – this corresponds to approximately 15 small drusen from stereo photographs or 5–10 small drusen

Intermediate drusen considered extensive if soft, indistinct drusen are present and the total area occupied by the drusen is equivalent to the area that would be occupied by 20 drusen each having a diameter of 100 μm. If no soft indistinct drusen are present, intermediate drusen are considered to be extensive when they occupy an area equivalent to at least $\frac{1}{5}$ of a disc area (approximately 65, 100 μm diameter drusen)

DDx of yellow foveal spot: solar maculopathy, adult vitelliform dystrophy, Best's disease, stage 1a macular hole, CSR, old subfoveal hemorrhage, CME, pattern dystrophy

FA: hyperfluorescence of drusen due to window defects (from degeneration of overlying RPE) and uptake of dye within drusen (staining)

Signs of CNV: subretinal blood, fluid, and/or lipid; RPE detachment (PED); gray-green subretinal discoloration

Types of CNV: historically defined by appearance of leakage on FA

Classic:

EARLY PHASE: bright, fairly uniform hyperfluorescence that progressively intensifies throughout the transit phase

LATE PHASE: progressive leakage of dye that extends beyond the margins of the CNV seen in early stages

Occult (2 types):

FIBROVASCULAR PED:

EARLY PHASE: irregular mottled hyperfluorescence at level of RPE

LATE PHASE: stippled hyperfluorescent leakage that is not as bright or extensive as classic lesions

LATE LEAKAGE OF UNDETERMINED ORIGIN:

EARLY PHASE: no apparent leakage

LATE PHASE: stippled hyperfluorescence at level of RPE

Can also be defined by lesion location:

TYPE 1: CNV under RPE; PCV is a variant of type 1

TYPE 2: CNV above RPE

TYPE 3: retinal angiomatous proliferation (RAP) = often bilateral with small intraretinal hemorrhages and associated PED; develop retinal-choroidal anastamosis

Location of CNV:

Extrafoveal: posterior border of CNV is 200–2500 μm from center of foveal avascular zone (FAZ)

Juxtafoveal: 1–199 μm from center of FAZ, or CNV 200–2500 μm from center of FAZ with blood or blocked fluorescence within 200 μm of FAZ center

Subfoveal: under center of FAZ

ICG: helpful for visualizing CNV that is not well seen on FA; CNV appears as focal hot spots or plaque of late hyperfluorescence; can demonstrate CNV under thin hemorrhage that would be blocked on FA; high-speed ICG useful to delineate feeder vessels of CNV

Treatment: follow Amsler grid, low-vision aids, vitamin supplements; consider intravitreal injections (anti-VEGF [vascular endothelial growth factor] agents), laser, or PDT for CNV

Age-related Eye Disease Study (AREDS):

Supplements with high-dose antioxidants and zinc are helpful in reducing vision loss and the progression of disease in patients with category 3 and 4 AMD; ongoing AREDS2 study is evaluating lutein, zeaxanthin, and omega-3 fatty acids in addition to the original AREDS formulation

Avoid beta-carotene in smokers

Vitamin C and E can increase risk of myocardial infarction (MI) in postmenopausal women

Zinc is associated with benign prostate hypertrophy in men and stress incontinence in women

Macular Photocoagulation Study (MPS):

Treatment of well-demarcated extrafoveal or juxtafoveal CNV with uniform laser. After 5 years, 64% of untreated eyes had >6 lines of vision loss; 46% of treated eyes had >6 lines of vision loss; >50% recurrence rate. However, many patients do not qualify owing to subfoveal CNV and occult lesions

Treatment of Age-Related Macular Degeneration with Photodynamic Therapy (TAP) Trial:

Photodynamic therapy with verteporfin (Visudyne) can prevent vision loss in eyes with subfoveal, predominantly classic and occult AMD, with no classic CNV

Verteporfin in Photodynamic Therapy (VIP) Trial:

Photodynamic therapy with verteporfin (Visudyne) can prevent vision loss in eyes with occult and no classic CNV, especially if less than 4 MPS Da in size or baseline vision worse than 20/50

Pegaptanib (Macugen) VISION Trial: FDA-approved aptamer that is a selective VEGF antagonist binding to the 165 isoform of VEGF-A while sparing other isoforms; no longer commonly used; intravitreal injection every 6 weeks.

Ranibizumab (Lucentis) MARINA and ANCHOR Trials: FDA-approved, humanized, antigen-binding fragment (Fab) designed to bind and inhibit all VEGF isoforms; intravitreal injection monthly or as needed (CATT finding was equal efficacy when delivered monthly or as needed).

Bevacizumab (Avastin): Off-label, full-length antibody that binds and inhibits all VEGF isoforms (FDA approved for colorectal cancer): the Complications of

Age Related Macular Degeneration treatment Trials (CATT) study reported that monthly avastin was non-inferior to monthly lucentis, but as needed avastin was not equal. There were significantly greater serious systemic adverse events in the avastin groups than lucentis; intravitreal injection monthly.

Aflibercept (VEGF Trap Eye) VIEW 1&2 Trials: fusion receptor decoy containing domain 2 from VEGF receptor 1 and domain 3 from VEGFR2 fused to human Fc fragment that blocks all isoforms of VEGF-A and placental growth factor (PLGF); injected every two months after a loading dose of 3 monthly injections.

Anti-VEGF safety: all anti-VEGF agents can get into the systemic circulation putting patients at risk of arteriothrombotic events (ATE) such as hypertension, MI, and stroke.

Combination treatment: Combination therapy with PDT and anti-VEGF agents has been shown to be safe with similar visual results and decreased injections (DENALI and MT BLANC studies). In particular, the best therapy for PCV is combination therapy PDT and anti-VEGF agents (EVEREST Study). In the future, combination therapy with radiation and other drugs will also likely be used.

Radiation: internal (strontium-90)(CABERNET Study) or external (low-dose X-ray radiation) combined with anti-VEGF agents (experimental)

Surgery: in certain cases, consider submacular surgery to remove CNV or displace hemorrhage in cases with large submacular hemorrhage, or macular translocation (experimental)

Prognosis:

Rate of Progression to Advanced AMD (AREDS) over 5 years
1.3% many small or few medium drusen (if both eyes have many intermediate drusen, but no large drusen, then patient score = 1 in scale below)
18% many medium or any large drusen
43% unilateral advanced AMD

AREDS Clinical Severity Scale (AREDS) for AMD
Based on giving 1 point for the presence of ≥1 large drusen and/or pigment changes (hyper, hypo, or non-central GA) per eye, or 2 points for advanced AMD in 1 eye, then total 2 eyes to come up with a point score that shows patient's risk of developing advanced AMD in 5 years:
0 points = 0.5%
1 point = 3%
2 points = 12%
3 points = 25%
4 points = 50%

Risk of CNV in fellow eye at 5 years: if drusen is present
Hard (nodular) = 10%
Soft = 30%
Pigmented = 30%
Soft and pigmented = 60%

Risk of fellow eye developing CNV: 4–12% per year; increased risk with multiple soft drusen, RPE clumping, densely packed drusen, PED

MAJOR AGE-RELATED MACULAR DEGENERATION CLINICAL STUDIES

Macular Photocoagulation Study (MPS)

Objective: to evaluate efficacy of laser photocoagulation in preventing visual loss from CNV

Methods: patients were randomly assigned to laser photocoagulation vs observation in the following groups:

Extrafoveal Study: well-demarcated CNV due to AMD or ocular histoplasmosis syndrome (OHS), or idiopathic, that was 200–2500 μm from center of foveal avascular zone (FAZ) with vision better than 20/100. Patients who received previous photocoagulation were excluded. Patients were randomly assigned to argon blue-green treatment to the entire CNV and 100–125 μm beyond the borders of the lesion vs observation

Juxtafoveal (Krypton) Study: well-demarcated CNV due to AMD or OHS, or idiopathic, that was 1–199 μm from center of foveal avascular zone (FAZ), or with a CNV more than 200 μm with blood or pigment extending within 200 μm and with vision better than 20/400. Patients were randomly assigned to Krypton red treatment of entire CNV and 100 μm beyond the borders of the lesion except on the foveal side of the lesion vs observation

Subfoveal, New CNV AMD Study: well-demarcated CNV due to AMD under the center of foveal avascular zone (FAZ) with vision between 20/40 and 20/320. The entire lesion had to measure less than 3.5 MPS disc areas in size and could be classic or occult CNV. Patients were randomly assigned to argon green or krypton red treatment of entire CNV and 100 μm beyond the borders of the lesion vs observation

Subfoveal Recurrent CNV Study: well-demarcated CNV due to AMD under the center of foveal avascular zone (FAZ) contiguous with previous laser treatment scar and with vision between 20/40 and 20/320. The entire lesion had to measure less than 6MPS disc areas in size and could be classic or occult CNV. Patients randomly assigned to argon green or krypton red treatment of entire CNV and 100 μm beyond the borders of the lesion vs observation

DEFINITIONS:
EXTRAFOVEAL: 200–2500 μm from center of foveal avascular zone (FAZ)
JUXTAFOVEAL: 1–199 μm from center of FAZ
SUBFOVEAL: extends beneath center of fovea

MAIN OUTCOME MEASURES: visual acuity, contrast sensitivity, reading speed, persistent and/or recurrent CNV, treatment complications

Results:

Extrafoveal Study:

After 18 months:
AMD: 25% of treated vs 60% of untreated eyes had lost ≥6 lines of vision (a quadrupling of the visual angle [i.e. 20/50 to 20/200])

POHS: 9.4% of treated vs 34.2% of untreated eyes had lost ≥6 lines of vision

IDIOPATHIC: sample size (67) was too small to reach clinical significance, but trend was similar to results for AMD and POHS

Recurrence of CNV after argon laser was 52% with AMD, 28% with POHS, 28% with idiopathic CNV

After 3 years:

Relative risk of severe vision loss (≥6 lines) for no treatment vs treatment was 1.4 for AMD, 5.5 for POHS, and 2.3 for idiopathic CNV

After 5 years:

AMD: treated eyes lost 5.2 lines of vision vs 7.1 lines in untreated eyes; recurrence in 54% of treated eyes; 26% developed CNV in fellow eye

POHS: treated eyes lost 0.9 line of vision vs 4.4 lines in untreated eyes; recurrence in 26% of treated eyes

IDIOPATHIC: treated eyes lost 2.7 lines of vision vs 4.4 lines in untreated eyes; recurrence in 34% of treated eyes

Juxtafoveal Study:

After 3 years:

POHS: 4.6% of treated vs 24.6% of untreated eyes had lost ≥6 lines of vision

IDIOPATHIC: 10% of treated vs 37% of untreated eyes had lost ≥6 lines of vision

After 5 years:

Relative risk of severe vision loss (≥6 lines) for no treatment vs treatment was 1.2 for AMD (hypertensive patients had little or no benefit), 4.26 for POHS, and intermediate between AMD and POHS for idiopathic CNV

Subfoveal New AMD Study:

After 3 months:

AMD: 20% of treated vs 11% of untreated eyes had lost ≥6 lines of vision

After 2 years:

AMD: 20% of treated vs 37% of untreated eyes had lost ≥6 lines of vision; recurrence in 51% of treated eyes

After 4 years:

AMD: 22% of treated vs 47% of untreated eyes had lost ≥6 lines of vision

Subfoveal Recurrent AMD Study:

After 3 years: 12% of treated vs 36% of untreated eyes had lost ≥6 lines of vision

Conclusions:

Treat extrafoveal CNV in patients with AMD, POHS, and idiopathic lesions

Patients with juxtafoveal CNV (AMD, POHS, and idiopathic) benefit from krypton laser photocoagulation, except for hypertensive AMD patients

AMD patients with subfoveal CNV (new or recurrent) benefit equally from argon green or krypton red laser treatment

For unilateral CNV, large drusen and focal hyperpigmentation are risk factors for development of CNV in fellow eye

Treatment of AMD patients with juxtafoveal CNV is beneficial when the lesion is classic, even though CNV recurs; treatment of classic CNV alone in lesions with both classic and occult CNV was not beneficial

Treatment of Age-Related Macular Degeneration with Photodynamic Therapy Trial (TAP)

Objective: to evaluate verteporfin (Visudyne) ocular photodynamic therapy (OPT) in the management of subfoveal CNV with some classic characteristics

Methods: patients with evidence of AMD, age >50 years, evidence of new or recurrent subfoveal 'classic' (can have occult features) CNV by fluorescein angiography with greatest linear dimension of CNV <5400 μm (9MPS disc areas), ETDRS visual acuity of 20/40 to 20/200, and the ability to return every 3 months for 2 years. Patients were excluded who had other ocular diseases that could compromise visual acuity, history of previous experimental treatment for CNV, porphyrin allergy, liver problems, or intraocular surgery within the previous 2 months. Two thirds of patients in both studies were randomly assigned (2:1 randomization scheme) to receive verteporfin (Visudyne 6 mg/m^2) and one third to control vehicle (D$_5$W IV infusion) infused over a 10-minute period. All patients were then irradiated with the use of a 689-nm diode laser (light dose: 50 J/cm^2; power density: 600 mW/cm^2; duration: 83 seconds) 15 minutes after the start of the infusion

Results: enrollment included 609 patients (311 in Study A and 298 in Study B). Vision was stabilized or improved in 61.4% of patients treated with Visudyne OPT compared with 45.9% treated with placebo at 12 months. The difference was sustained at 24 and 60 (TAP Extension Study) months. In subgroup analysis, the visual acuity benefit was most pronounced for lesions in which the area of classic CNV occupied more than 50% of the entire area of the lesion (predominantly classic). Specifically, 33% of the Visudyne-treated eyes compared with 61% of the placebo-treated eyes sustained moderate visual loss. No difference in visual acuity was noted when the area of classic CNV was greater than 0% but less than 50% of the entire lesion (minimally classic). Sixteen percent of patients experienced an improvement in vision (1 or more lines) in the Visudyne-treated group compared with 7.2% in the control group. Overall, the Visudyne group was 34% more likely to retain vision. Most patients required periodic retreatments with an average of 3.4 (of a possible 4) being required in the first year, 2.1 in the second year (5.5 total over 24 months), and 1.5 in the third year (7 total over 36 months)

Conclusions: Visudyne ocular photodynamic therapy is recommended for subfoveal, predominantly classic, CNV

Verteporfin in Photodynamic Therapy (VIP) Trial Verteporfin in Photodynamic Therapy–Pathologic Myopia (VIP-PM) Trial

Objective: to evaluate Visudyne ocular photodynamic therapy (OPT) in the management of subfoveal CNV not included in the original TAP investigation

Methods: patients with evidence of AMD, age >50 years, evidence of subfoveal 'occult' only CNV by FA with recent disease progression defined as evidence of hemorrhage, loss of ≥1 line of vision, or increased size of the lesion by 10% during the preceding 3 months, and Early Treatment Diabetic Retinopathy Study (ETDRS) visual acuity ≥20/100; or subfoveal 'classic' CNV with ETDRS visual acuity of ≥20/40, greatest linear dimension of CNV <5400 μm (9 MPS disc areas), and the ability to return every 3 months for 2 years. Patients were excluded who had other ocular diseases that could compromise visual acuity, history of previous experimental treatment for CNV, porphyrin allergy, liver problems, or intraocular surgery within the previous 2 months. Two-thirds of the patients in both studies were randomly assigned (2:1 randomization scheme) to receive verteporfin (Visudyne 6 mg/m^2) and one third to control vehicle (D$_5$W IV infusion) infused over a 10-minute period. All patients were then irradiated with the use of a 689 nm diode laser (light dose: 50 J/cm^2; power density: 600 mW/cm^2; duration: 83 seconds) 15 minutes after the start of the infusion

Results: 459 patients enrolled. The 1-year results showed no statistically significant difference between the Visudyne-treated patients and placebo (difference 4.2%). However, by 24 months, a statistically significant difference was seen that was due to a decline in vision in the control group (difference 13.7%). Moreover, this difference was most pronounced in patients with 'occult' only CNV lesions measuring <4MPS disk areas in size at baseline, or who had a baseline visual acuity of 20/50 or worse

Few ocular or other systemic adverse events were seen with Visudyne therapy. In 4.4% of patients, an immediate severe visual decrease within 7 days of treatment was observed

Conclusions: Visudyne ocular photodynamic therapy (OPT) is recommended in the management of subfoveal occult but not classic CNV when there is evidence of recent disease progression, especially if the baseline lesion size is smaller than 4 MPS DA, or the baseline vision is worse than 20/50

Age-Related Eye Disease Study (AREDS)

Objective: to evaluate the effect of high-dose supplements on the progression of AMD, and on the development and progression of cataracts

Methods: patients aged 55–80 years with 20/32 or better vision OU, or 20/32 or better in one eye and AMD in fellow eye, received antioxidants (vitamin C [500 mg], vitamin E [400 IU], beta-carotene [vitamin A, 15 mg]), zinc (80 mg plus 2 mg copper), both, or placebo
Categorized into 4 groups:
Category 1: fewer than 5 small (<63 μm) drusen
Category 2 (mild AMD): multiple small drusen or single or nonextensive intermediate (63–124 μm) drusen, or pigment abnormalities
Category 3 (intermediate AMD): extensive intermediate-sized drusen, or 1 or more large (>125 μm) drusen, or noncentral geographic atrophy
Category 4 (advanced AMD): vision loss (<20/32) due to AMD in 1 eye (due to either central/subfoveal geographic atrophy or exudative macular degeneration
Primary outcomes:
Progression to advanced AMD: treatment for CNV or photographic evidence (geographic atrophy of center of macula, nondrusenoid RPE detachment, serous or hemorrhagic RD, subretinal hemorrhage or fibrosis)
Moderate vision loss: ≥15-letter loss (doubling of visual angle)
Development and progression of lens opacities
Results: 4757 patients enrolled
Antioxidants plus zinc: reduced the risk of progression to advanced AMD and vision loss over 6 years in 25% of high-risk patients
HIGH-RISK PATIENTS: intermediate AMD (many intermediate drusen [63–124 μm] or 1 large drusen [≥125 μm] in 1 or both eyes) or advanced AMD (in 1 eye only)
Zinc alone: reduced risk of vision loss by 21%
Antioxidants alone: reduced risk of vision loss by 17%

Conclusions:

High-dose supplements are beneficial in reducing the risk of vision loss in patients with high-risk AMD (categories 3 and 4). Caution should be exercised in smokers or recent smokers in the use of high-dose beta-carotene because of the possible increased risk of lung cancer

Treatment is of no benefit in patients with no AMD or early AMD (several small or intermediate drusen)

Treatment does not affect development or progression of cataract

Age-Related Eye Disease Study (AREDS2)

Objective: to evaluate the effect of high-dose supplements, macular carotenoids, and omega-3-fatty acid on the progression of AMD

Methods: patients randomized to receive various combinations of vitamin C (500 mg), vitamin E (400 IU), beta-carotene (vitamin A, 15 mg), zinc (80 mg plus 2 mg copper), lutein (10 mg), zeaxanthin (2 mg), omega-3 long-chain polyunsaturated fatty acids (LCPUFA) in the form of docosahexaenoic acid (DHA) (350 mg) and eicosapentaenoic acid (EPA) (650 mg)

VEGF Inhibition Study in Ocular Neovascularization trial (VISION)

Objective: to evaluate intravitreal pegaptanib for subfoveal CNV due to neovascular AMD

Methods: 2 concurrent randomized, double-masked clinical trials, 1208 patients received either pegaptanib intravitreal injection (0.3 mg, 1.0 mg, or 3.0 mg) or a sham injection into study eye every 6 weeks for a total of 48 weeks. Patients were eligible for the trial if they were 50 years old or older and had subfoveal classic, minimally classic, and/or occult CNV due to wet AMD with a best-corrected visual acuity of 20/40 to 20/320 in the study eye.

Results: on average, patients treated with pegaptanib 0.3 mg and sham-treated patients continued to experience vision loss. However, the rate of visual acuity decline in the pegaptanib-treated group was slower than the rate in the patients who received sham treatment; 70% of patients treated with pegaptanib sodium injection (0.3 mg; $n = 294$) lost fewer than 15 letters of visual acuity compared with 55% in the control group ($n = 296$; $P < 0.001$); 10% of patients treated with pegaptanib sodium injection (0.3 mg; $n = 294$) had severe visual acuity loss (30 letters or more) compared with 22% in the control group ($n = 296$; $P < 0.001$). The beneficial effect was observed for all subtypes of neovascularization (NV). The beneficial effect was sustained for up to 2 years of follow-up

Conclusions: pegaptanib was better than sham and PDT for neovascular AMD

Minimally Classic/Occult Trial of the Anti-VEGF Antibody Ranibizumab in the Treatment of Neovascular AMD (MARINA) Trial

Objective: pivotal phase III, multicenter, double-blind 24-month study, which compared monthly intravitreal injections of ranibizumab 0.3 or 0.5 mg or sham injections (n = 716) in patients with subfoveal occult only or minimally classic CNV due to wet AMD

Results: enrolled 716 patients with minimally classic and occult subfoveal CNV associated with AMD. The primary outcome was prevention of moderate visual loss (≤15 letters loss of vision), which was seen in 94.5% with ranibizumab 0.3 mg, 94.6% with ranibizumab 0.5 mg and 62.2% of patients receiving sham injections ($P < 0.001$). Vision improved by ≥15 letters for a significantly ($P < 0.0001$) greater number of ranibizumab-treated patients (24.8% for 0.3 mg and 33.8% for 0.5 mg) versus sham-treated patients (5.0%). Mean increases in VA from baseline were +6.5 letters for the ranibizumab 0.3 mg group and +7.2 letters for the ranibizumab 0.5 mg group, whereas sham-injected patients had a mean decrease of −10.4 letters. This benefit in VA in ranibizumab-treated patients was maintained through 24 months. At 24 months, 90% of ranibizumab-treated patients in the MARINA study lost less than 15 letters of visual acuity; 33% gained 15 or more letters of visual acuity ($P < 0.01$). Ranibizumab-treated patients exhibited a statistically significant improvement compared with sham-treated patients in all subgroups for all outcome measures.

Conclusions: ranibizumab was better than sham for occult with no classic and minimally classic CNV due to neovascular AMD

Anti-vascular endothelial growth factor (VEGF) Antibody for the Treatment of Predominantly Classic Choroidal Neovascularization (CNV) in Age-related Macular Degeneration (ANCHOR) Trial

Objective: second pivotal phase III, multicenter, randomized, double-masked 24-month clinical trial, which compared ranibizumab with the active control verteporfin PDT in subfoveal predominantly classic CNV due to wet AMD

Results: enrolled 423 patients with predominantly classic subfoveal CNV associated with AMD. The primary outcome was prevention of moderate visual loss (≤15 letters loss of vision), which was seen in 94.3% with ranibizumab 0.3 mg, 96.4% with ranibizumab 0.5 mg and 64.3% of patients receiving PDT ($P < 0.001$). Vision improved by ≥15 letters in significantly more ranibizumab-treated patients (35.7% for 0.3 mg and 40.3% for 0.5 mg) than PDT-treated patients (5.6%; $P < 0.0001$). At 12 months, mean change in VA increased by +8.5 letters in the ranibizumab 0.3 mg group and by +11.3 letters in the 0.5 mg group, but decreased by −9.5 letters in the sham group ($P < 0.0001$)

Conclusions: ranibizumab was superior to verteporfin for treatment of predominantly classic CNV due to neovascular AMD

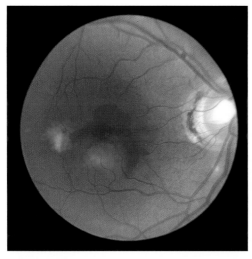

Figure 11-51. POHS demonstrating peripapillary scarring and macular, juxtafoveal choroidal neovascular membrane with surrounding subretinal hemorrhage. (From Noorthy RS, Fountain JS: Fungal uveitis. In: Yanoff M, Duker JS (eds) Ophthalmology. London, Mosby, 1999.)

Other Disorders Associated with Choroidal Neovascular Membrane (CNV)

Treatment for all CNV: consider laser only for extrafoveal lesions (MPS showed that laser treatment for juxtafoveal and extrafoveal CNV was beneficial); juxtafoveal and subfoveal lesions are treated with anti-VEGF agents or photodynamic therapy (see above)

Presumed Ocular Histoplasmosis Syndrome (POHS)

Due to *Histoplasma capsulatum,* a dimorphic fungus (mold in soil, yeast in animals and birds) endemic to Mississippi and Ohio River valleys; rare in Europe; rare among African Americans. Age of onset commonly 20–45 years; no sex predilection; 90% of patients with ocular signs have positive skin reaction (>5 mm) to intracutaneous 1 : 100 histoplasmin (test usually not used because it may incite macular disease)

Macular involvement associated with HLA-B7, HLA-DRw2; however, HLA typing is not commonly used

Primary infection involves inhalation of spores into respiratory tract and a self-limited flu-like illness; dissemination of the fungus then occurs to spleen, liver, and choroid. Primary choroidal infection causes granulomatous, clinically unapparent inflammation that resolves into a small, atrophic scar ('histo spot') that can disrupt Bruch's membrane

Findings: POHS consists of the triad of peripapillary atrophy, multiple punched-out chorioretinal scars ('histo spots,' may enlarge, 5–10% develop new spots), and maculopathy. No anterior or posterior segment cell; CNV can occur (different from that in AMD in that vessels penetrate Bruch's membrane and extend over RPE; a second

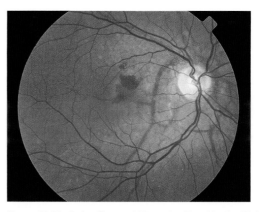

Figure 11-52. Peripapillary angioid streaks. (From Vander JF: Angioid streaks. In: Yanoff M, Duker JS (eds) Ophthalmology. London, Mosby, 1999.)

layer of RPE forms [basal side up] and attempts to encircle the CNV) (Figure 11-51)

Risk of CNV: 1% with normal disc and macula; 25% risk over 4 years if not normal

CXR: calcifications

Angioid Streaks

Peripapillary linear cracks in thickened, degenerated, and calcified Bruch's membrane (Figure 11-52)

Subretinal hemorrhage can occur with minor trauma; patients should consider safety glasses

Etiology: 50% associated with systemic condition, 50% idiopathic

Mnemonic **PEPSI**:
  Pseudoxanthoma elasticum (PXE) (AR ≫ AD): female > male; peau d'orange appearance to retina; redundant skin with waxy, yellow, papule-like lesions ('plucked chicken' skin); increased elastic tissue; vascular malformations; abnormal mucosal vasculature may cause GI bleeds; may have optic nerve head drusen; angioid streaks present in 85%
  Ehlers-Danlos syndrome (fibrodysplasia hyperelastica) (AD): hyperextensible skin due to deficient collagen matrix; other eye findings include subluxed lens, high myopia, keratoconus, blue sclera, retinal detachment
  Paget's disease: increased bone production and destruction; increased serum alkaline phosphatase; prone to basal skull and long bone fractures; other bone disorders (acromegaly, calcinosis)
  Sickle cell: risk for autoinfarction of spleen and thrombotic episodes; other hematologic diseases (thalassemia, hereditary spherocytosis, acanthocytosis [Bassen-Kornzweig syndrome]); angioid streaks present in 1%
  Idiopathic: 50%

DDx: lacquer cracks in myopia

Pathologic Myopia

High myopia = Axial length >26 mm; > −6 D of myopia; Pathologic myopia = Axial length >32.5 mm; > −8 D of myopia;

Approximately 2% of US population; female > male

CNV due to PM commonly occurs in young patients; bilateral common (12–40%)

Findings: long, oval disc, may be tilted, cup usually shallow; temporal crescent; posterior staphyloma; tigroid fundus with visible choroidal vessels; lacquer cracks (breaks in Bruch's membrane); Foerster-Fuchs' spot (macular hemorrhage); cataract; retinal holes and high risk of rhegmatogenous RD

Lacquer crack: sudden decrease in vision, metamorphopsia, often in teenagers; focal subretinal hemorrhage, dense, round, deep, and often centered on fovea; blood may obscure crack

Complications: CNV often near fovea (65%) worse prognosis; 60% with vision <20/200 at 2 years

Treatment: Same as CNV due to AMD

Other Causes of Macular CNV

Idiopathic, optic nerve head drusen, choroidal rupture, choroidal nevus, sympathetic ophthalmia, Vogt-Kayanagi-Harada disease, serpiginous choroiditis, other posterior uveitides (choroidal inflammation may enhance production of angiogenic factors; when coupled with RPE-Bruch's membrane disruption, CNV can develop)

Vascular Diseases

Damage to vessel walls causes leakage of serum and blood into plexiform layers, causing edema, exudates, and hemorrhages

Edema: histologically appears as clear cystoid spaces

Lipid: appears as yellow lesion; histologically, hard exudates are eosinophilic and PAS-positive

DDx: diabetes, hypertensive retinopathy, CNV, vein occlusion, parafoveal telangiectasia, Coats' disease, radiation retinopathy, CSR, trauma, macroaneurysm, papilledema, angiomatosis retinae

Microaneurysm: fusiform outpouching of capillary wall

Cotton wool spot: microinfarction of NFL (usually secondary to occlusion of retinal arteriole) with cessation of axoplasmic flow, mitochondria accumulate (resemble a nucleus, so lesion appears like a cell ['cytoid body'])

Hemorrhage: shape of intraretinal blood depends on layer in which it occurs (dot/blot in plexiform layer where cells are oriented vertically; flame-shaped/feathery border in NFL where cells are oriented horizontally)

Roth spot: white-centered hemorrhage

DDx: ischemia (anemia, anoxia, carbon monoxide poisoning), elevated venous pressure (birth trauma, shaken baby syndrome, intracranial hemorrhage), capillary fragility (hypertension, diabetes), infection (bacterial endocarditis, HIV), leukemia, collagen vascular disease

Neovascularization: growth of new vessels on vitreous side of ILM; new vessels grow along posterior hyaloid

Vascular tortuosity: may be congenital (arterial and venous) or acquired (venous)

DDx: hypertension, high venous pressure (occlusion), papilledema, high viscosity, AV fistula; associated with fetal alcohol syndrome, Peter's anomaly, optic nerve hypoplasia

Retinal Vasculitis

Involvement of retinal arterioles (arteritis), veins (phlebitis), or both (periphlebitis)

Findings: sheathing of vessels, hemorrhage

DDx: temporal arteritis, polyarteritis nodosa, lupus, Behçet's disease, inflammatory bowel syndrome, multiple sclerosis, pars planitis, Wegener's granulomatosis, Eales disease, sarcoidosis, syphilis, toxoplasmosis, viral retinitis (HSV, HZV), IV drug abuse, Lyme disease, tuberculosis

Cystoid Macular Edema (CME)

Intraretinal edema in honeycomb-like spaces; flower-petal pattern due to Henle's layer

Etiology: mnemonic DEPRIVEN

Diabetes
Epinephrine
Pars planitis
RP
Irvine-Gass syndrome
Venous occlusion
E_2 prostaglandin
Nicotinic acid maculopathy (does not leak)

Others: XRT, parafoveal telangiectasia, CNV (rare), juvenile retinoschisis (does not leak), Goldmann-Favre (does not leak), latanoprost (Xalatan), vitreous wick

Pathophysiology: abnormal perifoveal retinal capillary permeability; initial fluid accumulation may be within Müller's cells (rather than in spaces of outer plexiform and inner nuclear layers)

Findings: CME, optic nerve swelling, vitreous cell (Figure 11-53)

FA: multiple small focal fluorescein leaks early; late pooling of dye in cystoid spaces; classically, flower-petal ('petalloid') pattern; staining of optic nerve (Figure 11-54)

OCT: cystic intraretinal spaces (Figure 11-55)

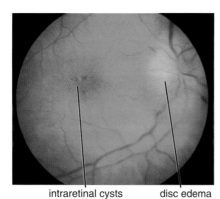

intraretinal cysts   disc edema

Figure 11-53. Cystoid macular edema with decreased foveal reflex, cystic changes in fovea, and intraretinal hemorrhages. (From Kaiser PK, Friedman NJ, Pineda R II: Massachusetts Eye and Ear Infirmary Illustrated Manual of Ophthalmology, 2nd edn. Philadelphia, Saunders, 2004.)

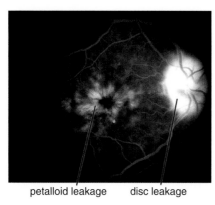

petalloid leakage   disc leakage

Figure 11-54. Fluorescein angiogram of same patient as in Figure 11-53, demonstrating characteristic petalloid appearance with optic nerve leakage. (From Kaiser PK, Friedman NJ, Pineda R II: Massachusetts Eye and Ear Infirmary Illustrated Manual of Ophthalmology, 2nd edn. Philadelphia, Saunders, 2004.)

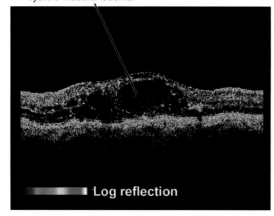

cystoid macular edema

Figure 11-55. Optical coherence tomography of cystoid macular edema, demonstrating intraretinal cystoid spaces and dome-shaped configuration of fovea. (From Kaiser PK, Friedman NJ, Pineda R II: Massachusetts Eye and Ear Infirmary Illustrated Manual of Ophthalmology, 2nd edn. Philadelphia, Saunders, 2004.)

DDx of cystic macular changes (looks like CME clinically, but no fluorescein filling of cysts):

1. Juvenile retinoschisis
2. Goldmann-Favre
3. Some types of RP
4. Nicotinic acid maculopathy

Treatment: depends on etiology; focal laser treatment, topical steroids and NSAID, oral Diamox, sub-Tenon's or intravitreal steroid injection

Congenital Retinal Telangiectasia / Coats' Disease (Leber's Miliary Aneurysms)

(See Ch. 5, Pediatrics / Strabismus.)

Parafoveal / Juxtafoveal Telangiectasia (PFT, JXT)

Microaneurysmal and saccular dilation of parafoveal vessels

Classification:

Type 1: unilateral, male > female (10 : 1); onset during middle age; in spectrum of Coats' disease

    TYPE 1A: congenital; confined to temporal half of fovea; macular edema and exudation (lipid)

    TYPE 1B: idiopathic; capillary telangiectasia confined to 1 clock hour at edge of FAZ; minimal leakage on FA; occasional hard exudates; vision usually better than 20/25; can be treated with laser

Type 2A (most common): bilateral, acquired; male = female; 5th–6th decade of life; symmetric, involving area <1 DD; minimal macular edema; occasionally, superficial glistening white dots (Singerman's spots); right-angle retinal venules dive deep into choroid; eventual develop RPE hyperplasia; occasionally, yellow lesion measuring $\frac{1}{3}$ DD centered on FAZ (pseudovitelliform macular degeneration); may develop macular edema that is due to ischemia (not amenable to laser treatment); $\frac{1}{3}$ abnormal glucose tolerance test

    FA: parafoveal capillary leakage; risk of CNV

Type 3: bilateral, idiopathic; male = female; capillary occlusion predominates

    TYPE 3A: occlusive idiopathic

    TYPE 3B: occlusive idiopathic; associated with central nervous system vasculopathy

Structural abnormalities in types 2 and 3 are similar to diabetic microangiopathy (but no risk of NVE)

DDx: diabetes, vein occlusion, radiation retinopathy, Coats' disease, Eales' disease, Best's disease, sickle cell, Irvine-Gass syndrome, ocular ischemia

Complications: macular edema, exudates, CNV, intraretinal neovascularization, retinal–retinal anastamosis

Retinal Arterial Macroaneurysm (RAM)

May bleed, then autoinfarcts

Usually, elderly females; most common along temporal arcades; 10% bilateral

Mechanism: arteriosclerosis (fibrosis, thinning, decreased elasticity of vessel wall), hypertension (increased pressure on thin wall)

Findings: blood in every retinal layer, lipid exudate, artery occlusion downstream (especially following laser treatment), CME (Figure 11-56)

DDx of blood in every retinal layer (subretinal, intraretinal, and preretinal)**:** macroaneurysm, trauma, sickle cell retinopathy, choroidal melanoma, vein occlusion (rare), CNV (rare)

Pathology: overall thickening of vessel wall with hypertrophy of muscularis

Treatment: observation; consider focal laser (risk of hemorrhage)

Hypertensive Retinopathy

Focal or generalized vasoconstriction, breakdown of blood–retinal barrier with subsequent hemorrhage and exudate

Associated with microaneurysms or macroaneurysms

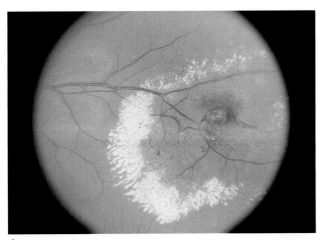

A

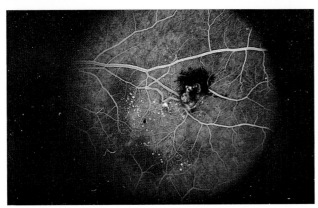

B

Figure 11-56. Macroaneurysm with surrounding dilated and telangiectatic capillary bed:. **A,** fundus photograph;, **B,** FA. (Courtesy Susan Fowell, MD. From Mittra RA, Mieler WF, Pollack JS: Retinal arterial macroaneurysms. In: Yanoff M, Duker JS (eds) Ophthalmology. London, Mosby, 1999.)

Classification systems:
Keith-Wagener-Barker Classification
  GROUP I: minimal constriction and tortuosity of arterioles
  GROUP II: Moderate constriction of arterioles; focal narrowing and arteriovenous nicking
  GROUP III: Group II plus cotton wool spots, hemorrhages, and exudates
  GROUP IV: Group III plus optic disc edema
Scheie Classification
  GROUP 0: no visible changes
  GROUP I: Diffuse arteriolar narrowing
  GROUP II: Pronounced arteriolar narrowing and focal constriction
  GROUP III: Grade II plus retinal hemorrhages
  GROUP IV: Grade III plus optic disc edema

Findings:
Retinopathy: AV nicking, 'copper or silver wire' arterial changes, hemorrhages, exudates, cotton wool spots
Choroidopathy: fibrinoid necrosis of choroidal arterioles; may have Elschnig's spots (zone of nonperfusion of choriocapillaris; pale white or red patches of RPE), Siegrist streak (reactive RPE hyperplasia along sclerosed choroidal vessel), and exudative RD; due to acute hypertensive episode (pre-eclampsia, eclampsia, or pheochromocytoma); FA shows early hypoperfusion and late staining
Optic neuropathy: florid disc edema with macular exudate, linear flame hemorrhages

Pathology: thickening of arteriolar walls leads to nicking of venules; endothelial hyperplasia

Complications: retinal vein occlusion, retinal macroaneurysm, nonarteritic AION, ocular motor nerve palsies, worsening of diabetic retinopathy

Diabetic Retinopathy (DR)

Leading cause of new blindness in United States, adults aged 20–74 years

Classification:
Background or nonproliferative (BDR, NPDR): hemorrhages, exudates, cotton wool spots, microaneurysms (MA), intraretinal microvascular abnormalities (IRMA), venous beading (Figure 11-57)
Severe NPDR ('4-2-1 rule') (15% progress to PDR in 1 year):
  Defined as any one of the following:
  4 quadrants of hemorrhages/MAs
  2 quadrants of venous beading
  1 quadrant of IRMA (Figure 11-58)
Very severe NPDR (50% progress to PDR in 1 year):
  Defined as 2 or more of the above
Proliferative (PDR): NV of disc or elsewhere (Figure 11-59)
High–risk proliferative (HR-PDR):
  Defined as any one of the following:

317

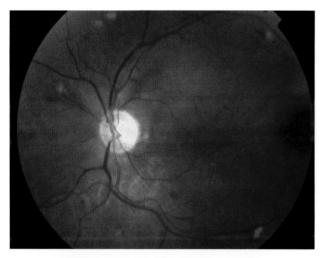

Figure 11-57. Nonproliferative diabetic retinopathy.

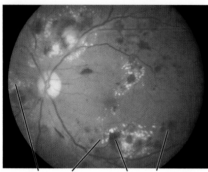

lipid exudate   intraretinal hemorrhages

Figure 11-58. Severe nonproliferative diabetic retinopathy with extensive hemorrhages, microaneurysms, and exudates. (From Kaiser PK, Friedman NJ, Pineda R II: Massachusetts Eye and Ear Infirmary Illustrated Manual of Ophthalmology, 2nd edn. Philadelphia, Saunders, 2004.)

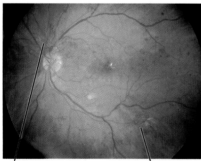

neovascularization   neovascularization
of the disc   elsewhere

Figure 11-59. Proliferative diabetic retinopathy demonstrating florid neovascularization of the disc and elsewhere. (From Kaiser PK, Friedman NJ, Pineda R II: Massachusetts Eye and Ear Infirmary Illustrated Manual of Ophthalmology, 2nd edn. Philadelphia, Saunders, 2004.)

1. NVD ≥ ¼ to ⅓ disc area
2. Any NVD with vitreous hemorrhage
3. NVE ≥ ½ disc area with vitreous hemorrhage

Epidemiology:
Type 1 DM:
   AT DIAGNOSIS: no BDR
   AT 5 YEARS: 25% BDR, PDR rare
   AT 20 YEARS: 98% BDR, 60% PDR, 30% CSME

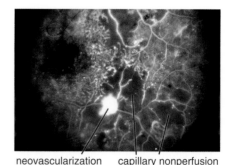

neovascularization   capillary nonperfusion

Figure 11-60. Fluorescein angiogram of a patient with proliferative diabetic retinopathy, showing extensive capillary nonperfusion, neovascularization elsewhere, and vascular leakage. (From Kaiser PK, Friedman NJ, Pineda R II: Massachusetts Eye and Ear Infirmary Illustrated Manual of Ophthalmology, 2nd edn. Philadelphia, Saunders, 2004.)

Type 2 IDDM:
   AT DIAGNOSIS: 30% BDR
   AT 5 YEARS: 40% BDR, 2% PDR
   AT 20 YEARS: 90% BDR, 25% PDR, 40% CSME
Type 2 NIDDM:
   AT DIAGNOSIS: 20% BDR
   AT 5 YEARS: 30% BDR, 2% PDR
   AT 20 YEARS: 50% BDR, 10% PDR, 20% CSME

Findings: cotton wool spots, lipid exudates (may appear as circinate exudate [ring of hard exudate surrounding leaky focus] or macular star [pattern reflects radial orientation of Henle's fibers]), hemorrhages (blot [outer plexiform layer], flame [tracks along NFL]), microaneurysms, IRMA (intraretinal microvascular abnormalities; shunts [arteriole to venule]), venous beading and loops, neovascularization (disc [NVD], elsewhere in retina [NVE], iris [NVI]) (Figure 11-60)

Clinically significant macular edema (CSME) definition: one of the following:
1. Thickening within 500 μm of the foveal avascular zone (FAZ)
2. Hard exudate within 500 μm of the FAZ with associated thickening of adjacent retina
3. Zone of retinal thickening 1 disk *area* in size, any part of which is within 1 disk *diameter* of the foveal center

Asymmetric diabetic retinopathy is usually due to carotid disease (on either side)

Main cause of vision loss in NPDR: macular edema or ischemia

Main causes of vision loss in PDR: tractional RD (TRD), neovascular glaucoma (NVG), vitreous hemorrhage (VH)

Other sequelae:
Diabetic cataract: aldose reductase pathway converts glucose into sorbitol and fructose; causes osmotic effect; aldose reductase also converts galactose into galactitol (which causes cataracts in galactosemia)

Diabetic iridopathy: iris NV; lacy vacuolization of iris pigment epithelium in 40%; glycogen-filled cysts in iris pigment epithelium (PAS+)

Papillitis: acute disc swelling; vision usually ≥20/50; 50% bilateral; may have VF defect; most recover to ≥20/30

Isolated cranial nerve palsies: CN 3, 4, 6 (including pupil-sparing CN 3 palsy)

Pupillary abnormalities: light-near dissociation

Fluctuation in refractive error: due to osmotic effect on crystalline lens from unstable blood sugar levels

Pathology: selective loss of pericytes, no endothelial cells or pericytes in nonperfused areas; thickening of retinal capillary basement membranes; microaneurysm formation; retinal capillary closure; breakdown of blood–retinal barrier; lacy vacuolization of iris pigment epithelium; intraepithelial vacuoles contain glycogen; gitter cells (lipid-laden macrophages) (Figures 11-61, 11-62)

DDx: ocular ischemic syndrome, radiation retinopathy, hypertensive retinopathy, retinal vein occlusion, proliferative retinopathies (sarcoidosis, sickle cell), juxtaoveal telangiectasia

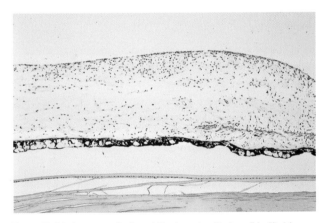

Figure 11-61. Lacy vacuolization of iris pigment epithelium. (Modified from Yanoff M et al: Am J Ophthalmol, 69:201, 1970. From Yanoff M, Fine BS: Ocular Pathology, 5th edn. St Louis, Mosby, 2004.)

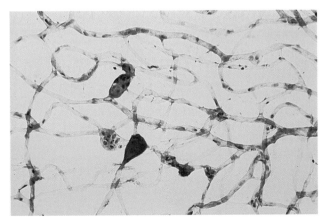

Figure 11-62. Microaneurysms, pericyte dropout, and acellular capillaries are seen. (From Benson WE: Diabetic retinopathy. In: Yanoff M, Duker JS (eds) Ophthalmology. London, Mosby, 1999.)

FA: to identify macular ischemia, localize microaneurysms to guide focal laser treatment, identify areas of NVE, identify areas of capillary nonperfusion

OCT: macular edema appears as increased retinal thickness, cysts, and subretinal fluid; can identify vitreous traction

B-scan ultrasound: to identify TRD if VH present

Treatment:
Based on results from several important studies:

Diabetes Control and Complications Trial (DCCT):
  Tight control of blood sugar slows progression of retinopathy, diabetic macular edema, and visual loss in type 1 diabetic patients; patients with HbA1c <8% had a significantly reduced risk of retinopathy
  Rapid normalization and tight control of blood sugar after a period of prolonged hyperglycemia can lead to worsening of retinopathy

United Kingdom Prospective Diabetes Study (UKPDS):
  Tight control of blood sugar and blood pressure slows progression of retinopathy and development of macular edema in type 2 diabetic patients

Early Treatment Diabetic Retinopathy Study (ETDRS):
  Focal laser decreases vision loss from macular edema by 50%
  No benefit from aspirin
  Focal laser: for CSME (visual acuity is not part of treatment criteria); argon green preferred; yellow (577 nm) is also used because it is well absorbed by hemoglobin within microaneurysms; re-examine every 3–4 months

Diabetic Retinopathy Study (DRS):
  PRP reduces incidence of severe vision loss in high-risk PDR by 60%
  CRITERIA: HR-PDR
    1. NVD ≥¼ to ⅓ disc area
    2. Any NVD with vitreous hemorrhage
    3. NVE ≥½ disc area with vitreous hemorrhage
  COMPLICATIONS: decreased night vision (destruction of extramacular rods), angle-closure glaucoma (choroidal effusion), retinal detachment (regression of NV fronds can cause contracture, leading to retinal tear and rhegmatogenous or traction RD), central scotoma (worsening of CSME), progression of cataract
  Up to 33% of patients will not respond to PRP

Anti-VEGF agents: For diabetic macular edema involving fovea (no CSME definition in the anti-VEGF trials) monthly ranibizumab injections with immediate or deferred laser were significantly better than laser therapy alone (DRCR.net, RISE, RIDE, RESOLVE, and RESTORE studies, see below)

Steroids: Triamcinolone acetonide intravitreal injections found to be effective in pseudophakic patients, but not in the overall group (see DRCR.net Protocol B below). Iluvien (Alimera) is a sustained drug delivery system that uses a drug matrix in a tiny cylindrical tube that is injected intravitreally via a 25 g needle, releasing 0.2 µg/day of the corticosteroid fluocinolone acetonide over 2–3 years (found to be effective in the Phase 3 FAME studies)

Diabetic Retinopathy Vitrectomy Study (DRVS):

Early vitrectomy for VH in type 1 diabetics only, can defer in type 2 (however indications for vitrectomy have changed from these DRVS study conclusions largely owing to better vitrectomy systems, improved instrumentation, and the use of endolaser)

INDICATIONS FOR VITRECTOMY:

Nonclearing vitreous hemorrhage

Combined tractional-rhegmatogenous RD

Traction retinal detachment of the fovea. If tractional detachment is extramacular, watch closely; if macula is threatened or detaches, perform vitrectomy

Anterior hyaloidal fibrovascular proliferation

Refractory macular edema: patients with taut posterior hyaloid face can have chronic macular edema that does not resolve with laser. Chronic traction of vitreous face on macula appears to produce persistent leakage; can resolve after traction is relieved with vitrectomy

Progressive fibrovascular proliferation despite complete PRP

Ghost cell glaucoma

Consider for refractory diabetic macular edema (also consider injecting steroids, or intravitreal anti-VEGF agents)

Prognosis: risk of progression without treatment from preproliferative to proliferative DR over 2 years is 50%

Severe NPDR has 50% risk of progression to proliferative disease in 12–18 months

Conditions that exacerbate diabetic retinopathy: hypertension, puberty, pregnancy (at conception, if no BDR, 88% have no retinopathy; if mild BDR, 47% worsen, 5% develop PDR; if PDR, 46% have progression), renal disease, anemia

Follow HbA1c (serum glycosylated hemoglobin [provides 3-month view of blood sugar levels])

MAJOR DIABETIC RETINOPATHY CLINICAL STUDIES

Diabetic Retinopathy Study (DRS)

Objective: to evaluate whether photocoagulation prevents severe visual loss in eyes with diabetic retinopathy

Methods: patients had PDR in at least 1 eye or severe NPDR in both eyes, or 20/100 or better vision in each eye, and were randomly assigned to treatment with scatter laser photocoagulation (randomly assigned to

either xenon arc [200–400, 4.5° spots] or argon blue-green laser [800–1600, 500 µm spots]) in 1 eye and no treatment in the fellow eye (protocol later amended to allow deferred laser photocoagulation). Surface neovascularization (NVE) treated directly with confluent burns, and NVD treated directly only in argon laser–treated eyes. Patients were excluded if they had previous panretinal photocoagulation or a traction retinal detachment threatening the macula

Severe NPDR defined as having at least 3 of the following:

Cotton wool spots

Venous beading

Intraretinal microvascular abnormalities (IRMA) in ≥2 of 4 contiguous overlapping photographic fields

Moderate to severe retinal hemorrhages and/or microaneurysms in ≥1 standard photographic field

Results: 1727 patients enrolled

PRP reduced the risk of severe vision loss (VA <5/200 on 2 consecutive visits 4 months apart) by 50% to 60% in patients with high-risk characteristics (see later)

Conclusions: perform PRP for patients with high-risk proliferative retinopathy (HR-PDR) regardless of vision

NVD (new vessels on or within 1 disc diameter of the disc) ≥ ¼–⅓ of disc area (standard photo 10A)

Any NVD with vitreous or preretinal hemorrhage

NVE (new vessels elsewhere) ≥½ of disc area (standard photo 7) with vitreous or preretinal hemorrhage

PRP is also indicated for NVI

DRS did not report a clear benefit for immediate PRP in patients with severe nonproliferative diabetic retinopathy and proliferative diabetic retinopathy without high-risk characteristics. However, older-onset diabetic patients should be considered for earlier PRP

Early Treatment Diabetic Retinopathy Study (ETDRS)

Objective: to evaluate
1. Whether photocoagulation is effective for diabetic macular edema
2. Effect of aspirin on the course of diabetic retinopathy
3. When to initiate PRP treatment for diabetic retinopathy

Methods: patients had mild, moderate, or severe NPDR or early PDR (does not meet high-risk criteria of PDR) in both eyes, and 20/200 or better vision in each eye, and were randomly assigned to receive 650 mg daily aspirin or not AND 1 of the following:
1. Moderate to severe NPDR or early PDR with no macular edema = immediate PRP (further randomly

assigned to full [1200–1600, 500 µm spots] scatter or mild [400–650, 500 µm spots] scatter PRP) vs deferred PRP until high-risk characteristics developed

2. Mild or moderate NPDR and macular edema = immediate laser (further randomly assigned to immediate focal laser photocoagulation and deferred full scatter or mild scatter when high-risk characteristics developed; or immediate mild or full scatter PRP and deferred focal laser photocoagulation) vs deferred laser photocoagulation

3. Severe NPDR or early PDR and macular edema = immediate laser (further randomly assigned to immediate mild or full PRP and immediate or deferred focal laser photocoagulation) vs deferred laser photocoagulation

Patients were excluded if they had high-risk proliferative diabetic retinopathy

Mild NPDR defined as:
At least 1 microaneurysm, but not enough to qualify as moderate NPDR

Moderate NPDR defined as:
Extensive intraretinal hemorrhages and/or microaneurysms, cotton wool spots, IRMA, venous beading, but not enough to qualify as severe NPDR

Severe NPDR defined with '4-2-1 rule' as any one of the following:
Intraretinal hemorrhages and/or microaneurysms in all 4 quadrants

Venous beading in at least 2 quadrants

IRMA in at least 1 quadrant

CSME defined as one of the following:
1. Retinal thickening at or within 500 µm of the foveal avascular zone (FAZ)
2. Hard exudates at or within 500 µm of the foveal avascular zone (FAZ) with associated thickening of the adjacent retina
3. Retinal thickening ≥1 disc *area* in size ≤1 disc *diameter* from the center of the fovea

Results: 3711 patients enrolled

Immediate focal laser decreased moderate vision loss in patients with clinically significant macular edema by ~50%

Early PRP reduced the risk of development of high-risk PDR in patients with NPDR and early PDR, but difference in severe visual loss was minimal

Immediate focal laser and deferred scatter PRP reduced moderate visual loss by 50% in patients with mild or moderate NPDR and macular edema

Immediate focal laser and scatter PRP reduced severe visual loss by 50% in patients with severe NPDR or early PDR and macular edema

Aspirin had no effect on progression or complications of diabetic retinopathy

Conclusions: treat all patients with CSME regardless of vision

Immediate PRP should be reserved for patients with high-risk PDR and possibly those with severe NPDR in both eyes

No benefit from aspirin (650 mg/day)

Diabetic Retinopathy Vitrectomy Study (DRVS)

Objective: to observe patients with severe DR in type 1 and type 2 diabetes over 2 years to determine visual outcomes

Methods: patients with severe NPDR or early PDR (do not meet high-risk criteria of PDR) were placed into 1 of 3 groups

Group N: natural history study with 744 eyes of 644 patients enrolled

Group NH: to evaluate early surgical intervention vs delayed surgery (for at least 1 year) in eyes with severe diabetic retinopathy and active neovascularization or fibrovascular proliferation but without severe visual loss (vision better than 10/200). 370 eyes enrolled. Amount of new vessel severity was quantified

NVC-1 (least severe): new vessel severity no worse than moderate in only 1 photographic field

NVC-2 (moderately severe): moderate new vessels in 2 or more fields, but not severe in any field

NVC-3 (severe): severe NVD or NVE in at least 1 field

NVC-4 (very severe): severe NVD and NVE in at least 1 field

Group H: to evaluate early surgical intervention (within days) vs delayed surgery (for at least 1 year, unless TRD of macula detected on ultrasound examination) in eyes with severe diabetic retinopathy and active neovascularization or fibrovascular proliferation, with history of sudden visual loss from severe vitreous hemorrhage within 6 months (vision worse than 5/200, not NLP). 616 eyes enrolled. (Note: endophotocoagulation was not used in the DRVS)

Patients were excluded if they had a previous vitrectomy, photocoagulation within 3 months, IOP >29 mmHg on medications, severe iris neovasularizataion, or neovascular glaucoma

Results:

Group NR:

4-YEAR RESULTS: patients in the early vitrectomy group had better vision than those in the deferral group

Up to 18 months, the early vitrectomy group had a higher risk of no light perception vision; this was not seen at later time points

Type 1 diabetic patients had an increased chance of obtaining good vision with early vitrectomy

Previous PRP increased chances of good vision

With increasing severity of vessels, early intervention was better than deferred intervention

Group H:

2-YEAR RESULTS: patients in the early vitrectomy group had better vision than those in the deferral group

Patients with type 1 DM had superior outcomes from early vitrectomy, no advantage seen in type 2 DM

Conclusions: early vitrectomy for eyes with severe visual loss due to nonclearing vitreous hemorrhage (at least 1 month) is helpful in type 1 diabetic patients and monocular patients despite the type of diabetes. Early vitrectomy is also recommended for eyes with useful vision and advanced active PDR, especially when extensive neovascularization is present. NLP was seen in 20% of eyes regardless of intervention once a severe vitreous hemorrhage had occurred. Eyes with traction retinal detachment not involving the fovea can be observed until the fovea becomes detached, provided that the fibrovascular proliferation is not severe

Diabetes Control and Complications Trial (DCCT)

Objective: to evaluate effect of tight vs conventional control of blood sugar on diabetic complications in type 1 diabetic patients

Methods: patients with insulin dependence defined by C-peptide secretion were randomly assigned to either

Intensive therapy: 3 or more daily insulin injections or implantation of an insulin pump

Self-monitoring of glucose levels at least 4 times a day

Adjust insulin dose based on glucose level

Preprandial glucose = 70–120 mg/dL (3.9 and 6.7 mmol/L)

Postprandial glucose <180 mg/dL (10.0 mmol/L)

Weekly 3 AM glucose >65 mg/dL (3.6 mmol/L)

Monthly HbA1c <6.05% (nondiabetic range)

Conventional therapy: 1 or 2 daily insulin injections

Daily self-monitoring of glucose levels

Did not adjust insulin dose daily

Education about diet and exercise

Followed every 3 months

No glycosuria or ketonuria

Absence of hyperglycemic or hypoglycemic symptoms

Results: 1441 patients included, study stopped after average follow-up of 6.5 years by independent safety and monitoring committee

Average difference in HbA1c was >2% between groups; however, <5% of intensive group kept <6.05%

Incidence of DR was the same up to 36 months

At baseline, 726 patients had no retinopathy, and 715 had mild retinopathy. After 5 years, the incidence of retinopathy was approximately 50% less with intensive therapy

Patients with HbA1c <8% had significantly reduced risk of retinopathy

Intensive control:

Reduced the risk of development of DR by 76%

Slowed the progression of DR by 54% and reduced the development of severe NPDR or PDR by 47%

Reduced the risk of macular edema by 23%

Reduced the risk of laser treatment by 56%

Reduced albuminuria by 54%

Reduced clinical neuropathy by 60%

Adverse effect: 2–3× increase in severe hypoglycemia

Conclusions: tight control is beneficial; however, rapid normalization and tight control of blood sugar after a period of prolonged hyperglycemia can lead to an initial worsening of retinopathy

Epidemiology of Diabetes Interventions and Complications (EDIC) Trial

Objective: to gain further follow-up of patients from the DCCT

Methods: 1208 patients from DCCT, all of whom received intensive therapy and were followed for an additional 4 years

Results: intensive therapy reduced the risk of

Progression of retinopathy by 75%

Any macular edema by 58%

Laser treatment by 52%

Conclusions: tight control is still beneficial

United Kingdom Prospective Diabetes Study (UKPDS)

Objective: to compare the effects on the risk of microvascular and macrovascular complications of intensive blood glucose control with oral hypoglycemics and/or insulin and conventional treatment with diet therapy

Methods: 4209 newly diagnosed patients with type 2 diabetes, median age 54 years (range, 25–65 years), were randomly assigned to intensive therapy with a sulfonylurea (chlorpropamide, glibenclamide (glyburide), or glipizide) or with insulin, or conventional therapy using diet control

Results: after a median duration of therapy of 11 years, intensive treatment with sulfonylurea, insulin, and/or metformin was equally effective in reducing fasting plasma glucose concentrations.

Over 10 years, HbA1c was 7.0% (range 6.2–8.2) in the intensive group compared with 7.9% (range, 6.9–8.8) in the conventional group – an 11% reduction. No difference in HbA1c was seen among agents in the intensive group.

Compared with the conventional group, the risk in the intensive group was 12% lower for any diabetes-related end point; 10% lower for any diabetes-related death; and 6% lower for all-cause mortality.

The reduction in HbA1c was associated with a 25% overall reduction in microvascular complications, including retinopathy (21% reduction) and nephropathy (34% reduction). 37% of patients had microaneurysms in 1 eye at diagnosis and random assignment

Conclusions: type 2 diabetic patients benefit from intensive glycemic control, as do type 1 diabetic patients

The United Kingdom Prospective Diabetes Study – Hypertension in Diabetes Study (UKPDS-HDS)

Objective: to compare the effects of intensive blood pressure control on the risk of microvascular and macrovascular complications

Methods: 1148 patients with type 2 diabetes and mild to moderate hypertension to determine if 'tight blood pressure control (150/85 mmHg)' using an angiotensin-converting enzyme (ACE) inhibitor or a β-blocker vs 'less tight control (<180/105 mmHg)' would prevent diabetic complications.

Patients were randomly assigned to captopril (ACE inhibitor) or atenolol (β-blocker) and followed for a median of 8.4 years.

Results: tight control of blood pressure in patients with hypertension and type 2 diabetes reduced the risk of death related to diabetes by 32%.

In addition, there was a 34% reduction in risk of deterioration of retinopathy by 2 or more ETDRS steps from baseline, and a 47% reduction in risk of deterioration of visual acuity by 3 ETDRS lines with tight blood pressure control.

Lowering of blood pressure with captopril or atenolol was similarly effective in reducing the incidence of diabetic complications, suggesting that blood pressure reduction in itself may be more important than the treatment used

Conclusions: tight blood pressure control reduced the risk of complications from diabetic retinopathy

RIDE

Objective: to compare efficacy of ranibizumab versus sham with laser rescue in patients with diabetic macular edema

Methods: multicenter, randomized, double-masked, sham injection-controlled, 36-month (sham injection-controlled for 24 months) Phase III study designed to assess the efficacy and safety profile of ranibizumab in 382 patients with diabetic macular edema (DME). Patients were randomized to receive monthly injections of either 0.3 mg ranibizumab (*n* = 125), 0.5 mg ranibizumab (*n* = 127) or monthly sham injections (*n* = 130). Beginning at three months, macular laser rescue treatment was made available to all patients, if needed, based on pre-specified criteria. After month 24, patients in the sham injection group were eligible to receive monthly injections of 0.5 mg ranibizumab, and all patients will continue to be followed and dosed monthly for a total of 36 months. The study then continues in an open-label extension phase.

Results: at 24 months, 33.6% of patients (42/125) who received 0.3 mg ranibizumab and 45.7 percent of patients (58/127) who received 0.5 mg ranibizumab were able to read ≥ 15 letters compared to baseline, compared to 12.3% of patients (16/130) who received sham injections with laser rescue.

Conclusions: ranibizumab injections are effective in diabetic macular edema

RISE

Objective: to compare efficacy of ranibizumab versus sham with laser rescue in patients with diabetic macular edema

Methods: multicenter, randomized, double-masked, sham injection-controlled, 36-month Phase III study designed to assess the safety and efficacy profile of ranibizumab in 377 patients with DME. The primary endpoint compared the proportion of ranibizumab and sham-treated patients who gained ≥15 letters in best corrected visual acuity (BCVA) at month 24, relative to baseline. Patients were randomized to receive monthly injections of either 0.3 mg ranibizumab (*n* = 125), 0.5 mg ranibizumab (*n* =125), or monthly sham injections (*n* = 127). At 3 months, rescue laser treatment was made available to all patients, if needed based on pre-specified criteria. After month 24, patients in the control group are eligible to receive monthly injections of 0.5 mg ranibizumab and all patients will continue to be followed for 36 months.

Results: patients receiving monthly ranibizumab achieved an improvement in vision (BCVA) of ≥ 15 letters at 24 months, compared to those in a control group, who received a placebo (sham) injection.

Conclusions: ranibizumab injections are effective in diabetic macular edema

RESTORE/RESOLVE

Objective: to compare efficacy of ranibizumab with or without laser versus laser alone in patients with diabetic macular edema

Methods: randomized, double-masked, multicenter, laser-controlled phase III trial (*n* = 345) with patients randomized to either ranibizumab 0.5 mg with 3 monthly loading dose followed by PRN ranibizumab alone; focal laser and ranibizumab 0.5 mg with 3 monthly loading dose followed by PRN ranibizumab; or focal laser alone. The primary outcome was mean change in vision from baseline at month 12.

Results: at month 12, the ranibizumab alone group (*n* = 115) gained +6.1 letters, ranibizumab plus laser (*n* = 118) gained +5.9 letters, and the laser alone (*n* = 110) gained +0.8 letters (*P* < 0.0001). There was a mean of 2.1 laser treatments in the laser alone group. The groups gained ≥15 letters in 22.6%, 22.9% and 8.2% respectively. Central retinal thickness improved in all groups: the ranibizumab alone group decreased −118.7 µm, ranibizumab plus laser decreased −128.3 µm, and the laser group decreased by −61.3 µm (*P* < 0.0001). A companion study RESOLVE reported that ranibizumab-treated patients achieved an average +11.7 letters gain in visual acuity at 12 months compared with sham-treated patients, some of who received laser treatment.

Conclusions: ranibizumab therapy with or without laser resulted in significant visual gain over laser treatment alone.

Diabetic Retinopathy Clinical Research Network (DRCR.net): Major Protocols Only

Protocol B

Objectives: to compare intravitreal triamcinolone acetonide injections at doses of 1 mg or 4 mg and macular laser photocoagulation in the treatment of diabetic macular edema

Methods: patients age ≥18 years. Study eye with center-involved DME present on clinical exam and on OCT based on a mean retinal thickness on two OCT measurements ≥250 microns in the central subfield, and best corrected E-ETDRS acuity ≥24 letters (20/320 or better) and ≤73 letters (worse than 20/40). Patients randomized to either 1 or 4 mg triamcinolone acetonide or focal laser photocoagulation. The primary outcome was ≥15-letter improvement in visual acuity from baseline at 2 years

Results: 840 eyes (693 subjects) enrolled at 88 clinical sites. The primary outcome was mean improvement in

vision at 24 months: +1 letters in the laser group (*n* = 330); −2 letters in the 1 mg triamcinolone group (*N*=256)(*p*=0.02); -3 letters in the 4 mg triamcinolone group (*n* = 254)(*P* = 0.002). Increased IOP >30 mmHg was seen in 4% of laser treated patients, 9% of 1 mg TA patients and 21% in the 4 mg TA group. Cataract surgery was required in 13% of laser treated patients, 23% of 1 mg TA patients and 51% in the 4 mg TA group.

Conclusions: triamcinolone acetonide injections were not superior to focal/grid photocoagulation, and resulted in more adverse events

Protocol I

Objectives: to evaluate the safety and efficacy of (1) intravitreal ranibizumab in combination with focal laser photocoagulation, (2) intravitreal ranibizumab treatment alone, and (3) intravitreal triamcinolone acetonide in combination with focal laser photocoagulation in eyes with center-involved DME

Methods: patients age ≥18 years. Study eye with center-involved DME present on clinical exam and on OCT based on a mean retinal thickness on two OCT measurements ≥250 µm in the central subfield, and best corrected acuity 20/32 or worse. Patients were randomized to one of the following 4 groups: Group A: Sham injection plus focal (macular) photocoagulation; Group B: 0.5 mg injection of intravitreal ranibizumab plus focal photocoagulation; Group C: 0.5 mg injection of intravitreal ranibizumab plus deferred focal photocoagulation; Group D: 4 mg intravitreal triamcinolone plus focal photocoagulation The primary outcome was ≥15-letter improvement in visual acuity from baseline at 1 year

Results: 854 patients randomized. The primary outcome was mean improvement in vision at 12 months: +3 letters in the laser group (*n* = 293); +9 letters in the ranibizumab with prompt laser group (*n* = 187)(*P* < 0.001); +9 letters in the ranibizumab with deferred laser group (*n* =188) (*P* < 0.001); and +4 letters in the triamcinolone plus laser group (*n* = 186)(*P* = 0.31). Only 28% of patients in the ranibizumab plus deferred laser group received laser in the first year and 42% by year 2. At 24 months, the mean improvement in vision was +2 letters in the laser group; +7 letters in the ranibizumab with prompt laser group (*P* = 0.01); +10 letters in the ranibizumab with deferred laser group (*P* < 0.001); and +0 letters in the triamcinolone plus laser group (*P* < 0.43). The mean change in retinal thickness was −102 µm in the laser group; −131 µm in the ranibizumab with prompt laser group (*P* < 0.001); −137 µm in the ranibizumab with deferred laser group (*P* < 0.001); and −-127 µm in the triamcinolone plus laser group (*P* < 0.001).

Conclusions: intravitreal ranibizumab with prompt or deferred (≥24 weeks) focal/grid laser had superior VA and OCT outcomes compared with focal/grid laser treatment alone. Although intravitreal triamcinolone combined with focal/grid laser did not result in superior VA outcomes compared with laser alone, an analysis limited to pseudophakic eyes showed that the triamcinolone group's outcome for VA appeared to be of similar magnitude to that of the 2 ranibizumab groups.

Sickle Cell (SC) Retinopathy

Proliferative retinopathy, usually equatorial or pre-equatorial

Most severe in HbSC disease; SC > S Thal > SS > SA

Incidence in African American population: SS = 1%; sickle trait = 8%; SC <0.5%;

20–60% autoinfarct, unlike DR, neovascularization can regress spontaneously and involute

Findings: salmon patch (intraretinal hemorrhage following peripheral retinal arteriolar occlusion), black sunburst (chorioretinal scar with RPE proliferation due to old hemorrhage), sea fan (peripheral NV), refractile spots (old, resorbed hemorrhages), silver wiring of peripheral vessels, angioid streaks, vascular occlusions (macular arteriolar occlusions [wedge sign], CRAO, RVO, choroid; CRAO can develop in patients with hyphema), venous tortuosity, comma-shaped conjunctival vessels, vitreous hemorrhage, rhegmatogenous and traction RD (due to contracture of NV fronds) (Figures 11-63 to 11-65)

   Stage 1: Peripheral arterial occlusions
   Stage 2: Peripheral anastomoses
   Stage 3: Neovascularization (sea fan) at posterior border of areas of non-perfusion
   Stage 4: Vitreous hemorrhage
   Stage 5: Vitreous traction with RD

Diagnosis: sickle cell prep, Hgb electrophoresis

FA: capillary nonperfusion, AV anastomoses, neovascularization (Figure 11-66)

Treatment: laser (PRP) or consider cryotherapy (controversial) for neovascularization; surgery for RD and chronic VH; risk of anterior segment ischemia if encircling scleral buckle placed or large volume of intraocular gas; try to avoid epinephrine in infusion fluid during surgery

Eales' Disease

Idiopathic retinal perivasculitis and peripheral nonperfusion with NV
Occurs in healthy young men; 90% bilateral
More common in Middle East and India
Increased risk of BVO

Findings: NV (80%, NVD or NVE), recurrent VH, rubeosis, neovascular glaucoma, cataract, vascular sheathing (80%) with leakage on FA, vascular tortuosity, collateral

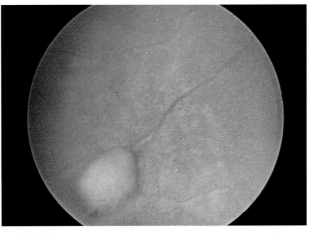

Figure 11-63. An equatorial 'salmon patch' intraretinal hemorrhage with periarteriolar hemorrhage. (Courtesy of William Tasman, MD. From Ho AC: Hemoglobinopathies. In: Yanoff M, Duker JS (eds) Ophthalmology. London, Mosby, 1999.)

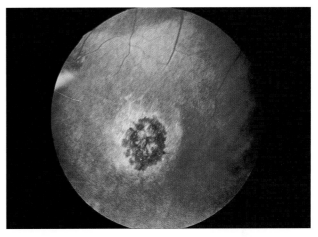

Figure 11-64. A black 'sunburst' retinal lesion. (From Ho AC: Hemoglobinopathies. In: Yanoff M, Duker JS (eds) Ophthalmology. London, Mosby, 1999.)

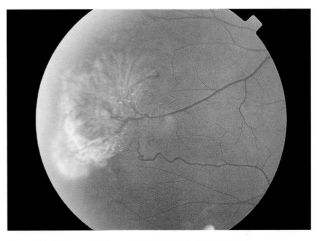

Figure 11-65. A sea fan in a sickle SC patient. (From Ho AC: Hemoglobinopathies. In: Yanoff M, Duker JS (eds) Ophthalmology. London, Mosby, 1999.)

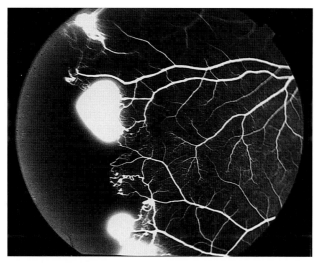

Figure 11-66. Fluorescein angiography of sea fans with peripheral nonperfusion. (From Ho AC: Hemoglobinopathies. In: Yanoff M, Duker JS (eds) Ophthalmology. London, Mosby, 1999.)

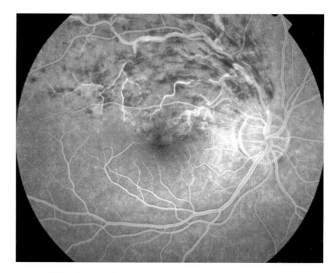

Figure 11-67. BVO. Early leakage.

formation around occluded vessels, peripheral nonperfusion; may have AC reaction, KP, vitreous cells, macular edema

Stage 1: sheathing of retinal venules, retinal edema, hemorrhages
Stage 2: more severe involvement and vitreous haze
Stage 3: peripheral NV
Stage 4: proliferative retinopathy with VH and TRD

Other findings: vestibulocochlear involvement (sensorineural hearing loss and vestibular dysfunction), PPD-positive, cerebral vasculitis (rare), epistaxis

DDx of peripheral neovascularization:
hemoglobinopathies, diabetes, retinal vein occlusions, ROP, FEVR, retinal emboli (talc), hyperviscosity syndromes, carotid-cavernous sinus fistula, ocular ischemia, sarcoidosis, lupus, inflammatory bowel disease, retinal vasculitis, uveitis, VKH syndrome, pars planitis, Norrie's disease, incontinentia pigmenti

Retinopathy of Prematurity (ROP; Retrolental Fibroplasia)

(See Ch. 5, Pediatrics/Strabismus.)

Familial Exudative Vitreoretinopathy (FEVR)

(See Ch. 5, Pediatrics/Strabismus.)

Branch Retinal Vein Occlusion (BVO)

Site of occlusion is at AV crossing (usually thickened artery compresses vein in common adventitial sheath); generally superotemporal (63%)
Associated with increased age (>60 years), cardiovascular disease, hypertension, increased BMI at age 20, glaucoma, papilledema, optic disc drusen, and high serum alpha$_2$-globulin. Note: diabetes is *not* a risk factor. Decreased

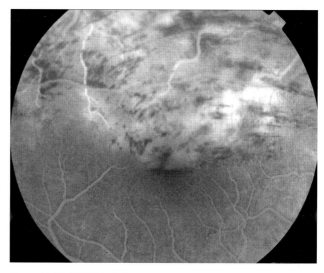

Figure 11-68. BVO. Late leakage.

incidence with high levels of HDL cholesterol and light to moderate alcohol consumption (especially after ophthalmology board exams)

Types:
Nonischemic: <5 DD of capillary nonperfusion
Ischemic: ≥5 DD of capillary nonperfusion

Findings: numerous deep and superficial hemorrhages (in a wedge-shaped distribution with the tip pointing toward the etiologic crossing), cotton wool spots, CME, disc edema (Figures 11-67, 11-68)

Treatment: sector PRP for NV and VH, grid laser for macular edema when vision <20/40 for at least 3 months and no macular ischemia on FA; recent studies with intravitreal anti-VEGF and steroids agents have shown better results than laser

Branch Vein Occlusion Study (BVOS):

Perform grid argon laser for macular edema and vision <20/40 for >3 months (treated eyes more likely to have improved vision: +6.7 letters vs. +1 letter with observation)

Perform PRP for ≥5 DD of nonperfusion if neovascularization develops (treated eyes less likely to develop NV and VH)

BRAVO

Intravitreal injection of ranibizumab (Lucentis, Genentech) for macular edema

GENEVA (Global Evaluation of Implantable Dexamethasone in Retinal Vein Occlusion with Macular Edema) Study

Intravitreal injection of sustained release dexamethasone intravitreal implant (Ozurdex, Allergan) for macular edema

Prognosis: 30% have spontaneous recovery; >50% maintain vision better than 20/40 after 1 year; 10% have episode in fellow eye

Complications:

Nonischemic BVO: macular edema can develop

Ischemic BVO: macular edema, ischemic maculopathy, neovascularization, vitreous hemorrhage, tractional or rhegmatogenous RD; 40% risk of developing NV (NVI rare)

Central Retinal Vein Occlusion (CVO)

Thrombosis of central retinal vein at or posterior to the lamina cribrosa

Types:

Perfused/non-ischemic (70%): vision >20/200, 16% progress to nonperfused; 50% resolve completely without treatment; defined as <10 DD of capillary nonperfusion (Figure 11-69)

Non-perfused/ischemic (30%): ≥10 DD non-perfusion; patients are older and have worse vision; 60% develop iris NV; up to 33% develop neovascular glaucoma (NVG; '90-day' glaucoma since it occurs 3–5 months after occlusion); extensive hemorrhage with marked venous dilation and cotton wool spots; very poor prognosis with only 10% having better than 20/400 vision (Figure 11-70)

10% combined with BRAO (usually cilioretinal artery due to low perfusion pressure of choroidal system)

Risk factors: age (>50 years old in 90%), hypertension (61%), diabetes (unlike BVO), heart disease, glaucoma, increased ESR in women, syphilis, sarcoidosis, vasculitis, increased intraorbital or intraocular pressure, hyphema, hyperviscosity syndromes (multiple myeloma, Waldenström's macroglobulinemia, leukemia), high homocysteine levels, sickle cell, HIV

Findings: venous dilation and tortuosity, hemorrhages in all 4 quadrants, may have disc edema and macular edema

High-risk characteristics: marked vision loss, numerous cotton wool spots, positive RAPD, dense central scotoma with peripheral field changes on VF, widespread capillary nonperfusion on FA, reduced b-wave-to-a-wave ratio on ERG

Pathology: marked retinal edema, focal retinal necrosis, gliosis; subretinal, intraretinal, and preretinal hemorrhages

Workup: younger patients require more extensive workup including systemic vascular disease (hypertension, diabetes mellitus, cardiovascular disease), blood dyscrasias (polycythemia vera, lymphoma and leukemia), clotting disorders (activated protein C resistance, lupus anticoagulant, anticardiolipin antibodies, protein C and protein S, antithrombin III) paraproteinemia and dysproteinemias, multiple myeloma, cryoglobulinemia, vasculitis, syphilis, sarcoidosis, autoimmune disease, systemic lupus erythematosus, oral contraceptive use in women, other rare associations (closed-head trauma, optic disc drusen, arteriovenous malformations of retina)

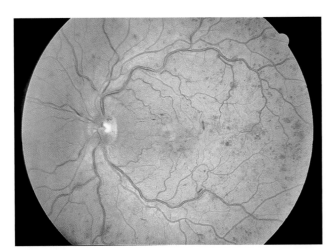

Figure 11-69. Nonischemic central retinal vein occlusion. (From Heier JS, Morley MG: Venous obstructive disease of the retina. In: Yanoff M, Duker JS (eds) Ophthalmology. London, Mosby, 1999.)

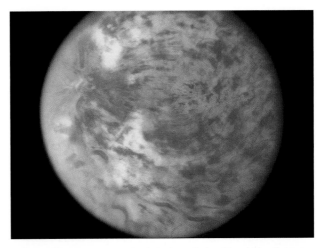

Figure 11-70. Ischemic central retinal vein occlusion. (From Heier JS, Morley MG: Venous obstructive disease of the retina. In: Yanoff M, Duker JS (eds) Ophthalmology. London, Mosby, 1999.)

Treatment: follow every month for first 6 months, including gonioscopy; Intravitreal steroids or anti-VEGF agents for macular edema

    Central Vein Occlusion Study (CVOS):

        No benefit from early PRP (to prevent iris NV) in ischemic CVO; therefore, wait until first sign of NV

        No benefit from focal laser for macular edema

    CRUISE:

        Intravitreal injection of ranibizumab (Lucentis, Genentech) for macular edema

    COPERNICUS/GALILEO Studies:

        Intravitreal injection of aflibercept (VEGF Trap Eye, Regeneron) for macular edema

    GENEVA (Global Evaluation of Implantable Dexamethasone in Retinal Vein Occlusion with Macular Edema) Study:

        Intravitreal injection of dexamethasone sustained-release intravitreal implant (Ozurdex, Allergan) for macular edema [as of 2011 the only FDA-approved treatment for macular edema from vein occlusion]; time to first gain of ≥15 letters was faster with the biodegradable implant compared with observation with 20–30% 3-line gainers. Watch IOP as 25% eyes increased.

Prognosis: >75% have disease progression.

Complications: iris NV (more common than NVD or NVE), NVG, TRD, VH, and macular edema

Hemiretinal Vein Occlusion (HRVO)

Risk factors: hypertension, diabetes, glaucoma

Ischemic HRVO: higher risk of NVD (30%) or NVE (40%) than with either an ischemic CVO or a BVO; NVI in 10%

MAJOR RETINAL VEIN OCCLUSION CLINICAL STUDIES

Branch Vein Occlusion Study (BVOS)

Objective: to evaluate photocoagulation in patients with branch vein occlusion (BVO) for:

1. Prevention of neovascularization
2. Prevention of vitreous hemorrhage
3. Improvement of vision in eyes with macular edema, reducing vision to 20/40 or worse

Methods:

    Group I (at risk for neovascularization): patients with BVO occurring within 3–18 months with an area of retinal involvement at least 5 DD in size, with no neovascularization present and vision better than 5/200, were randomly assigned to peripheral scatter laser photocoagulation vs observation

    Group II (at risk for vitreous hemorrhage): patients with BVO occurring within 3–18 months with disc or peripheral neovascularization and vision better than 5/200 were randomly assigned to peripheral scatter laser photocoagulation vs observation

    Group III (at risk for vision loss due to macular edema): patients with BVO occurring within 3–18 months with macular edema involving the fovea and vision worse than 20/40 were randomly assigned to grid pattern laser photocoagulation with argon laser vs observation

    Group X (at high risk for neovascularization): patients with BVO occurring within 3–18 months with at least 5 DD of capillary nonperfusion were followed. Note: This group was recruited after group I recruitment had ended

Results:

    Group 1: 319 patients enrolled. After an average follow-up of 3.7 years, the development of neovascularization was significantly less in laser-treated eyes. Treated eyes were less likely to develop NV (12% vs 24% of untreated)

    Group II: 82 eyes enrolled. After an average follow-up of 2.8 years, the development of vitreous hemorrhage was significantly less in the laser-treated eyes. Treated eyes were less likely to develop VH (29% vs 61% of untreated)

    Group III: 139 patients enrolled. After an average follow-up of 3.1 years, treated eyes were more likely to have improved vision (gain of ≥2 lines in 65% vs 37% of untreated), vision >20/40, and final average vision better than untreated eyes

    Group X: eyes with ≥5 DD of nonperfusion were considered nonperfused and showed a greater risk of developing neovascularization

Conclusions:

    Grid pattern laser photocoagulation recommended for eyes with a BVO of 3–18 months duration if visual acuity is 20/40 or worse *and* if fluorescein angiography documents macular edema without foveal hemorrhage as the cause of visual loss

    Perform PRP if retinal neovascularization develops, especially if ≥5 DD of nonperfusion exists

The Standard Care vs Corticosteroid for Retinal Vein Occlusion (SCORE) Study

Objective: to compare intravitreal triamcinolone to observation in retinal vein occlusion

Methods: Patients >18 years old with center-involved macular edema due to CVO or BVO of at least 3 months' duration but no longer than 18 months with central retinal thickness >250 µm on OCT and ETDRS visual acuity score 20/40–20/200 randomized to either 1 mg or

4 mg doses of preservative-free intravitreal triamcinolone acetonide (TA) versus standard of care (observation in CVO, and focal laser in BVO). The primary outcome was ≥3 line gainers at month 12. All patients will be followed and retreated as needed every 4 months for 3 years

Results: 271 patients enrolled. For CVO, the patients with ≥3 line gain in vision at month 12 (primary outcome) was 7% in the observation group ($n = 73$), 27% in the 1 mg TA group ($n = 83$) and 26% in the 4 mg TA group ($n = 82$). The mean change in vision at 12 months was −12.1 letters in the observation group, −1.2 letters in the 1 mg TA group and −1.2 letters in the 4 mg TA group. For BVO, the patients with ≥3 line gain in vision at month 12 (primary outcome) was 29% in the laser group, 26% in the 1 mg TA group and 27% in the 4 mg TA group. Overall, IOP lowering medications were required in 8% in the laser group, 20% in the 1 mg TA group and 35% in the 4 mg TA group. Cataract progression was seen in 18% in the standard of care group, 26% in the 1 mg TA group and 33% in the 4 mg TA group.

Conclusions: Triamcinolone acetonide was superior to observation in CVO (5 times greater chance of gaining 3 lines), but not to laser in BVO. The complications were higher in the 4 mg TA group than the 1 mg TA group, so 1 mg is preferred.

BRAVO Study

Objective: to assess the safety and efficacy profile of ranibizumab (Lucentis, Genentech) in macular edema secondary to branch retinal vein occlusion.

Methods: Multicenter, randomized, double-masked, sham injection-controlled Phase III study of 397 patients designed to assess the safety and efficacy profile of ranibizumab in macular edema secondary to branch-RVO. Patients were included if they were ≥18 years age with foveal center-involved ME secondary to branch/hemi RVO diagnosed within 12 months prior to screening. BCVA 20/40 to 20/400 and retinal thickness ≥250 μm. Patients were randomized to 0.3 mg ranibizumab, 0.5 mg, or sham injections. Laser rescue after 3 months. The primary endpoint was mean change in vision from baseline at 6 months. In the next 6 months, monthly ranibizumab PRN was allowed for all patients with rescue laser at month 9.

Results: At 6 months, the mean change in vision (primary outcome) was +7.3 letters in the sham group ($n = 132$), +16.6 letters in the 0.3 mg ranibizumab group ($n = 134$), and +18.3 letters in the 0.5 mg ranibizumab group ($n = 131$)($P < 0.0001$). In addition, 55% (74/134) of patients who received 0.3 mg of ranibizumab and 61% (80/131) who received 0.5 mg of ranibizumab had their vision improved by ≥15 letters, compared with 29% (38/132) of patients receiving sham injections. Mean gain in BCVA was observed beginning at day seven with a +7.6 and +7.4 letter gain in the 0.3 mg and 0.5 mg study arms of ranibizumab, respectively (compared with +1.9 letters in the sham injection arm).

Conclusions: Ranibizumab injections are safe and effective in branch retinal vein occlusion

Central Vein Occlusion Study (CVOS)

Objective: to evaluate patients with central retinal vein occlusion (CVO) for:
1. Natural history of eyes with perfused (<10 disc areas of nonperfusion) CVO
2. Improvement of vision in eyes with perfused macular edema
3. Eyes with nonperfused CVO; does early PRP prevent NVI?
4. Eyes with nonperfused CVO; is early PRP more effective than delayed PRP in preventing NVG?

Methods:

Group P (perfused): patients with CVO occurring for less than 1 year with intraretinal hemorrhages in all 4 quadrants and with capillary nonperfusion less than 10 DD in size and with no iris or angle neovascularization. These patients were observed; 547 patients enrolled

Group N (nonperfused): patients with CVO occurring for less than 1 year with intraretinal hemorrhages in all 4 quadrants and with capillary nonperfusion greater than 10 DD in size and with no iris or angle neovascularization were randomly assigned to immediate PRP or observation; 180 patients enrolled

Group I (indeterminate): patients with CVO occurring for less than 1 year with intraretinal hemorrhages in all 4 quadrants and with retinal hemorrhages that prevent measurement of the area of capillary nonperfusion and with no iris or angle neovascularization. These patients were followed; 52 eyes enrolled

Group M (macular edema): patients with CVO occurring for at least 3 months with macular edema that involves the fovea and with visual acuity of 20/50 to 5/200 were randomly assigned to grid pattern laser photocoagulation or observation; 155 eyes enrolled

Results:

Group P: 34% became nonperfused at 3 years
RISK FACTORS FOR PROGRESSION TO NONPERFUSED: CVO of less than 1 month duration, visual acuity less than 20/200, presence of greater than 5 disc areas of nonperfusion
Group N: prophylactic PRP did not prevent iris or angle NV (18 of 90 eyes [20%] with prophylactic PRP developed iris or angle NV, vs 32 of 91 eyes [35%] that did not receive prophylactic PRP), eyes

prophylactically treated with PRP did not respond well to supplemental PRP (18 of 32 [56%] observation eyes responded to PRP following development of iris or angle NV, vs 4 of 18 eyes [22%] that received prophylactic PRP responded to supplemental PRP).

RISK FACTORS FOR DEVELOPING NVI: amount of nonperfused retina, extent of retinal hemorrhages, male sex, CVO of less than 1-month duration

Group M: grid pattern photocoagulation did not preserve or improve visual acuity (but reduced angiographic evidence of macular edema)

Conclusions:

No benefit from early PRP in nonperfused CVO; therefore, wait until first sign of NVI before initiating PRP

PRP for nonperfused CVO when 2 clock hours of NVI or any angle NV present

Monthly follow-up with gonioscopy during first 6 months after CVO

No benefit from focal laser for treatment of macular edema after CVO

CRUISE Study

Objective: to assess the safety and efficacy profile of ranibizumab (Lucentis, Genentech) in macular edema secondary to central-RVO.

Methods: multicenter, randomized, double-masked, sham injection-controlled Phase III study designed to assess the safety and efficacy profile of ranibizumab in 392 patients with macular edema secondary to central-RVO. Patients were included if they were ≥18 years age with foveal center-involved ME secondary central RVO diagnosed within 12 months prior to screening. BCVA 20/40 to 20/400 and baseline retinal thickness ≥250 μm. Patients were randomized to 0.3 mg ranibizumab, 0.5 mg, or sham injections. The primary endpoint was mean change in vision from baseline at 6 months. In the next 6 months, monthly ranibizumab PRN was allowed for all patients.

Results: at 6 months, the mean change in vision (primary outcome) was +0.8 letters in the sham group ($n = 130$), +12.7 letters in the 0.3 mg ranibizumab group ($n = 132$), and +14.9 letters in the 0.5 mg ranibizumab group ($n = 130$)($P < 0.0001$). In addition, 46% (61/132) of patients given 0.3 mg of ranibizumab and 48% (62/130) given 0.5 mg of ranibizumab had their vision improved by ≥15 letters compared with 17% (22/130) of patients receiving sham injections. Mean gain in BCVA was observed beginning at day seven with a +8.8 and +9.3 letter gain in the 0.3 mg and 0.5 mg study arms of ranibizumab, respectively, compared with +1.1 letters in the sham injection arm.

Conclusions: ranibizumab injections are safe and effective in central retinal vein occlusion

Branch Retinal Artery Occlusion (BRAO)

90% caused by emboli (cholesterol, calcium, fibrin, platelets)

Most commonly at retinal arterial bifurcations

10% risk of episode in fellow eye

Central Retinal Artery Occlusion (CRAO)

Most common cause of cherry red spot (thin transparent foveal tissue surrounded by opacified ischemic retina)

Etiology:

Atherosclerosis: of CRA at lamina cribrosa

Emboli: cholesterol (73%), platelet fibrin (15%) from carotid plaque, calcific (from heart especially valves), tumor (atrial myxoma), lipid emboli (pancreatitis), talc

Vasculitis: GCA in elderly patient (always check ESR)

Trauma: retrobulbar injection, orbital surgery, penetrating injury

Coagulopathy: oral contraceptives, pregnancy, sickle cell (especially after hyphema), platelet or factor abnormalities, homocystinuria, hyperhomocysteinemia, protein S deficiency, antiphospholipid antibody (check anticardiolipin antibody panel; also at risk for DVT, pulmonary embolism, cardiac vessel blockage, and spontaneous abortion; treat with coumadin; steroids do not decrease risk of thromboembolism)

Ocular abnormalities: optic disc drusen, prepapillary loops, elevated IOP

Collagen vascular disease: lupus, polyarteritis nodosa, Wegener's granulomatosis

Migraine: in young patients

Orbital mucor

Fibromuscular hyperplasia

Behçet's disease

Leukemia

Findings: severe visual loss (LP to CF vision in 90%), retinal whitening in posterior pole with cherry red spot, box-carring (interruption of blood column), emboli, positive RAPD; whitening resolves after 4–6 weeks, and pale disc and attenuated vessels develop

Pathology: atrophy of inner retinal layers (those supplied by retinal circulation) (Figure 11-71)

DDx: ophthalmic artery occlusion, inadvertent intraocular injection of gentamicin, arteritic AION (check ESR and C-reactive protein)

DDx of cherry red spot: sphingolipidosis (Tay-Sachs, Niemann-Pick, Gaucher's, Farber's disease), quinine toxicity, commotio retinae, macular hole with surrounding RD, macular hemorrhage, subacute sclerosing panencephalitis, ocular ischemia, methanol toxicity

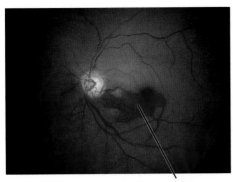

Retinal edema   Patent
                 cilioretinal
                 artery

Figure 11-71. Cilioretinal artery-sparing central retinal artery occlusion with patent cilioretinal artery, allowing perfusion (thus no edema) in a small section of the macula. (From Kaiser PK, Friedman NJ, Pineda R II: Massachusetts Eye and Ear Infirmary Illustrated Manual of Ophthalmology, 2nd edn. Philadelphia, Saunders, 2004.)

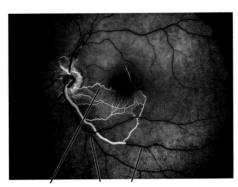

Patent   Absent flow
cilioretinal
artery

Figure 11-72. Fluorescein angiogram of the same patient as in Figure 11-71, demonstrating no filling of retinal vessels except in cilioretinal artery and surrounding branches. (From Kaiser PK, Friedman NJ, Pineda R II: Massachusetts Eye and Ear Infirmary Illustrated Manual of Ophthalmology, 2nd edn. Philadelphia, Saunders, 2004.)

Diagnosis:
Lab tests: CBC, ESR, complete cardiovascular workup; consider workup for clotting disorders: serum protein electrophoresis, protein C, activated protein C resistance (factor 5 Lieden deficiency), protein S, antithrombin III, anticardiolipin antibodies, lupus anticoagulant, plasma homocysteine, C-ANCA
FA: delayed filling, increased AV transit time, focal staining at obstruction, collateral or retrograde flow (Figure 11-72)
ERG: depressed b-wave (inner retina), normal/supernormal a-wave, loss of oscillatory potentials

Treatment: irreversible damage occurs after 90 minutes; therefore, emergent lowering of IOP to allow arterial pressure to re-establish blood flow: paracentesis, ocular massage, carbogen (95% O_2, 5% CO_2) or breath into paper bag, oral and topical ocular hypotensive agents may be tried; PRP for neovascular complications

Prognosis: 10% recover vision (usually from cilioretinal artery [in 25% of population]), 18% have vision ≥20/40, 66% have vision ≤20/400; <5% develop neovascular glaucoma; 1% with bilateral disease; 10% risk of episode in fellow eye

Complications: rubeosis (15%)

Ophthalmic Artery Occlusion

NLP vision and no cherry red spot; RPE pigmentary changes develop

May occur with orbital mucormycosis

FA: absent choroidal and retinal filling

ERG: absent a-wave

Ocular Ischemic Syndrome

Reduced blood flow to globe produces anterior and/or posterior segment ischemia

Etiology: carotid occlusion (most common, usually >90% obstruction), carotid dissection, arteritis (rare)
Associated with diabetes (56%), hypertension (50%), coronary artery disease (38%), CVA/TIA (31%)

Symptoms: amaurosis fugax, gradual or sudden visual loss, dull pain (improves on lying down); may experience transient visual loss, sometimes precipitated by exposure to bright light (due to impaired photoreceptor regeneration)

Findings:
Anterior segment: chronic conjunctival injection, rubeosis and neovascularization of the iris (NVI) common (IOP often not elevated due to ciliary body shutdown), PAS, AC cells and flare, corneal edema, cataract, altered IOP, hypopyon (rare)
Posterior segment: vitreous cells, NV, optic disc pallor (40%), optic nerve swelling (8%), superficial hemorrhages in midperiphery, CME, cherry red spot (18%), altered vessels (attenuated, box-carring, dilated, nontortuous veins) (Figure 11-73)

DDx: aortic arch disease, Takayasu's disease

Diagnosis: digital pressure on eye causes arterial pulsation
FA: delayed filling (retina and choroid), diffuse leakage (Figure 11-74)
Ophthalmodynamometry: decreased retinal arterial pressure
Carotid ultrasound: severe stenosis (>80%)

Treatment: lower IOP to increase perfusion pressure, carotid surgery; PRP (controversial because anterior segment

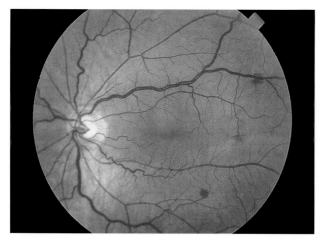

Figure 11-73. Retinal vascular changes in ocular ischemic syndrome. (From Fox GM, Sivalingham A, Brown CG: Ocular ischemic syndrome. In: Yanoff M, Duker JS (eds) Ophthalmology. London, Mosby, 1999.)

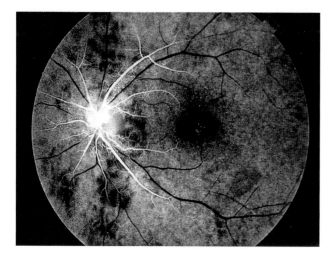

Figure 11-74. Fluorescein angiography, ocular ischemic syndrome. (From Fox GM, Sivalingham A, Brown CG: Ocular ischemic syndrome. In: Yanoff M, Duker JS (eds) Ophthalmology. London, Mosby, 1999.)

ischemia can possibly be due to uveal ischemia without retinal ischemia); carotid endarterectomy (CEA) beneficial when carotid stenosis 70–99% (not possible when 100%) – may lead to increased IOP from improved ciliary body perfusion

Radiation Retinopathy

Slowly progressive microangiopathy following exposure to radiation (6 months to 3 years after radiation treatment)

Threshold dose is 300 rads (3 Gy); occurs 4–32 months following plaque brachytherapy with mean dose of 15,000 rads (150 Gy); occurs 36 months after external beam radiation with mean dose of 5000 rads (50 Gy)

Findings: hemorrhage, exudate, microaneurysms, capillary nonperfusion, cotton wool spots, NV, optic disc swelling,

optic neuropathy; gradual occlusion of larger retinal vessels, eventually proliferative retinopathy

Pathology: vascular decompensation with focal loss of capillary endothelial cells and pericytes; radiation-induced optic neuropathy: ischemic demyelination with obliterative endarteritis of nerve sheath vasculature

Treatment: focal laser for macular edema, PRP for NV; hyperbaric O_2 (controversial)

Certain types of chemotherapy and pre-existing vascular compromise (e.g. diabetic or hypertensive retinopathy) can worsen radiation retinopathy

Hypercoagulable States

Etiology: antiphospholipid antibodies (lupus anticoagulant) and anticardiolipins, Waldenström's macroglobulinemia, leukemia

Findings: cotton wool spots, blot hemorrhages, box-carring, capillary nonperfusion, arteriolar attenuation

Disseminated Intravascular Coagulation

May cause fibrinoid necrosis of choriocapillaris, serous retinal detachments, and multiple areas of RPE changes

Phakomatoses

(See Ch. 5, Pediatrics/Strabismus.)

Inflammatory/Immune Disease

(See Ch. 8, Uveitis.)

Infections

(See Ch. 8, Uveitis.)

Neuroretinitis

Usually unilateral

50% have viral prodrome

Symptoms: decreased vision; colors appear washed out; rarely, retrobulbar pain, pain associated with eye movement, or headache

Findings: optic nerve swelling (optic atrophy can develop), peripapillary NFL hemorrhages, serous RD; iritis, vitritis, and/or scleritis (rare); vascular occlusions may develop

Etiology:

Noninfectious: cerebral AV malformation, elevated ICP, malignant hypertension, ischemic optic neuropathy, polyarteritis nodosa, Leber's idiopathic stellate neuroretinitis

LEBER'S IDIOPATHIC STELLATE NEURORETINITIS (LISN):

Affects individuals age 8–55 years old (usually in 3rd decade); male = female; >70% unilateral

Viral prodrome in 5%

FINDINGS: decreased vision; positive RAPD (75%); cecocentral or central scotoma; vitreous cells; optic disc edema (resolves over 8–12 weeks); optic atrophy is rare; macular star develops in 2nd week; exudative peripapillary RD can occur; RPE defects late; rarely develop chorioretinitis with elevated yellow-white spots in deep retina

FA: hot disc; no perifoveal capillary leakage or macular abnormalities

PROGNOSIS: excellent

Infectious (suggested by multiple areas of retinitis): syphilis, Lyme disease, viral (influenza A, mumps, coxsackie B, EBV), cat-scratch disease (*Bartonella henselae*), TB, *Salmonella typhi*, parasites (*Toxocara, Toxoplasma,* DUSN)

DIFFUSE UNILATERAL SUBACUTE NEURORETINITIS (DUSN):

Due to subretinal nematode: *Ancylostoma caninum* (dog hookworm), *Baylisascaris procyonis* (raccoon worm)

Chronic course

Does not have characteristic neuroretinitis appearance

FINDINGS: multifocal pigmentary changes due to movement of the worm, minimal intraocular inflammation, decreased vision (typically out of proportion to findings); may have positive RAPD. Late findings include visual field defects, optic nerve pallor, chorioretinal atrophy, and narrowed retinal vessels

DIAGNOSIS: stool for ova and parasites, CBC with differential (eosinophilia sometimes present); LDH and SGOT sometimes elevated

FA: early hypofluorescence and late staining of lesions, perivascular leakage, and disc staining; multifocal window defects in late disease

ERG: subnormal, loss of b-wave

TREATMENT: laser photocoagulation of the worm; rarely subretinal surgery to remove worm (controversial)

Systemic antihelmintic medications (thiabendazole, diethylcarbamazine, pyrantel pamoate) are controversial and often not effective; steroids are usually added because worm death may increase inflammation

PROGNOSIS: poor without treatment; variable if worm can be killed with treatment

DDx of optic nerve swelling and macular star:

Leber's idiopathic stellate neuroretinitis, syphilis, hypertension, trauma, acute febrile illness (measles, influenza), TB, coccidiomycosis, cat-scratch disease, papillitis, papilledema, AION (macular star rare), DUSN (macular star rare)

Diagnosis:

Lab tests: ESR, VDRL, FTA-ABS, Lyme titer, *Bartonella* serology, *Toxoplasma* and *Toxocara* titers, PPD

FA: diffuse leakage from disc, peripapillary capillary staining; 10% have disc leakage in fellow eye; no leakage in macula

Treatment: treat underlying disease, observe idiopathic form; most recover ≥20/50 after 3 months; only 3–5% have permanent severe visual loss

HIV Retinopathy

Microangiopathy in up to 50% of human immunodeficiency virus (RNA retrovirus) infected individuals due to complement deposition (not infectious)

Asymptomatic, non-progressive

Findings: cotton wool spots, Roth spots, hemorrhages, and microaneurysms in posterior pole; many HIV-positive patients have early presbyopia caused by inflammation of ciliary body with loss of accommodative amplitude

Diagnosis: HIV antibody test, CD4 count, HIV viral load

Treatment: none; spontaneous resolution within 1–2 months

Toxic Retinopathies

Aminoglycosides (Gentamicin / Tobramycin / Amikacin)

Findings: acute, severe, permanent visual loss after intraocular injection of toxic doses with marked retinal whitening (especially in macula) and retinal hemorrhages; optic atrophy and pigmentary changes occur later

Toxic dose: seen after injecting 0.1 mg of gentamicin (also described after diffusion through cataract wound from subconjunctival injection)

FA: sharp zones of capillary nonperfusion corresponding to the areas of ischemic retina

No effective treatment with poor visual prognosis

Chloroquine (Aralen) / Hydroxychloroquine (Plaquenil)

Binds to melanin in RPE; ganglion cells are also directly affected

Toxic dose: chloroquine >3.0 mg/kg/day or 300 g total; hydroxychloroquine >6.5 mg/kg/day or 700 g total; <400 mg/day appears safe; total dose is more important than daily dose

Findings: early, mild mottling of perifoveal RPE with decreased foveal reflex; progresses to bull's-eye maculopathy;

peripheral pigmentary retinopathy, eyelash whitening, and cornea vortex keratopathy may develop

DDx of bull's-eye maculopathy: cone dystrophy, AMD, Stargardt's disease, fundus flavimaculatus, Spielmeyer-Vogt disease, albinism, fenestrated sheen macular dystrophy, central areolar choroidal dystrophy, benign concentric annular macular dystrophy, clofazimine toxicity, fucosidosis

VF: decreased; small, paracentral scotoma to red test object on tangent screen

ERG: enlarged a-wave, depressed b-wave

EOG: depressed

OCT: ring of outer retinal thinning

Progression of retinopathy can occur after cessation of medication; vision loss rarely recovers

Thioridazine (Mellaril)

Concentrates in uveal tissue with RPE damage, decreased vision, nyctalopia, and sometimes altered color vision

Toxic dose: >1200 mg/day

Findings: peripheral pigmentary retinopathy, pigment deposition in eyelids, cornea, and lens (Figure 11-75)

ERG: depressed a and b-waves

Progression of retinopathy can occur after cessation of medication

Chlorpromazine (Thorazine)

Toxic dose: 1200–2400 mg/day for at least 12 months

Findings: pigment deposition in eyelids, cornea, lens, and retina

Chloramphenicol

Atrophy of maculopapillar bundle

VF: cecocentral scotoma

Quinine

Findings: fine RPE mottling, retinal vascular attenuation, disc pallor
  Toxicity causes blurred vision, visual field loss, photophobia, sometimes transient blindness; patient may become comatose
  Acute toxicity (single dose of 4 g): blurred vision, nyctalopia, nausea, loss of hearing, drowsiness, dilated pupils, retinal opacification with cherry red spot, dilated retinal vessels; after acute phase resolves, vision can improve

Tamoxifen

Toxic dose: >30 mg/day
Asymptomatic

Findings: fleck-like crystalline retinopathy with refractile retinal deposits, typically in ring around macula; may develop pigmentary retinal changes and mild CME (Figure 11-76)

FA: macular edema

Canthaxanthine

Toxic dose: >35 g (cumulative) of this oral tanning agent

Symptoms: asymptomatic, or mild metamorphopsia

Findings: refractile yellow deposits in a ring around the fovea; 'gold-dust' retinopathy (Figure 11-77)

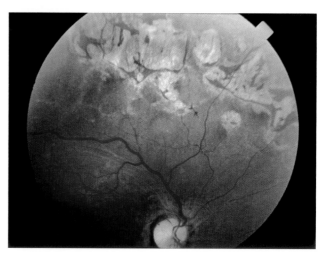

Figure 11-75. Thioridazine retinopathy associated with chronic use (nummular retinopathy). (From Weinberg DV, D'Amico DJ: Retinal toxicity of systemic drugs. In: Albert DM, Jakobiec FA (eds) Principles and Practice of Ophthalmology. Philadelphia, WB Saunders, 1994.)

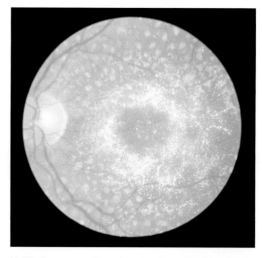

Figure 11-76. Severe tamoxifen retinopathy. (From McKeown CA, Swartz M, Blom J, et al: Tamoxifen retinopathy. Br J Ophthalmol 65:177–179, 1981.)

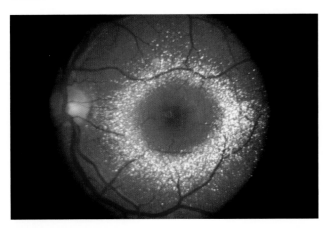

Figure 11-77. Canthaxanthine retinopathy. (From Weinberg DV, D'Amico DJ: Retinal toxicity of systemic drugs. In: Albert DM, Jakobiec FA (eds) Principles and Practice of Ophthalmology. Philadelphia, WB Saunders, 1994.)

Methoxyflurane

Crystalline retinopathy due to oxalate crystals

Methoxyflurane is metabolized to oxalate, which binds with calcium to form insoluble calcium oxalate salt

Crystals are permanent

Talc

Particles deposit in blood vessels of IV drug users; appear as tiny crystals

Talc deposits in lungs; with prolonged abuse pulmonary AV shunts develop and talc passes into systemic circulation

Talc emboli can cause arteriolar occlusions, resulting in ischemic maculopathy, retinal NV, and VH

Treatment: consider PRP for neovascularization

Nicotinic Acid Maculopathy

Atypical nonleaking CME due to intracellular edema of Müller's cells

Blurred vision with metamorphopsia

FA: CME does not leak

Digoxin

Direct effect on cones; causes visual disturbance with minimal fundus changes

Findings: xanthopsia (yellow vision), blurred vision, poor color vision, paracentral scotomas, and reduced vision with increased background light

Ergotamine

Vasoconstriction of retinal vessels, CME, CVO, papillitis, optic disc pallor; orthostatic hypotension, postpartum hemorrhages

Oral Contraceptives

Associated with thromboembolic disease

May develop CME, retinal hemorrhages, vascular occlusions

Gentamicin

Intraocular injection can cause rapid macular ischemia, optic atrophy, RPE changes, neovascular glaucoma

Macular infarction can occur with 400 μm

Interferon

Presumed to be due to immune complex deposition in retinal vasculature followed by white blood cell infiltration with eventual vascular closure

Findings: cotton wool spots, hemorrhages, macular edema, capillary nonperfusion, vascular occlusions

May exacerbate autoimmune thyroiditis and polyarthropathy

Sildenafil (Viagra) / Tadalafil (Cialis) / Vardenafil (Levitra)

May cause transient blue hue to vision 1–2 hours after ingestion, possibly by changing the transduction cascade in photoreceptors

ERG: mildly reduced photopic and scotopic b-wave amplitudes and less than 10% decrease in photopic a- and b-wave implicit times during acute episode, reverts back to normal over time

For Viagra, occurs in 3% of individuals taking a dose of 25–50 mg, 11% of patients taking 100 mg dose, and in 50% taking >100 mg; no permanent effects seen

Inherited Retinal Diseases

(See Ch. 5, Pediatrics/Strabismus.)

Metabolic Diseases

(See Ch. 5, Pediatrics/Strabismus.)

Vitreoretinal Disorders

(See Ch. 5, Pediatrics/Strabismus.)

Degenerations

(Table 11-5)

Oral Bay

Oval island of pars plana epithelium immediately posterior to ora serrata (Figure 11-78); retinal break may occur

Table 11-5. Classification of retinal degenerations

Benign	Predisposing to RD
White without pressure	Lattice degeneration
Pigment clumping	Snail track degeneration
Diffuse chorioretinal atrophy	Zonuloretinal traction tufts
Peripheral microcystoid changes	Snowflake degeneration
Pavingstone degeneration	
Oral pigmentary degeneration	
Degenerative 'senile' retinoschisis	

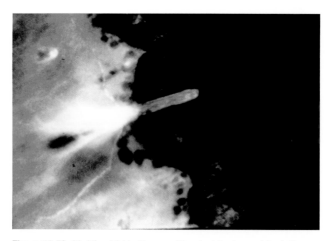

Figure 11-79. Meridional fold with a small break at the base of the fold. (From Tasman WS: Peripheral retinal lesions. In: Yanoff M, Duker JS (eds) Ophthalmology. London, Mosby, 1999.)

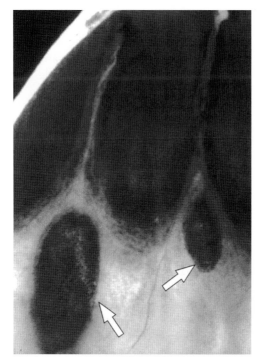

Figure 11-78. Enclosed oral bays. (From Tasman WS: Peripheral retinal lesions. In: Yanoff M, Duker JS (eds) Ophthalmology. London, Mosby, 1999.)

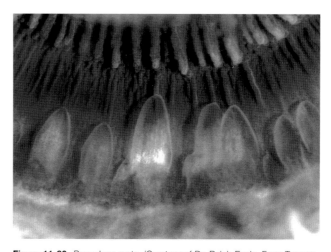

Figure 11-80. Pars plana cysts. (Courtesy of Dr. Ralph Eagle. From Tasman WS: Peripheral retinal lesions. In: Yanoff M, Duker JS (eds) Ophthalmology. London, Mosby, 1999.)

Meridional Fold

Elevated fold of retina in upper nasal quadrant

20% prevalence

Retinal break may occur (Figure 11-79)

Meridional Complex

Meridional fold extending to posterior aspect of a ciliary process

Retinal break may occur

Normal variation of anatomy at ora serrata

Vitreoretinal Tuft

Small internal projection of retinal tissue

Noncystic retinal tuft: short, thin (base <0.1 mm) projection of fibroglial tissue; can break off, leaving fragments in vitreous; usually inferonasal; not associated with retinal break; not present at birth

Cystic retinal tuft: chalky white, nodular projection (base 0.1–1.0 mm) of fibroglial tissue; usually nasal; may have pigment at base; increased vitreous adhesion predisposes to tractional tears from PVD; present at birth; occurs in 5% of population; <1% risk of RD, therefore no prophylactic treatment; associated with 10% of RDs; second to lattice degeneration as visible peripheral retinal lesion associated with RD

Zonular traction tuft: thin strand of fibroglial tissue extending from peripheral retina anteriorly to a zonule; usually nasal; present at birth; break occurs in 2–10%

Pars Plana Cyst (Figure 11-80)

Clear cystoid space between pigmented and nonpigmented ciliary epithelium of pars plana; filled with mucopolysaccharides (hyaluronic acid)

Not a true cyst (not lined with epithelium)

Occurs in 17% of autopsied eyes

Analagous to detachment of sensory retina from underlying RPE; caused by traction by vitreous base and zonules; no increased risk of RD

Stains with Alcian blue

Also seen in conditions with formation of abnormal proteins (multiple myeloma)

Ora Serrata Pearl

Glistening opacity over oral tooth

Increased prevalence with age

Resembles drusen

White With/Without Pressure

Geographic areas of peripheral retinal whitening

More common in young individuals, African Americans, and myopes

White with pressure: visible only with scleral depression

White without pressure: visible without scleral depression

Peripheral Microcystoid Degeneration

Typical/'senile' (Blessig-Iwanoff cysts): outer plexiform layer; bubble-like appearance behind ora serrata; lined by Müller's cells; may coalesce and progress to typical degenerative ('senile') retinoschisis

Reticular: nerve fiber layer; linear or reticular pattern, corresponding to retinal vessels; finely stippled internal surface; continuous with and posterior to typical type (therefore, does not reach the ora); may progress to reticular degenerative retinoschisis

Degenerative (Involutional) 'Senile' Retinoschisis

Occurs in 7–31% of individuals >40 years old, 50–80% bilateral, often symmetric; 70% inferotemporal, 25% superotemporal

Usually asymptomatic and nonprogressive; hyperopia in 70%

Findings: splits or cysts within neurosensory retinal layers; typical peripheral cystoid degeneration is precursor
  Inner wall: smooth, dome-shaped surface; may be markedly elevated in reticular type; sheathed retinal vessels; holes uncommon (small if present)
  Outer wall: pock-marked on scleral depression; holes (16–23%) are larger and well delineated, more common in reticular type, have rolled margins (Figure 11-81)
  Typical: splitting of OPL; bilateral; elderly patients; 1% of adult population; follows coalescence of cavities of microcystoid degeneration; beaten metal appearance;

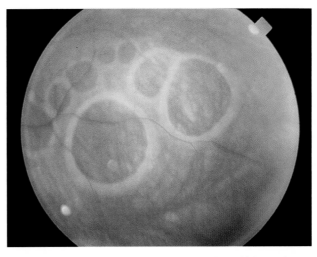

Figure 11-81. Degenerative retinoschisis demonstrating multiple outer layer breaks. (From Tasman WS: Peripheral retinal lesions. In: Yanoff M, Duker JS (eds) Ophthalmology. London, Mosby, 1999.)

white spots (Müller's cell remnants [Gunn's dots]) in stippled pattern along edge appear as glistening dots or snowflakes; inner layer holes can occur; no risk of RD unless outer layer hole is also present; intact outer retinal layer whitens/blanches with scleral depression
  Reticular: splitting of NFL; 41% bilateral; 18% of adult population; always posterior to peripheral cystoid; fine delicately stippled surface

Differentiate from RD: no underlying RPE degeneration, no tobacco dust; absolute scotoma (relative scotoma in RD); laser treatment blanches underlying RPE (RD will not blanch); no shifting fluid; dome shaped

Pathology: cavity contains hyaluronic acid, Müller's cell remnants on inner and outer surfaces of cavity, fibrous thickening of vessel walls with patent lumen

Treatment: laser barrier, treat tears and RD

Complications: RD (from outer layer holes; slowly progressive, unless both outer and inner holes), progression (toward posterior pole; rare through fovea), hemorrhage (into vitreous or schisis cavity)

Pavingstone/Cobblestone Degeneration

Usually inferior; 33% bilateral

Occlusion of choriocapillaris causes loss of outer retinal layers and RPE

Increased incidence with age and myopia (27% in those >20 years old)

No symptoms or complications

Findings: yellow-white spots ½–2 DD in size adjacent to ora; traverse retinal and choroidal vessels; may have irregular black pigmentation at margins

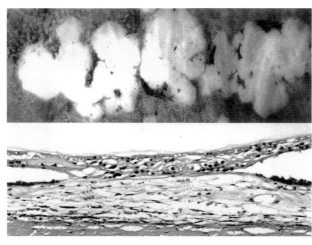

Figure 11-82. Pavingstone degeneration. (Courtesy of Dr. Ralph Eagle. From Tasman WS: Peripheral retinal lesions. In: Yanoff M, Duker JS (eds) Ophthalmology. London, Mosby, 1999.)

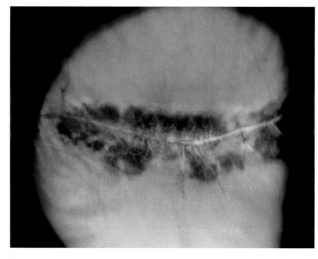

Figure 11-83. Lattice degeneration showing the typical white lines. (From Tasman WS: Peripheral retinal lesions. In: Yanoff M, Duker JS (eds) Ophthalmology. London, Mosby, 1999.)

Pathology: degeneration of choroid and retina; loss of outer retinal layers; RPE absent; firm adhesion between retina and Bruch's membrane/choroid (no predisposition to RD) (Figure 11-82)

Lattice Degeneration

Occurs in 7% of population; more common in myopic eyes; no sex predilection

Often bilateral; usually superotemporal

Present in 20–35% of eyes with RD; 0.5% risk that patient with lattice will develop an RD

Findings: peripheral circumferential cigar-shaped atrophic retinal patches; criss-crossing pattern of sclerosed vessels (fine white lines) within lesion in 12%; superficial white dots in 80% (ILM and inner retina); pigmentary disturbance in 82%; firm adhesions of vitreous at margins; clear pockets of vitreous fluid over central thin portion; retinal breaks (round or atrophic holes) in 18%, horseshoe tear in 1.4% at posterior or lateral edge due to severe vitreous traction (Figure 11-83)

Pathology: discontinuity of ILM, overlying pocket of liquid vitreous, condensation and adherence of vitreous at margin of lesion, focal area of retinal thinning with loss of inner retinal layers, melanin-laden macrophages, fibrous thickening of retinal vessel walls

Treatment: no proof that prophylactic treatment prevents RD; consider treatment of fellow eye if history of RD from lattice

Detachments

Rhegmatogenous Retinal Detachment (RD)

Etiology: retinal break allows liquid vitreous access to subretinal space (Figures 11-84 and 11-85)

1 in 10,000/year; retinal break can be found in 97%

Most tears (70%) are located superiorly between 10 and 2 o'clock positions

Types of breaks:

Horseshoe tear

Atrophic hole: myopia, increasing age

Dialysis: splitting of vitreous base (usually inferotemporally, second most common site is superonasal); traumatic or idiopathic

Giant tear: greater than 3 clock hours or 90°; trauma (≥90%), myopia; 50% risk of RD in fellow eye

Operculated hole: fragment of retinal tissue found in overlying vitreous

Risk factors: age, history of RD in fellow eye (15%), high myopia/axial length (7%), family history, lattice degeneration, trauma, cataract surgery (1% after ICCE; 0.1% after ECCE with intact posterior capsule), diabetes, Nd:YAG laser posterior capsulotomy

After blunt trauma, dialysis is most common form of tear, followed by giant retinal tear, flap tear, and tear around lattice degeneration

Symptoms: flashes and floaters in 50%

Findings: retinal break; detached retina is opaque, corrugated, and undulates; tobacco dust (pigment in vitreous); decreased IOP; VH; nonshifting subretinal fluid

Long-standing RD: thin retina, small breaks or dialysis, demarcation lines, underlying RPE atrophy, subretinal precipitates, macrocysts; may have increased IOP, PVR

DDx: exudative or traction RD

Treatment:

Pneumatic retinopexy: ideal if RD caused by single break in superior 8 clock hours or multiple breaks within

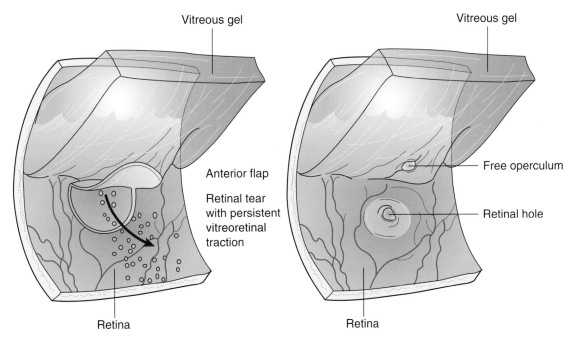

Figure 11-84. Retinal breaks demonstrating horseshoe tear and operculated hole. (From Wilkinson CP: Rhegmatogenous retinal ophthalmology. In: Yanoff M, Duker JS (eds) Ophthalmology. London, Mosby, 1999.)

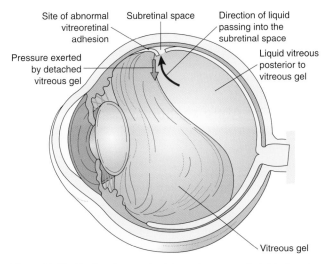

Figure 11-85. Classic pathogenesis of rhegmatogenous retinal detachment. (From Wilkinson CP: Rhegmatogenous retinal ophthalmology. In: Yanoff M, Duker JS (eds) Ophthalmology. London, Mosby, 1999.)

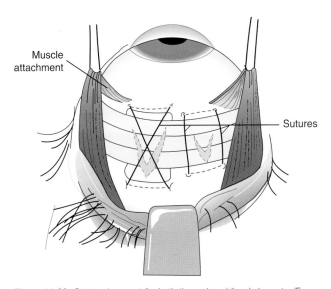

Figure 11-86. Suture placement for both tire and meridional elements. (From Williams GA: Scleral buckling surgery. In: Yanoff M, Duker JS (eds) Ophthalmology, 2nd edn. St Louis, Mosby, 2004.)

1–2 clock hours; phakic patients tend to do better than aphakic patients

Injection of inert gas or sterile air into vitreous cavity; strict positioning of patient's head allows gas bubble to contact retinal break and form barrier (RPE pumps subretinal fluid into choroid, allowing retina to reattach), break is sealed with cryo at time of gas injection or sealed with laser once subretinal fluid has resorbed

INTRAOCULAR GASES (in order of decreasing time gas remains in eye): perfluoropropane (C_3F_8), perfluoroethane (C_2F_6), sulfur hexafluoride (SF_6), air

Surgery: scleral buckle and/or vitrectomy, with laser therapy or cryotherapy

GOALS:

Identify all retinal breaks

Close all retinal breaks

Place scleral buckle to support all retinal breaks and bring retina and choroid into contact; retinal tears should be flat on buckle (Figure 11-86)

Reduce vitreous traction on retinal breaks

Complications of cryotherapy: proliferative vitreoretinopathy (PVR), uveitis, CME, intraocular hemorrhage, chorioretinal necrosis

339

Complications of scleral buckle surgery: ischemia (anterior or posterior segments), infection, perforation, strabismus, erosion or extrusion of explant, change in refractive error (induced myopia from increased axial length), macular pucker, cataract, glaucoma, new retinal tears (1.6%), PVR (4%), failure (5–10%)

Complications of SRF drainage: hemorrhage, retinal tear, retinal incarceration, hypotony, vitreous loss, infection

Silicone oil: specific gravity less than water; surface tension less than that of all gases; buoyant when placed in eye; therefore, make iridectomy inferiorly; complications: cataract (100%), band keratopathy (24%), glaucoma (19%), corneal decompensation (8%)

Prognosis: scleral buckle has 91% success rate;
Final vision depends on macular involvement: worse prognosis if macular detached; timing of macular detachment is also important: if <1 week, 75% recover vision >20/70; if >1 week, 50% >20/70

Complications: PVR

Proliferative Vitreoretinopathy (PVR)

(Figure 11-87)

Retinal break allows cells (RPE, glial, myofibroblasts) to proliferate on inner and outer surfaces of retina along scaffold of detached vitreous

Membranes contract, causing fixed folds and tractional RD

Risk of PVR: following ocular perforation = 43%, following rupture = 21%, following penetration = 15%; associated with intraocular foreign body in 11%

Most common reason for failure of retinal reattachment surgery; usually occurs 4–6 weeks after initial repair

Classification system: 3 grades (A–C) in order of increasing severity

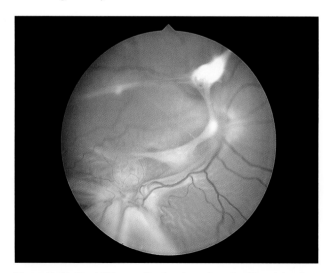

Figure 11-87. Star fold from proliferative vitreoretinopathy. (From Aylward GW: Proliferative vitreoretinopathy. In: Yanoff M, Duker JS (eds) Ophthalmology. London, Mosby, 1999.)

B-scan ultrasound: detached retina with triangle sign (transvitreal membrane connecting the 2 sides)

Treatment: vitreoretinal surgery is successful in approximately 70% of cases, leading to anatomic success

Exudative RD

Etiology: uveitis (VKH syndrome, sympathetic ophthalmia, pars planitis, viral retinitis), tumors, glomerulonephritis, hypertension, eclampsia/pre-eclampsia, hypothyroidism, Coats' disease, nanophthalmos, scleritis, CSR (Figure 11-88)

Findings: shifting fluid, smooth retinal surface, no retinal break, retina behind the lens (pathognomonic)

Traction RD

Etiology: penetrating trauma (PVR), proliferative retinopathies, PHPV, toxoplasmosis, vitreous degenerations

Findings: taut retinal surface, immobile, concave shape, no retinal break; does not extend to the ora serrata

Pathology: subretinal fluid, photoreceptor degeneration, cystoid degeneration, glial membrane formation

Folds of Neurosensory Retina

Due to epiretinal membrane or rhegmatogenous RD

Not visible on FA; can be seen on OCT

Choroidal Abnormalities

Choroidal Folds

Results from shrinkage of inner choroid or Bruch's membrane, causing undulations of overlying RPE and outer retina

Etiology: (mnemonic THIN RPE): tumors, hypotony, inflammation/idiopathic, neovascular membrane, retrobulbar mass, papilledema, extraocular hardware

Findings: yellow elevated crests alternating with darker bands between crests

FA: light bands/crests contain thinner RPE, producing prominent choroidal fluorescence; dark bands/troughs contain compressed RPE, producing relative hypofluorescence

Choroidal Detachment

Due to fluid (choroidal effusion) or blood (choroidal hemorrhage) in suprachoroidal space

Etiology: hypotony, uveitis, idiopathic, uremia, nanophthalmos (thickened sclera impedes vortex venous drainage), intraocular surgery (rapid change in IOP shears choroidal perforating arteries), intense PRP

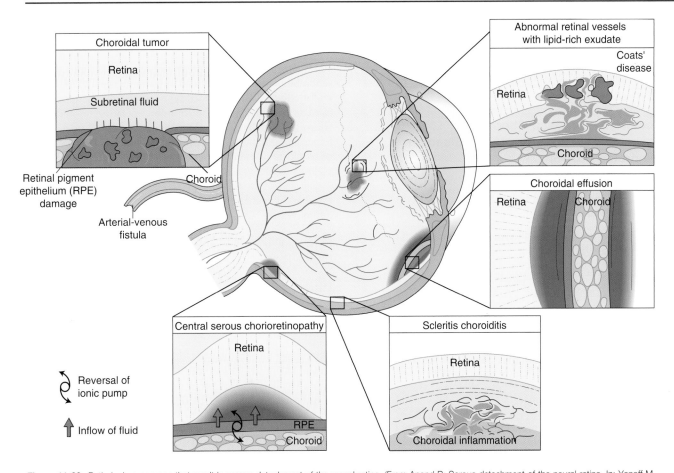

Figure 11-88. Pathologic processes that result in serous detachment of the neural retina. (From Anand R: Serous detachment of the neural retina. In: Yanoff M, Duker JS (eds) Ophthalmology, 2nd edn. St Louis, Mosby, 2004.)

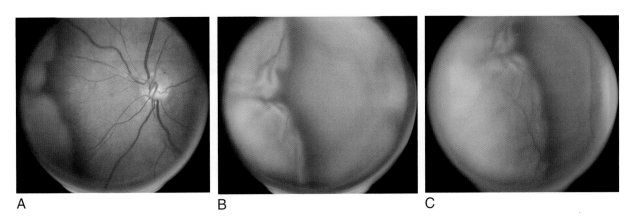

A   B   C

Figure 11-89. A–C, Hemorrhagic choroidal detachment viewed ophthalmoscopically. (From Kapusta MA, Lopez PF: Choroidal hemorrage. In: Yanoff M, Duker JS (eds) Ophthalmology. London, Mosby, 1999.)

Hemorrhage is caused by rupture of small vessels with sudden decrease of IOP (opening globe for surgery); may be expulsive with loss of intraocular contents through wound

Findings:
dark dome-shaped appearance (Figure 11-89)

B-scan ultrasound: echogenic convexity attached at scleral spur and vortex veins (not at optic nerve)

Treatment: treat underlying disorder; consider partial-thickness scleral windows near vortex vein exit sites in 3 or 4 quadrants; if it occurs during surgery, immediately close globe and give mannitol IV; may require drainage (sclerotomies)

Choroidal Ischemia

May occur with hypertensive retinopathy

Elschnig's spot: zone of nonperfusion of choriocapillaris, which appears as atrophic area of RPE overlying infarcted choroidal lobule

Siegrist streak: reactive RPE hyperplasia along sclerosed choroidal vessel

Posterior Polypoidal Choroidal Vasculopathy/Posterior Uveal Bleeding Syndrome (PUBS)

Idiopathic peripapillary CNV; may bleed or leak fluid

Miscellaneous

Albinism, Aicardi's syndrome, color blindness (see Ch. 5, Pediatrics/Strabismus)

Tumors

Benign Tumors

Choroidal Nevus

Neoplasm of choroidal melanocytes; most common primary intraocular tumor

Can also arise within iris, ciliary body, or optic disc

Usually unilateral and unifocal; increased frequency with age; prevalence of 6.5% in US population >49 years old

Multifocal nevi: associated with neurofibromatosis

Findings: flat slate-gray to dark brown choroidal lesion with ill-defined margins; surface drusen common; subretinal fluid and orange clumps of pigment rare (Figure 11-90)

Features that suggest benign nevus may grow and evolve into choroidal melanoma:
thickness (>2 mm), orange pigment (lipofuscin), juxtapapillary location, subretinal fluid, visual symptoms

Pathology: benign spindle cells with pigment

DDx: CHRPE, melanoma, melanocytoma

FA: hyperfluorescence

Choroidal Cavernous Hemangioma

Congenital, unilateral vascular tumor

Types:
Diffuse: associated with Sturge-Weber syndrome
Circumscribed: not associated with systemic disease

Symptoms: blurred vision, micropsia, metamorphopsia; vision loss due to cystic macular retinal degeneration or adjacent exudative RD

Findings:
Diffuse type: generalized red-orange choroidal thickening ('tomato catsup' fundus); may have elevated IOP

Circumscribed type: red-orange dome-shaped choroidal mass within 2 DD of optic disc or fovea

Pathology: lakes of erythrocytes separated by thin, fibrous septa; large-caliber vascular channels lined by mature endothelium. Circumscribed type has sharply demarcated borders and compresses surrounding melanocytes and choroidal lamellae (seen clinically as ring of hyperpigmentation at periphery of lesion and on FA as ring of blockage of underlying choroidal fluorescence) (Figure 11-91)

FA: early hyperfluorescent filling of lesion at same time as retinal vessels, and late leakage/staining of entire lesion

ICG: early hyperfluorescent filling of intralesional vessels (Figure 11-92)

Ultrasound: A-scan shows high initial spike with high internal reflectivity; B-scan shows sonoreflective tissue, often with choroidal thickening (Figure 11-93)

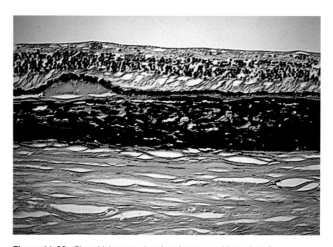

Figure 11-90. Choroidal nevus showing drusen overlying a heavily pigmented choroidal nevus composed almost completely of plump polyhedral nevus cells. (Modified from Naumann G, et al: Arch Ophthalmol 76:784, 1966. From Yanoff M, Fine BS: Ocular Pathology, 5th edn. St Louis, Mosby, 2002.)

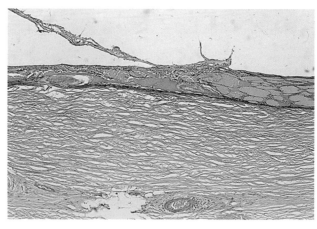

Figure 11-91. Hemangioma of choroid. (From Yanoff M, Fine BS: Ocular Pathology, 5th edn. St Louis, Mosby, 2002.)

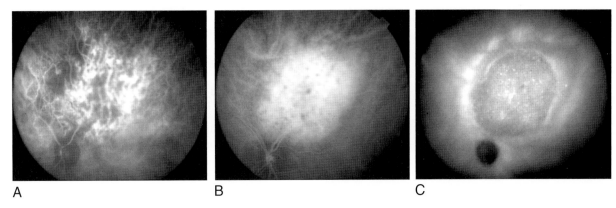

Figure 11-92. A—C, Indocyanine green angiography of circumscribed choroidal hemangioma. (From Augsburger JJ, Anand R, Sanborn GE: Choroidal hemangiomas. In: Yanoff M, Duker JS (eds) Ophthalmology. London, Mosby, 1999.)

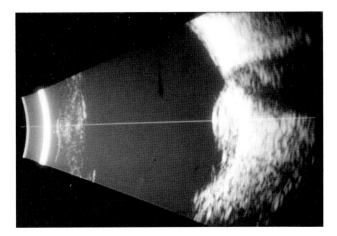

Figure 11-93. B-scan ultrasonography of circumscribed choroidal hemangioma. (From Augsburger JJ, Anand R, Sanborn GE: Choroidal hemangiomas. In: Yanoff M, Duker JS (eds) 1999 Ophthalmology. London, Mosby, 1999.)

Treatment: laser therapy, photodynamic therapy, or low-dose external beam XRT for exudative RD

Choroidal Osteoma

Tumor composed of bone
Sporadic, unifocal, bilateral in 20%
Arises in late childhood to early adulthood; more common in women (90%)

Symptoms: blurred vision, central scotoma

Findings: yellow-white to pale orange circumpapillary lesion with well-defined pseudopod-like margins; CNV and RPE disruption can cause progressive visual impairment

Pathology: plaque of mature bone involving full-thickness choroid, usually sparing RPE

FA: patchy early hyperfluorescence and late staining of lesion

ICG: hypofluorescence of lesion with hyperfluorescent intralesional vessels, late leakage of lesion

B-scan ultrasound: highly reflective plate-like lesion with orbital shadowing beyond lesion (Figure 11-94)

CT scan: plate-like thickening of eye wall

Treatment: for CNV if present

Retinal Capillary Hemangioma

Vascular tumor (hemangioblastoma); AD, sporadic, or associated with von Hippel-Lindau disease (bilateral retinal capillary hemangiomas [40–60%], cystic cerebellar hemangioblastoma [60%, most common cause of death], renal cell carcinoma, pheochromocytoma, liver, pancreas, and epididymis cysts = chromosome 3p26-p25; mutation in the VHL tumor suppressor gene)
Arises in older children and young adults

Symptoms: blurred vision, visual field loss

Findings: red globular mass with prominent dilated tortuous afferent and efferent retinal blood vessels, exudative RD may develop

FA: feeding arteriole fills rapidly; dye leaks into vitreous and subretinal space

Treatment: slowly progressive if untreated; can treat with laser, cryotherapy, or photodynamic therapy (PDT)

Retinal Cavernous Hemangioma

Vascular tumor; probably congenital; occasionally associated with similar CNS or skin vascular lesions
Usually unilateral, unifocal; rarely progressive

Findings: cluster of dark red intraretinal vascular sacs ('bunch of grapes' appearance), typically associated with an anomalous retinal vein; associated overlying retinal gliosis; no intraretinal exudates or detachment; may have VH

FA: fluid levels within the vascular sacs

Treatment: vitrectomy for nonclearing VH

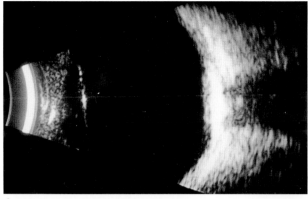

A

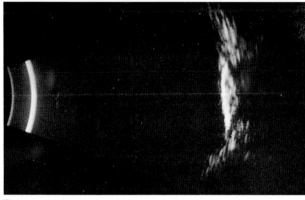

B

Figure 11-94. B-scan ultrasonography of choroidal osteoma. **A,** At 77 dB the osteoma appears as an intensely white plate in the posterior eye wall. **B,** At 55 dB the lesion persists but most of the normal tissues are no longer evident. (From Yanoff M, Duker JS (eds) Ophthalmology. London, Mosby, 1999.)

Retinal Astrocytoma (Astrocytic Hamartoma)

Glioma arising from retinal glial cells

Occurs in older children and young adults; can be unilateral or bilateral, unifocal or multifocal; usually stable

Rarely associated with tuberous sclerosis (multifocal, bilateral) and NF

Symptoms: blurred vision, visual field loss, or asymptomatic

Findings: 1 or more yellow-white masses that obscure retinal vessels; occasionally exudative RD; calcification in some larger lesions; may have glistening, mulberry appearance or softer, fluffy appearance

Combined Hamartoma of the Retina and RPE

Tumor composed of neurosensory retina and RPE; probably congenital; associated with neurofibromatosis type 2

Usually unilateral, unifocal; minimal progression

Symptoms: blurred vision

Findings: gray, juxtapapillary lesion with surface gliosis and prominent intralesional retinal vascular tortuosity; amblyopia (Figure 11-95)

Pathology: cords of proliferated pigment epithelium with excess blood vessels and glial tissue

Treatment: none

Adenoma and Adenocarcinoma

Tumor composed of RPE cells, rarely arise from nonpigmented ciliary epithelium; seldom undergoes malignant transformation

Findings: elevated dark black lesion, may resemble deeply pigmented melanoma; may have iridocyclitis, secondary cataract, subluxated lens

Pathology: massive proliferation of RPE cells

Treatment: excision

Racemose Hemangioma

Congenital AV malformation

Associated with Wyburn-Mason syndrome when associated with AVM of midbrain

No exudate or leakage

Malignant Tumors

Retinoblastoma (RB)

(See Ch. 5, Pediatrics/Strabismus.)

Choroidal Malignant Melanoma

Malignant neoplasm of uveal melanocytes; unilateral, unifocal; 75% arise in choroid, less common in CB or iris

Most common primary intraocular malignant tumor in Caucasian adults (1 in 2000)

Uncommon before age 40 years

Risk factors: ocular melanocytosis, sunlight exposure, uveal nevi, race (Caucasian; only 1–2% in African Americans or Asians), cigarette smoking, neurofibromatosis, dysplastic nevus syndrome, bilateral diffuse uveal melanocytic proliferation (BDUMP) syndrome

Symptoms: blurred vision, visual field loss, flashes and floaters

Findings: brown, domed-shaped or mushroom-shaped tumor; orange pigment clumps (accumulation of lipofuscin in RPE), adjacent exudative RD, sentinel vessel (dilated tortuous episcleral vessel); secondary glaucoma; may be amelanotic and appear as a pale mass

Pathology: Callender classification (Figures 11-96 to 11-99)

Spindle A cells: slender, cigar-shaped nucleus with finely dispersed chromatin; low nuclear-to-cytoplasmic ratio; absent or inconspicuous nucleolus; no mitotic figures; tumors composed exclusively of spindle A cells are considered benign nevi

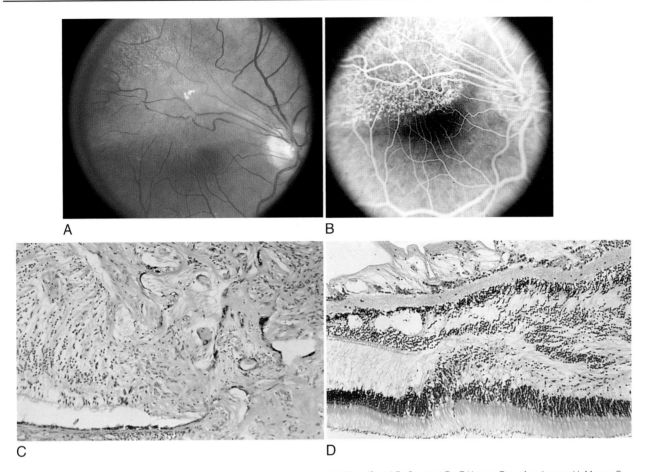

A

B

C

D

Figure 11-95. A–D, Combined hamartoma of neural retina and retinal pigment epithelium. (C and D, Courtesy Dr. E Howes. From Augsburger JJ, Meyers S: Combined harartoma of retina. In: Yanoff M, Duker JS (eds) Ophthalmology. London, Mosby, 1999.)

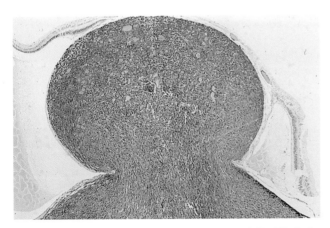

Figure 11-96. Uveal mushroom melanoma. (From Yanoff M, Fine BS: Ocular Pathology, 5th edn. St Louis, Mosby, 2002.)

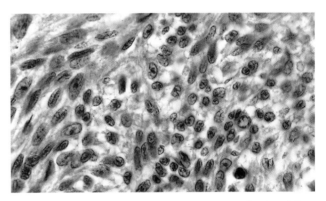

Figure 11-97. Callender classification. Spindle A cells, identified by a dark stripe parallel to the long axis of the nucleus, are seen in longitudinal section. They are identified in transverse cross section by the infolding of the nuclear membrane that causes the dark stripe. (From Yanoff M, Fine BS: Ocular Pathology, 5th edn. St Louis, Mosby, 2002.)

Spindle B cells: oval (larger) nucleus with coarser chromatin and prominent nucleolus; mitotic figures; tumors with spindle A and B cells are called spindle cell melanomas. Spindle A and B cells grow as a syncytium with indistinct cytoplasmic borders

Epithelioid cells: polyhedral with abundant cytoplasm; poorly cohesive; distinct borders; most malignant; large, round-to-oval nucleus with peripheral margination of chromatin; prominent eosinophilic or purple nucleolus (epithelioid cells 'look back at you'); worst prognosis

Mixed cell melanoma: composed of spindle and epithelioid cells

Gross examination requires identification of vortex veins to rule out tumor extension

Transillumination: most melanomas cast shadow

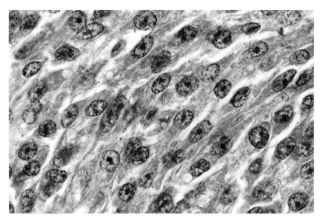

Figure 11-98. Callender classification. Histologic section of spindle B cells. (From Yanoff M, Fine BS: Ocular Pathology, 5th edn. St Louis, Mosby, 2002.)

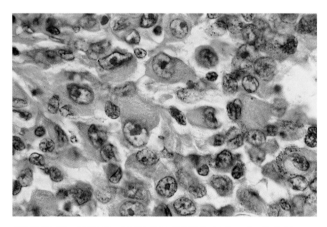

Figure 11-99. Callender classification. Histologic section of epithelioid cells. (From Yanoff M, Fine BS: Ocular Pathology, 5th edn. St Louis, Mosby, 2002.)

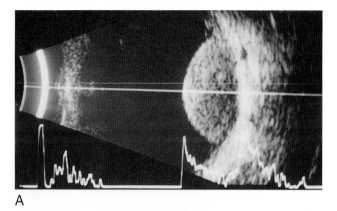

A

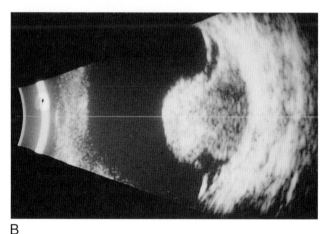

B

Figure 11-100. A, B, Ultrasonography of posterior uveal melanoma. (From Augsburger JJ, Damato BE, Bornfield N: Uveal melanoma. In: Yanoff M, Duker JS (eds) Ophthalmology. London, Mosby, 1999.)

Ultrasound: A-scan shows low internal reflectivity with characteristic reduction in amplitude from front to back, high-amplitude spikes consistent with break in Bruch's membrane; B-scan shows solid tumor with mushroom shape or biconvex shape (Figure 11-100)

FA: 'double' circulation (choroidal and retinal vessels), mass is hypofluorescent early, pinpoint leakage late (Figure 11-101)

MRI: bright on T1; dark on T2

Treatment:

Enucleation: large tumor, optic nerve invasion, macular location, painful eye with poor visual potential

Plaque brachytherapy: most eyes with medium-sized tumors with visual potential, or failure of laser
   HIGH ENERGY: cobalt-60, iridium-192
   LOW ENERGY: iodine-125 (sphere of radiation), palladium-106 (25% less energy than I-125), ruthenium-106 (β-particles, travel only 5 mm; therefore, use for small tumors)

Charged particle radiation: proton beam (cylinder of radiation); large anterior segment dose, low macular dose (reverse of plaque)

Resection: most irido and iridociliary tumors; some ciliary body and choroidal tumors

Transpupillary thermotherapy: small tumors

Zimmerman hypothesis: manipulation of tumor during enucleation causes metastasis and increases mortality; not true. Derived from plotting of life table data, which showed Bell-shaped curve for death rate; specifically, mortality rate increased to 8% following enucleation (vs 1% per year in patients with untreated tumors)

Complications of treatment: radiation retinopathy (if severe, treat with PRP to prevent NVG); cataracts (PSC in 42% within 3 years of proton beam therapy); dry eye

Collaborative Ocular Melanoma Study (COMS):
   SMALL TUMOR TRIAL (height = 1–3 mm; diameter >5 mm): 1/3 grew; 5-year mortality = 6%
   MEDIUM TUMOR TRIAL (height = 2.5–10 mm; diameter <16 mm): survival rates similar between enucleation and iodine-125 plaque brachytherapy; I-125 brachytherapy has a high risk of substantial visual loss (up to 49%)

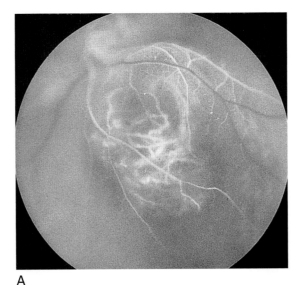

A

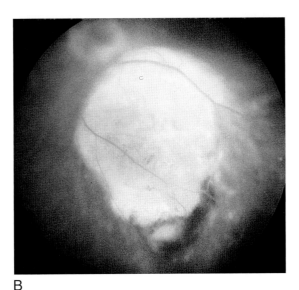

B

Figure 11-101. A, B, Fluorescein angiograms of mushroom-shaped choroidal melanoma. (From Augsburger JJ, Damato BE, Bornfield N: Uveal melanoma. In: Yanoff M, Duker JS (eds) 1999 Ophthalmology. London, Mosby, 1999.)

LARGE TUMOR TRIAL (height >10 mm; diameter >16 mm; without mets): pre-enucleation radiation does not change the survival rate in patients with large choroidal melanomas with or without metastases over enucleation alone

Prognosis:

Factors:

CELL TYPE: epithelioid has worst prognosis (5-year survival <30%); presence of epithelioid cells is important in survivability; 5-year survival rate for spindle A cell is 95%, 15-year survival rate for mixed tumor is 37%, 15-year survival for pure spindle cell melanoma with no epithelioid cells is 72%

SIZE: larger and diffuse tumors have a worse prognosis
LOCATION
VARIABILITY IN NUCLEOLAR SIZE
PRESENCE OF INTRATUMOR VASCULAR NETWORKS
PRESENCE OF NECROSIS
METALLOTHIONEIN LEVELS: may indicate metastatic potential and poor survival

Approximately 50% with large tumors have metastasis within 5 years

Mean survival after metastasis is 9 months

Metastasis: hematogenous spread via vortex veins; risks include elevation (>2 mm), proximity to optic nerve, visual symptoms, growth; 92% of metastases are to liver, also skin, lungs, other organs; local extension into optic nerve and brain

Metastatic workup: abdominal examination (hepatosplenomegaly), liver function tests (LFTs), CXR; 2% have evidence of metastasis at diagnosis; if any abnormal then liver/abdomen/chest CT and MRI

MAJOR CLINICAL STUDY

Collaborative Ocular Melanoma Study (COMS)

Objective: To Evaluate Treatment Options For Choroidal Malignant Melanomas

Methods:

Small tumor study (not large enough for COMS trial) (apical height = 1–3 mm; basal diameter 5–16 mm): not randomized; observation vs treatment at discretion of investigator

Medium tumor trial (apical height = 2.5–10 mm; basal diameter <16 mm): randomized to enucleation vs radiation (I-125 plaque brachytherapy)

Large tumor trial (apical height >10 mm; basal diameter >16 mm; no mets): randomized enucleation alone vs 20 Gy external beam radiation for 5 days and then enucleation (PERT)

Primary outcome was survival; secondary outcomes included tumor growth, visual function, time to metastasis, and quality of life

Results:

Small tumor study: 21% grew by 2 years and 31% by 5 years; 6 deaths were due to metastatic melanoma; 5-year all-cause mortality was 6%, and 8-year was 14.9%; risk factors for growth included initial tumor thickness and diameter, presence of orange pigment, absence of drusen, and absence of adjacent RPE changes

Medium tumor trial: after 3 years, 43–49% of I-125–treated eyes had poor vision outcomes (loss of ≥6

lines of visual acuity or VA of 20/200 or worse), and this was strongly associated with larger tumor apical height and smaller distance from the foveal avascular zone; other risk factors for poor visual outcome included diabetes, tumor-related retinal detachment, and tumors that were not dome-shaped; estimated 5-year survival rates were 81% for the enucleation group and 82% for the I-125 group

Large tumor trial: 1003 patients enrolled. Estimated 5-year survival rates were 57% for enucleation alone and 62% for radiation followed by enucleation, and for patients with metastases at the time of death, the 5-year survival was 72% vs 74%; prognostic risk factors were age and basal diameter

Conclusions:

Small tumor study: otherwise healthy patients with small choroidal melanomas have a low risk of death within 5 years

Medium tumor trial: there is a high risk of substantial visual loss from I-125 brachytherapy (up to 49%); I-125 brachytherapy does not change the survival rate (for up to 12 years) in patients with medium choroidal melanomas

Large tumor trial: pre-enucleation radiation does not change the survival rate in patients with large choroidal melanomas with or without metastases

Primary Intraocular Lymphoma (Reticulum Cell Sarcoma)

Non-Hodgkin's B-cell lymphoma, large cell type

Affects elderly patients; usually bilateral and multifocal

No systemic involvement outside of CNS

Increased risk of development of concurrent primary CNS lymphoma

Symptoms (precede CNS signs in 80%): blurred vision, floaters; dementia may occur

Findings: creamy white, diffuse sub-RPE and vitreous infiltrates; AC reaction, hypopyon, vitritis, secondary glaucoma; may have multifocal atrophic or punched-out lesions, and exudative RD; choroidal form manifests with choroidal nodules or detachments of RPE and is associated with systemic lymphoma (Figure 11-102)

Diagnosis: CT scan, LP (positive in 25%), vitreous biopsy (low yield; atypical lymphocytes with prominent nucleoli, mitoses; cellular necrosis) (Figure 11-103)

FA: leopard spots

Treatment: chemotherapy or XRT

Prognosis: poor, mortality often within 2 years (mean survival is 22 months)

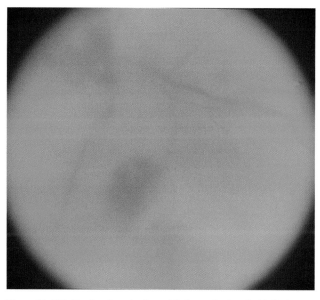

Figure 11-102. Fundus view of yellow-white hemorrhagic retinal infiltrates. (From Burnier MN, Blanco G: Intraocular lymphoma. In: Yanoff M, Duker JS (eds) Ophthalmology. London, Mosby, 1999.)

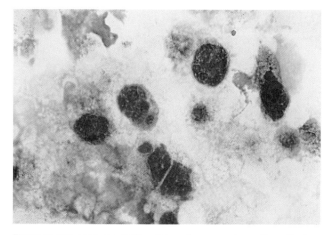

Figure 11-103. Large neoplastic cells in a vitreous specimen. (From Burnier MN, Blanco G: Intraocular lymphoma. In: Yanoff M, Duker JS (eds) Ophthalmology. London, Mosby, 1999.)

Reactive lymphoid hyperplasia of the choroid

benign counterpart

Findings: diffuse or multiple yellow choroidal lesions; overlying RD may occur; often similar infiltrates in conjunctiva and orbit (check conjunctiva for salmon patch)

Associated with systemic lymphoma (vs retinovitreous lymphoma, which is associated with CNS lesions)

Pathology: mass of benign lymphocytes, plasma cells, and Dutcher bodies

Treatment: low-dose XRT

Intraocular Leukemia

(See Ch. 5, Pediatrics/Strabismus.)

Metastases

Most common intraocular tumor (including cases evident only at autopsy)

Most commonly breast carcinoma in women (most have previous mastectomy), lung carcinoma in men (often occult)

Bilateral and multifocal in 20%; 25% have no previous history of cancer

93% to choroid; 2% to ciliary body; 5% to iris; can also metastasize to optic nerve; retina is rare

Symptoms: blurred vision, visual field defects, flashes and floaters

Findings: 1 or more golden-yellow, thin, dome-shaped choroidal tumors or creamy yellow amelanotic tumors with placoid or nummular configuration; may produce extensive exudative RD; usually metastasize to macula (richest blood supply)

DDx of amelanotic choroidal mass: amelanotic melanoma, old subretinal hemorrhage, choroidal osteoma, granuloma, posterior scleritis

FA: early hyperfluorescence with late staining of lesions

Ultrasound: A-scan shows medium to high internal reflectivity; B-scan is sonoreflective (Figure 11-104)

Treatment: chemotherapy, external beam XRT, or combination

Carcinoma-Associated Retinopathy (CAR)/Melanoma-Associated Retinopathy (MAR)

Rare, paraneoplastic syndrome; antiretinal antibodies (recoverin, enolase, heat shock cognate protein 70); loss of photoreceptors without inflammation

Findings: decreased vision, nyctalopia that clinically appears normal in early cases, but may develop uveitis, chorioretinal atrophy, retinal pigment degeneration, narrowed retinal vessels, optic atrophy, and vitreous cells later

ERG: extinguished

Treatment: steroids, treatment of primary cancer (usually small cell lung carcinoma)

Prognosis: poor

Bilateral Diffuse Uveal Melanocytic Proliferation Syndrome (BDUMPS)

Paraneoplastic syndrome

Diffuse uveal thickening

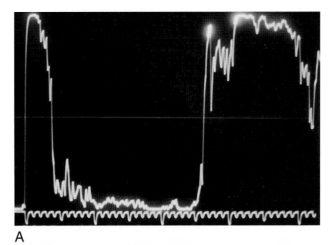

Figure 11-104. Ultrasonography of metastatic carcinoma to choroid. **A**, A-scan. **B**, B-scan. (From Augsburger JJ, Guthoff R: Metastatic cancer to the eye. In: Yanoff M, Duker JS (eds) Ophthalmology. London, Mosby, 1999.)

Findings: orange or pigmented fundus spots, iris thickening and pigmentation

ERG: markedly reduced

FA: orange spots hyperfluoresce

Treatment: none

LASER TREATMENT

Thermal burn (photocoagulation) of inner retina will occur with argon blue-green or xenon arc

Retinal structures that absorb laser:
   Melanin: primary site of light absorption and heat emission; absorbs argon blue-green, argon green, and krypton red
   Hemoglobin: absorbs argon blue-green, argon green; does not absorb krypton (used to penetrate hemorrhage)
   Xanthophyll: absorbs blue wavelengths

Wavelengths:

Blue-green (488 and 514 nm): blue light is absorbed by cornea and lens, heavily absorbed by nuclear sclerotic cataracts and absorbed by xanthophyll pigment

Green (514 nm): absorbed by blood, melanin; preferred for treatment of CNV in cases in which RPE has little pigment

Yellow (577 nm): may be better for treatment of microaneurysms; be careful of blood vessels

Red (647 nm): penetrates cataracts better; not absorbed by blood; causes less inner retinal damage; absorbed by melanin; poorly absorbed by xanthophyll (safer near fovea); passes through mild vitreous hemorrhage and nuclear sclerotic cataracts better than argon

Infrared (810 nm): has similar characteristics as red, but with deeper penetration

Xenon arc: polychromatic white light; not as precisely focused as monochromatic light; emits considerable amount of blue light, which can be harmful to retina and lens

Panretinal Photocoagulation (PRP)

Indications: treatment of NV and peripheral nonperfusion, most commonly in retinal vascular diseases (PDR, CVO, BVO, sickle cell, radiation, and hypertensive retinopathy)

Parameters: 500 μm spot size, 0.1-0.5 s duration, 1200–2000 spots; moderate white burn, 1 burn-width apart, 2 DD from fovea and 1 DD from optic nerve; 2 or more sessions

Adverse effects: decreased acuity (worsened by 1 line in 11%; worsened by 2 lines in 3%), constricted visual field, loss of color vision in 10%
Retreat at 4 weeks if NVD fails to regress or develops, new NVE develops, iris or angle NV develops, further regression of NV desired

Complications: choroidal effusion, exudative RD, permanent mydriasis and impairment of accommodation (ciliary nerve damage), vitreous hemorrhage, lens or corneal damage, foveal or optic nerve damage, CME, CNV, retinal vascular occlusion, angle closure

Focal Laser

Indication: treatment of macular edema (CSME, BVO, JXT)

Parameters: 50–100 μm spot size, 0.1 s duration; burns that slightly blanch the RPE, should be barely visible immediately after treatment, grid pattern 1 burn-width apart, in areas of diffuse edema; focal treatment of leaking vessels and microaneurysms; whiten/darken microaneurysms and/or cause mild depigmentation of RPE; do not treat over hemorrhage; identify leaking microaneurysms by FA

Decreases risk of moderate visual loss over 3 years by 50% in CSME

Retreat at 3 months if CSME still present, or treatable areas seen on repeat FA

REVIEW QUESTIONS (Answers start on page 370)

1. Which substance does not cause crystalline deposits in the retina?
   a. thioridazine
   b. canthaxanthine
   c. tamoxifen
   d. talc
2. What is the chance that a child of a patient with Best's disease will inherit the disorder?
   a. 25%
   b. 50%
   c. 75%
   d. 100%
3. The MPS showed the best prognosis for laser treatment of CNV in which disorder?
   a. AMD
   b. myopia
   c. idiopathic condition
   d. POHS
4. Which of the following is not a feature of Stickler's syndrome?
   a. Pierre-Robin malformation
   b. autosomal dominant inheritance
   c. retinoschisis
   d. marfinoid habitus
5. Sites at which the uvea is attached to the sclera include all of the following except
   a. vortex veins
   b. optic nerve
   c. scleral spur
   d. ora serrata
6. The inheritance of gyrate atrophy is
   a. sporadic
   b. X-linked recessive
   c. autosomal dominant
   d. autosomal recessive
7. All 3 types of retinal hemorrhage (preretinal, intraretinal, and subretinal) may occur simultaneously in all of the following conditions except
   a. macroaneurysm
   b. AMD
   c. diabetes
   d. capillary hemangioma
8. Characteristics of choroidal melanoma include all of the following except
   a. choroidal excavation
   b. high internal reflectivity
   c. double circulation
   d. orbital shadowing
9. Which of the following statements regarding the ETDRS is false?
   a. The ETDRS concluded that PRP reduces the risk of severe visual loss in patients with high-risk PDR
   b. The ETDRS identified the risk factors for development of PDR

c. The ETDRS defined CSME

d. The ETDRS showed that aspirin does not affect disease progression

10. The DRVS found that early vitrectomy for vitreous hemorrhage was helpful in
    a. type 1 diabetic patients
    b. type 2 diabetic patients
    c. type 1 and 2 diabetic patients
    d. none of the above

11. Which of the following treatments is a CVOS recommendation?
    a. focal laser for macular edema of >3 to 6 months' duration with VA <20/40
    b. PRP for >10 disc areas of nonperfusion
    c. PRP for iris or angle neovascularization
    d. macular grid photocoagulation for CME

12. Which peripheral retinal lesion has the greatest risk of a retinal detachment?
    a. cystic retinal tuft
    b. aymptomatic retinal hole
    c. senile retinoschisis
    d. lattice degeneration

13. The intraocular structure most commonly affected by leukemia is
    a. iris
    b. choroid
    c. retina
    d. optic nerve

14. Which is not a function of the RPE?
    a. conversion of vitamin A alcohol to aldehyde
    b. concentration of taurine
    c. inactivation of toxic products of oxygen metabolism
    d. phagocytosis of rod outer segments

15. Which of the following best describes the cellular reaction when light strikes a photoreceptor?
    a. increased cGMP, closed Na channel
    b. increased cGMP, open Na channel
    c. decreased cGMP, closed Na channel
    d. decreased cGMP, open Na channel

16. Prognostic factors for choroidal melanoma include all of the following except
    a. size
    b. location
    c. cell type
    d. pigmentation

17. Which of the following does not involve the outer plexiform layer of the retina?
    a. degenerative retinoschisis
    b. cystoid macular edema
    c. Henle's fiber layer
    d. diabetic microaneurysm

18. The best test for distinguishing between a subretinal hemorrhage and a choroidal melanoma is
    a. FA
    b. B-scan
    c. A-scan
    d. ERG

19. Which of the following is the least radiosensitive lesion?
    a. metastases
    b. lymphoma

c. RB

d. melanoma

20. Which of the following is the least common complication of PRP?
    a. iritis
    b. increased IOP
    c. RD
    d. narrow angle

21. A cluster of pigmented lesions is seen in the peripheral retina of a patient's left eye during routine ophthalmoscopy. Which of the following tests would be most helpful in detecting an associated hereditary disorder?
    a. EKG
    b. colonoscopy
    c. brain MRI
    d. chest CT scan

22. Which of the following is not associated with a typical angiographic appearance of CME?
    a. nicotinic acid
    b. epinephrine
    c. Irvine-Gass syndrome
    d. pars planitis

23. The least likely finding in a patient with a chronic detachment of the inferotemporal retina is
    a. retinal thinning
    b. macrocysts
    c. fixed folds
    d. RPE atrophy

24. In a patient with AMD, which type of drusen is most associated with development of CNV?
    a. soft
    b. basal laminar
    c. hard
    d. calcific

25. The ERG oscillatory potential is caused by which cell type?
    a. Müller's
    b. amacrine
    c. bipolar
    d. RPE

26. Chloroquine retinopathy
    a. is reversible with discontinuation of the medication
    b. can be associated with other CNS reactions
    c. is best diagnosed with red-free photographs
    d. is more likely with higher cumulative doses, rather than higher daily doses

27. Proven systemic control for diabetic retinopathy includes
    a. lowering serum cholesterol
    b. aspirin use
    c. ACE inhibitors
    d. blood pressure control

28. Retinal artery macroaneursysms
    a. are usually located in the macula
    b. produce multilayered hemorrhages
    c. are best seen on ICG angiography
    d. should be treated with focal laser photocoagulation to prevent bleeding

29. The Branch Vein Occlusion Study reported that
    a. aspirin prevented recurrent episodes
    b. focal laser photocoagulation decreased visual loss
    c. panretinal photocoagulation should be applied in ischemic patients
    d. photocoagulation should be delayed in the presence of extensive macular ischemia

30. True statements about ocular photodynamic therapy include all of the following except
    a. requires light precautions for 48 hours after treatment
    b. is indicated for occult with no classic CNV lesions
    c. often requires retreatment every 6 weeks
    d. stabilizes but rarely improves vision

31. Cystoid macular edema
    a. does not leak fluorescein when associated with nicotinic acid
    b. responds to nonsteroidal anti-inflammatory drops
    c. is associated with beta-blockers
    d. has a petalloid appearance on fluorescein angiography

32. PDR is most likely to develop if which one of the following findings is present on fundus exam?
    a. exudates
    b. hemorrhages
    c. microaneurysms
    d. venous beading

33. Which of the following is the biggest risk factor for AMD?
    a. smoking
    b. elevated serum cholesterol level
    c. dark iris color
    d. myopia

34. The most important visual prognostic factor for a rhegmatogenous RD is
    a. size of the break
    b. extent of the detachment
    c. macular involvement
    d. type of surgery

35. The earliest sign of a macular hole is
    a. RPE atrophy in the fovea
    b. vitreous detachment at the fovea
    c. yellow spot in the fovea
    d. partial-thickness eccentric hole in the fovea

36. Focal laser treatment is indicated for diabetic macular edema when there is
    a. hard exudates with retinal thickening 1000 μm from the center of the fovea
    b. neovascularization elsewhere greater than 1/3 disc area in size
    c. ischemia within 250 μm of the center of the fovea
    d. retinal edema within 500 μm of the center of the fovea

37. Reduced IOP would be most unexpected in a patient with
    a. choroidal effusion
    b. choroidal hemorrhage
    c. serous retinal detachment
    d. rhegmatogenous retinal detachment

38. Which of the following is the correct indication for treating macular edema from a Branch Retinal Vein Occlusion?
    a. ≥5 DD of capillary nonperfusion
    b. thickening within 500 μm of the fovea
    c. exudates in the fovea
    d. vision worse than 20/40 for greater than 3 months

39. Which test is best for distinguishing a choroidal melanoma from a choroidal hemangioma?
    a. transillumination
    b. red free photo
    c. ultrasound
    d. CT scan

40. The etiology of vitreous hemorrhage in Terson's syndrome is
    a. intracranial hypertension
    b. hypercoagulability
    c. embolus
    d. neovascularization

41. The most common site of metastasis for a choroidal melanoma is
    a. brain
    b. liver
    c. lungs
    d. skin

42. Which of the following is least characteristic of Eales' disease?
    a. vascular sheathing
    b. vitreous hemorrhage
    c. neovascularization
    d. macular edema

43. Crystalline retinopathy is not associated with
    a. tamoxifen
    b. methoxyflurane
    c. thioridazine
    d. canthaxanthine

44. Combined hamartoma of the retina and RPE has been associated with all of the following except
    a. neurofibromatosis
    b. tuberous sclerosis
    c. Gorlin syndrome
    d. Gardner syndrome

45. All of the following statements regarding uveal metastases are true except
    a. most common primary sites are breast and lung
    b. most common ocular location is anterior choroid
    c. often have an exudative RD
    d. fluorescein angiography usually demonstrates early hyperfluorescence

SUGGESTED READINGS

American Academy of Ophthalmology, vol 12. San Francisco, AAO, 2012.

Bell WJ, Stenstrom WJ: Atlas of the Peripheral Retina. Philadelphia, WB Saunders, 1998.

Byrne SF, Green RL: Ultrasound of the Eye and Orbit, 2nd edn. St Louis, Mosby, 1992.

Gass J: Stereoscopic Atlas of Macular Diseases: Diagnosis and Treatment, 4th edn. St Louis, Mosby, 1997.

Guyer DR, Yannuzzi LA, Chang A, et al: Retina-Vitreous-Macula. Philadelphia, WB Saunders, 1999.

Ryan SJ: Retina, 3rd edn. St Louis, Mosby, 2001.

Shields JA, Shields CL: Intraocular Tumors: A Text and Atlas, 2nd edn. Philadelphia, Lippincott Williams & Wilkins, 2007.

Wilkinson CP, Rice TA: Michels's Retinal Detachment, 2nd edn. St Louis, Mosby, 1997.

Yannuzzi LA: The Retinal Atlas. Philadelphia, Saunders, 2010.

Answers to Questions

CHAPTER 1 OPTICS

1. Prince's rule is helpful in determining all of the following except
   d. accommodative convergence

2. A myope who pushes his spectacles closer to his face and tilts them is
   d. increasing effectivity, increasing cylinder

3. The Prentice position refers to
   a. glass prism perpendicular to visual axis

4. The purpose of Q-switching a laser is to
   b. decrease energy, increase power

5. A 50-year-old woman with aphakic glasses wants a new pair of spectacles to use when applying make-up. How much power should be added to her distance correction so that she can focus while sitting 50 cm in front of her mirror?
   c. +1.00 D—with a plane mirror, the image is located as far behind the mirror as the object is in front of the mirror; therefore, the distance between her eye and the image of her eye is 100 cm=1 m, and this requires +1.00 D of extra magnification

6. How far from a plano mirror must a 6-ft-tall man stand to see his whole body?
   b. 3 feet—to view one's entire body, a plane mirror need be only half one's height

7. A 33-year-old woman with a refraction of $-9.00 +3.00 \times 90$ OD at vertex distance 10 mm and keratometry readings of 46.00@90/43.00@180 is fit for a rigid gas-permeable (RGP) contact lens 1 D steeper than flattest K. What power lens is required?
   c. −7.00 D—step 1: change refraction to minus cylinder form (because the tear lake negates the minus cylinder) and use this sphere (−6.00); step 2: adjust to zero vertex distance $(-6+0.01[-6]^2=-5.64)$; step 3: adjust for tear lens (SAM-FAP rule) (add −1.00=−6.64)

8. What is the size of a 20/60 letter on a standard 20-ft Snellen chart (tangent of 1 minute of arc=0.0003)?
   d. 27 mm—20/60 letter subtends 5 minutes at 60 ft (18 m); therefore, size of letter=18 (tan 5′)=18 (0.0015)=0.027 m or 27 mm

9. A Galilean telescope with a +5 D objective and a −20 D eyepiece produces an image with what magnification and direction?
   a. 4×, erect—magnification=−(−20)/5=+4, meaning 4× magnification and erect image

10. An object is placed 33 cm in front of an eye. The image formed by reflection from the front surface of the cornea (radius of curvature equals 8 mm) is located
    b. 4 mm behind cornea—reflecting power of the cornea is −2/0.008=−250 D; thus, the focal point is 1/−250= −4 mm, or 4 mm behind the cornea

11. A convex mirror produces what type of image?
    d. virtual, erect, minified—remember VErMin

12. In general, the most bothersome problem associated with bifocals is
    a. image jump—therefore, choose bifocal segment type to minimize jump; flat-top segments minimize image jump because the optical center is near the top; this also reduces image displacement in myopes

13. A refraction with a stenopeic slit gives the following measurements: +1.00 at 90° and −2.00 at 180°. The corresponding spectacle prescription is
    c. $-2.00 + 3.00 \times 180$—this is the correct spherocylindrical notation for a power cross diagram with +1.00 along the 90° meridian and −2.00 along the 180° meridian

14. A point source of light is placed 1/3 of a meter to the left of a +7 D lens. Where will its image come to focus?
    a. 25 cm to the right of the lens—the light has vergence of −3 D and encounters a +7 D lens; thus, the exiting light has vergence of +4 D, and the image will come to focus 25 cm to the right of the lens

15. What is the equivalent sphere of the following cross cylinder: -3.00×180 combined with $+0.50 \times 90$?
    b. −1.25—the cross cylinder has a spherocylindrical notation of $-3.00 + 3.50 \times 90$; so the spherical equivalent is −3.00 + (3.50/2)=−1.25

16. What is the size of a letter on a standard 20-ft Snellen chart if it forms an image of 1/2 mm on a patient's retina?
    d. 18 cm—using the reduced schematic eye and similar triangles, 0.5/17 mm=object size/6 m; solving for object size yields 18 cm

17. The image of a distant object is largest in which patient?
    b. hyperope with spectacles

18. What type of image is produced if an object is placed in front of a convex lens within its focal length?
    b. erect and virtual

19. What is the correct glasses prescription if retinoscopy performed at 50 cm shows neutralization with a plano lens?
    a. −2.00—remember to subtract for working distance (1/0.5 m=2 D); thus, a plano lens minus 2 D yields a −2.00 D glasses prescription

20. An anisometropic patient experiences difficulty while reading with bifocals. Which of the following is not helpful for reducing the induced phoria?
    c. progressive lenses—this problem is due to the prismatic effect of the underlying lens and will occur with all bifocal styles, including progressive lenses

21. A Geneva lens clock is used to measure what?
    d. base curve

22. What is the induced prism when a 67-year-old woman reads 10 mm below the upper segment optical center of her bifocals, which measure +2.50 + 1.00×90 OD and −1.50 + 1.50×180 OS add +2.50 OU?
    c. 2.5 prism diopters—using Prentice's rule, the induced prism is (+2.50×1) OD and ([−1.50 +1.50]×1) OS (cylinder power acts in the vertical meridian, so it must be used in the calculation); the total is +2.5 PD BU OD; the effect is due to the underlying lens; the power of the bifocal segment can be ignored because it is the same for both lenses (5 PD BU OD and 2.5 PD BU OS=2.5 PD BU OD)

23. The optimal size of a pinhole for measuring pinhole visual acuity is approximately
    c. 1.25 mm—limited by diffraction if smaller than 1.2 mm

24. A person looking at an object 5 m away through a 10^Δ prism placed base-in over the right eye would see the image displaced
    b. 50 cm to the right—a 10^Δ prism displaces light 10 cm/1 m or 50 cm at 5 m, and the image is displaced to the apex

25. Calculate the soft contact lens power for a 40-year-old hyperope who wears +14.00 D glasses at a vertex distance of 11 mm.
    b. +16.00 D—using the simplified formula, new power=$14+0.011\ (14)^2=16.156$

26. After cataract surgery, a patient's refraction is −0.75+1.75×10, in what meridian should a suture be cut to reduce the astigmatism?
    d. 10°—the steep meridian corresponds to the axis of the plus cylinder (plus cylinder acts to steepen the flat meridian, which is 90° away from the cylinder axis)

27. What is the appropriate correction in the IOL power if the A constant for the lens to be implanted is changed from 117 to 118?
    b. increase IOL power by 1.0 D—the change in A constant is equivalent to the change in IOL power

28. An IOL labeled with a power of +20 D has a refractive index of 1.5. If this lens were removed from the package and measured with a lensometer, what power would be found?
    d. +59 D—using the formula for calculating the power of a thin lens immersed in fluid $(D_{air}/D_{aqueous})=(n_{iol}-n_{air})/(n_{iol}-n_{aqueous})$, $D_{air}=20$ $([1.5-1.0]/[1.5-1.33])=+58.8$ D

29. The spherical equivalent of a 0.50 D cross cylinder is
    a. plano—by definition, all cross cylinders have a spherical equivalent of zero; this is evident by writing the cross cylinder in spherocylindrical notation
    example: +0.50−1.00×90

30. To minimize image displacement in a hyperope, the best type of bifocal segment style is
    c. round top—to minimize image displacement, the prismatic effects of the bifocal segment and the distance lens should be in opposite directions; a round top acts like a base-down prism and the underlying hyperopic lens acts like a base-up prism

31. The logMAR equivalent to 20/40 Snellen acuity is
    b. 0.3

32. A patient who is pseudophakic in one eye and phakic in the other eye will have what amount of aniseikonia
    b. 2.5%

33. A patient with 20/80 vision is seen for a low vision evaluation. What add power should be prescribed so the patient does not have to use accommodation to read the newspaper
    b. +4—the add power is calculated from the inverse of the distance Snellen acuity: 80/20=4

34. The spherical equivalent of a −2.00+1.50×90 lens is
    c. −1.25—the spherical equivalent is obtained by adding half the cylinder power to the sphere: −2.00+0.75=−1.25

35. After extracapsular cataract extraction a patient is found to have 2 D of with-the-rule astigmatism and a tight suture across the wound at 12 o'clock. Corneal topography is obtained and the placido disc image shows an oval pattern with the mires closest together at
    a. 12 o'clock with the short axis at 90 degrees—WTR astigmatism refers to steep meridian (short axis) at 90 degrees (12 o'clock) which corresponds to the tight suture. The pattern of projected placido rings is oval in astigmatism with the lines closest together in the steepest meridian (short axis)

36. A 57-year-old woman has a 0.25 mm macular hole in her left eye. The size of the corresponding scotoma on a tangent screen at 1 meter is approximately
    b. 1.5 cm—using similar triangles and the model eye with a nodal point of 17 mm, the resulting equation is: 0.25/17=x/1000

37. During retinoscopy, when neutralization is reached, the light reflex is
    d. widest and fastest—at neutralization, the retinoscopic reflex is fastest, widest, and brightest

38. A patient undergoing fogged refraction with an astigmatic dial sees the 9 to 3 o'clock line clearer than all the others. At what axis should this patient's minus cylinder correcting lens be placed?
    c. 90 degrees—with an astigmatic dial, the axis of the minus cylinder correcting lens is found by multiplying the lower number of the clearest line by 30 (i.e., for the 9 to 3 o'clock line: $3 \times 30 = 90$)

39. Myopia is associated with all of the following conditions except
    a. nanophthalmos—nanophthalmos is associated with hyperopia.

40. What is the ratio of the magnification from a direct ophthalmoscope to the magnification from an indirect ophthalmoscope with a 20 D lens at a distance of 25 cm if the patient and examiner are both emmetropic?
    c. $5:1$—the magnification for the direct is $60/4 = 15$ and the magnification for the indirect is $60/20 = 3$, so the ratio of the magnifications is $15:3 = 5:1$

41. A patient with anisometropia wears glasses with a prescription of +5.00 OD and +1.25 OS. Which of the following actions will not reduce the amount of aniseikonia?
    b. decrease center thickness of left lens—this will have the opposite effect (increase the anisometropia)

42. The principal measurement determined by a Prince's rule and +3 D lens in front of the patient's eye is the
    b. amplitude of accommodation—the Prince's rule is primarily designed to measure the amplitude of accommodation

43. The 10× eyepiece of the slit lamp biomicroscope is essentially a simple magnifier. Using the standard reference distance of 25 cm, what is the dioptric power of the 10× eyepiece?
    d. +40 D—magnification = D/4, so 10 = D/4 and D = 40

44. When refracting an astigmatic patient with a Lancaster dial, the examiner should place the
    d. entire conoid of Sturm in front of the retina—the patient must be fogged so that the entire conoid of Sturm is in front of the retina

45. To increase the magnification of the image during indirect ophthalmoscopy, the examiner should:
    a. move closer to the condensing lens—this causes the image to subtend a larger angle on the examiner's retina thereby increasing the magnification

CHAPTER 2 PHARMACOLOGY

1. Which antibiotic results in the highest intravitreal concentration when administered orally?
    a. ciprofloxacin

2. Which anesthetic agent would most interfere with an intraocular gas bubble?
    d. nitrous oxide

3. Which of the following is not an adverse effect of CAIs?
    c. iris cysts

4. Which β-blocker has the least effect on β_2 receptors?
    b. betaxolol—this is a cardioselective β_1-blocker

5. Which drug has the least effect on uveoscleral outflow?
    d. Trusopt—this is a CAI that decreases aqueous production; Xalatan and atropine increase and pilocarpine decreases uveoscleral outflow.

6. Which enzyme is inhibited by steroids?
    b. phospholipase A_2

7. Which of the following steroid formulations has the best corneal penetrability?
    a. prednisolone acetate—order of corneal penetrability is acetate > alcohol > phosphate

8. Adverse effects of foscarnet include all of the following except
    b. infertility

9. Which glaucoma medication is not effective when IOP is >60 mmHg?
    c. pilocarpine—because of iris ischemia, which occurs at IOP >40 mmHg

10. Which medicine is not associated with OCP-like conjunctival shrinkage?
    d. timoptic

11. Which β-blocker is β_1-selective?
    c. betaxolol

12. The most appropriate treatment for neurosyphilis is
    a. penicillin G—IV penicillin is used to treat neurosyphilis

13. The correct mechanism of action of botulinum toxin is
    a. prevents release of acetylcholine

14. Fluoroquinolones are least effective against
    c. anaerobic cocci

15. Hydroxychloroquine toxicity depends most on
    b. cumulative dose

16. Calculate the amount of cocaine in 2 mL of a 4% solution.
    d. 80 mg—a 1% solution indicates 1 g/100 mL; therefore, a 4% solution is 4000 mg/100 mL = 40 mg/mL

17. NSAIDs block the formation of all of the following substances except
    b. leukotrienes—NSAIDs block the conversion of arachidonic acid by cyclooxygenase into endoperoxides (thus inhibiting the formation of prostaglandins, thromboxane, and prostacyclin); leukotrienes are formed from arachidonic acid by lipoxygenase; steroids block the formation of arachidonic acid (and therefore, all subsequent end products) by inhibiting phospholipase A_2

18. Systemic effects of steroids may include all of the following except
    d. renal tubular acidosis

19. Which drug does not produce decreased tear production?
    a. pilocarpine

20. Natamycin is a
    c. polyene

21. Which glaucoma medicine does not decrease aqueous production?
    b. pilocarpine—miotics increase aqueous outflow

22. β-blockers may cause all of the following except
    a. constipation

23. Idoxuridine may cause all of the following except
    c. corneal hypesthesia

24. Which of the following antifungal agents has the broadest spectrum against yeast-like fungi?
    d. amphotericin

25. All of the following medications are combination antihistamine and mast cell stabilizers except
    a. Alomide—is only a mast cell stabilizer

26. The antidote for atropine toxicity is
    b. physostigmine

27. Which of the following agents is contraindicated for ruptured globe repair?
    d. succinylcholine—this nicotinic receptor antagonist causes muscle contraction and is therefore contraindicated in ruptured globe repair since EOM contraction could result in extrusion of intraocular contents

28. The duration of action of one drop of proparacaine is
    b. 20 minutes—the duration of proparacaine is 10–30 minutes

29. Which of the following medications is not commercially available as a topical formulation?
    d. vancomycin—must be compounded, the others are available as Zirgan, Azasite, and Restasis, respectively

30. All of the following are complications of carbonic anhydrase inhibitors except
    c. metabolic alkalosis—CAIs cause metabolic acidosis

31. Topirimate is associated with
    d. angle-closure glaucoma without pupillary block

32. A patient with ocular hypertension and an allergy to sulfonamides should not be treated with
    b. dorzolamide—CAIs are sulfa drugs and are contraindicated in patients with a sulfa allergy

33. Infectious keratitis due to *Candida albicans* is best treated with topical
    a. amphotericin B

34. Which of the following oral agents should be used to treat a patient with ocular cicatricial pemphigoid?
    c. cyclophosphamide—this cytotoxic agent is used to treat patients with OCP

35. The glaucoma medication contraindicated in infants is
    b. brimonidine—selective alpha-agonists can cause death in infants

36. Which systemic antibiotic is used to treat Chlamydia during pregnancy?
    d. erythromycin—erythromycins are the preferred antibiotic for Chlamydia infection and are safe during pregnancy

37. The local anesthetic with the longest duration of action is
    c. bupivacaine

38. A 33-year-old man has had follicular conjunctivitis with a watery discharge for 5 weeks. Elementary bodies are present on a conjunctival smear, therefore, the most appropriate treatment is
    a. oral azithromycin—the patient has chlamydial conjunctivitis and requires oral antibiotics

39. The most appropriate treatment for *Fusarium* keratitis is topical
    b. pimaricin—this antifungal, also known as natamycin, is used to treat fungal keratitis

40. All of the following are associated with vitamin A toxicity except
    d. band keratopathy

CHAPTER 3   EMBRYOLOGY/PATHOLOGY

1. Which stain is the most helpful in the diagnosis of sebaceous cell carcinoma?
   c. Oil-red-O, which stains lipid

2. Pagetoid spread is most commonly associated with
   c. sebaceous cell carcinoma—this is invasion of intact epithelium by nests of cells and is characteristic of sebaceous cell carcinoma; pagetoid spread can also occur in the rare superficial spreading form of melanoma that occurs on unexposed skin areas (back, legs)

3. A melanoma occurring in which of the following locations has the best prognosis?
   a. iris—often can be completely excised

4. Calcification in retinoblastoma is due to
   a. RPE metaplasia

5. The type of organism that causes Lyme disease is a
   b. spirochete

6. Characteristics of ghost cells include all of the following except
   d. biconcave

7. A moll gland is best categorized as
   b. apocrine

8. Which of the following is not a Gram-positive rod?
   c. *Serratia*—this bacterium is Gram-negative

9. Trantas' dots are composed of what cell type?
   c. eosinophil

10. Types of collagen that can be found in the cornea include all of the following except
    b. II—is found in vitreous; type I is found in normal coneal stroma, III in stromal wound healing, and IV in basement membranes

11. Lens nuclei are retained in all of the following conditions except
    d. Alport's syndrome

12. Vogt-Koyanagi-Harada syndrome is best described by which type of hypersensitivity reaction?
    d. IV

13. Lacy vacuolization of the iris occurs in which disease?
    b. diabetes—lacy vacuolization is a pathologic finding of glycogen-filled cysts in the iris pigment epithelium

14. Antoni A and B cells occur in which tumor?
    a. neurilemmoma (schwannoma)

15. Which tumor is classically described as having a 'Swiss cheese' appearance?
    b. adenoid cystic carcinoma

16. Which iris nodule is correctly paired with its pathology
    b. Lisch nodule, neural crest hamartoma—this is correct. JXG nodules are composed of histiocytes and Touton giant cells, Koeppe nodules are collections of inflammatory cells, and Brushfield spots are stromal hyperplasia.

17. Which of the following statements is true concerning immunoglobulin
    a. IgG crosses the placenta

18. A retinal detachment caused by fixation artifact can be differentiated from a true retinal detachment by all of the following except
    a. a fold at the ora serrata—is a fixation artifact found in newborn eyes called Lange's fold. It is not related to an artifactual or true retinal detachment.

19. Which of the following epithelial changes in the eyelid refers to thickening of the squamous cell layer
    b. acanthosis

20. Intraocular hemorrhage may cause all of the following sequelae except
    c. asteroid hyalosis—is calcium soaps suspended in the vitreous and is unrelated to hemorrhage.

21. Intraocular calcification may occur in all of the following except
    b. medulloepithelioma—this tumor may contain cartilage.

22. The histopathology of which tumor is classically described as a storiform pattern of tumor cells
    d. fibrous histiocytoma

23. Which of the following findings is a histologic fixation artifact
    a. Lange's fold—is a fold at the ora serrata that is a fixation artifact in newborn eyes.

24. The corneal stroma is composed of
    b. neural crest cells

25. *Neisseria* is best cultured with which media
    d. chocolate agar

26. Which of the following stains is used to detect amyloid
    c. crystal violet—stains used to detect amyloid are Congo red, crystal violet, and thioflavin T

27. HLA-B7 is associated with
    b. presumed ocular histoplasmosis syndrome—POHS is associated with HLA-B7; the other associations are

Behçet's disease with B51, iridocyclitis with B27, and sympathetic ophthalmia with DR4

28. Which of the following conjunctival lesions should be sent to the pathology lab as a fresh unfixed tissue speciment?
    a. lymphoma—fresh tissue is required for immunohistochemical staining

29. Subepithelial infiltrates in the cornea from epidemic keratoconjunctivitis are thought to be
    c. macrophages containing adenoviral particles

30. Which is the correct order of solutions for performing a Gram stain?
    d. crystal violet stain, iodine solution, ethanol, safranin

CHAPTER 4   NEURO-OPHTHALMOLOGY

1. The visual field defect most characteristic of optic neuritis is
    b. central—all of these may occur in optic neuritis, but a central scotoma is most characteristic

2. Which cranial nerve is most prone to injury in the cavernous sinus?
    d. 6—travels in middle of sinus and is not protected by lateral wall as are CN 3, 4, and 5

3. Which of the following agents is least toxic to the optic nerve?
    b. dapsone

4. Seesaw nystagmus is produced by a lesion located in which area?
    c. suprasellar—also associated with bitemporal hemianopia; chiasmal gliomas can cause spasmus nutans—like eye movements in children; lesions in the posterior fossa cause dissociated nystagmus, and those in the cervicomedullary junction cause downbeat nystagmus

5. What is the location of a lesion that causes an ipsilateral Horner's syndrome and a contralateral CN 4 palsy?
    a. midbrain—this is due to a nuclear/fascicular lesion at the level of the midbrain

6. The least useful test for functional visual loss is
    c. HVF—the other tests can commonly be used to trick the patient

7. Optociliary shunt vessels may occur in all of the following conditions except
    d. ischemic optic neuropathy

8. Which is not a symptom of pseudotumor cerebri?
    b. entoptic phenomena

9. A 63-year-old woman reports sudden onset of jagged lines in the right peripheral vision. She has experienced 3 episodes in the past month, which lasted approximately 10 to 20 minutes. She denies headaches and any history or family history of migraines. The most likely diagnosis is
    c. migraine variant—this is a characteristic visual disturbance that occurs in acephalgic migraines and is

called a fortification phenomenon; the other common visual alteration is a scintillating scotoma (appears as flickering colored lights that grow in the visual field)

10. A 60-year-old man with optic disc swelling in the right eye and left optic atrophy most likely has
    a. ischemic optic neuropathy—these findings are consistent with Foster-Kennedy syndrome; however, the most common cause is pseudo-Foster-Kennedy syndrome due to ION

11. Which of the following findings may not be present in a patient with an INO?
    c. absent convergence—this occurs only in an anterior INO, not in a posterior INO (convergence is preserved); thus if the patient has a posterior INO, then absent convergence will not be found; the other 3 findings occur in both anterior and posterior forms of INO

12. A paradoxical pupillary reaction is not found in which condition?
    b. albinism—foveal hypoplasia occurs but pupillary reactivity is normal; paradoxical pupillary response is found in CSNB, achromatopsia, Leber's congenital amaurosis, optic atrophy, and optic nerve hypoplasia

13. Inheritance of Leber's optic neuropathy is
    c. mitochondrial DNA

14. An OKN strip moved to the left stimulates what part of the brain?
    a. right frontal, left occipital

15. The smooth pursuit system does not involve the
    d. frontal motor area—this area is involved with fast eye movements

16. Dorsal midbrain syndrome is not associated with
    a. absent convergence—convergence is present and results in convergence-retraction nystagmus

17. The location of Horner's syndrome is best differentiated by which drug?
    b. paredrine—distinguishes between preganglionic and postganglionic lesions

18. The blood supply to the prelaminar optic nerve is
    c. short posterior ciliary arteries

19. Optic nerve hypoplasia is associated with all of the following except
    d. spasmus nutans

20. A lesion in the pons causes
    b. miosis

21. Which of the following syndromes is characterized by abduction deficit and contralateral hemiplegia?
    c. Millard-Gubler—Foville's and Gradenigo's involve CN 6 but do not cause hemiparesis; Weber's does cause hemiparesis but involves CN 3, not CN 6

22. All of the following are features of progressive supranuclear palsy except
    b. loss of oculovestibular reflex

23. Pituitary apoplexy is characterized by all of the following except
    a. nystagmus

24. Which of the following is most likely to produce a junctional scotoma?
    d. meningioma—a junctional scotoma is caused by a lesion at the junction of the optic nerve and chiasm; this is most commonly due to a meningioma

25. All of the following are characteristics of an optic tract lesion except
    b. decreased vision—visual acuity is not affected

26. The saccade system does not involve the
    a. occipital motor area

27. A 22-year-old man sustains trauma resulting in a transected left optic nerve. Which of the following is true regarding the right pupil?
    c. it is equal in size to the left pupil—because of the intact consensual response in the left eye

28. Characteristics of spasmus nutans include all of the following except
    d. signs present during sleep—spasmus nutans disappears during sleep

29. A congenital CN 4 palsy can be distinguished from an acquired palsy by
    a. vertical fusional amplitude >10 prism diopters

30. Characteristics of a diabetic CN 3 palsy may include all of the following except
    d. aberrant regeneration—this does not occur with vasculopathic causes of CN 3 palsy, only with compression (aneurysm, tumor) or trauma

31. A CN 3 lesion may cause all of the following except
    a. contralateral ptosis—depending on location of the lesion, the ptosis may be ipsilateral (complete or superior division CN 3 paresis), bilateral (nuclear), or no ptosis present (inferior division CN 3 palsy)

32. Optic nerve drusen is associated with all of the following except
    c. CME

33. A lesion causing limited upgaze with an intact Bell's phenomenon is located where?
    a. supranuclear—if Bell's phenomenon is intact, then the lesion must be supranuclear

34. An acute subarachnoid hemorrhage due to a ruptured aneurysm may produce all of the following except
    b. orbital hemorrhage—does not result from a subarachnoid hemorrhage, but vitreous hemorrhage (Terson's syndrome), ptosis, and an afferent pupillary defect (CN 3 palsy) can occur

36. The length of the canalicular portion of the optic nerve is approximately
    b. 10 mm

36. Findings in ocular motor apraxia include all of the following except
    b. abnormal pursuits

37. Which of the following statements is true regarding the optic chiasm?
    c. 55% of nasal retinal fibers cross to the contralateral optic tract

38. Which of the following statements is false regarding the lateral geniculate body (LGB)?
    d. P cells are important for motion detection—this is false, P cells are involved with fine spatial resolution and color vision. M cells are important for motion detection, stereoacuity, and contrast

39. A patient with a homonymous hemianopia is found to have an asymmetric OKN response. The location of the lesion is
    a. parietal lobe—this is Cogan's dictum: for homonymous hemianopia, asymmetric OKN indicates parietal lobe lesion and symmetric OKN indicates occipital lobe lesion

40. The only intact eye movement in one-and-a-half syndrome is
    c. abduction of contralateral eye

41. A pineal tumor is most likely to cause
    d. Parinaud's syndrome

42. Metastatic neuroblastoma is most likely to be associated with
    a. opsoclonus

43. Which of the following statements regarding pupillary innervation is true?
    d. sympathetic innervation of the iris dilator involves three neurons and the ciliospinal center of Budge

44. The most important test to order in a patient with chronic progressive external ophthalmoplegia is
    b. EKG—to rule out heart block from Kearns-Sayre syndrome

45. Pseudotumor cerebri is most likely to cause a palsy of which cranial nerve?
    d. 6

46. CT scan of a patient with visual loss shows a railroad-track sign. The most likely diagnosis is
    c. optic nerve meningioma

47. The most likely etiology of homonymous hemianopia with macular sparing is
    a. vascular—the most common cause of occipital lobe lesions

48. All of the following findings can occur in optic neuritis except
    d. metamorphopsia

49. Which of the following findings is not associated with an acoustic neuroma
    b. light-near dissociation

50. A superior oblique muscle palsy is most commonly caused by
    d. trauma—the most common etiology of a CN 4 palsy

51. A 29-year-old obese woman with headaches, papilledema, and a normal head CT scan is diagnosed with idiopathic intracranial hypertension. All of the following findings are consistent with her diagnosis except
    b. homonymous hemianopia

52. Transection of the left optic nerve adjacent to the chiasm results in
    a. visual field defect in the right eye—junctional scotoma due to crossing fibers in knee of von Willebrand

53. The Amsler grid tests how many degrees of central vision?
    b. 10

54. Aberrant regeneration of CN 3 may cause all of the following except
    c. monocular dampening of the OKN response

55. A 42-year-old woman admitted to the hospital with severe headache and neck stiffness suddenly becomes disoriented and vomits. On examination her left pupil is dilated and does not react to light. She most likely has
    d. subarachnoid hemorrhage—this scenario represents a CN 3 palsy due to a ruptured aneurysm (posterior communicating artery)

CHAPTER 5 PEDIATRICS/STRABISMUS

1. The approximate age of onset for accommodative ET is closest to
   b. 3 years old

2. A 15-year-old girl with strabismus is examined, and the following measurements are recorded: distance deviation of 10 prism diopters, near deviation of 35 prism diopters at 20 cm, and interpupillary distance of 60 mm. Her AC/A ratio is
   a. 11 : 1—to calculate the AC/A ratio with this information, use the heterophoria method: $IPD + [(N - D)/Diopt] = 6 + [(35 - 10)/5] = 11$ (remember to convert IPD to cm, and 20 cm = 5 D)

3. Duane's syndrome is thought to be due to a developmental abnormality of
   d. abducens nucleus

4. The most helpful test in a patient with aniridia is
   b. abdominal ultrasound—to rule out Wilms' tumor in sporadic cases

5. The best test for an infant with a normal fundus and searching eye movements is
   a. VER—can be used to determine acuity

6. The most common congenital infection is
   c. CMV

7. ARC is most likely to develop in a child with
   a. congenital esotropia

8. Which of the following most accurately reflects what a patient with harmonious ARC reports when the angle of anomaly is equal to the objective angle?
   c. simultaneous macular perception

9. The inferior oblique muscle is weakened most by which procedure?
   d. anteriorization

10. The test that gives the best dissociation is
    b. Worth 4 Dot

11. The 3-step test shows a left hypertropia in primary position that worsens on right gaze and with left head tilt. The best surgical procedure is
    d. LIO weakening—this is an LSO palsy, so possible treatments include LIO weakening, RIR recession, LSO tuck, and LIR resection

12. In the treatment of a superior oblique palsy, Knapp recommended all of the following except
    d. resection of the contralateral SR—the contralateral SR should be weakened with a recession, not strengthened with a resection

13. The best results of cryotherapy for ROP occur for treatment of disease in which location?
    b. anterior zone 2

14. Characteristics of congenital ET include all of the following except
    c. amblyopia

15. The contralateral antagonist of the right superior rectus
    a. passes under another muscle—the contralateral antagonist of the right superior rectus is the left superior oblique (the antagonist [LSO] of the yoke muscle [LIO] of the paretic muscle [RSR]); the SO passes under the SR, is an incyclotorter (therefore causes excyclotorsion when paretic), abducts the eye, and is innervated by CN 4

16. With respect to Panum's area, physiologic diplopia occurs at what point?
    c. in front of Panum's area—physiologic diplopia occurs in front of and behind Panum's area; within Panum's area binocular vision occurs with fusion and stereopsis, on the horopter only fusion

17. The best treatment of an A pattern ET with muscle transposition is
    d. LR resection with downward transposition—appropriate surgery for the ET is LR resection or MR recession; to fix the A pattern, the LRs are moved toward the empty space of the pattern (down for ET) or the MRs are moved toward the apex of the pattern (up for ET)

18. A superior rectus Faden suture is used for the treatment of which condition?
    b. dissociated vertical deviation

19. Which medication should be administered to a child who develops trismus under general anesthesia?
    d. dantrolene—because trismus is a sign of malignant hyperthermia

20. Congenital superior oblique palsy is characterized by all of the following except
    d. <10 D of vertical vergence amplitudes—usually, these amplitudes are >10 D

21. Which of the following statements regarding monofixation syndrome is false?
    c. Fusional vergence amplitudes are absent

22. Iridocyclitis is most commonly associated with which form of JRA?
    d. pauciarticular

23. Congenital rubella is most commonly associated with
    a. retinal pigment epitheliopathy

24. The most common cause of proptosis in a child is
    b. orbital cellulitis

25. Which form of rhabdomyosarcoma has the worst prognosis?
    c. alveolar—is the most malignant and has the worst prognosis; embryonal is the most common, botryoid is a subtype of embryonal, and pleomorphic is the rarest and has the best prognosis

26. Which of the following conditions is the least common cause of childhood proptosis?
    a. cavernous hemangioma—this is the most common benign orbital tumor of adults and occurs most commonly in middle-aged women

27. A child with retinoblastoma is born to healthy parents with no family history of RB. The chance of RB occurring in a second child is approximately
    a. 5%

28. The best chronologic age to examine a baby for ROP is
    c. 36 weeks

29. All of the following are associated with trisomy 13 except
    c. epiblepharon

30. Paradoxical pupillary response does not occur in
    d. albinism

31. An infant with bilateral cataracts is diagnosed with galactosemia. Which enzyme is most likely to be defective?
    b. galactose-1-P-uridyl transferase

32. All of the following are associated with optic nerve drusen except
    c. increased risk of intracranial tumors

33. The etiology of torticollis and intermittent, fine, rapid, pendular nystagmus of the right eye in a 10-month-old baby is most likely
    d. none of the above—this infant has spasmus nutans which is usually benign and rarely due to optic nerve glioma

34. The most common malignant tumor of the orbit in a 6-year-old boy is
    b. rhabdomyosarcoma

35. Retinitis pigmentosa and deafness occur in all of the following disorders except
    c. Refsum's disease—there is no deafness in this RP variant

36. Which of the following agents is most likely to increase IOP during an EUA (examination under anesthesia)?
    d. ketamine—ketamine and succinylcholine raise IOP, chloral hydrate has no effect, and halothane and thiopental decrease IOP

37. α-galactosidase A deficiency is associated with
    a. cornea verticillata—this is the enzyme defect in Fabry's disease

38. Congenital cataracts and glaucoma may occur in all of the following disorders except
    b. Alport's syndrome—glaucoma is not a finding in Alport's syndrome

39. RPE degeneration and optic atrophy are found in all of the following mucopolysaccharidoses except
    d. MPS type IV—findings in MPS type IV include corneal clouding and optic atrophy, not RPE degeneration

40. Which vitamin is not deficient in a patient with abetalipoproteinemia (Bassen-Kornzweig syndrome)?
    b. C—the fat soluble vitamins A, D, E, and K cannot be absorbed in abetalipoproteinemia

41. Hearing loss is not found in
    b. Refsum's disease—this is a form of RP without hearing loss

42. Pheochromocytoma may occur in all of the following phakomatoses except
    a. Louis-Bar syndrome

43. Maternal ingestion of LSD is most likely to result in which congenital optic nerve disorder
    c. hypoplasia—ON hypoplasia is associated with maternal ingestion of alcohol, LSD, quinine, and dilantin

44. A patient with strabismus wearing −6 D glasses is measured with prism and cover test. Compared to the actual amount of deviation, the measurement would find
    b. more esotropia and more exotropia—remember, minus measures more

45. Prism glasses are least helpful for treating
    c. sensory esotropia

46. A 4-year-old boy has bilateral lateral rectus recessions for exotropia. Two days after surgery he has an esotropia measuring 50^Δ. The most appropriate treatment is
    d. surgery—this indicates a slipped muscle which requires surgical repair

47. The most common cause of a vitreous hemorrhage in a child is
    b. shaken baby syndrome—trauma is the most common etiology followed by regressed ROP (which is the most common cause of a spontaneous VH)

48. A 5-year-old girl with 20/20 vision OD and 20/50 vision OS is diagnosed with an anterior polar cataract OS. The most appropriate treatment is
    a. start occlusion therapy

49. Chronic iritis in a child is most commonly caused by
    a. JRA

50. All are features of ataxia-telangiectasia except
    b. thymic hyperplasia—the thymus is hypoplastic

51. All of the following vitreoretinal disorders are inherited in an autosomal dominant pattern except
    d. Goldmann-Favre disease—this is autosomal recessive

52. The most common location for an iris coloboma is
    d. inferonasal

53. Von Hippel-Lindau disease has been mapped to which chromosome?
    a. 3

54. Which X-linked disorder is not associated with an ocular abnormality in the female carrier?
    c. juvenile retinoschisis—female carriers have normal fundus; in the other 3 disorders, female carriers have retinal changes: midperipheral pigment clusters and mottling in macula in albinism, equatorial pigment mottling in choroideremia, golden reflex in posterior pole in retinitis pigmentosa

55. Which tumor is not associated with von Hippel-Lindau disease?
    a. hepatocellular carcinoma

CHAPTER 6   ORBIT/LIDS/ADNEXA

1. The most common causitive organism of canaliculitis is
    c. *Actinomyces israelii*

2. Sequelae of a CN 7 palsy may include all of the following except
    b. ptosis—CN 7 palsy causes inability to close the lid and exposure keratopathy; CN 3 palsy causes ptosis

3. Which procedure is the best treatment option for the repair of a large upper eyelid defect?
    a. Cutler-Beard—is a lid-sharing procedure for repair of large upper eyelid defects, Bick is a horizontal lid-shortening procedure, Hughes is a lid-sharing procedure for repair of large lower eyelid defects, and Fasanella-Servat is a tarsoconjunctival resection for ptosis repair

4. The extraocular muscle with the largest arc of contact is the
    b. IO—which is 15 mm; next is LR at 12 mm, then SO at 7–8 mm, and MR at 7 mm

5. The risk of systemic involvement is highest for an ocular lymphoid tumor in which location?
    b. eyelid—67% have systemic involvement; for orbit, it is 35% and for conjunctiva, 20%

6. The rectus muscle with the shortest tendon of insertion is the
    c. MR—the IO has the shortest tendon (1 mm), but of the rectus muscles, the MR has the shortest tendon at 4.5 mm; the others are SR=6 mm, IR=7 mm, and LR=7 mm

7. Which of the following bones does not make up the medial orbital wall?
    d. palatine—is part of the orbital floor; the medial wall is composed of the other 3 bones and the sphenoid

8. Which of the following clinical features is least commonly associated with a tripod fracture?
    a. restriction of the inferior rectus—tripod fractures include disruption of the orbital floor, but entrapment

of ocular tissues is rare and is usually associated with large floor fractures (blow-out fracture); the other 3 findings are much more common in a tripod fracture

9. A carotid-cavernous fistula can be differentiated from a dural-sinus fistula by all of the following characteristics except
   a. proptosis—this can occur in both types of AV fistula; the other signs are seen with C-C fistulas

10. Basal cell carcinoma is least likely to occur at which site?
    d. lateral canthus—the order (in decreasing frequency) is as follows: lower lid > medial canthus > upper lid > lateral canthus

11. All of the following are sites of attachment of the limbs of the medial canthal tendon except
    c. orbital process of the frontal bone

12. Which muscle is most commonly responsible for vertical diplopia after 4-lid blepharoplasty?
    b. inferior oblique—because it lies below the IR and is encircled by the capsulopalpebral fascia

13. Congenital and involutional ptosis can be distinguished by all of the following except
    c. width of palprebal fissure

14. Congenital obstruction of the lacrimal drainage system usually occurs at the
    d. valve of Hasner

15. What is the correct order of structures that would be encountered when the upper eyelid is penetrated 14 mm above the lid margin?
    a. preseptal orbicularis muscle, orbital septum, levator aponeurosis, Müller's muscle

16. What is the best treatment option for a child who develops recurrent proptosis after upper respiratory infections?
    a. observation—this scenario is common with an orbital lymphangioma, and spontaneous regression often occurs

17. All of the following are features of mucormycosis except
    b. ipsilateral CN 7 palsy—mucor may cause an orbital apex syndrome, but CN 7 is not involved

18. All of the following are associated with blepharophimosis except
    c. AR inheritance—blepharophimosis may be part of an AD syndrome (chromosome 3q), as well as trisomy 18; findings include blepharophimosis, ptosis, telecanthus, ectropion, and epicanthus inversus

19. Which of the following is the most important test to perform in a patient with a capillary hemangioma?
    d. bleeding time—to look for Kassabach-Merritt syndrome (consumptive coagulopathy)

20. For entropion repair, the lateral tarsal strip is sutured
    c. above and anterior to the rim

21. Staged surgery for a patient with severe thyroid-related ophthalmopathy is best done in what order
    a. decompression, strabismus, lid repair—because decompression may affect ocular alignment and lid

position, and strabismus surgery may affect lid position

22. Which of the following best explains why when a ptotic lid is lifted, the contralateral lid falls?
    d. Hering's law—equal and simultaneous innervation to synergistic muscles; thus, lifting a ptotic lid decreases the innervation to the levator bilaterally so the contralateral lid will fall slightly

23. Which study is most helpful in the evaluation of a patient with opsoclonus?
    b. MRI—to rule out neuroblastoma or visceral carcinoma

24. What is the most appropriate treatment for a benign mixed tumor of the lacrimal gland?
    b. excision—must excise completely en bloc to prevent recurrence and malignant transformation

25. What is the most appropriate treatment for a biopsy-positive basal cell carcinoma of the lower eyelid?
    d. excision with frozen section control of the margins

26. CT enhancement is most associated with which lesion?
    d. meningioma—produces characteristic railroad track sign

27. Which of the following factors is least likely to contribute to the development of entropion?
    a. preseptal orbicularis override—this can occur but is less common than the other factors

28. A 24-year-old woman presents after blunt trauma to the left orbit with enophthalmos and restriction of upgaze. Which plain film radiographic view would be most helpful?
    c. Waters view—gives best view of orbital floor

29. All of the following may cause enophthalmos except
    b. lymphoma—may cause proptosis but not enophthalmos; breast cancer can cause either, and phthisis and floor fractures may cause enophthalmos

30. All of the following nerves pass through the superior orbital fissure except
    c. CN V_2—passes through the inferior orbital fissure

31. Blepharospasm is associated with
    d. Parkinson's disease

32. The anatomic boundaries of the superior orbital fissure are
    b. the greater and lesser wings of the sphenoid

33. Which of the following is most likely to exacerbate the symptoms of thyroid-related ophthalmopathy
    b. cigarettes

34. a 44-year-old woman develops a left lower eyelid ectropion following a severe facial burn. The most appropriate procedure includes
    a. horizontal tightening—and revision of the cicatrix is performed for cicatricial ectropion repair, and a vertical lengthening procedure with full-thickness graft may also be required

35. All of the following are methods of treating spastic entropion except
    c. Wies marginal rotation—is used to treat involutional entropion

36. The most common complication of a hydroxyapatite orbital implant is
    d. conjunctival erosion

37. Which collagen vascular disease is associated with malignancy?
    a. dermatomyositis

38. Oral antibiotics are indicated for
    b. dacryocystitis—dacryocystitis is treated with topical and systemic antiobiotics, while dacryoadenitis may sometimes require systemic antibiotics.

39. The levator muscle inserts onto all of the following structures except
    d. trochlea

40. When performing a DCR, the osteum is created at the level of the
    b. middle turbinate

CHAPTER 7   CORNEA/EXTERNAL DISEASE

1. Which is the least desirable method for corneal graft storage?
   b. glycerin—does not preserve endothelial cells and can be used only for lamellar or patch grafts; moist chamber at 4°C preserves tissue for 48 hours, Optisol for up to 10 days, and cryopreservation potentially for years

2. Presently in the United States, phlyctenule is most commonly associated with
   c. Staphylococcus

3. Which blood test is most helpful in the evaluation of a patient with Schnyder's crystalline corneal dystrophy?
   d. cholesterol—may be elevated

4. Which disease has never been transmitted by a corneal graft?
   a. CMV—the others have been transmitted in humans or experimentally in animals

5. Which corneal dystrophy does not recur in a corneal graft?
   d. PPMD

6. A conjunctival map biopsy is typically used for which malignancy?
   c. sebaceous cell carcinoma

7. Corneal clouding does not occur in which mucopolysaccharidosis?
   a. Hunter

8. All of the following may cause follicular conjunctivitis except
   b. Neisseria

9. Which of the following tests is least helpful in determining the etiology of enlarged corneal nerves?
   a. EKG—the others are all helpful in detecting disorders that are associated with enlarged corneal nerves: calcitonin for medullary thyroid carcinoma (MEN 2b), urinary VMA for pheochromocytoma (MEN 2b), acid-fast stain for atypical Mycobacteria (leprosy)

10. Corneal filaments are least likely to be present in which condition?
    b. Thygeson's SPK

11. Which of the following is not an appropriate treatment for SLK?
    c. silver nitrate stick—may cause globe perforation; therefore, use only silver nitrate solution

12. In what level of the cornea does a Kayser-Fleischer ring occur?
    d. Descemet's membrane

13. Cornea verticillata—like changes are associated with all of the following except
    b. thorazine

14. The least common location for a nevus is
    a. bulbar conjunctiva

15. All of the following ions move across the corneal endothelium by both active transport and passive diffusion except
    a. Cl⁻—moves across endothelium only by passive diffusion

16. Which organism is associated with crystalline keratopathy?
    d. S. viridans

17. Which of the following conditions is associated with the best 5-year prognosis for a corneal graft?
    b. Fuchs' dystrophy

18. The best strategy for loosening a tight contact lens is to
    c. decrease the diameter—decreasing the curvature will also loosen a tight lens but not as well; increasing the diameter or curvature will tighten a lens

19. The type of contact lens that causes the least endothelial pleomorphism is
    a. soft daily wear

20. Which of the following conditions is associated with the worst prognosis for a corneal graft?
    c. Reis-Bucklers' dystrophy—this dystrophy commonly recurs in the graft

21. Which is not a treatment of acute hydrops?
    d. corneal transplant—eventually, this may be an option, but short-term treatment is medical only

22. Which organism cannot penetrate intact corneal epithelium?
    c. P. aeruginosa—cannot penetrate intact corneal epithelium; the others and Listeria can

23. Which organism is most commonly associated with angular blepharitis?
    b. Moraxella

24. Which of the following medications would be the best choice in the treatment of microsporidial keratoconjunctivitis?
    a. fumagillin

25. All of the following agents are used in the treatment of *Acanthamoeba* keratitis except
    b. natamycin

26. Goblet cells are most abundant in which location?
    a. fornix

27. Thygeson's superficial punctate keratopathy is best treated with topical
    c. loteprednol—steroids are the best treatment

28. EKC is typically contagious for how many days?
    d. 14 days

29. A shield ulcer is associated with
    c. VKC

30. Ulcerative blepharitis is most likely to be caused by
    b. Herpes

31. Which of the following is most likely to be associated with melanoma of the conjunctiva and uvea?
    c. Nevus of Ota—increased risk of melanomas in Caucasians. This is rarer for congenital melanosis oculi (ocular melanocytosis), and acquired melanosis oculi (PAM) is not associated with uveal melanoma.

32. Which of the following is not associated with *N. gonorrheae* conjunctivitis?
    a. pseudomembrane—GC conjunctivitis causes a true membrane

33. Even spreading of the tear film depends most on which factor?
    c. mucin

34. A neurotrophic ulcer should not be treated with
    b. antiviral—this can cause more toxicity

35. Which layer of the cornea can regenerate?
    c. Descemet's membrane—can regenerate if endothelium is intact

36. The most appropriate treatment for a patient with scleromalacia is
    d. oral immunosuppressive agent—scleromalacia is caused by severe rheumatoid arthritis

37. The HEDS recommendation for treating stromal (disciform) keratitis is
    b. topical steroid and topical antiviral—oral acyclovir was not found to be useful

38. A satellite infiltrate with feathery edges is most characteristic of a corneal ulcer caused by
    d. Fusarium—these characteristics are associated with fungal ulcers

39. PTK would be most appropriate for treating which of the following corneal disorders?
    a. superficial granular dystrophy

40. A 62-year-old woman with keratoconjunctivitis sicca is most likely to demonstrate corneal staining in which location?
    b. middle third (interpalpebral)—due to exposure between the eyelids

41. Which of the following findings is most commonly associated with SLK?
    a. filaments—found in 50%

42. Which lab test is most helpful to obtain in a 38-year-old man with herpes zoster ophthalmicus?
    d. HIV test—herpes zoster is rare in healthy individuals younger than 40 years old and may indicate immunosuppression

43. A patient with conjunctival intraepithelial neoplasia is most likely to have
    d. HPV—this virus is associated with CIN, and patient who have HIV are also more likely to develop CIN

44. Which of the following disorders is most likely to be found in a patient suffering from sleep apnea?
    c. follicular conjunctivitis—secondary to floppy eyelid syndrome

45. A patient with graft-vs-host disease is most likely to have which eye finding?
    b. symblepharon—due to cicatrizing conjunctivitis

CHAPTER 8 UVEITIS

1. The most effective antibiotic for the treatment of *P. acnes* endophthalmitis is
   c. vancomycin

2. For the diagnosis of granulomatous inflammation, which cell type must be present?
   d. epithelioid histiocyte

3. All of the following are true concerning sarcoidosis except
   a. Touton giant cells are common—sarcoidosis is characterized by Langhans' giant cells

4. Which of the following is not characteristic of Fuchs' heterochromic iridocyclitis?
   c. posterior synechiae

5. The most common organism causing endopthalmitis following cataract surgery is
   d. *S. epidermidis*

6. MEWDS can be differentiated from APMPPE by
   b. female predilection

7. All of the following disorders are correctly paired with their HLA associations except
   a. POHS, B9—POHS is associated with HLA-B7, DR2

8. Decreased vision in a patient with intermediate uveitis is most likely due to
   b. macular edema

9. A 71-year-old woman with a 6-month history of fatigue, anorexia, and 10-pound weight loss is found to have

left-sided weakness, visual acuity of 20/80 OD and 20/60 OS, and vitreous cells. The most helpful workup is
   a. LP and vitrectomy—to rule out CNS lymphoma

10. The most common organisms causing endophthalmitis following trauma is
    b. *Bacillus* species and *S. epidermidis*

11. All of the following are features common to both sympathetic ophthalmia and Vogt-Koyanagi-Harada syndrome except
    c. pathology localized to choroid—retina is also involved in VKH

12. Which disorder is more common in males?
    b. uveal effusion syndrome

13. EVS findings include all of the following except
    b. intravitreal corticosteroids were helpful—intravitreal steroids were not evaluated in the EVS

14. Which of the following is not characteristic of MEWDS?
    b. bilaterality

15. The most common cause of posterior uveitis is
    d. toxoplasmosis

16. All of the following are causes of HLA-B27-associated uveitis except
    d. psoriasis—is not associated with uveitis, but psoriatic arthritis is

17. Which of the following is not part of the classic triad of findings in Reiter's syndrome?
    a. iritis—iritis occurs but the classic triad of Reiter's is arthritis, conjunctivitis, and urethritis

18. Which of the following laboratory tests is most commonly found in JRA-related iritis?
    c. RF−, ANA+—which occurs in early-onset pauciarticular JRA

19. Phacoantigenic endophthalmitis is characterized by which pattern of granulomatous inflammation?
    a. zonal

20. Which combination of findings is least likely to occur in rubella?
    b. glaucoma and cataract—each occurs but rarely together

21. A 35-year-old man with decreased vision OD is found to have ON edema and a macular star. The causative organism most likely is
    b. *Bartonella henselae*—which causes cat-scratch disease and a neuroretinitis; *O. volvulus* causes onchocerciasis, *T. pallidum* causes syphilis, and *B. burgdorferi* causes Lyme disease

22. Which is least helpful for the diagnosis of toxocariasis?
    d. stool examination—no ova or parasites are found in the stool

23. A person living in which area of the US would be most likely to develop POHS?
    c. Midwest—in the US, histoplasmosis is most prevalent in the Ohio River valley and Eastern states

24. All of the following are true of birdshot choroidopathy except
    a. more common in males—birdshot choroidopathy is more common in females

25. Which of the following is least commonly associated with *Treponema pallidum* infection?
    d. glaucoma—is not associated with ocular involvement of syphilis

26. The HLA association for pars planitis with multiple sclerosis is
    d. DR15

27. Retinal S antigen is found in
    c. photoreceptors—retinal S antigen is found in outer segments of receptor cells

28. Features of Harada's disease include all of the following except
    b. deafness—only eye findings are seen in Harada's disease

29. Larva cause all of the following infections except
    d. Cat-scratch disease—is caused by the bacteria *Bartonella henselae*

30. Which of the following signs of pars planitis is most associated with multiple sclerosis
    c. periphlebitis

31. CSF abnormalities are associated with all of the following disorders except
    b. ocular sarcoidosis

32. All of the following can present as uveitis except
    b. choroidal hemangioma

33. Which of the following is not associated with inflammatory bowel disease?
    c. interstitial keratitis

34. Anterior vitreous cells are least likely to be found in
    a. retinitis pigmentosa

35. Gastrointestinal disorders associated with uveitis include all of the following except
    c. diverticulitis

36. All of the following may occur in ocular sarcoidosis except
    d. low serum gamma globulin—serum gamma globulin level is elevated

37. The choroid is the primary location of the pathologic process in
    d. VKH syndrome

38. Which of the following is least likely to be found in a patient with sympathetic ophthalmia
    b. granulomatous nodules in the retina—nodules occur in the choroid

39. Band keratopathy is least likely to occur in a patient with
    c. Behçet's disease

40. A patient with APMPPE is most likely to have
    c. viral prodrome

CHAPTER 9   GLAUCOMA

1. Which form of glaucoma is associated with Down's syndrome?
   c. Axenfeld-Rieger

2. What is the most appropriate initial treatment of pupillary block in a patient with microspherophakia?
   d. cyclopentolate—which helps pull the anteriorly displaced lens back to its normal position

3. Which of the following statements is true? Uveoscleral outflow is
   c. increased by atropine—cycloplegics and prostaglandin analogues (Xalatan, Lumigan, Travatan) increase (and miotics decrease) uveoscleral outflow; fluorophotometry measures the rate of aqueous formation; uveoscleral outflow accounts for 15% to 20% of total outflow and is independent of pressure

4. Risk factors for angle-closure glaucoma include all of the following except
   b. myopia—this is a risk factor for open-angle glaucoma, not angle-closure glaucoma

5. Which of the following would cause the greatest elevation in IOP?
   a. blinking—IOP is lowered by decreased blood cortisol levels (reduces aqueous formation) and elevation of the head (changing from supine to sitting position); darkening the room may increase IOP in patients with narrow angles

6. The most likely cause of a large filtering bleb and a shallow chamber is
   d. overfiltration—which causes both findings; a leak would cause a flat or low bleb; pupillary block and aqueous misdirection would not change the size of the blebs

7. A change in Goldmann visual field stimulus from I4e to II4e is equivalent to
   a. 1 log—the Roman numeral indicates the size of the test object in mm^2 (0=1/16, I=1/4, II=1, III=4, IV=16, V=64) and is a logarithmic scale; therefore, changing from size I to II is 1 log unit

8. An Amsler grid held at 33 cm measures approximately how many degrees of central vision?
   b. 10

9. The most decreased sensitivity in an arcuate scotoma occurs in which quadrant?
   c. superotemporal

10. The best gonioscopy lens for distinguishing appositional from synechial angle closure is
    b. Zeiss—this is the only lens of the 4 that can be used for indentation gonioscopy (indenting the cornea forces aqueous into the angle pushing the iris backward and allowing one to view the angle)

11. Which is not a risk factor for POAG?
    d. CRAO

12. ALT would be most effective in a patient with which type of glaucoma?
    c. pigmentary—patients with pigmentary glaucoma often respond well to ALT, whereas those with inflammatory, congenital, and aphakic glaucoma do not

13. In which direction should a patient look to aid the examiner's view of the angle during Zeiss gonioscopy?
    b. toward the mirror—this allows for a better view of the portion of the angle being inspected

14. The best parameter for determining the unreliability of a Humphrey visual field is
    a. fixation losses

15. Which of the following does not cause angle-closure glaucoma?
    c. RD—does not cause angle closure; the others do: PHPV and choroidal effusion by a posterior pushing mechanism and ICE syndrome by an anterior pulling mechanism

16. Factors producing increased IOP 2 days postoperatively include all of the following except
    d. steroid drops—steroid response does not occur this quickly (it usually takes at least 7–10 days)

17. Treatment of malignant glaucoma may include all of the following except
    b. pilocarpine—miotics are contraindicated in malignant glaucoma because the aim of medical therapy is to pull the lens/iris diaphragm posteriorly (cycloplegics)

18. The most common organism associated with bleb-related endophthalmitis is
    a. Streptococcus species—are most common (~50%) followed by coagulase-negative Staph and then H. flu

19. Which visual field defect is least characteristic of glaucoma?
    c. central scotoma—central vision is not affected until late in the disease

20. The type of tonometer most greatly affected by scleral rigidity is
    c. Schiøtz—low scleral rigidity yields falsely low readings (i.e., high myopia, thyroid disease, previous ocular surgery, miotic therapy), and high scleral rigidity yields falsely high readings (i.e., high hyperopia, vasoconstrictor therapy)

21. As compared with plasma, aqueous has a higher concentration of
    c. ascorbate—has a concentration 15× higher in aqueous than in plasma, whereas the concentrations of sodium, calcium, and protein are lower in aqueous

22. The rate of aqueous production per minute is approximately
    b. 2 μL

23. The location of the greatest resistance to aqueous outflow is
    c. juxtacanalicular connective tissue

24. Facility of aqueous outflow is best measured by
   a. tonography—manometry measures episcleral venous pressure, tonometry measures intraocular pressure, fluorophotometry measures rate of aqueous formation (via decreasing fluorescein concentration)

25. A patient recently had an acute angle closure attack in the right eye. What is the most appropriate treatment for her left eye?
   b. laser peripheral iridotomy—iridotomies must be performed in both eyes

26. The most likely gonioscopic finding in a patient with glaucoma and radial midperipheral spoke-like iris transillumination defects is
   a. concave peripheral iris—this is the characteristic iris configuration in pigment dispersion syndrome and pigmentary glaucoma

27. A 60-year-old myope with early cataracts and enlarged cup-to-disc ratios of 0.6 OU is found to have an abnormal Humphrey visual field test OS. He has no other risk factors for glaucoma. What is the most appropriate next step for this patient?
   a. repeat visual fields—any initial abnormal glaucoma field test or interval change in field should be confirmed by repeating the test

28. Bilateral scattered PAS in an elderly hyperope with no past ocular history is most likely due to
   c. chronic angle-closure glaucoma

29. According to the CIGTS 5-year results, initial treatment of POAG with which two methods had similar visual field outcomes?
   b. medicine or trabeculectomy

30. Which of the following medications should not be used to treat a patient with HSV keratouveitis and elevated IOP?
   a. pilocarpine—miotics can exacerbate the inflammation and increase the risk of developing posterior synechiae

31. A patient undergoes multiple subconjunctival injections of 5-FU after glaucoma filtration surgery. The most common reason for discontinuing these injections is if the patient develops toxicity of which tissue?
   c. cornea—corneal epithelial toxicity (i.e., SPK, epithelial defects, ulcers) is the most common complication of subconjunctival 5-FU injections

32. A patient with retinoblastoma develops glaucoma. The most common mechanism is
   c. neovascular—NVG (due to retinal ischemia) is the cause of ~75% of RB-associated glaucoma cases; the other mechanism is secondary angle closure due to anterior displacement of the lens-iris diaphragm

33. Glaucoma due to elevated episcleral venous pressure occurs in all of the following except
   b. hyphema—glaucoma is caused by red blood cells clogging the trabecular meshwork

34. The earliest color deficit in glaucoma is loss of
   d. blue-yellow axis

35. Blood in Schlemm's canal is not associated with
   a. Fuchs' heterochromic iridocyclitis—there is no blood in Schlemm's canal, but fine-angle neovascularization occurs and may cause spontaneous hyphema

CHAPTER 10   ANTERIOR SEGMENT

1. The most helpful test for evaluating macular function in a patient with advanced cataract is
   b. 2-light separation—the others test gross function

2. Ectopia lentis is least likely to be associated with
   a. cleft palate—is not associated with lens subluxation; the other abnormalities are pectus excavatum in Marfan's syndrome, short stature in Weill-Marchesani syndrome, and mental retardation in homocystinuria, sulfite oxidase deficiency, and hyperlysinemia

3. Anterior segment signs of ciliary body melanoma include all of the following except
   a. corneal edema—does not occur; however, ciliary body melanoma can cause increased IOP from angle closure (posterior pushing mechanism), and astigmatism and cataract from mechanical effects on the crystalline lens

4. Which of the following is least characteristic of ICE syndrome?
   b. increased IOP

5. The crystalline lens is formed from which embryologic tissue?
   b. ectoderm

6. A stellate anterior subcapsular cataract is most likely to be found in a patient with
   d. electrical injury—the other entities cause different types of cataract: atopic dermatitis (ASC), myotonic dystrophy (Christmas tree cataract), Fabry's disease (spoke-like cataract)

7. The most useful diagnostic test in an infant with an oil-droplet cataract is
   d. urine-reducing substances—to check for galactosemia

8. Which of the following does not occur in siderosis bulbi?
   c. sunflower cataract—is seen in conditions with abnormal copper (not iron) deposition (i.e., Wilson's disease and chalcosis)

9. A patient has a history of increased IOP with exercise; which finding is associated with this condition?
   a. Krukenberg spindle—these are both signs of pigment dispersion syndrome

10. Separation between the longitudinal and circumferential fibers of the ciliary muscle is called
   b. angle recession—this is the definition; iridoschisis is separation of the iris surface, iridodialysis is separation of the iris root from its insertion, and cyclodialysis is separation of the ciliary body from the scleral spur

11. Characteristics of pigment dispersion syndrome include all of the following except
   c. phacodenesis

12. Genetics of aniridia are best summarized as
    d. 1/3 sporadic, 2/3 AD

13. A sickle cell patient with a hyphema develops increased IOP; which of the following treatment choices is best?
    d. timoptic—is the safest medication because it does not affect sickling; miotics destabilize the blood-aqueous barrier, CAIs decrease aqueous pH (leading to sickling), and hyperosmotics cause hemoconcentration and sickling

14. A pigmentary retinopathy occurs in which mesodermal dysgenesis syndrome?
    b. Alagille's syndrome

15. Of the following causes of iris heterochromia, the involved iris is hyperchromic in
    a. ICE syndrome—pigmented iris nodules (pseudonevi) can occur; the involved iris is hypochromic in the other 3 conditions

16. Which of the following iris lesions is a true tumor?
    c. Lisch nodule—is an iris hamartoma associated with neurofibromatosis; Kunkmann-Wolffian body is composed of normal iris stroma, Koeppe nodule is composed of inflammatory cells, and nodules in JXG are granulomatous infiltrates

17. At which location is the lens capsule thinnest?
    b. posterior capsule

18. The iris sphincter is derived from what embryologic tissue?
    c. neural ectoderm

19. Which of the following is not associated with sunset syndrome?
    d. hyphema—is not associated with inferior decentration of an IOL; polyopia can occur if the edge of the lens is within the pupil; asymmetric haptic placement and weak zonules (which occur in pseudoexfoliation) are risk factors

20. Lens epithelial cells differentiate into lens fibers
    a. anterior to the equator

21. Light of which wavelength is absorbed greatest by a dense nuclear sclerotic cataract?
    d. blue—this is why patients notice that blues and purples are especially vibrant after cataract surgery

22. A patient with background diabetic retinopathy and clinically significant macular edema desires cataract surgery. The most appropriate management is
    b. focal laser treatment then cataract surgery—it is important to treat and stabilize the preexisting macular edema prior to cataract surgery, which can exacerbate it

23. After finishing phacoemulsification on a dense cataract, the surgeon notes whitening of the clear corneal incision. The most likely cause is
    a. tight incision—causes reduced irrigation and insufficient cooling of the phaco needle resulting in a wound burn

24. Nuclear brunescence increases with higher concentrations of which lens protein?
    d. main intrinsic polypeptide

25. Lens fibers contain nuclei in all of the following conditions except
    b. syphilis

26. The most likely cause of an intraoperative complication during cataract surgery in a patient with pseudoexfoliation syndrome is
    c. weak zonules

27. The majority of glucose metabolism in the lens is by
    a. glycolysis

28. The most appropriate systemic treatment for a patient with a sunflower cataract is
    b. penicillamine—to reduce serum copper levels

29. Which of the following is the least likely cause of decreased vision 2 years after cataract surgery?
    d. cystoid macular edema—occurs in the first 2 months after surgery

30. Which type of cataract is most closely associated with UV-B exposure?
    b. cortical

CHAPTER 11   POSTERIOR SEGMENT

1. Which substance does not cause crystalline deposits in the retina?
   a. thioridazine

2. What is the chance that a child of a patient with Best's disease will inherit the disorder?
   b. 50%—Best's is autosomal dominant

3. The MPS showed the best prognosis for laser treatment of CNV in which disorder?
   d. POHS—The MPS studied laser treatment of CNV in patients with AMD, POHS, and idiopathic membranes; POHS patients had the best response to laser treatment; patients with CNV secondary to myopia and angioid streaks were not studied

4. Which of the following is not a feature of Stickler's syndrome?
   c. retinoschisis

5. Sites at which the uvea is attached to the sclera include all of the following except
   d. ora serrata

6. The inheritance of gyrate atrophy is
   d. autosomal recessive

7. All 3 types of retinal hemorrhage (preretinal, intraretinal, and subretinal) may occur simultaneously in all of the following conditions except
   c. diabetes—diabetic retinopathy can cause preretinal and intraretinal hemorrhages but does not cause subretinal hemorrhage

8. Characteristics of choroidal melanoma include all of the following except
   b. high internal reflectivity

9. Which of the following statements regarding the ETDRS is false?
   a. The ETDRS concluded that PRP reduces the risk of severe visual loss in patients with high-risk PDR—this conclusion is from the DRS

10. The DRVS found that early vitrectomy for vitreous hemorrhage was helpful in
    a. type 1 diabetic patients

11. Which of the following treatments is a CVOS recommendation?
    c. PRP for iris or angle neovascularization

12. Which peripheral retinal lesion has the most risk of a retinal detachment?
    d. lattice degeneration

13. The intraocular structure most commonly affected by leukemia is
    d. optic nerve

14. Which is not a function of the RPE?
    b. concentration of taurine

15. Which of the following best describes the cellular reaction when light strikes a photoreceptor?
    c. decreased cGMP, closed Na channel

16. Prognostic factors for choroidal melanoma include all of the following except
    d. pigmentation

17. Which of the following does not involve the outer plexiform layer of the retina?
    d. diabetic microaneurysm

18. The best test for distinguishing between a subretinal hemorrhage and a choroidal melanoma is
    a. FA—blockage occurs from the hemorrhage, and tumor circulation is visible in the melanoma

19. Which of the following is the least radiosensitive lesion?
    d. melanoma

20. Which of the following is not a complication of PRP?
    c. RD

21. A cluster of pigmented lesions is seen in the peripheral retina of a patient's left eye during routine ophthalmoscopy. Which of the following tests would be most helpful in detecting an associated hereditary disorder?
    b. colonoscopy—check for polyps (FAP, Gardner's disease)

22. Which of the following is not associated with a typical angiographic appearance of CME?
    a. nicotinic acid—this maculopathy clinically appears like CME, but there is no fluorescein filling of the cysts; other entities that fall into this category are juvenile retinoschisis, Goldmann-Favre disease, and some types of RP

23. The least likely finding in a patient with a chronic detachment of the inferotemporal retina is
    c. fixed folds—may occur from PVR, whereas the other 3 findings are common with chronic RD

24. In a patient with AMD, which type of drusen is most associated with development of CNV?
    a. soft

25. The ERG oscillatory potential is caused by which cell type
    b. amacrine

26. Chloroquine retinopathy
    b. can be associated with other CNS reactions—including tinnitus

27. Proven systemic control for diabetic retinopathy include
    d. blood pressure control—shown in the United Kingdom Prospective Diabetes Study

28. Retinal artery macroaneursysms
    b. produce multilayered hemorrhages

29. The Branch Vein Occlusion Study reported that
    b. focal laser photocoagulation decreased visual loss—especially when vision worse than 20/40

30. True statements about ocular photodynamic therapy include all of the following except
    c. often requires retreatment every 6 weeks—actually it is every 3 months, early retreatment was not shown to be beneficial

31. Cystoid macular edema
    a. does not leak fluorescein when associated with nicotinic acid

32. PDR is most likely to develop if which one of the following findings is present on fundus exam?
    d. venous beading

33. Which of the following is the biggest risk factor for AMD?
    a. smoking

34. The most important visual prognostic factor for a rhegmatogenous RD is
    c. macular involvement—macula-on has a better prognosis than macula-off

35. The earliest sign of a macular hole is
    c. yellow spot in the fovea—stage 1a hole

36. Focal laser treatment is indicated for diabetic macular edema when there is
    d. retinal edema within 500 μm of the center of the fovea

37. Reduced IOP would be most unexpected in a patient with
    b. choroidal hemorrhage—choroidal hemorrhage causes increased IOP

38. Which of the following is the correct indication for treating macular edema from a Branch Retinal Vein Occlusion?
    d. vision worse than 20/40 for greater than 3 months

39. Which test is best for distinguishing a choroidal melanoma from a choroidal hemangioma?
    c. ultrasound

40. The etiology of vitreous hemorrhage in Terson's syndrome is
    a. intracranial hypertension—from a subarachnoid or subdural hemorrhage

41. The most common site of metastasis for a choroidal melanoma is
    b. liver—92% of metastases are to liver

42. Which of the following is least characteristic of Eales disease?
    d. macular edema

43. Crystalline retinopathy is not associated with
    c. thioridazine—causes a pigmentary retinopathy

44. Combined hamartoma of the retina and RPE has been associated with all of the following except
    d. Gardner syndrome

45. All of the following statements regarding uveal metastases are true except
    b. most common ocular location is anterior choroid—usually metastasize to macula because of richest blood supply

Index

Page numbers followed by "f" indicate figures, "t" indicate tables, and "b" indicate boxes.